Saunders
Nursing Guide to
Laboratory and Diagnostic Tests

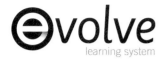
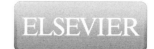
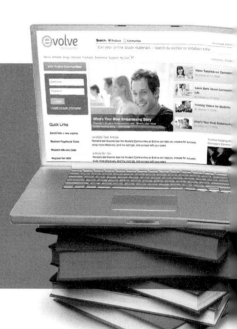

SECOND EDITION

Saunders
Nursing Guide to
Laboratory and
Diagnostic Tests

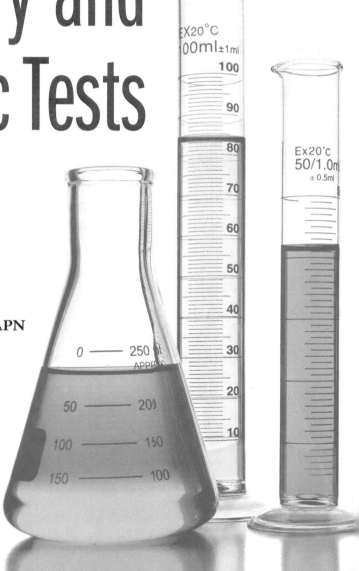

Louise M. Malarkey, EdD, RN
Professor Emeritus
Department of Nursing
College of Staten Island
City University of New York
Staten Island, New York

Mary Ellen McMorrow, EdD, RN, APN
Professor
Department of Nursing
College of Staten Island
City University of New York
Staten Island, New York

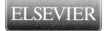

3251 Riverport Lane
St. Louis, Missouri 63043

SAUNDERS NURSING GUIDE TO LABORATORY AND DIAGNOSTIC TESTS   ISBN: 978-1-4377-2712-8

Notice

Knowledge and best practice in this field are constantly changing. As new research and experience broaden our understanding, changes in research methods, professional practices, or medical treatment may become necessary.

Practitioners and researchers must always rely on their own experience and knowledge in evaluating and using any information, methods, compounds, or experiments described herein. In using such information or methods they should be mindful of their own safety and the safety of others, including parties for whom they have a professional responsibility.

With respect to any drug or pharmaceutical products identified, readers are advised to check the most current information provided (i) on procedures featured or (ii) by the manufacturer of each product to be administered, to verify the recommended dose or formula, the method and duration of administration, and contraindications. It is the responsibility of practitioners, relying on their own experience and knowledge of their patients, to make diagnoses, to determine dosages and the best treatment for each individual patient, and to take all appropriate safety precautions.

To the fullest extent of the law, neither the Publisher nor the authors, contributors, or editors, assume any liability for any injury and/or damage to persons or property as a matter of products liability, negligence or otherwise, or from any use or operation of any methods, products, instructions, or ideas contained in the material herein.

Nursing Diagnosis - Definitions and Classification 2009-2011. Copyright © 2009, 2007, 2005, 2003, 2001, 1998, 1996, 1994 by NANDA International. Used by arrangement with Wiley-Blackwell Publishing, a company of John Wiley & Sons, Inc. In order to make safe and effective judgments using NANDA-I diagnoses it is essential that nurses refer to the definitions and defining characteristics of the diagnoses listed in this work.

Library of Congress Cataloging-in-Publication Data
Malarkey, Louise M.
    Saunders nursing guide to laboratory and diagnostic tests / Louise M.
Malarkey, Mary Ellen McMorrow. -- 2nd ed.
        p. ; cm.
    Nursing guide to laboratory and diagnostic tests
    Includes bibliographical references and index.
    ISBN 978-1-4377-2712-8 (pbk. : alk. paper)
    1. Diagnosis, Laboratory--Handbooks, manuals, etc. 2. Nursing--Practice--Handbooks, manuals, etc.
3. Diagnosis--Handbooks, manuals, etc. I. McMorrow, Mary Ellen. II. Title. III. Title: Nursing guide to laboratory and diagnostic tests.
    [DNLM: 1. Nursing Care. 2. Diagnostic Techniques and Procedures--nursing. 3. Laboratory Techniques and Procedures--nursing. WY 100.1]
    RB38.2.M345 2012
    616.07'5--dc23
                                                                                    2011023965

Senior Editor: Tamara Myers
Managing Editor: Jean Sims Fornango
Developmental Editor: Tina Kaemmerer
Publishing Services Managers: Radhika Pallamparthy and Deborah L. Vogel
Project Managers: Sivaraman Moorthy and John W. Gabbert
Designer: Maggie Reid

Printed in the United States of America

Last digit is the print number: 9   8   7   6   5   4   3   2   1

Reviewers

Amy J. Key, RN, BSN
Nursing Instructor
Tennessee Technology Center at Pulaski
Pulaski, Tennessee

Pamela D. Korte, RN, MS
Professor of Nursing
Monroe Community College
Rochester, New York

Stephen D. Krau, PhD, RN, CNE, CT
Associate Professor
School of Nursing
Vanderbilt University Medical Center
Nashville, Tennessee

Rebecca LaMont, MSN, APN, RN
Instructor of Nursing
Family Practitioner
Heartland Community College
Normal, Illinois

Carla Lynch, MS, RN
Nursing Faculty
Rogers State University
Claremore, Oklahoma

Elaine Maruca, MSN, RN, FNP-BC, CNE
Saint Francis Medical Center School
  of Nursing
Trenton, New Jersey

Kristine A. Rose, MSN, RN
Instructor
Saint Francis Medical Center College
  of Nursing
Peoria, Illinois

Stephen M. Setter, PharmD, DVM, CGP, CDE
Associate Professor
College of Pharmacy
Washington State University
Spokane, Washington

Bonnie Welniak, MSN, RN
Assistant Professor of Nursing
Monroe County Community College
Monroe, Michigan

Kathleen S. Whalen, PhD, RN, CNE
Assistant Professor of Nursing
Loretto Heights School of Nursing
Regis University
Denver, Colorado

Paige Wimberley, MSN, APN, CNE, CNS
Assistant Professor of Nursing
Arkansas State University
Jonesboro, Arkansas

Marcia Wojcik, MS, RN
Assistant Professor of Nursing
Fulton-Montgomery Community College
Johnstown, New York

Alan H.B. Wu, PhD, DABCC
Professor, Laboratory Medicine
University of California, San Francisco
San Francisco, California

This book is dedicated to our families

To my sons, Frank and Charlie
Louise Malarkey

To my sisters, Lydia, Peggy, and Ruth
and my daughter, Mary
Mary Ellen McMorrow

Preface

This edition of the *Saunders Nursing Guide to Laboratory and Diagnostic Tests* provides the nursing student and the nurse in clinical practice with easily accessible information about laboratory tests and diagnostic procedures that are frequently encountered in patient care settings. The major strength of the book is its emphasis on the nursing care related to the specific tests and procedures.

PART 1

Chapter 1 addresses the overall responsibilities of the nurse in laboratory and diagnostic testing. The discussion emphasizes the nursing role and the nurse-patient interactions in the pretest period, during the test, and in the posttest period. The content is written in the nursing process format so that the reader can use critical thinking abilities to provide accurate nursing care. Chapter 2 addresses the procedures used by the nurse to accurately collect the various specimens of blood, feces, or urine. The nurse's interactions with the physician and laboratory personnel ensure timely and accurate specimens and help produce valid test results.

PART 2

The largest section of the book contains the specific laboratory tests and diagnostic procedures, presented in alphabetical order. The tests and procedures are comprehensive in scope, including those used in cardiopulmonary, gastrointestinal, renal, hepatobiliary, gynecological, obstetrical, pediatric, hematological, vascular, orthopedic, neurological, oncological, and endocrine disorders, as well as infectious diseases and genetic testing.

The specific tests and procedures include the new tests approved for clinical use, familiar tests that have been approved for expanded use, and additional tests that were not included in previous editions, some of which include the following:

- Computed tomography angiography of targeted vascular locations and specific organs
- Positron emission tomography combined with computed tomography (PET-CT)
- Rapid antigen tests for suspected infectious disorders
- DNA testing to identify bacteria and viruses, influenza testing
- Expanded prenatal screening for genetic abnormality of the fetus
- Genetic sonogram
- Newborn screening tests
- Fetal fibronectin
- Carboxyhemoglobin
- CT colonography
- Fecal immunochemical testing (FIT) for detection of blood in the lower gastrointestinal tract
- Cardiac troponin
- Allergy testing
- Hepatitis E
- Sentinel node biopsy
- Angiography, carotid arteries
- Angiography Torso, extremities

In this edition, older tests have been deleted from discussion because they are becoming obsolete or have been replaced by improved, more accurate alternatives.

SPECIAL FEATURES

- Reference values are provided for a range of age groups from fetus or newborn to adults in old age. Critical values are identified when applicable.
- Explanations for elevated, decreased, or abnormal values are based on altered anatomy and physiology.
- Explanations of the purpose of the test or procedure and how it is performed provide a succinct overview of what the patient will experience.
- Significance of test results is presented as a list of medical conditions that are diagnosed by or associated with the altered test value.
- Interfering factors for the specific test are identified. During the pretest phase of testing, the patient is taught to eliminate or avoid them.
- Nursing care is presented for pretest, during the test, and posttest phases with emphasis on what actions the nurse takes with the patient to ensure safety and an accurate outcome.
- Patient teaching provides instructions to the patient in the pretest phase and in preparing for the patient's discharge in the posttest phase. Often the patient is at home until just before the test and he or she returns home directly after the test is completed. Patient teaching improves the patient's ability to perform accurate and confident self-care.
- Health promotion discussions are included for those tests or procedures that are recommended for health screening and preventative health care. The content of each discussion is based on the most current national recommendations. Current screening tests include Papanicolaou smear, fecal blood testing, colonoscopy, prostatic specific antigen, mammography, lead levels in the blood, electrocardiogram, cholesterol, dual energy X-ray absorptiometry, prenatal screening, and newborn screening.
- Critical values are now prevalent because accredited hospitals across the nation have determined which tests have defined critical values, what the numeric values should be in their institution, and the protocol that is used when a patient's laboratory result is in the critical value range. In this text, nursing responses to a critical value are identified including notification of the physician, nursing assessments of the patient, and preparation for possible interventions in the emergency situation.
- Nursing response to complications during the procedure or in the posttest phase of the procedure include nursing assessments that monitor for possible complications and early nursing interventions that can be implemented while awaiting medical evaluation of the patient. Depending on the specific procedure, possible complications can include hypersensitivity reaction, anaphylaxis, stroke, thrombosis, infection, cardiac arrhythmia, respiratory impairment, bleeding, perforation, shock, or other problems.
- Illustrations appear throughout the text. There are more than 100 line drawings of procedures and diagnostic images of abnormal findings from ultrasound images, nuclear scans, CT scans, MRI, X-rays, PET scans, and EKG tracings. The illustrations help the nurse to visualize how the procedure is performed, where the abnormal finding is located in the body, and what it looks like. The combination of written explanation and illustration enables the reader's understanding of the test and the significance of the test results to grow.

A COMMENTARY ON CURRENT AND FUTURE TRENDS

In the past 10 years, there has been extraordinary growth in the fields of laboratory and diagnostic testing. The changes have evolved because of factors that include, but are not limited to, the patient's shorter stay in a hospital, increases in patient care delivered on an outpatient basis, greatly improved technology particularly in ultrasound, PET scans, computed tomography, and new innovations in automated laboratory equipment. The imaging is sharper and more complete. Many laboratory results are obtained more quickly, with more definitive results. DNA identification of bacteria and viruses provides a faster method than the culture of a specimen and is more accurate than tests based on antigen or antibody detection. Genetic testing is rapidly expanding in use and ability to detect potential or actual inherited abnormalities in offspring. Improvements in diagnostic methods favor the use of non invasive or minimally invasive procedures that increase patient safety and limit the occurrence of complications. Medical care of the patient will continue to evolve and change based, in part, on the additional information provided by laboratory and diagnostic testing. New laboratory tests will likely be developed with a goal of improved sensitivity and specificity, thus improving the interpretation of test results.

The nurse needs up-to-date information about his or her patient's condition, including the significance of laboratory and diagnostic test results. Patient teaching by phone contact and written instruction is frequently used when the patient will not be in contact with professionals until the time of the test. The development and implementation of critical values define a new emphasis for nursing practice in hospitals, with the need for the nurse to act quickly to notify the physician and to perform accurately during the patient's crisis. Nurses also have a role in the community and can help provide education regarding health promotion screening tests, why they are valuable, when they are recommended, what is involved, and what to do if the results are abnormal. As in all other aspects of nursing practice, the nurse grows by learning about new laboratory tests and diagnostic procedures. Finally, in this highly technical world of laboratory and diagnostic testing, the nurse uses communication and interpersonal skills to help the patient understand what the purpose and test results mean. The nurse also provides support, information, and guidance as the patient must make difficult decisions that are based upon the results and the physician's recommendations.

We have written this book for nursing students and nurses who practice in clinical settings. Their learning needs were always in our minds as this new edition was developed. As nursing educators, we have endeavored to write for this audience to best enhance their learning process while ensuring satisfying results.

Louise M. Malarkey
Mary Ellen McMorrow

Acknowledgments

This edition was written with the support and encouragement of many people, including our families, friends and colleagues. The authors wish to thank them for being there, whenever we looked up from our computers or from behind a tower of papers and texts.

With over 70 years of teaching experience between us, we wish to thank our many students, who have taught us that nursing is a challenging and fulfilling profession. Our students continuously rejuvenate our spirits by their enthusiasm for learning and their commitment to quality nursing care.

Special thanks to Tamara Myers, Senior Editor; Jean Sims Fornango, Managing Editor; Tina Kaemmerer, Developmental Editor; and Johnny Gabbert, Project Manager for their help in bringing this book to fruition. Their support and encouragement was always there. This book was an enjoyable collaboration because of their responsiveness, vision, and communication ability.

List of Figures

Contents

PART I:
Nursing Responsibilities in Laboratory Tests and Diagnostic Procedures, 1

PART II:
Laboratory Tests and Diagnostic Procedures, 39

Tests presented in alphabetical order

APPENDIXES

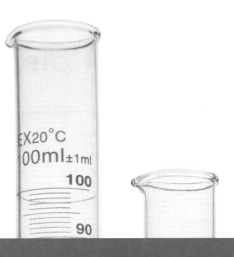

PART

I

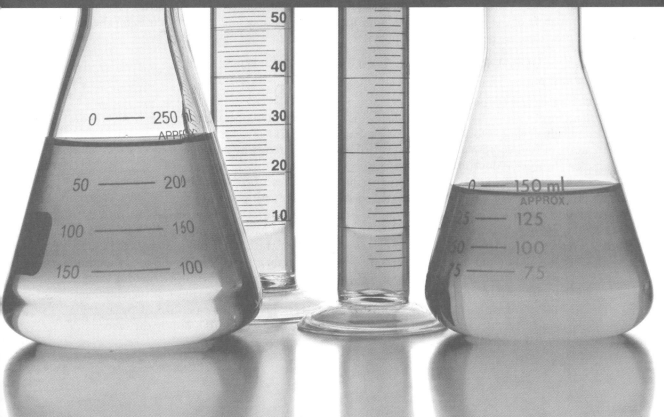

Nursing Responsibilities in Laboratory Tests and Diagnostic Procedures

The Nursing Role

In this chapter, the content is organized to address two broad areas of nursing performance related to laboratory tests and diagnostic procedures. The first area pertains to the testing procedures and the nursing role in the process of testing in an accurate and timely manner. The second area concerns the nursing interactions with the patient who must undergo a diagnostic test or procedure. The nursing process is used to organize patient care and meet the patient's needs.

In some instances, diagnostic work is an interdisciplinary function that involves coordination and communication among the nurse, several physicians, and technicians of the laboratory, radiology department, or diagnostic specialty units. The nurse's role is often pivotal in the transmission of information to and from the testing center. Particularly for diagnostic procedures, pertinent needs or problems of the patient are explained to the testing center personnel, such as limited mobility, weakness, or mental status of the patient. The nurse also explains the pretest laboratory or diagnostic requirements to the patient, such as dietary restrictions and other specific pretest preparations. The goal for all participants is to accomplish the diagnostic work accurately, safely, and in a timely manner.

The process of laboratory or diagnostic testing can be conceptualized as a cycle that has four phases of operation: (1) the pretest phase, (2) the test phase, (3) the posttest phase, and (4) analysis of the results (Figure 1). Appropriate nursing roles and responsibilities for the test or procedure are pertinent in each phase.

PROCEDURAL ROLE AND NURSING RESPONSIBILITIES

Pretest Phase

Scheduling of a Diagnostic Test

This involves communication among the individual who prescribes the test, the patient, and the individual who performs the test. When diagnostic testing involves different departments, the nurse or unit coordinator may be involved with coordination of the scheduling of the tests so that the work is done in a timely way.

When multiple tests in various departments are prescribed, it is sometimes necessary to prioritize the test schedule because the method of conducting one test can interfere with the results of another. For example, x-ray studies that use contrast medium are performed before x-ray studies that use barium contrast material. Residual barium remains in the intestine for several days, and its opacity would obscure the view of the other tissues, such as the biliary tract and abdominal vasculature. Likewise, blood tests that use a radioimmunoassay method of analysis must be performed before or 7 days after a nuclear scan because the radioisotopes of the scan would interfere with the radioimmunoassay method of analysis of the blood and alter the test results. When these interfering factors involve tests performed by a single department, such as the laboratory, the priorities are routinely sorted out by the laboratory personnel.

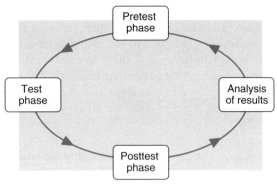

Figure 1. **The cycle of laboratory testing.** Both the nurse and the patient are involved in each phase of the cycle. After analysis of the test results, the cycle may be restarted for additional testing as needed.

Some priorities in scheduling are determined by the acuity of the patient. Particular test results may be needed rapidly for the assessment of the patient's status, for correct medical diagnosis and treatment, or for evaluation of the patient's response to treatment. Blood tests may be prescribed serially, for example, every hour for 4 hours; daily; or immediately (Stat). The nurse monitors to ensure that the tests are completed, as requested. The results are reported to the physician, as needed, and are posted manually or electronically in the patient's record. When a test is needed urgently, the laboratory or diagnostic unit is notified, the scheduling arrangements are confirmed, and the test or procedure is completed immediately.

Some tests can be performed at the bedside with immediate results provided by point-of-care testing. Other tests, such as a culture, require time to obtain results and the results may not be available for several days or more. Nonroutine or special tests must be scheduled in advance. For example, positron emission tomography (PET) is a nuclear scan using a radioisotope that is made by splitting atoms in a cyclotron. This special and costly radioisotope is created on the day of the test, but has a short half-life of only 7.5 hours. When the person lives at home and is scheduled to come to the nuclear medicine department for the PET scan, it is essential that the scan starts on time. Prior to the day of the test, the radiology nurse phones the patient to review pretest instructions, answer any questions, and remind the person of the appointment.

Requisition Forms
The laboratory requisition form is the major way to request the needed tests for the patient. The physician or health care provider who orders the test is also responsible to complete the requisition form. This simplified method avoids potential transcription errors that can occur when someone else completes the written request (McPherson & Pincus, 2007). Usually, the requisition is sent to the laboratory electronically, but it may be written manually.

The form must contain the same patient's identifying information that is on the patient's identification wristband and all hospital records. The information includes the patient's name, identification number, birth date, gender, age, social security number (if possible), and physician's name. Additional identifying data may be included, based on the institution's preferences.

The needed tests are selected by the physician or health care provider. Specific information may be included, such as pertinent medical history, suspected diagnosis, date of last menstrual period, or pregnancy status. This additional information is used to help with diagnosis and to establish the correct reference values based on age, gender, or other biologic variables.

Once the data of the requisition form is entered into the laboratory information system, an individual bar code is created. This bar code is automatically printed on the labels for the collected specimens, along with the identifying patient information. The bar code is used to identify the specimen as it moves through laboratory analysis and also is a tracking device that ensures that all specimens are identified, analyzed, and the results are entered in the patient's record.

Test Phase

The procedural responsibilities of the nurse vary considerably with different tests, and they vary somewhat among different institutions or units within the institution. When the specimen collection is performed by the physician or other health care provider, the nurse may have only indirect responsibility for ensuring that the test is performed, the specimen is labeled properly, and sent to the laboratory. Laboratory technicians, phlebotomists, or radiology technicians are supervised by personnel in their respective departments. The nurse has no official role in their work, unless patient safety becomes an issue.

If the hospitalized patient must go to the radiology department or to a special diagnostic unit, the nurse ensures that patient care is completed and that the patient is prepared for transport to the unit. Equipment, such as an intravenous line or a urine drainage system, must be functional and secured properly.

In some cases, the nurse is directly involved in the collection of specimens. This may include the collection of blood, urine, stool, and culture specimens, as well as assisting with the collection of a sample of tissue or body fluids. In these processes, the nurse shares in the responsibility for maintenance of quality controls, proper performance of the equipment, accurate identification of the patient, and correct labeling of the specimen. Along with the patient identification data and bar code on the label, the nurse includes the date and time of the collection procedure and identification of the tissue or fluid that was obtained.

Identification Procedures

It is essential to perform a correct identification before collecting the specimen or starting a diagnostic procedure, such as bone marrow or other biopsy, culture, or any other specimen. The Joint Commission (2010) requires that the person who collects the specimen must obtain the patient's identification from two different sources. One source is the name on the patient's wristband and it is the same name as that on the requisition. The second source is that the patient states his or her full name. The patient's room number or physical location cannot be used for identification purposes.

If the patient cannot respond, the staff nurse or a relative of the patient verifies the identity. There must be an exact match of identification among the two name identifications and the requisition information. The label also contains the same identifying information and after the specimen is obtained, the label is applied directly to the specimen container before leaving the patient.

Infection Control: Standard Precautions

Standard precautions must be used when obtaining or handling a blood or body fluid specimen. Gloves must be worn during the collection procedure. If splashing or contact with a mucous membrane is anticipated, the nurse wears a mask, protective eyewear, and a gown or protective clothing in addition to the gloves.

All specimens of blood or body fluids are placed in the correct containers with tightly fitted lids to prevent leakage during transport of the specimen to the laboratory. After the completion of the procedure, the gloves and disposable clothing are removed and discarded. Hands are washed with soap and water.

Precautions are taken to prevent the puncture or cutting of one's own skin with a contaminated needle, scalpel blade, or sharp instrument. To prevent needlestick injury, the needle-and-syringe unit is disposed of in a puncture-resistant container. The needle is not recapped, broken, bent, or removed from the syringe because of the risk of accidentally puncturing the hand.

Special reusable needles, such as those for a spinal tap or aspiration of a joint, are placed in puncture-resistant containers for transport to the area where they are cleansed and sterilized. Reusable instruments and diagnostic equipment are also cleansed and sterilized or disinfected according to established protocol.

The use of standard precautions is based on the premise that all patients are potentially infectious and that there is a risk of transmission of infection after exposure to blood or other body fluids. The precautions are used to protect all health care workers against blood-borne pathogens, including HIV.

Point-of-Care Testing

Point-of-care (POC) testing refers to methods of testing and analysis that bring the laboratory services nearer to the patient. This type of testing also is known as bedside testing, near-patient testing, or a rapid test. Satellite laboratories may be established near operating rooms, intensive care units, and emergency departments. Desktop analyzers may be used in these sites as well and in a clinic, an ambulatory care setting, a physician's office, and long-term care facility. There is rapid turn-around time between obtaining the specimen and receiving the test results. Medical diagnosis and treatment is based on real-time values and will be more accurate, avoiding a long delay before the central laboratory results could be available. There has been a dramatic expansion of these rapid tests during the past decade and this trend is likely to continue in the future (Lewandrowski, 2009a; Nichols, 2007). A partial list of the point-of-care tests is presented in Box 1.

When electronic charting is used, the laboratory results are transferred electronically from the point-of-care analyzer to a central computer system and entered automatically in the patient's record. If manual entry is used, the nurse must ensure that all the test results are charted in the correct order and time sequence.

With point-of-care methodology, reference values are different from the values of the same tests analyzed in the central laboratory. Different reagents, test equipment, and method of analysis create the differences in the reference values. The nurse refers to the point-of-care reference values provided by the central laboratory or the manufacturer of the point-of-care equipment for correct interpretation of the data.

Another category of point-of-care testing refers to the testing that is performed with small handheld instruments that analyze the patient's blood in a few minutes. The specimen is obtained and the blood analyzed wherever the patient is located, including the home or the workplace. The patient is usually the person who performs the test as part of self-care responsibilities. Blood testing monitors are used for timely measurement of glucose levels in diabetics and more recently for monitoring the prothrombin time-international normalized ratio (INR) in those who are maintained on anticoagulant medication.

BOX 1	Partial List of Tests Available With Point-of-Care Testing

Chemistry
Glucose
Blood gases and electrolytes
Lactate
Cholesterol
Hemoglobin A_{1c}
Microalbumin
Basic metabolic panel
Lipid panel
Liver function panel
Cardiac markers (including natriuretic
    peptides)
Urinalysis
Urea nitrogen
Creatinine
Ionized calcium
Drugs of abuse
Pregnancy testing
Infertility testing
Fetal fibronectin

Hematology
Prothrombin time
Partial thromboplastin time
Activated clotting time
Platelet function
D-dimer
Complete blood count

Microbiology
Physician-performed microscopy
Helicobacter pylori testing
Influenza, A, B testing
Respiratory syncytial virus
Gonorrhea, chlamydia
Streptococcus A
HIV

Other
Fecal occult blood
Gastric occult blood
Immunochemical methods for occult blood

From Lewandrowski, K. (2009). Point of care testing: An overview and a look to the future (circa 2009, United States). *Clinics in Laboratory Medicine, 29*(3), 427.

Expanded Nursing Role

Point-of-care testing involves an expanded role for nurses that overlaps with that of laboratory technicians. The nurse may collect the blood sample, perform the analysis, and produce the test results. When the patient monitors his or her own glucose levels or prothrombin-INR levels, patient teaching is an essential component of nursing care. The teaching begins in the hospital and continues by appointment in the specific clinic or office, until the patient can use the monitor, recalibrate the equipment accurately, interpret the results, and based on the results, adjust the medication according to the physician's guidelines. Repetition of the teaching-learning activities continue until the patient can perform these functions with consistent accuracy.

The laboratory is responsible for point-of-care testing, policies, procedures, and maintenance of the equipment. Nurses, as the providers of direct patient care, may use the automated analyzers. Alternatively, multitasked nursing assistants may perform the point-of-care testing. As part of laboratory accreditation requirements, the person who uses this equipment must have formal training for each test, certification that the training has been completed satisfactorily, and an annual reevaluation of performance (Ehrmeyer & Laessig, 2009). Without the training there is a high incidence of inconsistent performance and inaccurate test results.

Posttest Phase

Transport of the Specimen

The specimen is generally transported to the laboratory as quickly as possible. Some laboratory or pathology specimens become unstable shortly after they are collected. Specific factors, such as exposure to sunlight, warming, refrigeration, and exposure to air, can cause alteration or deterioration of particular specimens. For many blood tests, the unprocessed specimen will begin to deteriorate within a few hours. The phlebotomist and laboratory technician have responsibility for their own specimens. When needed, messengers may be used to deliver other specimens promptly, as from the operating room, emergency department, or patient care units.

When a fresh tissue sample must be analyzed for cytologic features, the specimen cannot be placed in fixative or preservative. Because the specimen will dry out after some exposure to the air, it may be delivered directly into the hands of the pathologist as soon as it is obtained. This coordination of activity provides immediate transport and tissue preparation so that the quality of the specimen is maintained.

Rejection Criteria

When an unsatisfactory specimen is delivered to the laboratory, rejection criteria are applied. The causes of rejection are presented in Box 2. When the specimen is rejected, the test must be repeated. The nurse or staff member who performs the specimen collection can help ensure acceptance of the specimen by collecting a sufficient quantity, by complying with the written protocol of the test, and by labeling the specimen container accurately.

Analysis of the Results

Reference Values

The outdated term, once called "normal values," is now more correctly called reference values. The values are usually in a range from the lower to the upper limits of normal. The reference values are used to interpret the results of the test, assist in making an accurate diagnosis, and to evaluate the patient's response to treatment.

BOX 2   Criteria for Rejection of an Unsatisfactory Laboratory Specimen

- Improper labeling of the specimen
- Lack of a label on the specimen
- Improperly completed requisition form
- Discrepancies between the specimen label and the requisition form
- Hemolysis/lipemia
- Clots in an anticoagulated specimen
- Improper collection of the specimen
- Delay in delivery of the specimen to the laboratory
- Improper preservation of the specimen
- Insufficient volume or quantity of the specimen
- Inadequate pretest preparation of the patient
  (Nonfasting when the test requires fasting)

The reference values for a specific test will vary with the different methods of chemical laboratory analysis and with different sources of specimen. For example, the reference value of chloride in a specimen of blood or plasma is different from the reference value of chloride in a sample of cerebrospinal fluid. The reference values usually vary with age of the patient, and sometimes vary with gender and race. The numeric values are different when reported in conventional reference values or international reference units. The nurse can use the reference values in this text as a general guide, but the reference values provided by the laboratory that performed the test are the most appropriate values for interpreting the findings in the clinical setting.

For some tests, the particular substance should not be present at all, such as cocaine or mercury. When it is not present, the result is described as negative. When it is present, the result is abnormal and the finding may be described as "present" or "positive," or it may be measured with a numeric value that quantifies the amount of substance found.

SI units refers to the International System of Units (Système International d'Unites), a system that reports laboratory data in terms of standardized international measurements. This system of measurement is currently used in a number of countries, with the eventual goal of worldwide use. Throughout this text, the reference values are presented in conventional units and their SI equivalents.

False Negatives and False Positives

A *false-negative* result means that the test result is negative, but the patient actually is positive and that the problem was not detected. The possible consequences of a false negative are that the patient and physician do not investigate further, treatment is delayed, and that the patient's symptoms continue unabated until additional tests identify the correct result and its cause.

A *false-positive* result means that the test result is positive, but the patient actually has no disease or problem. The possible consequences of a false positive can mean that additional tests will be done to investigate a problem that does not exist. Occasionally, treatment is started when there is no need to do so. When additional testing verifies that there is no problem, the patient is relieved, but sometimes becomes annoyed or angry because of needless worry about a nonexistent problem.

Sensitivity and Specificity

In laboratory terms, *sensitivity* means the probability that the person having the disease will be correctly identified by a positive result. *Specificity* means that the person who does not have the disease will be correctly identified by a negative result. In a perfect world, the perfect test has a proven performance of 100% sensitivity and specificity. However, no laboratory test is perfect and tests have lower than 100% sensitivity and specificity percentages (Jackson, 2008). The test with lower than desired sensitivity or specificity scores will have a higher rate of error because of false-positive or false-negative findings. Physicians generally order several tests or follow-up tests to verify the findings and eliminate errors.

Critical Values

The phrase "critical value" refers to a laboratory or diagnostic test result that is very abnormal and may indicate a life-threatening situation. The critical value may be a markedly elevated or decreased test result or it may identify a serious pathogen. Identification of critical values helps the nurse, physician, and nurse practitioner to differentiate between abnormal results and the extremes that indicate a possible crisis. Medical diagnosis and treatment are needed to correct the problem quickly before the patient's acute condition worsens.

The Joint Commission (2010) requires that all hospitals have an established critical values list, with the individual hospital's determination of which tests and diagnostic procedures demonstrate life-threatening results and the numerical values or diagnostic procedure findings that indicate the severity. Thus there is some variation among institutions as to the selection of laboratory tests, the numerical values, and diagnostic test findings that indicate a critical condition. Each hospital has its own written protocol of the laboratory's rapid notification. The policy must identify the reporting process "by whom" and "to whom" a critical result is reported. Generally, the physician in the laboratory reports by phone to the patient's physician. If the physician cannot be located, the nurse has the responsibility to receive the phone report from the laboratory, locate the physician as quickly as possible, and provide the needed information.

Verbal Reports

When a laboratory test result is in the critical value range or when the laboratory test or diagnostic procedure was ordered on a stat basis (to be done immediately), the laboratory or diagnostic unit physician will phone the patient's physician or the nurse to report the results immediately. With a verbal report, there is risk of error because of a potential misunderstanding of what was heard. The procedure the nurse follows is to write down the name of the test and the results and then to read back the information to the caller. The "read-back" process provides for confirmation of the accuracy of the received message or opportunity to correct a misunderstanding. The nurse must then contact the physician without delay and report the information. The physician uses the same read-back process.

PATIENT-NURSE INTERACTIONS

Dimensions of Nursing Care

The range of interactions between the patient and the nurse varies considerably with the complexity of the test or procedure. Laboratory tests that use specimens of blood, urine, or feces require some nursing intervention to ensure adequate patient preparation and accuracy in the collection of the specimen. Diagnostic procedures, however, require increased interaction with the patient, particularly when the procedures are invasive. Nursing responsibilities involve physical and psychosocial dimensions of patient care, with particular concern for the patient's safety.

Patient-nurse interactions involve direct or indirect care in the pretest, test, and posttest phases of the diagnostic procedure. The nursing process is applicable as a guide to the identification of the patient's needs and the development of the appropriate nursing interventions that lead to a positive outcome (Figure 2).

Changes in Health Care Delivery

These changes have resulted in shorter hospital stays for patients. Shorter periods of hospitalization limit the time for direct care during the acute phase of illness. For the acutely ill hospitalized patient, numerous diagnostic tests or procedures are often scheduled during a concentrated period. In addition to the routine pretest and posttest assessments of the patient, the nurse assesses for actual or potential complications related to the invasive diagnostic procedures.

Changes in health care delivery have resulted in many diagnostic tests being performed on an outpatient basis. The patient has been given greater self-care responsibility for pretest preparation

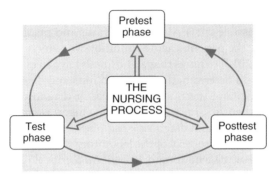

Figure 2. Application of the nursing process. In each phase of diagnostic testing, the nursing process is applied to provide safe, accurate, complete, and effective nursing care.

and posttest recovery. When outpatient testing occurs, the direct nursing interactions with the patient are often limited, unless the nurse works in radiology or the unit where invasive diagnostic testing is done.

When a diagnostic procedure is performed in the outpatient setting, the patient receives pretest planning information and instructions regarding special requirements necessary before and after the procedure. The clearly stated instructions are given to the patient or the family member who assists with the patient's care. If the instructions are complex, they should be given in writing so that the patient can refer to them as needed. Also, the patient needs the address and location of the laboratory or diagnostic unit, as well as the time and date for which the test is scheduled.

In procedures requiring sedation or light anesthesia, the patient is instructed in advance that a responsible individual will be required to provide transportation home at the end of the test. When a delayed complication in the posttest period is possible, the patient receives instruction so that he or she will recognize abnormal symptoms and notify the physician if they occur. All these measures are designed to provide continuity of care, even when the patient is some distance from the health care provider.

Pediatric Patients

Modifications in communication and safety measures are required for pediatric patients. These measures should be compatible with the age and behavior of the child. When explanations can be understood, time should be taken to prepare the young child for the test or procedure. Honest, friendly explanations help the child cope with the test. The child may fear pain, injections, the large equipment of the radiology department, or even the strangers who perform the test. Explanations are given simply and briefly. In some cases, the parents help prepare the child and provide calming reassurance.

Infants or active small children usually require restraints to protect them from harm and to maintain immobility during the test or procedure. The choice of restraint is based on the particular need and is used for tests of short duration. The choices include a sheet restraint, a mummy-style restraint, or a commercial restraint that holds the patient in a particular position.

When the procedure requires a prolonged period of immobility, sedation is often used for infants and small children. Because of their young age, children cannot be expected to remain still for a long time. The procedures that use sedation in children include nuclear medicine scans, computed tomography, magnetic resonance imaging, electroencephalography, echocardiography, and some ultrasound procedures.

Geriatric Patients

Older adult individuals may have certain needs that are age related or caused by a specific disease process. For the confused or depressed patient, instructions may need to be given slowly or repeated several times. The patient may have a hearing deficit or difficulty understanding speech or language. When indicated, alternative communication measures may include written pretest and posttest instructions, inclusion of a family member in the communications, or providing an interpreter to help the patient.

The elderly patient may take a wide range of medications, and some of them can interfere with particular laboratory tests. The physician is consulted regarding any alteration in the medication schedule, such as withholding the medication for a specified period.

Frail, elderly patients are at risk for injury from a fall. The common underlying problems include visual impairment, stiffness, weakness, mental confusion, dizziness, and the effects of medication. Care is taken to prevent accidental injury or a fall by assisting the patient out of the wheelchair and onto or off a gurney, examining table, radiography table, or toilet.

The elderly individual is often uncomfortable when lying on an x-ray table for a long time. The table is hard and the patient's joints are often stiff with arthritis. The room is usually cool, and some older patients complain that they feel cold. It may not be possible to change the patient's position during x-ray studies or other diagnostic procedures because of the requirements of the test; however, warm blankets are usually provided so that at least the discomfort of chilling is removed.

Pretest Phase

Nursing Assessment

This assessment consists of the appraisal of the patient's physical and psychosocial status in relation to the requirements of the test. Pertinent findings in the psychosocial and physical history include any problems with the patient's vision, hearing, mobility, and comprehension of instructions. Current medications are listed. When contrast medium is used in a radiologic study, the nurse assesses for any history of a sensitivity reaction, particularly a reaction to contrast medium during a previous radiology test. Allergies to foods and medications are also documented. If a female of childbearing age needs an x-ray study, she is questioned to determine whether there is any possibility of pregnancy. A rapid urinary pregnancy test may be done for verification before the radiologic procedure is done.

Vital signs are taken to establish baseline values, particularly for an invasive procedure or when contrast medium, sedation, or anesthesia is used. The infant's or child's weight is recorded when the dose of medication or contrast medium must be calculated according to body weight. In radiology imaging, contrast medium is often used. Because contrast medium is excreted in the urine, pretest, rapid urea nitrogen (BUN), and creatinine testing is often done, using point-of-care technology. Normal results ensure that renal function is normal and the healthy kidneys will be able to eliminate the contrast.

The nurse assesses the patient for signs of anxiety or fear. The cause can be apprehension about the test or procedure or fear of abnormal test results. If signs of distress are noted, the nurse asks the patient about the cause or source of the anxiety and provides reassurance, as appropriate.

The nurse also reviews the laboratory and other diagnostic test results and ensures that they are in the patient's record. Tests, such as prothrombin time, complete blood cell count, chest radiograph, electrocardiogram, BUN, and creatinine verify a health clearance before some of the more invasive diagnostic tests are undertaken.

Nursing Diagnoses

Once the nursing assessment is completed, the nurse formulates nursing diagnoses that are appropriate to the patient who will undergo a procedure. The pretest-phase nursing diagnoses are presented in Table 1.

Expected Outcomes

During the pretest period, the expected outcomes include the following:

1. When conscious sedation or anesthesia is anticipated, the patient arranges for a family member or friend to provide transportation home from the outpatient setting.
2. The patient shows no symptoms of infection.
3. The patient communicates any history of a sensitivity reaction to radiology contrast and allergies to specific foods and medications.
4. The patient's vital signs, test results for coagulation studies, and other blood profiles remain within normal limits.
5. The patient requests information or clarification regarding the test and any special measures required in preparation for the test.

Nursing Intervention

The nurse notifies the physician of abnormal pretest results that indicate infection, clotting abnormality, abnormal renal function, fever, or irregularity in the vital signs. The diagnostic procedure may have to be postponed until the abnormality is corrected.

TABLE 1 Pretest-Phase Nursing Diagnoses	
Nursing Diagnosis	**Defining Characteristics**
Risk for injury	Presence of risk factors such as developmental age, psychological factors, or physical factors such as sensory or motor deficit
Risk for infection or allergic reaction	Presence of risk factors, such as altered immune function, history of chronic illness, impaired oxygenation of tissues; external factors, such as allergens or infectious agents
Protection, ineffective	Presence of risk factors, such as altered clotting factors, immunosuppression, myelosuppression, altered cardiovascular or renal status, or disorientation
Impaired verbal communication	Unable to speak dominant language, speaks with difficulty, difficulty in comprehension, altered mental status
Anxiety	Presence of increased tension, uncertainty, fear of unspecific consequences, cardiovascular excitation, facial tension, insomnia, confusion

If the patient has allergies to food, medication, or contrast medium, the nurse posts an allergy warning in the patient's record. Other various types of allergy warning are determined by hospital policy, such as use of an allergy wristband.

Before the day of the test, the nurse provides or implements pretest instructions that can be understood by the patient. Pretest instructions often include the discontinuation of food and fluids for a specified period. They may also involve modification of activity or the temporary stoppage of one or more medications for a specified period. Some abdominal or intestinal tests require a cleansing of the bowel by enema or cathartic, or both.

When indicated, the nurse witnesses the patient's signature of consent for the test or procedure. The patient should have received the physician's explanation of the procedure, the method of performing the test, and the potential risks involved. If the patient cannot give consent because of age or physical or mental impairment, the nurse obtains the signature of the person who is legally responsible for the patient's health care decisions. Once the consent form is signed and witnessed, the nurse enters it into the patient's record.

The nurse provides reassurance or information, as needed, to help reduce the patient's anxiety. This is best done by communication with and assistance to the patient in an attentive and caring manner.

Nursing Outcomes

The pretest phase is completed successfully when the following have been accomplished:
1. Pretest instructions were completed accurately.
2. The patient's blood values, vital signs, and temperature measurement remain within normal limits.
3. The patient appears calm and accepting about the test.

Test Phase

Nursing Assessment

The nursing assessment during the test phase begins with the correct identification of the patient and the verification of the procedure and the area to be tested (such as right or left leg, arm, breast, or lung).

Monitoring of the physiologic status of the patient is carried out by a variety of measurements, depending on the complexity of the procedure and the use of conscious sedation or light anesthesia. Ongoing assessment of the patient may be performed through observation of the level of consciousness, repeated monitoring of vital signs, pulse oximetry, cardiac monitoring, or, in pregnant patients, fetal monitoring.

The skin is assessed for signs of infection or trauma, particularly at the site of intended venipuncture. The patient's chart is also reviewed for the most recent laboratory findings and the pretest vital signs.

The nurse observes the patient for signs of discomfort, including shivering, trembling, pain, and tension. To encourage communication of any problems or concerns, the patient is asked how he or she feels.

Nursing Diagnoses

Once the nursing assessment is completed, the nurse formulates nursing diagnoses that are appropriate to the patient who undergoes the procedure. The test-phase nursing diagnoses are presented in Table 2.

TABLE 2 Test-Phase Nursing Diagnoses	
Nursing Diagnosis	**Defining Characteristics**
Risk for impaired skin integrity	Disruption of the skin surface
	Presence of internal or external risk factors, including skin compression, immobility, or altered circulation
Decreased cardiac output	Variations in blood pressure readings, arrhythmias, color changes of the skin, decreased peripheral pulses, dyspnea, increased heart rate
Impaired gas exchange	Cyanosis, restlessness, dyspnea, hypoxemia
	Risk factors: administration of sedative analgesic medications, contrast medium, and potential sensitivity reaction
Risk for infection	Presence of risk factors such as inadequate primary defenses and performance of invasive procedures
Pain	Verbal report or expressive behavior, such as moaning, crying
	Observed evidence, such as guarding behavior or grimacing
Anxiety	Verbalization of feelings about the test or its potential findings, changes in cardiovascular and respiratory rates

Nursing Diagnoses-Definitions and Classification 2009-2011. **Copyright © 2009, 2007, 2005, 2003, 2001, 1998, 1996, 1994 by NANDA International. Used by arrangement with Wiley-Blackwell Publishing, a company of John Wiley & Sons, Inc.**

Expected Outcomes

During the test period, the patient's outcomes include the following:

1. The patient will maintain adequate skin circulation and tissue perfusion.
2. Cardiopulmonary stability will be maintained. Vital signs and the results of the monitoring devices continue in a normal range.
3. The puncture wound or incision will remain clean and free from infection.
4. The patient will express any pain or discomfort, including the location and characteristics of the sensation.
5. The patient will verbalize any feelings of apprehension and will help identify the cause of those feelings.

Nursing Intervention

The nurse positions the patient correctly for the procedure. Use padding, supportive devices, or restraints to promote safety and protect the patient's tissue against injury.

The patient's cardiopulmonary status is monitored continuously, including assessment of skin color and integrity, vital signs, breathing status, and level of consciousness.

The nurse keeps the emergency cart in a nearby location.

The nurse ensures that all invasive equipment is sterile or has been properly cleaned and disinfected. Before the skin is punctured or opened, ensure that the skin is appropriately cleansed. Draping the area with sterile towels may also be indicated.

Verbal or physical support is offered to the patient by the nurse, particularly when the patient appears distressed by the procedure.

The nurse administers prescribed pain medication as indicated.

Nursing Outcomes

The test phase is completed when the following has been accomplished:

1. The patient demonstrates normal cardiopulmonary function, as measured by normal vital signs and normal readings on all monitoring devices.
2. Normal skin color and tone are present and palpable peripheral pulses are present.
3. The patient experiences a lessening of pain, anxiety, or discomfort.
4. The patient has a clean, dry dressing with no signs of renewed bleeding, hematoma, swelling, or redness.

Posttest Phase

Nursing Assessment

The assessment after the test is completed is focused on the patient's physiologic, emotional, and mental status. Physiologic assessment is essential after an invasive procedure, conscious sedation, or anesthesia. The nurse assesses the expected alterations that occur because of the procedure or medications and the potential complications that may occur.

When cardiac monitoring, fetal monitoring, and pulse oximetry are used during procedures, they are usually continued into the posttest period until the results are stable and remain in a normal range. Alternatively, vital signs are taken manually to ensure that the hemodynamic status remains stable.

A risk of complications from a sensitivity response to the contrast medium in radiology imaging exists. Vital signs also are monitored frequently to identify any untoward changes in cardiorespiratory status. In addition, a risk of an embolus exists when invasive neurologic, cerebrovascular, or peripheral arterial imaging is performed. Neurovascular assessments are performed to assess the integrity of the distal arterial blood flow and the responses of the neurologic tissues that are supplied by that blood flow. The nurse also uses observation to perform many assessments. When the diagnostic procedure is invasive, the nurse examines the site of the incision, penetration of the needle, or insertion of the instrument. The dressing should be clean, dry, and intact. The tissue is examined for signs of swelling, discharge, bleeding, or discoloration. Some pain or soreness may be present because of the incision or the manipulation of internal tissue. The nurse asks the patient to describe and locate the pain or tenderness.

The assessment of mental status is appropriate when the patient has received conscious sedation or anesthesia or after a cerebrovascular invasive test. The nurse assesses the level of consciousness as well as clarity of thinking and speech. During the initial recovery from conscious sedation or anesthesia, the patient may be somewhat confused or drowsy, with diminished affect. As the medications are metabolized and excreted, increasing responsiveness and clarity of thinking are noted.

Before discharge, the patient who has had an invasive procedure is assessed for knowledge about continued requirements for care at home until healing is complete. The patient may be able to perform self-care, or there may be a need for family assistance for the remainder of the day. Assessment for infection or inflammation continues for several days, because the symptoms take time to develop. The patient or family member is taught to continue this assessment at home.

Nursing Diagnoses

Once the nursing assessment has been completed, the nurse formulates nursing diagnoses that are appropriate to the patient during the posttest phase of care. The posttest-phase nursing diagnoses are presented in Table 3.

Expected Outcomes

During the posttest period, the expected outcomes include the following:
1. The patient will be conscious and alert.
2. Oxygenation and tissue perfusion will be normal, including circulation to the extremities.
3. Adequate cardiac output will be maintained.
4. The skin and tissue will have no evidence of swelling or bleeding.
5. After medication is given, the patient will express relief from pain.
6. The site of puncture or incision will remain free from infection.
7. The patient or family member will verbalize understanding of discharge instructions regarding patient care.

Nursing Intervention

After the completion of a diagnostic procedure in which conscious sedation or a light anesthesia was used, position the patient on his or her side to maintain a patent airway.

Oxygen may be administered, and the intravenous fluid replacement continues until the patient is able to drink fluids.

Administer the prescribed pain medication as needed. To help relieve discomfort, encourage the patient to change positions. Provide support with pillows.

TABLE 3 Posttest-Phase Nursing Diagnoses	
Nursing Diagnosis	**Defining Characteristics**
Altered tissue perfusion: cerebral, cardiopulmonary, peripheral	Changes in skin temperature, blood pressure changes, arrhythmias, dyspnea, decreased peripheral pulses, altered mental status
Pain	Verbal report about pain or discomfort
	Alteration in muscle tone, movement, or facial expression
	Expressive behavior, such as moaning, grimacing, and crying
Risk for injury	Presence of risk factors such as immobility, developmental age, or sensory-motor deficit
Risk for infection	Presence of risk factors such as exposure to pathogens, immunosuppression, or broken skin
Knowledge deficit regarding care after procedure	Verbalization of the problem, inaccurate follow-through on instructions
Anxiety	Expressed concerns or uncertainty about the findings of the test or procedure, sleep disturbance, increased tension, worry

Maintain sterile technique in the assessment of the wound or in changing the dressing.

Inform the patient that the physician will discuss the diagnostic results as soon as the information is available. The patient with sutures is instructed to make an appointment with the physician for the evaluation of the incision and removal of the sutures.

Before discharge, instruct the patient about any recommended restrictions, such as instructions regarding activity, bathing, resumption of medication, the intake of fluids, or care of the incision.

Nursing Evaluation

The posttest phase is completed when the following have been accomplished.

1. Normal vital signs, responsiveness to questions, and normal skin color and temperature are evident.
2. The patient experiences a lessening of pain, anxiety, or discomfort.
3. The patient has a clean, dry dressing with no signs of renewed bleeding, hematoma, swelling, or redness.
4. The patient verbalizes his or her understanding of the discharge instructions.

Analysis of the Results and the Significance in Nursing Practice

The nurse who cares for the patient reads the laboratory results and reports of the diagnostic procedures that provide additional objective assessment information. The information helps confirm the patient's medical diagnosis and severity of the pathophysiologic changes. When repeat testing is done, the results are compared with previous results to monitor the patient's response to treatment.

In the diagnostic workup, the physician or health care provider uses the tests to confirm the medical diagnosis and estimate the severity of the condition. Often several tests are needed to identify the specific illness and exclude other possible conditions. Also, many illnesses cause alterations of more than one organ or body system. When repeat tests are used to monitor the patient's response to treatment, the nurse monitors the changes that indicate an improving condition.

The nurse also can use his or her knowledge of the significance of test findings to help patients. The patient may be apprehensive about the possibility of abnormal findings or in need of counseling, clarification, or reassurance regarding abnormal test results that are now known. The nurse can help the patient with emotional support by listening and providing calm and caring responses. The nurse also can try to determine what the patient understands about the meaning of the test results. Finally, the nurse also provides hope by encouraging the patient to consider treatment options and plan for follow-up care.

2 CHAPTER

Specimen Collection Procedures

Three major sources of specimen samples are blood, stool, and urine, with most tests performed on blood. The laboratory performs biochemical, DNA, cellular, and microscopic analysis of these body substances to provide objective data about the patient's health and to identify disease processes. For some specimens, point-of-care testing is used to analyze the specimens at or near the patient's bedside.

In collection procedures, accurate technique is essential for obtaining a valid specimen and to prevent patient injury. In addition, quality control measures are used in maintaining accuracy in the identification of the patient and the specimen, in the method of obtaining the specimen, and in the transportation of the specimen to the laboratory or site of analysis.

In all instances, the person who collects the specimen has the potential to be in contact with the patient's blood or body fluids. Gloves must be worn and the person washes his or her hands after the collection is completed.

BLOOD COLLECTION PROCEDURES

Arterial Puncture

SPECIMEN OR TYPE OF TEST: Arterial Blood

PURPOSE OF THE TEST

Arterial puncture is used to obtain a sample of arterial blood for analysis of blood gases and acid-base balance.

BASICS THE NURSE NEEDS TO KNOW

Arterial blood specimens are obtained for blood gas studies, including the measurement of oxygen, carbon dioxide, and pH. The assessment of arterial blood is usually performed on the patient who has an actual or potential problem with oxygenation. The nursing diagnoses may include ineffective airway clearance, ineffective breathing pattern, impaired gas exchange, and altered tissue perfusion: cardiopulmonary.

The procedure of arterial puncture is technically more difficult than that of venipuncture, but arterial blood is far more accurate for the measurement of oxygenation throughout the body. The usual puncture site is either the radial or the brachial artery, with the radial artery being preferred. The femoral artery can be used; however, the risk of hemorrhage at that site is greater.

Before an arterial puncture of the radial artery is carried out, the *Allen test* is performed to verify the presence of collateral circulation to the hand. If arterial occlusion of the radial artery occurs after arterial puncture, the presence of collateral circulation protects the hand from ischemic damage. The Allen test procedure is presented in the content on Arterial Blood Gases (p. 139).

Some institutions and settings permit the nurse with specialized training to draw blood through an arterial puncture. Refer to the institutional or laboratory protocol to determine who may do this procedure.

HOW THE TEST IS DONE

A heparinized syringe and needle is used to collect 3 mL of arterial blood. For radial artery puncture, a 23- to 25-gauge needle is used. For brachial artery puncture, an 18- to 20-gauge needle is used. In many institutions, a prepackaged kit provides the equipment for blood gas studies.

INTERFERING FACTORS

- Poor collateral circulation to the extremities
- Inability to puncture the artery or withdraw blood
- Air mixed in with the blood specimen

NURSING CARE

Pretest
- Identify the patient by asking his or her name, checking the identification bracelet, and comparing the two identifications with the name on the requisition form.
- When the radial artery is to be used, palpate the pulse of each wrist to select the site with the stronger circulation. Perform the Allen test to assess the collateral circulation to the hand. Position the hand so that the wrist is in slight dorsiflexion.
- Explain to the patient that a sharp pain will be felt as the needle punctures the blood vessel. In some cases, a local anesthetic may be given beforehand.

During the Test
- The interior of the syringe and needle must be coated with heparin. The syringe in the blood gas kit may be heparinized already. If heparin must be added, 1 mL (1000 or 5000 units/mL) is drawn into a 10-mL syringe. After the syringe is rotated to coat the entire interior surface, the heparin is expelled. A small amount of heparin remains in the dead space and within the shaft of the needle.
- Clean the skin over the pulse point with povidone-iodine, using sterile gauze. Remove this solution by wiping the skin with 70% alcohol. Allow the skin to dry.
- With the bevel of the needle up and the syringe placed at a 45- to 60-degree angle, slowly insert the needle into the artery (Figure 3). Blood will pulse into the syringe without your having to draw back on the plunger.
- Once the required amount of blood is in the syringe, remove the needle. The amount is usually 3 mL, but the volume can vary according to the type of syringe and the test protocol.

Posttest
- Use sterile gauze to apply immediate pressure to the puncture site for 5 minutes. Blood flow from the artery and hematoma formation can develop because of the pressure within the arterial walls. Pressure on the puncture point lessens the tendency of excess bleeding.

Continued

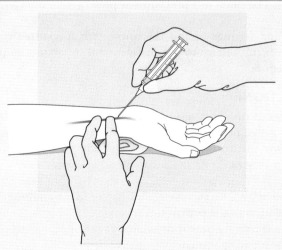

Figure 3. **Technique for arterial puncture.** Puncture of the radial artery can be performed only when both the radial and ulnar arteries provide adequate circulation to the hand.

- Remove the needle from the syringe. If there is air in the syringe, expel it. Place the airtight cap on the tip of the syringe. These measures limit or eliminate possible alteration of blood gas values because of contamination of the blood by the oxygen and carbon dioxide gases in the air.
- Place the syringe on ice and arrange for immediate transport of the specimen to the laboratory.
- Once the bleeding from the puncture site has stopped, the nurse applies a small sterile bandage and continues to assess the wrist and hand for signs of complications. It is common for the patient to complain of some temporary discomfort, such as aching, throbbing, or tenderness at the puncture site.

◆ **Nursing Response to Complications**

The three complications of arterial puncture are bleeding, infection, and thrombus formation, but the incidence is low.

Bleeding. The most common sign of bleeding is hematoma formation. The tissue becomes tense and somewhat swollen in the area of bleeding and spreads through the tissue by gravity. The nurse looks for bruising around the puncture site and at the tissue on the underside of the extremity.

Infection. If the patient develops an infection, the puncture site may become tender, reddened, and swollen. Systemically, the patient develops a fever and the white blood count rises above normal values.

Thrombus formation. The nurse assesses for signs of an obstruction in the circulation distal to the puncture site. This may include loss of a distal pulse when a brachial or femoral puncture site is used. In addition, the distal parts, such as fingers, feel cool or cold and appear pale or cyanotic. The patient complains of pain in the area where there is loss of circulation.

Capillary Puncture

Also called: Finger-stick; Heel-stick

SPECIMEN OR TYPE OF TEST: Capillary Blood

PURPOSE OF THE TEST

Capillary blood collection is used when a small amount of blood is sufficient or the venipuncture method is not feasible.

BASICS THE NURSE NEEDS TO KNOW

The capillary puncture is used for patients with small or inaccessible veins. This method is useful in burn patients, in those who are extremely obese, and in patients who have a tendency toward thrombus formation. It is the method of choice for obtaining blood samples from premature infants, neonates, and young children. It may be used to preserve the total blood volume of the infant or small child, particularly when there is a need for repeated blood testing.

Because capillary blood is similar in composition to venous blood, capillary blood collection may be performed for a complete blood cell count, hematocrit determination, blood smear, coagulation studies, and most blood chemistry tests. The specimen source is always identified on the requisition form, because there may be differences between venous and capillary blood values for calcium, glucose, potassium, and total protein.

Site of Collection

The available sites for collection of capillary blood are the finger and heel. The finger is often used for adults or older children. The locations most often used are the distal tips of the third and fourth fingers, slightly to the side (Figure 4). Few calluses are located on the sides of the fingers,

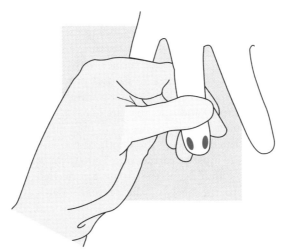

Figure 4. Capillary puncture sites in the finger. In adults the middle or ring finger is the preferred site for a capillary blood sample. The sterile lancet punctures the skin in the distal tip, slightly to the side of the finger pad.

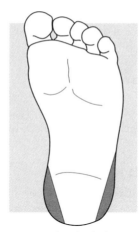

Figure 5. Heelstick sites for capillary puncture. The shaded areas are appropriate sites in neonates and infants. The central portion of the sole of the foot is never used.

and the lancet can puncture the skin more easily. The frontal tips or pads of the fingers are not used because many nerve endings are located there, and the puncture would be more painful.

The heel is used for premature infants, neonates, infants, and small children and for special cases, such as patients with thermal injury. With the heelstick technique, the medial or lateral plantar surface of the heel is used (Figure 5). The central area of the plantar surface of the foot is never used. There is a risk of damage to the calcaneus bone, Achilles tendon, or other tendons, nerves, and cartilage that are located in the central area of the foot.

In the selection of the skin puncture site, the tissue should not be edematous, inflamed, or recently punctured. These factors cause increased interstitial fluid to mix with the blood, and they also increase the risk of an infection.

The heelstick method is preferred for sampling blood in the premature baby and infant. It is technically easier to perform and avoids the significant complications that can occur with arterial or venous puncture. Some special considerations including noninvasive alternatives for monitoring must be made when a large number of heelstick punctures are needed. Each puncture is painful and stressful to the baby and the available tissue surface for the capillary punctures is very small. On average, the premature infant experiences 10 painful procedures per day (Berde & Stevens, 2009). The premature infant may weigh as little as 500 g and the heels are small, with little depth to the tissue for the many punctures and tests that are needed. Additionally, blood flow is often inadequate, and two or three punctures may be needed to obtain the required amount.

To help prevent injury to the calcaneus, the depth of the lancet must be controlled, and careful selection of the tissue site must be carried out. To help prevent infection and hematoma, aseptic technique and gentle handling of the tissue are needed whenever blood is drawn. Because of repeated trauma to the heels of the premature infant, the nurse assesses this tissue for signs of localized complications. These complications can occur during the stay in the neonatal unit, or they can develop years later.

HOW THE TEST IS DONE

A sterile lancet is used to collect capillary blood from a skin puncture site. The blood is blotted onto special filter paper (Figure 6) or collected in a narrow-diameter glass tube called a micropipette, microtube, or capillary tube.

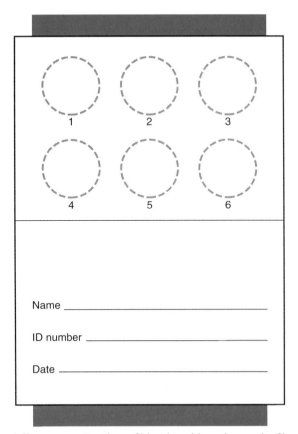

Figure 6. Capillary blood filter paper. Droplets of blood are blotted onto the filter paper at each circle. Each circle must be filled before moving on to fill the next circle. Do not partially fill some circles and then return to complete them later. To promote blood flow, the hand is kept lower than the heart, and the finger is stroked in a distal direction.

INTERFERING FACTORS
- Reduced cardiac output
- Vasoconstriction

NURSING CARE

Pretest
- Identify the patient using the patient's identification bracelet. For infants or small children, the parent or nurse can be the second identifier. Check the requisition form to be certain that the identifiers are the same as the name on the form.
- Particularly with small children, provide reassurance to help limit anxiety.
- If pretest fasting or dietary restriction is required, verify that the instructions were followed for the correct time period.
- The patient may be seated or in the supine position.

Continued

▌NURSING CARE—cont'd

During the Test

- Assess the skin site for color and temperature and the absence of infection and edema. If the skin is cool or pale, the circulation may be diminished. Put the hand in warm water or apply a warm, moist compress to the site for a few minutes. This helps increase circulation to the skin.
- Use gauze and 70% alcohol to cleanse the skin site. Allow the skin to dry.
- Holding the tissue between the thumb and the forefinger, use a firm, quick stroke to puncture the skin with the sterile lancet.
- Wipe away the first drop of blood, because it contains tissue fluids. Collect the subsequent drops of blood in capillary tubes or on the blotting paper.
- To help obtain more blood, the finger or heel may be massaged gently. The tissue near the puncture should not be squeezed because tissue fluids will mix with the blood, and the blood will clot quickly.
- The capillary tubes are held horizontally to prevent air bubbles. They should be filled two-thirds to three-quarters full and then sealed with clay.
- The circles on the filter paper are filled one at a time, until they are fully saturated. Allow the blood on the paper to air-dry for 10 minutes before it is placed in a collection envelope.

Posttest

- Once the specimen collection is completed, wipe the puncture site with alcohol.
- Place sterile gauze on the site and instruct the patient to apply pressure until the bleeding stops.
- If the infant or small child is crying, the nurse or family member provides comfort, such as by rocking, cuddling, or pacifier, as appropriate.
- Before leaving the patient's side, the label is applied directly to the specimen container. The specimen is promptly transported to the laboratory.

◆ **Nursing Response to Complications**

The nurse inspects the infant's feet daily for damage to the skin in the sites of capillary punctures. The laboratory findings are documented in the patient's record and abnormal results are reported to the physician.

Infection. The most serious but infrequent complication of heelstick puncture is infection. The infection is usually localized in the soft tissue, and the most common causative organism is *Staphylococcus aureus*. Weeks later, the infection can develop into osteomyelitis. The source of the infection is poor aseptic technique, a contaminated lancet, or injury to the bone during the skin puncture.

Infection is characterized by localized redness and swelling. The area is tender or painful. In more advanced infection, there may be purulent drainage or abscess formation. Because of the risk that the infection could spread to the bone, x-rays of the heel and foot may be ordered.

Hematoma and Bruising. Bruising, pain, scarring, and hematoma formation are more frequent complications. They occur from frequent skin punctures or excessive squeezing of the tissues during the collection of the blood samples.

When blood has leaked from the puncture site into tissue, the area becomes bruised and discolored. There may be leakage of blood onto the skin. The nurse should handle the baby's foot gently during the examination because the heel tissue will be painful.

Venipuncture

Also called: Phlebotomy; Venous Blood Collection

SPECIMEN OR TYPE OF TEST: Whole Blood, Serum, Plasma

PURPOSE OF THE TEST

Venipuncture is used to obtain a venous blood sample for laboratory analysis. The serum component of the blood is used for most of the chemistry analyses.

BASICS THE NURSE NEEDS TO KNOW

Venipuncture is performed by drawing and collecting a specimen of blood from a superficial vein. It is a quick method of obtaining a larger sample of blood, and the specimen can be used to perform many different laboratory analyses. Depending on the test to be performed, the analysis is carried out on whole blood, serum, or plasma.

Whole blood contains all the blood components. A centrifuge is used to separate the blood components and obtain either serum or plasma. If the blood has been collected in a tube containing anticoagulant, the centrifuge process produces plasma. If whole blood is collected in a tube without anticoagulant, the centrifuge process yields serum. Plasma is serum that contains fibrinogen.

Site of Collection

The most common site for venipuncture is the antecubital fossa, because several large superficial veins are available. The most commonly used veins are the median cubital, the basilic, and the cephalic veins (Figure 7). Veins of the wrists, hands, or ankles may also be used. One exception is that the ankle venipuncture site should not be used for the patient with diabetes.

Intervening Variables

When an intravenous line, shunt, or other intravenous device has been placed in one arm, the venipuncture should not be performed on that arm. The opposite arm or another venous site must be selected. The reason for avoiding these sites is that the administration of intravenous fluids alters the composition of the blood specimen. Additionally, venous shunts are established for specific treatments, and they can be damaged by excessive punctures.

For a variety of physiologic and age-related reasons, locating a suitable vein is sometimes difficult. When the patient is severely dehydrated or hypotensive, or both, the veins have less fluid volume. They are less visible and less palpable and may be partially collapsed. Reduced cardiac output also diminishes the volume of blood in the peripheral veins.

Severe obesity can be a problem because the overlying layers of fat interfere with the location and palpation of a suitable vein. In the elderly, the superficial veins of the hands are highly visible and prominent, but it is difficult to use these sites. The veins are fragile, and venipuncture can cause a hematoma to form. Additionally, these veins move during the venipuncture process, making it difficult to enter the lumen of the vein. The excess movement is caused by the loss of supportive muscle and connective tissue associated with aging.

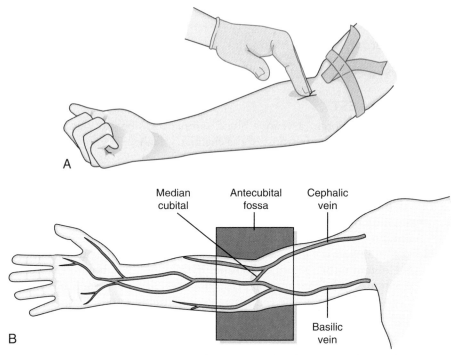

Figure 7. **Preferred sites for venipuncture. A,** Observation and palpation are done in the antecubital fossa to locate the most prominent vein for venipuncture. **B,** The three primary veins in the shaded area are preferred choices because they are usually visible and fixed in place by surrounding tissue. (**A,** From Pfeffinger JL: *Pfeffinger and Fowler's procedures for primary care,* ed 3, St. Louis, 2011, Mosby. **B,** From Lehmann, C.A. *Saunders manual of clinical laboratory science,* Philadelphia, 1998, Saunders.)

If any of these factors cause difficulty with venipuncture, capillary puncture may be an acceptable alternative. If the hand veins are selected for venipuncture, a butterfly needle and a syringe may be used to obtain the blood.

HOW THE TEST IS DONE

Either a vacuum tube system or a needle, syringe, and test tube containers are used to collect the blood sample. The selection of the color-coded specimen tube is based on the requirements of the specific test.

INTERFERING FACTORS

- Dehydration
- Hypotension
- Obesity
- Fragility of veins
- Prematurity and infancy

NURSING CARE

Pretest

- Identify the patient with two identifiers. These are usually the patient's wristband and the patient who states his or her name. Check that the requisition form and label also have the same information as the identifiers.
- Inform the patient that blood needs to be drawn from the designated site. Provide reassurance to help limit anxiety.
- If pretest fasting or dietary restriction is required, verify that the instructions were followed for the correct time period.
- Assemble the equipment and put on a pair of gloves.
- The patient may be seated or in the supine position. The patient's arm is in extension, with easy access to the antecubital fossa.

During the Test

- Inspect the antecubital fossae of both arms to select the best vein for the venipuncture. Ask the patient to open and close the hand a few times to help make the veins more visible.
- Gently palpate the vein to determine its location, direction, width, and depth.
- Cleanse the skin with 70% alcohol and allow it to air-dry.
- Apply the tourniquet about 2 to 3 inches above the antecubital fossa.
- Using your fingertips, anchor the vein above and below the puncture site.
- With the bevel up, insert the needle at a 15-degree angle along the pathway of the vein (Figure 8).

   Syringe method. Once the needle is in the vein, gently aspirate blood into the syringe. Collect the volume of blood that is needed.

   Vacuum tube system method. Once the needle is in the vein, hold it firmly in place. Push the blood collection tube fully into the holder so that the blood flows through the needle and into the vacuum tube (Figure 9). When multiple specimens are needed, remove each full tube and insert the next tube firmly into the holder. After all blood has been collected, release the tourniquet. Place sterile gauze over the puncture site. Remove the needle. Use the gauze and your finger to compress the puncture site.

   When blood is drawn by syringe or the vacuum tube system method, the tourniquet should not remain tied for more than 1 minute. The prolonged compression of the vein and stasis of the blood flow results in clumping or hemolysis of the erythrocytes. Hemolysis and clumping interfere with the laboratory analysis and alter some test results.

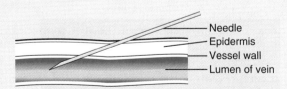

Figure 8. Needle placement during venipuncture. To obtain good blood flow into the collection tube or syringe, the needle tip must be positioned correctly in the vein lumen. The needle should not rest against the upper wall of the vein or puncture through the vein wall on the opposite side.

Continued

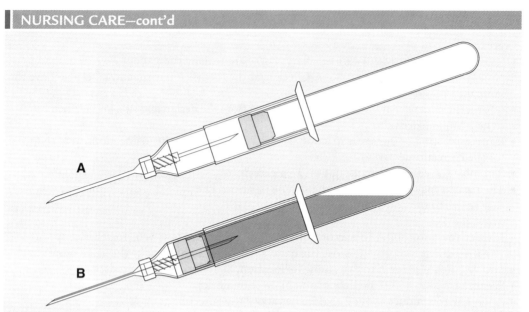

Figure 9. Function of the vacuum tube collection system. **A,** Before venipuncture, the vacuum tube is placed in the holder, resting gently on top of the sterile needle. **B,** Once the needle enters the vein, the tube is pushed to the front of the holder, and the needle penetrates the stopper of the collection tube. Because of the negative pressure in the tube, the blood will pull from the vein, through the needle, and fill the vacuum tube.

Posttest

- Instruct the patient to continue compression of the puncture site for 2 to 5 minutes or until the bleeding stops.
- If a syringe and needle were used, transfer the blood to the appropriate test tube containers.
- Label every vial of blood with the patient's name and identification number, the time, and the date.
- Assess the patient's arm to ensure that the bleeding has ceased. Apply an adhesive bandage as needed.
- Remove gloves and wash your hands.
- Arrange for prompt transport of the specimen to the laboratory.

◆ Nursing Response to Complications

Hematoma. Hematoma formation occurs when the vein continues to leak blood under the skin.

The nurse assesses for a bruised area in the site of the venipuncture. The problem can be prevented by continued compression of the puncture site until clotting occurs. The patient can also elevate the arm and rest it on top of the head. This reduces the blood volume and pressure on the walls of the vein, promoting clotting.

STOOL COLLECTION PROCEDURE

Stool Collection

Also called: Stool Specimen

SPECIMEN OR TYPE OF TEST: Feces

PURPOSE OF THE TEST

Analysis of feces is used to screen for intestinal disease in an asymptomatic individual and to help identify abnormal intestinal function or abnormal function of the gallbladder, liver, or pancreas. It is also used to detect microbes or parasites that reside in the intestinal tract and cause infection.

BASICS THE NURSE NEEDS TO KNOW

The laboratory testing of fecal matter may involve chemical analysis that identifies the abnormal composition of the feces or may involve microbiologic analysis that identifies infectious organisms. Once the abnormality has been identified, additional diagnostic tests or procedures are often needed to determine the cause and location of the problem.

One group of abnormal fecal test results is caused by diseases that damage the intestinal mucosa, alter the integrity of the intestinal tissue, or interfere with the functions of digestion, absorption, and elimination. The fecal changes may include the presence of blood or an alteration in the composition of the feces. Examples of these diseases include malignancy of the stomach or colon, peptic ulcer, regional ileitis, celiac disease, or scleroderma.

A second group of abnormal fecal test results is caused by abnormality in the organs and ducts that secrete into the intestinal tract. These organs include the liver, pancreas, and gallbladder. The fecal changes can include excess fat in the stool or a lack of fecal urobilinogen. Examples of these conditions include cystic fibrosis, pancreatic cancer, hepatitis, and bile duct obstruction.

A third category of abnormal fecal test results is caused by infectious organisms that infect the intestinal tract. The organisms are discovered by microscopic examination of the stool or stool culture. The infection may be of bacterial, viral, parasitic, or other origin, often infecting the small or large intestine. Sometimes the infection causes damage to the intestinal mucosa or underlying tissue, resulting in blood in the stool.

HOW THE TEST IS DONE

A half-pint waterproof container that is clean and dry and has a wide mouth with a tight-fitting lid is used to collect approximately 1 to 2 oz of fecal matter.

INTERFERING FACTORS
- Improper specimen collection
- Contamination of the specimen with water or urine
- Delay in transport of the specimen
- Failure to follow pretest dietary instructions
- Pretest ingestion of antibiotics, cathartics, or barium, or administration of an enema

| **NURSING CARE** |

Pretest

- Identify the patient by the use of two identifiers: the identification bracelet and the patient's statement of name. Check that the requisition form and the specimen label are the same name as the identifiers.
- Ask the patient if he or she has had a recent barium x-ray study or recent treatment with oral antibiotics. After ingestion, barium sulfate interferes with the analysis of feces for approximately 2 weeks. Stool culture is less likely to demonstrate the causative organism when antibiotics have been taken during the preceding 3 to 4 weeks. Schedule the stool collection accordingly.

○ *Patient Teaching.* The nurse instructs the patient about any dietary restrictions that are part of specific test preparations. For some of the tests, such as those looking for fecal fat and fecal occult blood, pretest dietary modifications are required or recommended. The patient is also instructed not to ingest castor oil, mineral oil, antacids, or antidiarrheal medications or to administer an enema before the test. These substances would appear in the fecal matter and interfere with the chemical or microscopic analysis.

During the test

○ *Patient Teaching.* The nurse instructs the patient to evacuate directly into the container or a clean, dry bedpan. Tongue blades can be used to transfer a small amount of feces from the bedpan into the collection container. Urine, water, or toilet paper must not be mixed in with the fecal specimen.

- Once the specimen is obtained, place the lid on the container and wash hands.

Posttest

- The person who collects the specimen places the label on the container (not the lid) with the patient's name and other appropriate data. Mark the time and date of the collection on the container and requisition form.
- Arrange for transport of the specimen within 30 minutes. If there is a delay before transport, store the specimen in the refrigerator. The cool temperature preserves any microorganisms that may be present.

URINE COLLECTION PROCEDURES

BASICS THE NURSE NEEDS TO KNOW

Urine provides a major source of data about the status and function of the urinary tract. In addition, because urine is an ultrafiltrate of the plasma, it is used to assess various homeostatic and metabolic processes of the body. Urine is easily collected, but the procedure must be performed completely and accurately. If there is an error in procedure, false or invalid test results can occur.

The four basic urine collection procedures, which are based on the time or duration of the collection period, are as follows: the first morning specimen, the random specimen, the fractional specimen, and the timed specimen. Because the purposes and methods vary, each of these procedures is discussed separately in subsequent sections of this chapter.

In addition to spontaneous voiding, several other possible methods of collection are available. A description of the special collection methods is presented here. When urine cannot be collected by normal voiding, these special methods are used for any of the basic collection procedures.

Special Collection Methods

Catheterization

A catheterized specimen is used when the patient cannot void or when an indwelling catheter is already in place. For straight catheterization, a sterile catheter is inserted through the urethra and into the bladder. The urine flows from the bladder, through the catheter, and into the specimen container. Once the bladder has been emptied, the catheter is removed.

For a patient with an indwelling catheter, fresh urine is collected directly from the catheter in all types of tests except the timed specimen. For the single urine specimen collection, the catheter is clamped below the port temporarily. After a short interval, a sterile needle and syringe are used to remove the urine sample through a special port in the catheter. Once the sample is obtained, the clamp is removed, and the urine flow to the collection bag resumes. A timed specimen has a much longer collection period and requires a larger volume of urine. At the start of the test, a new, empty collection bag is attached to the indwelling catheter and its tubing. The urine is removed from the collection bag at intervals and is added to the specimen collection container until the time period is completed.

Pediatric Specimens

If the child is toilet trained and can follow directions, the nurse can provide instructions to the parent or assist the child in the collection of the urine. For the infant or child who cannot control the release of urine voluntarily, a pediatric collection bag is used. The perineum is cleansed and dried, and then the bag is applied and fixed with an adhesive strip. For the male infant, the bag is placed over the penis. For the female infant, the bag is applied over the labia and perineum. In each gender, the rectum must be excluded to prevent the mixing of fecal matter with urine. Once the bag is in place, it is checked every 15 minutes until the urine is collected.

Suprapubic Aspiration

This method is used when an anaerobic culture is required or when there is a problem with external contamination of the urine culture, such as in infancy. With the use of sterile technique, the suprapubic aspiration is performed by the physician. A sterile needle is inserted through the abdominal wall above the symphysis pubis and then is advanced into the full bladder. A syringe is used to aspirate the urine specimen. The specimen is placed into a culture container, and the needle is removed.

First Morning Specimen

SPECIMEN OR TYPE OF TEST: Urine

PURPOSE OF THE TEST

The first morning specimen is used for routine urinalysis that includes chemical and microscopic analysis. This specimen is also used to identify orthostatic proteinuria.

BASICS THE NURSE NEEDS TO KNOW

The first morning specimen is the first urine to be voided after the patient awakens from sleep. This urine has been retained in the bladder for about 6 to 8 hours. Because of the lack of fluid intake or exercise during the period of sleep, the urine is concentrated and somewhat acidic.

This type of specimen is preferred for routine screening. It is also preferred for the detection of specific substances, including nitrites, protein, and microorganisms. Concentrated urine or an incubation period is needed to readily detect these substances in the urine.

HOW THE TEST IS DONE

A clean, dry plastic or glass container with a lid is used to collect a midstream urine specimen.

INTERFERING FACTORS

- Menstrual secretions
- Delay in the analysis of the urine
- Inadequate labeling of the specimen

NURSING CARE

Pretest
- The nurse provides the patient with a urine container with a lid.
- ○ *Patient Teaching.* Instruct the patient to collect a midstream voided specimen. A midstream void means that the patient begins to urinate, and about halfway through the process the specimen is collected. With this method, the initial urine flow washes the bacteria out of the distal urethra before the specimen is collected.
- ○ *Patient Teaching.* In some protocols, a midstream clean-catch method is used. If this is the case, provide the patient with the materials and instructions, as presented in Box 3.

Posttest
- The nurse seals the lid of the container completely to prevent leakage.
- The container must be labeled appropriately with the patient's name and other pertinent information, including the date and time of the collection. The information should not be placed on the lid.
- The nurse ensures that the specimen is delivered to the laboratory immediately. If a delay is anticipated, the specimen must be refrigerated or a preservative added to the urine container. If there is a delay of 2 hours or longer before analysis is performed, a warm, unpreserved specimen will undergo a number of changes. The changes vary among the individual specimens, but almost every laboratory value can be altered.

Video-Male and Female Mid-stream Urine Collection

Random Specimen

SPECIMEN OR TYPE OF TEST: Urine

PURPOSE OF THE TEST

The random specimen is used for routine urinalysis that includes chemical and microscopic examination. This method of collection is also used for bacterial culture and cytologic studies to help identify the cause of disease in the urinary tract.

| BOX 3 | Midstream Clean-Catch Urine Procedure |

Purpose

This method of urine collection reduces the external sources of contamination before the urine is collected. The contaminants are the bacteria and secretions of the skin that surround the urethra and reside in the distal portion of the urethra.

Procedure

Cleansing process: Male

The glans is exposed and cleansed with the use of three sterile cotton balls or gauze squares moistened with a mild antiseptic solution.

The first cotton ball cleanses the tissue from the urethral meatus to the ring of the glans in a single stroke. The cotton ball is then discarded. The process is repeated with the other two cotton balls, cleansing the remaining areas of the glans.

If the male is uncircumcised, the foreskin must be retracted and the tissue under the foreskin cleansed thoroughly before the preceding steps are taken.

Cleansing process: Female

The labia minora are separated to expose the urinary meatus. They must then remain separated throughout the cleansing process and urine collection phase.

The exterior mucous membranes and the meatus are cleansed with the use of three sterile cotton balls or gauze squares moistened with a mild antiseptic.

The first moist cotton ball cleanses the tissue on one side of the urinary meatus with a single stroke from front to back. The cotton ball is discarded. The second cotton ball cleanses the other side of the meatus with the same motion and direction. The third cotton ball cleanses the center of the meatus wiping in a single motion from front to back.

Midstream collection

The patient begins to void into the toilet or bedpan. The urine washes residual bacteria and secretions from the distal urethra.

At about the midpoint of voiding, the urine stream is interrupted. On release of the urine, 1 to 3 oz of urine is collected in the specimen container.

The container must not touch the perineal tissues or hair either during or after collection. The patient's fingers must not touch the inside of the container or lid.

Once the amount of urine in the container is sufficient, the patient finishes voiding into the toilet or bedpan, and that remaining amount is discarded.

BASICS THE NURSE NEEDS TO KNOW

The random urine specimen can be collected at any time. It is easy and convenient for the patient because there is no need to plan or schedule the test. Even though the daytime activities of fluid intake and exercise alter the composition of the urine, there is no need to control these variables. The specimen is usually satisfactory for the purposes of screening or routine urinalysis.

Cytologic studies are also performed on random urine samples. For this test, the patient must drink extra fluids before each of several urine sample collections. The goal is to flush out an increased number of cells so that the detection of abnormal cells is enhanced. Random samples are also used for urine cultures, with the goal of identifying microbial growth and the presence of infection.

HOW THE TEST IS DONE

For routine urinalysis or a random urine screen, a clean plastic or glass container with a lid is used to collect a urine sample at any time. A midstream clean-catch method is used (see Box 3).

For a bacterial, fungal, or viral culture, a sterile plastic or glass container with a lid is used to collect the random urine sample. The midstream clean-catch method is used. For cytologic studies, the midstream clean-catch method is used to collect each specimen in a clean plastic or glass container with a lid. Daily specimens are collected for 3 to 5 consecutive days.

INTERFERING FACTORS

- Menstrual secretions
- Delay in the analysis of the specimen
- Inadequate labeling of the specimen
- Contamination of the specimen

NURSING CARE

Pretest

○ *Patient Teaching.* The nurse provides written and verbal instructions regarding how to cleanse the urethral meatus and surrounding tissue and how to collect the specimen. The patient is given the appropriate collection container or containers.

○ *Patient Teaching.* For cytologic studies, the nurse instructs the patient to drink 24 to 32 oz of water each hour for 2 hours before voiding. In some laboratory protocols, the patient is also instructed to exercise for 5 minutes by skipping or jumping rope before voiding. The activity and fluid volume should increase the yield of cells needed for the study. This process is repeated daily for 3 to 5 days to provide for the analysis of three to five consecutive urine specimens.

Posttest

- The lid of the container must be closed completely to prevent leakage.
- The nurse labels the container appropriately with the patient's name and other pertinent information, including the date and time of the collection. The information is not placed on the lid.
- The nurse ensures that the specimen is delivered to the laboratory immediately. If there is an anticipated delay, the specimen must be refrigerated or a preservative added to the urine container. If a delay of 2 hours or longer occurs before analysis is performed, the warm, unpreserved specimen can undergo a number of changes. The changes vary among the individual specimens, but almost every laboratory value can be altered.

Fractional Specimen

Also called: Double-Voided Specimen

SPECIMEN OR TYPE OF TEST: Urine

PURPOSE OF THE TEST

Fractional collection is used to compare blood and urine values in screening for diabetes mellitus and in the diagnosis of some liver and kidney disorders.

BASICS THE NURSE NEEDS TO KNOW

A fractional collection of urine is a method used to compare a particular component of the urine with the serum level of that component. Blood samples and urine samples are collected at specific times, and the laboratory analysis measures the amount of the component found in each specimen.

The serum sample is measured for the blood level during controlled conditions, such as in a fasting state or after administration of a dye or solute. The urine samples are measured for the baseline and renal threshold values. One example of fractional collection is the Glucose Tolerance Test (p. 345).

HOW THE TEST IS DONE

Generally, baseline blood and urine specimens are obtained first. The patient then receives a measured intravenous or oral substance such as food, dye, or glucose. Thereafter, timed blood and urine specimens are collected according to the test protocol.

INTERFERING FACTORS

- Failure to complete the pretest preparation
- Failure to collect all urine specimens
- Failure to obtain all urine specimens at the correct times
- Failure to label all specimens accurately

NURSING CARE

Pretest

○ *Patient Teaching.* The nurse provides the patient with written and verbal instructions. Some of these tests require nothing-by-mouth (NPO) status for 6 to 8 hours before the test. Some have instructions to void and discard the first morning specimen. The instructions are specific to the test.

During the Test

- The nurse administers the prescribed oral glucose solution, injectable dye, or other measured substance used in the test.
- Each urine specimen is collected in a separate container at the specific time interval required by the protocol.

Continued

- The nurse labels each container with the patient's name and other appropriate identifying information. The time of each voided specimen is also recorded on the container (e.g., ½-hour specimen, 1-hour specimen). The information is not written on the lid.

Posttest

- The nurse sends all specimens to the laboratory together without delay. If a delay of more than 2 hours occurs, the specimens must be preserved by refrigeration. Many components of urine are altered when the specimen remains warm and a delay occurs in performing the analysis. In particular, the level of urinary glucose becomes falsely decreased because of cellular and bacterial glycolysis.

Timed Specimen

SPECIMEN OR TYPE OF TEST: Urine

PURPOSE OF THE TEST

The timed collection is used to perform quantitative urine assays and clearance tests and to identify abnormal cytology, or ova and parasites in the urine.

BASICS THE NURSE NEEDS TO KNOW

Timed collection is used for the quantitative analysis of a specific urinary component. Circadian rhythms, diurnal rhythms, metabolism, exercise, and hydration all affect the excretion rate of substances in the urine. At certain times during a 24-hour period, the excretion of substances such as electrolytes, hormones, proteins, and urobilinogen increases, and at other times excretion decreases. By collecting the quantity of urine over a specified period, accuracy of measurement is greater than that with a random specimen.

Sometimes, an abnormal substance is not present consistently in the urine. Thus the urine is collected for a longer period to try to identify the small amounts of the component that are occasionally present. Urine cytologic testing requires a 2-hour collection period repeated over several days. The parasites *Schistosoma* and *Onchocerca* are detected in urine that is collected over a 24-hour period.

Time Intervals

The designated time period for a urine collection depends on the specific component to be tested. Some tests are for a *predetermined length of time*, such as a 2-hour, 12-hour, or 24-hour urine collection. Other tests are for a *specific time of day*, such as 12 PM to 4 PM. In these instances, the time frame reflects when the substance is maximally excreted in the urine each day.

HOW THE TEST IS DONE

A large (3000-mL) clear or brown glass or plastic container with a lid is used to collect all urine within the designated period.

INTERFERING FACTORS

- Failure to discard the first voided specimen before the procedure begins
- Failure to collect all the urine voided during the test period
- Failure to refrigerate or preserve the urine specimen
- Improper labeling

▌ NURSING CARE

Pretest

◯ *Patient Teaching.* The nurse provides both written and verbal instructions regarding the collection of the urine. These instructions must include the specific times for the collection period. For a 24-hour urine collection, the nurse instructs the patient to moderately limit fluid intake during the collection period. Alcohol intake should be avoided for 24 hours before and during any timed collection of urine. Other restrictions are part of specific test protocols. Some tests have specific dietary restrictions, and some medications need to be withheld for a specific period. Any special restrictions or modifications are included in the patient's pretest instructions.

◯ *Patient Teaching.* When the patient works or is in school, the nurse advises that the easiest time to collect the specimen is on the weekend.

During the Test

- For all timed collections, the nurse or the patient maintains the specimen and container on ice or in the refrigerator during the collection period. Such measures prevent deterioration of the specimen.
- During the time period, all urine is added to the collection container. If any urine spills or if a specimen is discarded accidentally, the test is invalid. The stored specimen is discarded, and a new collection period is started the next day.
- For the 24-hour urine collection, the first void of the morning is discarded, and the urine collection period begins at 8 AM. Place all urine for 24 hours into the container. This includes the first voided specimen of the next morning.

Posttest

- The nurse labels the container with the patient's name and other appropriate identifying data. Include the time and date of the start and the completion of the urine collection period. No information is placed on the lid of the container. The nurse also arranges for prompt delivery of the specimen to the laboratory.

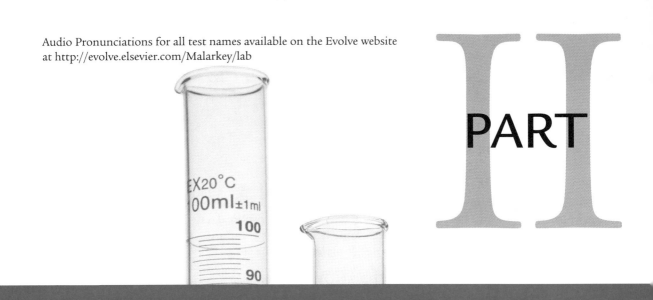

Audio Pronunciations for all test names available on the Evolve website at http://evolve.elsevier.com/Malarkey/lab

PART II

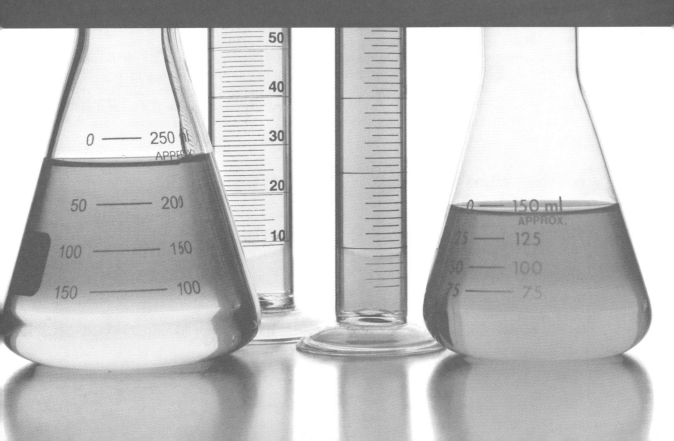

Laboratory Tests and Diagnostic Procedures

Activated Clotting Time

Also called: (ACT); Activated Coagulation Time

SPECIMEN OR TYPE OF TEST: Whole blood

PURPOSE OF THE TEST

The activated clotting time is used to measure the anticoagulation effect of high-dose heparin therapy during cardiac bypass surgery with extracorporeal circulation, angioplasty, and hemodialysis. It is also used to determine the dose of protamine sulfate needed to reverse the anticoagulant effect of heparin after completion of the surgical procedure.

BASICS THE NURSE NEEDS TO KNOW

When the patient receives very high doses of heparin medication, frequent monitoring of the anticoagulation effect is required. If the anticoagulant effect of the heparin is insufficient, the clotting time will be lower than the therapeutic value and the patient may form a blood clot. If the anticoagulant effect of the heparin therapy is beyond the therapeutic range, the patient may develop a hemorrhage. This blood test measures the time it takes for the blood to form a clot.

When high doses of heparin are given, the therapeutic values are elevated because it takes a longer time for the blood to coagulate. This is a desirable goal because the patient is protected from formation of a thrombus or embolus during the surgery or procedure. The therapeutic values vary with the type of procedure and coagulation risk that is involved. Generally, the therapeutic goal of anticoagulation during cardiopulmonary bypass surgery is longer than 400 to 500 seconds and during cardiac angioplasty, the therapeutic value is longer than 350 seconds.

The specimen for the activated clotting time is analyzed in point-of-care testing. This means that the analyzer instrument is at the patient's bedside or near the patient care unit so that test results can be obtained without delay. Several types of analyzer instruments are available. The test method and the test values vary with the analyzer instrument used. The nurse should refer to the instructions and normal values determined by the institution's laboratory and the manufacturer.

REFERENCE VALUES   70 to 180 seconds

HOW THE TEST IS DONE

Venipuncture is performed to collect a sample of venous blood.

SIGNIFICANCE OF TEST RESULTS

Elevated Values
Anticoagulation with heparin
Severe deficiency of coagulation factors of the intrinsic pathway (except Factors VII and VIII)

INTERFERING FACTORS

- Contamination with heparin in the intravenous line
- Hemodilution/hemoconcentration

NURSING CARE

Nursing actions are similar to those used in other venipuncture procedures (see Chapter 2), with the following additional measures.

Pretest

- The nurse uses a flow sheet that provides for documentation of the time, amount, and route of heparin administration, as well as the time and result of ACT testing.

During the Test

- If the nurse collects the specimen of blood, the intravenous line that contains heparin or heparin infusion should not be used. Select a vein in the opposite arm because the heparin in the intravenous line or catheter would falsely elevate the test result. Some specimen tubes require vigorous shaking to mix the blood with the activator in the tube. Other tubes require gentle mixing. The nurse should refer to the specific manufacturer's instructions for reference information. Once obtained, the specimen should be placed in the analyzer, without delay.

Posttest

- Using sterile gauze, the nurse applies pressure on the venipuncture site until bleeding ceases. There is a tendency to bleed for a longer time than usual because the patient is very anticoagulated.
- The nurse frequently assesses for signs of abnormal bleeding, as into the urine or from the gingivae and mucosa in the mouth. The skin is assessed for bruising, bleeding, and petechiae.
- Each ACT test result is posted in the patient's record and on the flow sheet.

▽ **Nursing Response to Critical Values**

When the activated clotting time result is elevated, the patient may begin to bleed or hemorrhage. The nurse performs frequent assessment for signs of bleeding and monitors the values of ACT test results.

The nurse keeps protamine sulfate on hand for use in case of hemorrhage. The action of protamine sulfate is to neutralize heparin, usually within 5 minutes after it is administered. If prescribed, this medication in its undiluted state is injected very slowly, intravenously. When protamine sulfate is administered, the nurse monitors the vital signs because if it is administered too rapidly, this medication can result in severe hypotension, bradycardia, and dyspnea. Thereafter, ACT values are monitored because of a potential heparin rebound effect that can occur several hours later. Protamine sulfate would lower the ACT value; a heparin rebound effect would again raise the ACT value.

A

Activated Partial Thromboplastin Time

Also called: (APTT); Partial Thromboplastin Time (PTT)

SPECIMEN OR TYPE OF TEST: Plasma

PURPOSE OF THE TEST

This test helps identify bleeding or clotting disorders that are hereditary or acquired. It is used to monitor the effect of heparin anticoagulant therapy and to adjust the dosage of heparin based on the test results.

BASICS THE NURSE NEEDS TO KNOW

The activated partial thromboplastin time measures the number of seconds needed for a clot to form. The test results include the patient's value and the control value. The control value of the test is the reference or normal value that is used to evaluate the patient's test result. The APTT is used to monitor the results of anticoagulation therapy with heparin, hirudin, or argatroban. The goal of anticoagulation therapy is to maintain the APTT in a therapeutic range of about 1.5 to 2.5 times the normal value. For example, if the control (normal) value is 30 seconds, the anticoagulated patient's therapeutic value should be in the range of 45 to 75 seconds. With a prolonged APTT, the patient takes longer to make a clot, and a thrombus or embolus is less likely to develop.

If the patient has an impairment of the intrinsic coagulation system that causes a prolonged APTT, the medical treatment may be a transfusion of whole blood or plasma so that the clotting factors are increased and the APTT value returns to normal.

REFERENCE VALUES*	Average value: 25 to 35 seconds Newborn: <90 seconds Premature infants: <120 seconds
▽ Critical Value	Adult: 100 to 150 seconds

*The reference values vary with the type of laboratory method and equipment that are used.

HOW THE TEST IS DONE

Venipuncture or capillary puncture is used to obtain a sample of venous blood.

SIGNIFICANCE OF TEST RESULTS

Elevated Values
Anticoagulant therapy
Deficiency of one or more coagulation factors
Hemophilia
Disseminated intravascular coagulation (DIC)
Circulatory anticoagulants such as lupus anticoagulants
Liver failure
Vitamin K deficiency

Decreased Values
Hypercoagulable states (with thrombus formation)

INTERFERING FACTORS
- Inadequate blood sample

NURSING CARE

Nursing actions are similar to those used in other venipuncture procedures (see Chapter 2), with the following additional measures.

Pretest
- When heparin is given in intermittent doses, the time for APTT monitoring is 6 hours after the anticoagulant is given. This timing provides accurate information and allows the physician to adjust the heparin dose as needed.
- When a continuous intravenous infusion of heparin is started, the APTT is drawn every 6 hours after the initial dose of anticoagulant for the first day and 6 hours after changing the medication dosage. Once the therapeutic range of anticoagulation is achieved, the APTT is tested once a day.

Posttest
- For the patient receiving anticoagulants, assess the venipuncture site for signs of bleeding or ecchymosis. To promote clotting at the venipuncture site, the nurse uses sterile gauze to apply pressure to the site or raises the patient's arm above the head while maintaining pressure on the site. Prolonged pressure is often needed because of the anticoagulant effect.
- When the patient receives heparin anticoagulation therapy, the nurse monitors each APTT result for a value in the therapeutic range. If the result is elevated beyond the therapeutic range, the nurse notifies the physician. The physician may lower the dose of the anticoagulant or the intravenous infusion with heparin may be discontinued for a short time. Protamine sulfate, the antidote to heparin, is kept available in case of a severe, excess anticoagulation result. When prescribed, the nurse injects the protamine sulfate subcutaneously.

○ *Patient Teaching.* The nurse teaches the anticoagulated patient how to protect against a bleeding episode. The patient should use an electric razor for shaving and a soft toothbrush to avoid scraping of the gingiva (gums) of the oral cavity. Over-the-counter medications such as aspirin and remedies that contain aspirin are to be avoided because they interfere with platelet aggregation. The patient is taught to observe signs of abnormal bleeding in the skin, gingiva, vomitus, stool, and urine.

▽ **Nursing Response to Critical Values**
If the APTT value is in the critical value range, the physician must be notified. The patient is at risk for spontaneous bleeding or hemorrhage.

The nurse assesses the patient for spontaneous bleeding, oozing of blood, bruising, and petechiae. The nurse observes the skin, mucus membranes, and gingiva of the oral cavity, and the urine and stool for manifestations of bleeding. The vital signs are taken, observing for hypotension and tachycardia. The nurse asks the patient if he or she has a headache because this can be an early sign of an intracranial bleeding episode. Until the physician is contacted, the nurse must withhold the next dose of heparin.

Adrenocorticotropic Hormone, Plasma

Also called: (ACTH); Corticotropin

SPECIMEN OR TYPE OF TEST: Plasma

PURPOSE OF THE TEST

A plasma ACTH determination is obtained to diagnose Cushing's disease and differentiate primary and secondary adrenal insufficiency.

BASICS THE NURSE NEEDS TO KNOW

Adrenocorticotropic hormone (ACTH) is produced and secreted by the anterior pituitary gland. Its secretion is under the control of the hypothalamus and the central nervous system by neurotransmitters and corticotropin-releasing hormone (CRH). ACTH, in turn, regulates the secretion of the glucocorticoids and androgens from the adrenal cortex.

The mechanisms of regulation of CRH, ACTH, and the adrenal hormones are multiple, and patterns of secretion of these hormones vary within the individual and among individuals. CRH and ACTH are excreted episodically and by circadian rhythm (remember crossing multiple time zones can affect a person's circadian rhythm). Increases in ACTH levels cause increased levels of glucocorticoids and androgens in the blood within minutes. Generally, CRH, ACTH, and cortisol (the major glucocorticoid) levels are low in the evening and continue to decline for the first few hours of sleep. After 3 to 5 hours of sleep, the levels of the hormones increase and then peak after 6 to 8 hours of sleep. On waking, the hormone levels begin to decline. Superimposed on this circadian rhythm are episodic secretions. The hormone levels increase with exercise, eating, and stress.

A negative feedback mechanism also regulates the hypothalamic-pituitary-adrenal hormonal responses. As the cortisol level increases in the plasma, it inhibits both ACTH secretion by the pituitary gland and CRH secretion by the hypothalamus (Figure 10). The nurse needs to be aware of the feedback inhibition of CRH and ACTH, which occurs with exogenous administration of glucocorticoids.

An increase or decrease in the production of ACTH will cause an increase or decrease in the glucocorticoid levels. A deficiency of ACTH will cause secondary adrenal insufficiency. An increase in ACTH will cause Cushing's disease (Cushing's syndrome is a primary adrenal disorder).

REFERENCE VALUES*

Adult
In morning (6 AM-10 AM): 25-100 pg/mL or SI: 25-100 pmol/L
In evening (9 PM-12 AM): 0-50 pg/mL or SI: 0-50 pmol/L

*Values vary depending on laboratory.

HOW THE TEST IS DONE

A venipuncture is done with chilled syringe and blood placed on ice and sent immediately to the lab.

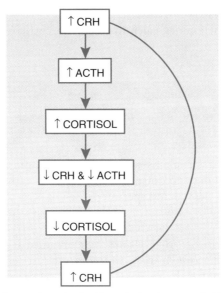

Figure 10. Hypothalamic-pituitary-adrenal axis. Hypothalamic control of adrenal hormone secretion occurs through release of corticotropin-releasing hormone (CRH), which stimulates the secretion of adrenocorticotropic hormone (ACTH) by the pituitary gland. ACTH stimulates the adrenals to increase their secretion of cortisol. By a negative feedback mechanism, the increase in serum cortisol level suppresses the release of CRH and ACTH.

SIGNIFICANCE OF TEST RESULTS

Elevated Values
Primary adrenal insufficiency
Cushing's disease
Congenital adrenal hyperplasia
Ectopic ACTH syndrome
Stress
Trauma

Decreased Values
Primary adrenal hypersecretion
Cushing's syndrome
Tumors of the adrenal gland may suppress the ACTH level if they produce glucocorticoids; however, not all adrenal tumors do.

INTERFERING FACTORS
- Noncompliance with medication, diet, or activity restrictions
- Administration of radioactive scans within 7 days
- Pregnancy
- Traumatic venipuncture

A

- Delay in specimen being tested or frozen
- Ingestion of alcohol, amphetamines, calcium gluconate, corticosteroids, estrogen, lithium, or spironolactone

NURSING CARE

Nursing actions are similar to those used in other venipuncture procedures (see Chapter 2), with the following additional measures.

Pretest

○ *Patient Teaching.* The nurse explains to the patient the need to obtain two specimens of blood, one in the early morning and one in the evening. The early morning specimen reflects the peak secretion time and the evening specimen, the low secretion time for ACTH. Instruct the patient to ingest nothing by mouth for 12 hours before the test. Some physicians recommend a low-carbohydrate diet for 2 days before the test.

- Check with the physician if cortisol levels are to be obtained at the same time.
- The nurse obtains a medication history and asks the physician if any interfering drugs should be withheld. The nurse also inquires and notes on the requisition slip if the patient is pregnant because this may affect test results.

During the Test

- After blood is obtained by venipuncture, place the specimen on ice and immediately send it to the laboratory.
- Write the time of the collection on the test tube.
- The nurse notifies laboratory personnel that the specimen is being transported because it should be frozen until a radioimmunoassay analysis (RIA) can be performed.

Posttest

- The patient resumes a normal diet, activity, and medication regimen. The nurse notifies the dietary department to bring the patient his or her meal.

Adrenocorticotropic Hormone Stimulation Test

Also called: ACTH Stimulation Test; Rapid or Short ACTH Test; Corticotropin Stimulation Test; Cosyntropin Test; Cortrosyn Stimulating Test

SPECIMEN OR TYPE OF TEST: Plasma, serum

PURPOSE OF THE TEST

The ACTH stimulation test is performed to diagnose primary and secondary adrenal insufficiency. It may also be done to assess outcome in patients in septic shock. A small increase in corticotropin in the simulation test indicates a poor outcome for patients in septic shock.

BASICS THE NURSE NEEDS TO KNOW

ACTH is secreted by the pituitary gland. Its target organ is the adrenal cortex, where it stimulates the secretion of glucocorticoids, aldosterone, and androgens. Synthetic ACTH, known as cosyntropin (Cortrosyn), normally has the same effect. It causes an increase in adrenal cortex hormones. A normal response excludes the diagnosis of primary adrenocorticoid insufficiency, because the gland was able to respond. A normal response will also rule out complete ACTH deficiency (secondary adrenocorticoid failure) because complete lack of ACTH causes adrenal atrophy, and the gland is unable to respond.

In an abnormal response, primary or secondary adrenal insufficiency may be present. Aldosterone levels may be measured to distinguish between the two forms. If no change occurs in the aldosterone levels after cosyntropin is given, primary adrenal insufficiency is present. With secondary adrenal insufficiency, aldosterone levels will increase by more than 4 µg/dL.

ACTH will also be secreted in response to insulin-induced hypoglycemia; therefore, insulin is another means to stimulate its secretion.

REFERENCE VALUES   Within 30 to 60 minutes, plasma cortisol increases to 18 to 20 µg/dL
or SI: 500 to 550 npmol/L.

HOW THE TEST IS DONE

After the baseline plasma cortisol level is obtained, cosyntropin or insulin is given intravenously. Cosyntropin may be given intramuscularly if the patient is not hypotensive. After 30 to 60 minutes, another plasma cortisol level is obtained.

SIGNIFICANCE OF TEST RESULTS

Elevated Values

Normal response

Unchanged Values

Addison's disease
Adrenal atrophy
Hypopituitarism

INTERFERING FACTORS

• See section on Cortisol, Total on p. 227.

NURSING CARE

See section on Cortisol, Total on p. 227.

Pretest

• The nurse explains to the patient the need for more than one venipuncture procedure.
• If insulin is being used as the stimulant, the nurse instructs the patient to fast overnight.

During the Test

• If insulin is used as the stimulant, the nurse observes the patient for clinical manifestations of hypoglycemia.
• Have a glucose source available to treat hypoglycemia.

Posttest

• The nurse ensures that the patient eats, especially if insulin was used as the stimulant.

Alanine Aminotransferase

Also called: (ALT); Glutamic-Pyruvic Transaminase (SGPT)

SPECIMEN OR TYPE OF TEST: Serum

PURPOSE OF THE TEST

The alanine aminotransferase (ALT) test is used to detect hepatocellular injury or necrosis (injury or death of liver cells). It is the most specific of the transaminase enzyme tests to detect acute hepatitis from a viral, toxic, or drug-induced cause. It is used to help determine the source of jaundice. After an acute episode of hepatitis has abated, the persistence of an elevated ALT level suggests that the illness has not resolved and the patient is at high risk to progress to chronic hepatitis. Serial measurements are used to track the course of the hepatitis.

BASICS THE NURSE NEEDS TO KNOW

Alanine aminotransferase is a transaminase enzyme that is found in the cells of the liver and kidneys, and to lesser extents in the cells of the heart, skeletal muscle, and red blood cells. When cellular injury or necrosis occurs in the liver and other tissues that contain this transaminase enzyme, the enzymes leave the cytoplasm, pass through damaged cell membranes, and enter the serum. In acute hepatitis, the serum level rises dramatically, to a level of 20 times the normal value. In cases of obstructive jaundice, cirrhosis, and liver tumor, the ALT level rises mildly or moderately, from two to four times the normal value.

   The ALT value also rises moderately as a result of myocardial infarction, heart failure, and shock. Mild skeletal muscle injury, as from trauma or surgery also causes a mild to moderate rise in the ALT level. A mildly elevated ALT level may be present because of obesity, particularly when there is fat accumulation in the abdomen. Fatty liver disease is the most common cause of liver disease in the pediatric population.

REFERENCE VALUES

Male and female (newborn-1 year): 13-45 IU/L
Male (1-60 years):10-40 IU/L
Female (1- 60 years): 7-35 IU/L
Male 60-90 years: 10-28 IU/L
Female 60-90 years: 10-28 IU/L
Male >90 years: 6-38 IU/L
Female >90 years: 5-24 IU/L

HOW THE TEST IS DONE

Venipuncture is performed to collect a sample of venous blood.

SIGNIFICANCE OF TEST RESULTS

Elevated Values
Acute or chronic hepatitis
Liver cell necrosis

Acute pancreatitis
Cirrhosis
Infectious mononucleosis
Biliary obstruction
Obstructive jaundice
Liver tumor
Fatty liver
Chronic alcohol abuse
Myocardial infarction
Heart failure
Shock
Muscle trauma
Recent surgery
Pregnancy-induced hypertension
Hemolytic anemia
Hemodialysis

INTERFERING FACTORS

• Hemolysis

NURSING CARE

Nursing actions are similar to those used in other venipuncture procedures (see Chapter 2), with the following additional measures.

Pretest

• Many medications cause an elevated test result. If they cannot be discontinued for 12 hours, list the medications on the laboratory request form.

Albumin, Serum

See Protein, Total, Serum on p. 522

Albumin, Urinary

Also called: Protein Screen; Urine Screen for Albumin; Urinary Albumin, 24-hour collection

SPECIMEN OR TYPE OF TEST: Urine

PURPOSE OF THE TEST

Urinary excretion of albumin is evaluated to assess renal function and to determine effectiveness of therapy in the management of urinary disease. Studies have shown that albumin in urine also can be used as a predictor of complications associated with diabetes mellitus.

A

BASICS THE NURSE NEEDS TO KNOW

Evaluation of protein in the urine is done as part of routine urinalysis or it may be done as a specific test to measure or monitor for proteinuria. In the healthy adult, the excretion of protein is so small that it is undetectable by routine methods of analysis. Proteinuria does not always mean there is renal disease. The proteinuria may be transient, as the result of factors such as strenuous exercise, dehydration, muscle injury, pregnancy, or severe viral infection. When the test is positive, retesting is done at intervals to determine if the result is transitory.

In urinary disorders, the origin of proteinuria may be from glomerular damage in the kidneys that alters filtration. Large protein molecules are filtered from the plasma by leaking through damaged glomerular membranes. It may also be due to tubular damage that alters reabsorption of small protein molecules. Additionally, protein may enter the urine from the lower urinary tract as in infection, inflammation, or bleeding from trauma or menstrual flow. The abnormal value of 30/mg/dL/24 hr or SI: 300 mg/L/24 hr or higher is considered a clinically significant abnormal value.

REFERENCE VALUES   Random specimen (microalbumin): <2 mg/dL
24-hour specimen: 10 mg/dL or less *or* SI: 100 mg/L or less
Reagent strip: Negative

HOW THE TEST IS DONE

Various methods are available for assessing urinary excretion of albumin. Reagent strips are sensitive to albumin, but not at very low levels. For a reagent strip analysis of albumin, a random urine specimen is collected in a clean container. A first voided urine specimen is preferred.

For microalbuminuria measurement, a 24-hour specimen of urine is used with no preservative in the collection container. The specimen is kept refrigerated and should be sent to the lab within 2 hours of its collection.

SIGNIFICANCE OF TEST RESULTS

Elevated Values
Glomerulonephritis
Nephrotic syndrome
Lupus nephritis
Pyelonephritis
Amyloidosis
Cystic kidney
Diabetes mellitus nephropathy
Heavy metal poisonings
Preeclampsia
Eclampsia
Multiple myeloma
Renal transplant rejection
Urinary tract malignancies
Cystitis
Proteinuria, pregnancy

INTERFERING FACTORS

- *With reagent strips:* Highly concentrated urine; highly alkaline urine; specimen contaminated with bacteria, blood, ammonium compounds (detergents), chlorhexidine (cleansers), or fabric softeners
- *With turbidimetric method:* Ingestion of cephalosporin, penicillin, sulfonamides, or tolbutamide; recent administration of radiocontrast dyes

NURSING CARE

Nursing actions are similar to those used in other urine collection procedures (see Chapter 2), with the following additional measures.

Health Promotion

The nurse may need to instruct patients who have renal disorders or possible diabetes mellitus complications to test their urine daily for albumin using a reagent strip.

Pretest

- Care is dependent on the method of analysis. Check with the laboratory regarding the method and specimen required. A laboratory urine specimen container should be used. Ordinary household jars or containers can have residual detergent or cleanser contaminants.

Posttest

○ *Patient Teaching.* If the patient is going to monitor his or her own urinary albumin at home, the nurse will assess the patient's understanding of the purpose of home testing, the reading of the test results when compared with the manufacturer's color chart of test results, and the need to notify the physician if albumin is present or if its concentration increases. Abnormal results are usually investigated in a follow-up by laboratory analysis and specific measurement of the protein amount.

- Instruct the patient to use the first voided urine in the morning. Warn the patient that any vigorous exercise before urine collection will increase the excretion of albumin in the urine and cause a false positive result. Teach the patient how to follow the manufacturer's instructions for using the reagent strip. Timing varies by the manufacturer. Instruct the patient to keep the top on the reagent strip container.

Aldosterone, Serum

SPECIMEN OR TYPE OF TEST: Serum, plasma

PURPOSE OF THE TEST

The aldosterone level is used in the workup for hypertension and in the diagnosis of aldosteronism.

BASICS THE NURSE NEEDS TO KNOW

Aldosterone is a mineralocorticoid produced by the adrenal cortex and controlled primarily by the renin-angiotensin system. Renin secreted by the kidneys acts on angiotensinogen to convert it to angiotensin I. Later, angiotensin I is converted to angiotensin II. Angiotensin II stimulates

A

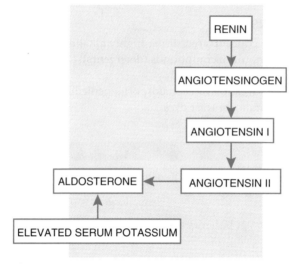

Figure 11. Primary regulation of aldosterone secretion.

the adrenal cortex to produce and secrete aldosterone. The aldosterone acts on the renal tubules to (1) increase sodium retention and thus increase fluid retention, which increases plasma fluid volume and blood pressure, and (2) to increase potassium excretion in urine (Figure 11).

Another stimulant for aldosterone secretion is the serum potassium level. When serum potassium levels are elevated, increased secretion of aldosterone occurs, promoting greater urinary excretion of potassium.

The presence of high levels of aldosterone is called aldosteronism. Primary aldosteronism often is caused by adrenal adenoma (Conn's syndrome). This condition is characterized by hypertension with hypokalemia and urinary potassium loss. Secondary aldosteronism is caused by nonadrenal disease that stimulates the adrenal cortex to produce and secrete excessive aldosterone.

In testing for serum aldosterone levels, a number of variables must be controlled to provide accurate results. A low-salt diet, an upright position, and stress all produce increased levels of aldosterone. A high-salt diet and a supine position decrease the serum levels.

If serum aldosterone levels are elevated, primary aldosteronism can be confirmed with a *captopril, fludrocortisone,* or *saline stimulation test.* With the administration of captopril, fludrocortisone acetate (Florinef) *or* intravenous saline, the secretion of aldosterone is suppressed in normal patients and in patients with secondary aldosteronism, but serum levels rise in patients with primary aldosteronism.

REFERENCE VALUES* **Child**
1 week-1 year: 1-160 ng/dL or SI: 0.03-4.43 nmol/L
1-3 years: 5-60 ng/dL or SI: 0.14-1.7 nmol/L
3-11 years: <5-80 ng/dL or SI: <0.14-2.22 nmol/L
11-15 years: <5-50 ng/dL or SI: <0.14-1.39 nmol/L

*Values vary depending on laboratory.

Adult (average sodium diet)
Peripheral blood, supine position: 3-10 ng/dL or SI: 0.08-0.27 nmol/L
Peripheral blood, upright position: 5-30 ng/dL or SI: 0.14-0.83 nmol/L
After fludrocortisone acetate (Florinef) suppression or intravenous
saline infusion: <4 ng/dL or SI: <0.11 nmol/L
Adrenal vein: 200-800 ng/dL or SI: 5.54-22.16 nmol/L

HOW THE TEST IS DONE

A venipuncture is done and the specimen is immediately placed on ice and sent to the lab. The vascular site may be any peripheral vein. The patient may be in a supine or an upright position. Using interventional radiographic techniques, a blood sample from the adrenal vein may be done to confirm the diagnosis of adrenal adenoma.

Other diagnostic methods include administering 2 L of normal saline over 4 hours before the blood test or drawing the blood on the third day after the administration of fludrocortisone acetate, a synthetic mineralocorticoid.

SIGNIFICANCE OF TEST RESULTS

Elevated Values
Primary Aldosteronism
Adrenal adenoma (Conn's syndrome)
Adrenal hyperplasia
Secondary Aldosteronism
Laxative abuse
Excessive diuretic therapy
Nephrotic syndrome
Renal juxtaglomerular hyperplasia
Renin-producing renal tumor
Bartter's syndrome
Toxemia of pregnancy

Decreased Values
Addison's disease
Turner's syndrome
Aldosterone deficiency
Diabetes mellitus
Renin deficiency
Acute alcoholic intoxication

INTERFERING FACTORS

- Licorice intake
- Uncontrolled sodium intake
- Postural changes
- Warming of the specimen
- Recent radioisotope administration
- Loop diuretics

A

NURSING CARE

Nursing actions are similar to those used in other venipuncture procedures (see Chapter 2), with the following additional measures.

Pretest

○ *Patient Teaching.* The nurse instructs the patient to follow a normal sodium intake (3 g/day) for 2 to 4 weeks, if not contraindicated by clinical status. The nurse also instructs the patient to discontinue all diuretics, antihypertensives, cyclic progesterone, estrogens, and licorice for 2 to 4 weeks if ordered by the physician.

- The nurse administers potassium replacement, as ordered.
- Any radioactive scans are scheduled for a time after the aldosterone level is obtained.

During the Test

- The nurse needs to make sure the position used and the site of the sample is standardized.
- *Supine position:* On the morning of the test, instruct the hospitalized patient to remain flat in bed until the specimen is drawn.
- *Upright position:* On the morning of the test, the nurse instructs the patient to remain seated in a chair for 2 hours until the blood is drawn.

Posttest

- Place the blood specimen on ice and arrange for its immediate transport to the laboratory.
- The nurse ensures that the requisition slip contains the following information: the time and date of the test, the venous source of the blood, the patient's position, the pretest diet, and the time and date of administration of fludrocortisone acetate or intravenous saline infusion.
- Since hepatic perfusion is the primary determinant of aldosterone metabolism, the nurse knows that interpretation of test results is influenced by any disorder that can interfere with liver blood flow, such as congestive heart failure.

Aldosterone, Urinary

SPECIMEN OR TYPE OF TEST: Urine

PURPOSE OF THE TEST

The main use of the urine aldosterone test is to help identify primary hyperaldosteronism caused by adrenal adenoma.

BASICS THE NURSE NEEDS TO KNOW

Aldosterone is a mineralocorticoid produced by the adrenal cortex. Its synthesis and release are controlled primarily by the renin-angiotensin system. Aldosterone acts on the renal tubules to resorb greater quantities of sodium, and therefore water, and increases the excretion of potassium into the urine. Elevated levels of urinary aldosterone may be caused by excess secretion of aldosterone by the adrenal glands, excessive secretion of renin, or conditions that result in decreased kidney perfusion.

REFERENCE VALUES*   2-26 µg/24 hr or SI: 6-72 nmol/24 hr

*Values for this test vary among laboratories.

HOW THE TEST IS DONE

A 24-hour urine specimen is collected in a clean plastic container. Some laboratories add a measured quantity of preservative (boric, acetic, or hydrochloric acid) to the container before the start of the collection period.

Unlike serum aldosterone levels, positioning does not affect urinary aldosterone levels.

SIGNIFICANCE OF TEST RESULTS

Elevated Values

Aldosterone-producing adrenal adenoma (Conn's syndrome)
Adrenal hyperplasia
Nephrotic syndrome
Renin-producing renal hyperplasia or tumor
Renal hypertension
Bartter's syndrome
Preeclampsia

Decreased Values

Addison's disease
Aldosterone deficiency
Renin deficiency
Diabetes mellitus
Acute alcoholic intoxication

INTERFERING FACTORS

- Excess salt intake
- Recent administration of radioisotopes
- Licorice intake
- Failure to collect all the urine
- Warming of the specimen
- Diuretics (loop or thiazides)
- Lithium
- Oral contraceptives

NURSING CARE

Nursing actions are similar to those used in other 24-hour urine collection procedures (see Chapter 2), with the following additional measures.

Pretest

○ *Patient Teaching.* The nurse instructs the patient to follow a normal (3 g/day) sodium diet for 2 to 4 weeks. Excessive sodium intake suppresses aldosterone secretion and causes a false decrease in the aldosterone value. Instruct the patient to discontinue all diuretics, antihypertensives, and oral contraceptives for 2 weeks, if ordered. These medications interfere with the test results.

- The nurse checks the patient's serum potassium level and administers prescribed potassium to correct any deficiencies that may be present.
- Schedule any radioisotope scan for after completion of the urine test.

During the Test

- At the start of the test, the nurse instructs the patient to void at 8 AM and discard this urine. The collection period starts at this time, and the patient collects all the urine for 24 hours, including the 8 AM specimen from the following morning.
- On the requisition slip and specimen label, the nurse writes the patient's name, and the time and date of the start and finish of the test period.
- The nurse ensures that the urine is kept refrigerated or on ice throughout the collection period.

Posttest

- On the requisition slip, write the pretest sodium diet.
- Arrange for prompt transport of the cooled specimen to the laboratory.

Alkaline Phosphatase

Also called: (ALP)

SPECIMEN OR TYPE OF TEST: Serum

PURPOSE OF THE TEST

Serum alkaline phosphatase (ALP) testing is a nonspecific indicator of liver disease, biliary tract obstruction, bone disease, or hyperparathyroidism. It is part of a battery of tests that evaluate liver function. It also serves as a tumor marker by indicating rapid cell growth or accelerated function caused by malignancy of the liver or bone.

BASICS THE NURSE NEEDS TO KNOW

ALP is an enzyme located primarily in the osteoblast cells of the bone, in the hepatocytes of the liver, and to a lesser extent in the intestines, kidney, and placenta. A high level of ALP usually means that a specific organ or tissue has increased the manufacture or release of the enzyme. The ALP enzyme is normally excreted via the biliary tract, but if there is any blockage in the biliary tree, the hepatocytes of the liver produce more ALP.

The ALP level will rise with increased activity from liver disease, biliary tract obstruction, or bone disease. In serious or advanced liver or bone disease, the ALP value can rise dramatically to

10 to 12 times the normal value. Additional transaminase enzyme tests can help identify the source of the ALP elevation. When the cause of an elevated ALP arises from liver disease, the alanine aminotransferase (ALT) and aspartate aminotransferase (AST) test results are also mildly elevated. With an elevated ALP result that is caused by bone disease, however, there is no associated elevation of the ALT or AST levels.

The normal values for children vary widely because of growth activity. During adolescence, the normal value of ALP may be 3 times higher than that of a normal adult. During normal skeletal growth, additional ALP leaks into the serum from the active osteoblast cells of the bones and causes elevated ALP results.

REFERENCE VALUES*	Children 4-15 years: 54-369 U/L
	Males 20-50 years: 53-128 U/L
	Females: 20-50 years: 42-98 U/L
	Males 60 years and older: 56-119 U/L
	Females 60 years and older: 53-141 U/L

*Note: These normal values are based on the IFCC laboratory methodology at 37° C.

HOW THE TEST IS DONE
Venipuncture is performed to collect a sample of venous blood.

SIGNIFICANCE OF TEST RESULTS
Elevated Values
Cancer of the liver
Cirrhosis
Acute fatty liver
Infiltrating liver disease (abscess, sarcoidosis, tuberculosis)
Cholangitis
Biliary obstruction (gallstones or pancreatic cancer)
Cholestasis
Paget's disease
Osteogenic sarcoma
Bone metastases
Rickets
Hyperparathyroidism
Healing bone fracture
Acromegaly
Infectious mononucleosis
Hyperthyroidism

Decreased Values
Malnutrition (deficiency of protein, zinc, or magnesium)
Hypophosphatemia
Hypothyroidism

INTERFERING FACTORS

- Pregnancy
- Fatty food intake, 2 to 4 hours before the test
- Healing bone fracture

NURSING CARE

Nursing actions are similar to those used in other venipuncture procedures (see Chapter 2), with the following additional measures.

Pretest

○ *Patient Teaching.* Instruct the patient to discontinue food intake for 12 hours before the test, as indicated by laboratory policy. Food in general and fatty food in particular can elevate the test results in some individuals.

Allergy Tests, Skin

Also called: Skin prick or skin puncture test, Intradermal skin test

PURPOSE OF THE TEST

Skin testing is done to identify a sensitivity response to specific allergens in the environment, food, or medications. Once sensitivity to a specific allergen is identified, the information is considered along with the clinical history to determine if an allergy exists. With accurate diagnosis, medical treatment will be more specific and effective.

BASICS THE NURSE NEEDS TO KNOW

Allergens are substances in the environment that have the potential to cause an allergic reaction when they enter the body or touch the skin of a sensitized person (Box 4). Sensitization means that specific IgE antibodies are present, but an allergic reaction depends on other variables such as whether the individual comes in contact with that specific allergen. If an allergic reaction starts, there is a rapid release of Immunoglobin E (IgE) antibody and histamine from the mast cells and symptoms emerge. This response will continue until all allergens are destroyed by the IgE antibody and cleared from the body. Allergy skin testing is a very effective method to identify which allergen is the cause of the sensitivity reaction. There are several methods of skin testing available. The two methods discussed in this section are the skin prick method and the intradermal method. Each of these tests uses very small doses of antigens that are introduced into the skin; then the examiner measures the amount of allergic response. In addition, the patch skin test can be done by placing suspected allergens on the skin surface and measuring the allergic response from the contact. (See Patch Test on p. 480). Additionally, allergy testing may be done on a specimen of blood; it involves a quantitative measure of the IgE antibody response to specific allergens. (See Immunoglobin E Antibody on p. 394).

The *skin prick method* is preferred for the initial testing of the skin. It is safer because it causes fewer systemic reactions. This method can screen for a number of suspected allergens at the

BOX 4	Common Allergens that Can Cause an Allergic Reaction

Environmental allergens may be in the home, work setting or outdoors. They are inhaled, ingested, or touched. Food allergens are ingested.

Environmental Allergens
Dust mites
Animal proteins in dander, saliva, and urine of pets with fur.
Mold spores
Pollens (tree, weed, grass)
Cockroach body parts and feces
Insect stings (bee, wasp, fire ant, yellow jacket)
Latex
Some medications

Food Allergens
Eggs
Peanuts
Fish (salmon)
Shellfish (crab, lobster, shrimp)
Tree nuts (pecan, walnut, etc.)
Wheat
Soy
Gluten

same time. The *intradermal test method* is more sensitive and accurate than the skin prick method. It is used in follow-up when a previously negative result occurs with the less sensitive skin prick method. It is also often used to test for an allergy to particular medications and for an allergy to insect venom, such as bee or wasp stings. There is a potential for a systemic reaction to the allergen that includes risk of anaphylaxis.

A positive skin test result is a wheal and flare response. The wheal is a localized area of very pale or white raised tissue that itches. The flare is the erythematous area around the wheal. A positive response is a raised wheal with a diameter of 3 mm or more and a flare of 10 mm or more across the longest diameter. The skin reactions are visible and measured after 15 to 20 minutes.

REFERENCE VALUES *Skin prick method*: Negative in response to the specific allergens tested
Intradermal method: Negative in response to the specific allergens tested

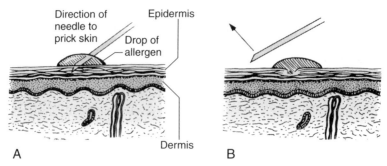

Figure 12. Allergy skin testing. The percutaneous skin prick method of testing. **A,** The drop of allergen is placed on the skin and the 27-gauge needle (bevel up) is placed through the allergen drop into the superficial epidermis. **B,** The needle pricks the skin at a 45-degree angle, allowing the allergen to come into contact with the sensitized mast cells in the epidermis, and then lifted up. The dermis is not penetrated and bleeding at the site is nonexistent or minimal. (From Pfenninger JL, Fowler GC: *Pfenninger and Fowler's procedures for primary care*, ed 3, St Louis, 2011, Mosby.)

HOW THE TEST IS DONE

For either skin prick or intradermal methods of testing, negative and positive control samples are implanted at the beginning of the test. The control samples ensure accuracy in the interpretation of the result. The inner aspect of the forearm is the preferred site for skin testing. Each antigen inoculation is identified with a label on the skin near the site.

Skin prick method: A drop of commercially prepared antigen solution is placed on the test stylus device. The stylus device is pushed down gently to prick the skin and allow the allergen to barely penetrate the epidermis. The stylus may have a single point for single allergen testing, or it may be a multitest device with up to 10 points to test the corresponding number of different allergens. Alternatively, a droplet of allergen is placed on the skin and a very small sterile needle is used (Figure 12).

Intradermal method: A small dose of very diluted allergen preparation is injected intradermally with a fine needle and 0.5 to 1.0 mL syringe.

SIGNIFICANCE OF THE TEST RESULTS

Positive Values

Sensitivity to specific allergens

INTERFERING FACTORS

• Current use of antihistamine medication

NURSING CARE

Pretest

- Perform a detailed clinical history, including the age of the person, his or her living environment, occupation, and preferred activities. All of these factors can give clues about the type of allergen that may be responsible for the allergy. The patient may be able to describe previous allergy-related symptoms, when the episode occurred, and possibly what caused it to occur.
- In the history, include a list of current medications the patient takes because some of the medications will alter the skin response in allergy testing. Additionally, some of the medications may have already caused an allergic response.
- A physical examination is performed, particularly noting any skin reactions, rashes, or other allergy symptoms that may be present.
- Instruct the patient to discontinue the use of antihistamine medications, such as diphenhydramine (Benadryl) or chlorpheniramine (Chlor-Trimeton), at least 24 hours before having the skin tests performed because these drugs would mute the test results.
- Obtain a signed, informed consent.
- Because anaphylaxis can occur during or shortly after the allergens are administered, the nurse ensures that a crash cart and emergency medications/equipment are nearby.

During the Test

- Observe the patient for complications during and after the testing period, particularly when using the intradermal test method. The allergic responses can be moderate to severe or fatal. The adverse reactions can be of rapid onset or delayed until after completion of the tests. Mild or moderate reactions consist of the onset of erythema (overall redness of the skin from inflammation), edema, induration (a hard area of tissue) and dysesthesia (a change in any sense, such as pain on gentle touching of the skin). A severe reaction is rare. It is usually a hypersensitivity reaction and is associated with drug (medication) testing. Shock, respiratory distress, and cardiac arrest can occur. Oxygen, emergency drugs, and CPR may be needed.

Posttest

○ *Patient Teaching.* Once the allergen is identified, the primary approach to patient teaching is that the patient should avoid exposure to the substance that will act as an "allergy trigger" and cause an allergic response. For a food allergy, the nurse can teach the patient to identify any hidden sources of allergens, such as by reading labels on canned or prepared food and making inquiries if ordering food in a restaurant.

If the patient has already had a life-threatening reaction to a particular allergen as a venomous sting or a particular medication, instruct the patient to carry an injectable device that contains epinephrine. The patient needs to learn how to use it, when to use it, and where to get additional medical care as quickly as possible. Some patients may choose to wear a medical bracelet that identifies the severe allergy and provides other pertinent information.

- For hospitalized patients, the information about any allergy must be posted in the patient's record and on a special allergy identification bracelet worn by the patient.

Alpha 1 Antitrypsin

See Protein Electrophoresis, serum on p. 520.

Alpha-Fetoprotein

Also called: (AFP), α-fetoprotein; fetoprotein

SPECIMEN OR TYPE OF TEST: Serum

PURPOSE OF THE TEST

In the nonpregnant patient, AFP is a tumor marker for primary cancer of the liver (hepatoma). It is used to help with the diagnosis and to monitor the effect of chemotherapy treatment on that tumor. It is also used as a tumor marker and to help with diagnosis and staging of some types of testicular cancer.

In a pregnant woman, serum AFP serves as a screening test for neural tube defects in the fetus. Neural tube defects in the fetus include spinal bifida, myelomeningocele, and anencephaly. It is also part of the multiple marker screening test that detects fetal Down syndrome in the pregnant woman.

BASICS THE NURSE NEEDS TO KNOW

In the blood of healthy, nonpregnant adults, AFP is present in very small amounts. If the liver has been injured by trauma, exposure to chemical toxins or the hepatitis virus, the AFP level will rise moderately as healing and regeneration of liver cells occurs.

As a tumor marker for primary hepatoma, the serum level rises to values of 1000 ng/mL (SI: 1000 µg/mL) or dramatically higher. When the test is used to monitor the response of the testicular tumor to chemotherapy treatment, a rising AFP value indicates additional growth of the tumor and a falling value indicates a favorable response to the chemotherapy treatment.

In a pregnant woman, the fetus produces the AFP and it is, therefore, present in the amniotic fluid and the maternal serum. The maternal serum level increases throughout the pregnancy and in the third trimester rises to 500 ng/mL (SI: 500 µg/L). The pregnant African American woman has a normal value that is 10% to15% higher than the Caucasian woman throughout the pregnancy. The normal value for the pregnant woman who has insulin-dependent diabetes is 20% lower than the average normal value.

For prenatal screening, the best time to draw the maternal blood is in the 16th to 18th week of the pregnancy, but the specimen can be drawn during the 15th to 21st week. An abnormally elevated value occurs with open neural tube defect and some other congenital defects in the fetus. The test, however, can have false positive results because the calculation of the normal value is based on the gestational age of the fetus.

The gestational age is best measured by ultrasound. Often, however, the calculation is based on the mother's estimate of when her last menstrual period occurred and this may not be precise. Because of the possibility of error, a positive screening test result is considered only suggestive of an abnormality in the fetus. Additional evaluation by ultrasound is recommended, and based on the results of the pregnancy ultrasound, amniocentesis may be needed. With a follow-up pregnancy ultrasound, the examination focus is on the fetal spine and cranium. With amniocentesis, the

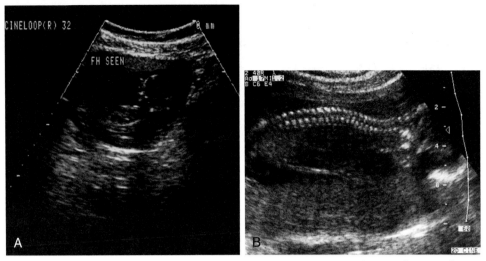

Figure 13. Pregnancy ultrasound. The varying densities and compositions of tissue allow visualization of the uterine contents. **A,** A normal 4-month-old fetus. The fetal heart (FH) is identified. **B,** The normal spinal structure of a 4-month-old fetus.

analysis of the amniotic fluid would provide accurate information about the condition of the fetus. Normal findings of these additional tests demonstrate that no neural tube defect exists (Figure 13).

Multiple Marker Screening for Down's Syndrome

Pregnant women can be tested for fetal Down syndrome in the first or early in the second trimester. The combined first trimester screen consists of human chorionic gonadotrophin, pregnancy associated plasma protein-A (PAPP-A), and nuchal translucency measurement. The quadruple marker screening test consists of alpha-fetoprotein human chorionic gonadotrophin, unconjugated estriol, and Inhibin A.

When Down syndrome affects the fetus, the quadruple marker screening test demonstrates characteristic changes in the second trimester of pregnancy. The alpha-fetoprotein result is 25% lower than normal and the unconjugated estriol result is 30% lower than normal. Both human chorionic gonadotrophin and inhibin A rise to twice the normal value. Pregnancy ultrasound must be done first to obtain an accurate gestational age. The quadruple marker screening test detects 80% of fetal Down syndrome pregnancies, with a 5% false positive rate of error. It is a very useful test for pregnant women younger than age 35, because there is a high rate of Down syndrome that occurs in pregnancies of younger females and amniocentesis is not done routinely to detect the problem. (See also: Amniocentesis and Amniotic Fluid Analysis, p. 66)

REFERENCE VALUES   Adult: <15 ng/mL *or* SI: <15 µg/L
Pregnancy: <15-500 ng/mL *or* SI: <15-500 µg/mL (result rises
    to the high-end value in the third trimester of pregnancy)
Pregnancy 16th-18th week gestation: 34.8-47.3 ng/mL or
    SI: 34.8-47.3 µg/L

A

HOW THE TEST IS DONE

Venipuncture is performed to collect a sample of venous blood.

SIGNIFICANCE OF TEST RESULTS

Nonpregnant State

Elevated Values

Liver cancer
Gonadal germinal tumor
Liver trauma
Hepatitis
Cirrhosis

Pregnant State

Elevated Values

Spina bifida
Myelomeningocele
Anencephaly
Esophageal or duodenal atresia
Multiple pregnancy
Underestimated gestational age

Decreased Values

Down syndrome (Trisomy 21)
Trisomy 18
Fetal death
Spontaneous abortion
Molar pregnancy
Overestimated gestational age

INTERFERING FACTORS

- Recent radioisotope scan

NURSING CARE

Health Promotion

The nurse teaches the patient that all pregnant females are encouraged to have the AFP blood test screening during the 15th to 18th week of gestation to help ensure that the fetus is healthy and developing normally. Generally, the blood is drawn during a routine prenatal visit.

For the AFP test itself, nursing actions are similar to those used in other venipuncture procedures (see Chapter 2), with the following additional measures.

Pretest

- For the pregnant woman, include the following data on the laboratory request form: gestational age, maternal weight, maternal race, and diabetic status. These are variables that affect the interpretation of the test results.

Posttest
- If there is an elevated AFP value that is suggestive of fetal abnormality, prospective parents often react with fear and anxiety. The physician gives the initial explanation of the findings and stresses the importance of follow-up testing with fetal ultrasound and amniocentesis. There is the possibility that the screening test result is a false positive because of an error in determining the gestational age of the fetus. The prospective parents, however, experience emotional distress and may not be listening or understanding the information. A one-time explanation by the physician may not be sufficient.
- The nurse can help the expectant parents to minimize maternal anxiety, particularly during the waiting time before performance of follow-up testing. The expectant mother often seeks more information and clarification. The nurse can help the patient understand the information that was provided by the physician and prepare a list of additional questions to ask the physician.
- Emotional support is necessary when the prospective parents think about possible abnormality of the fetus. They may consider possible decisions and outcomes prematurely. The nurse should remind the parents that this AFP test is a screening test and no plans should be made until additional test results and complete information are known. Prompt scheduling for follow-up testing with ultrasound and possible amniocentesis will be very helpful.

Ammonia

Also called: NH_3

SPECIMEN OR TYPE OF TEST: Plasma

PURPOSE OF THE TEST

The ammonia level is used to evaluate or monitor severe liver failure, hepatic encephalopathy, and the effects of impaired portal vein circulation. It also may be used to monitor patients on hyperalimentation therapy. It may help identify some rare forms of inborn errors of metabolism that can affect a neonate and may be used to help diagnose Reye's syndrome, a childhood disorder that results in an acute fatty liver and encephalopathy.

BASICS THE NURSE NEEDS TO KNOW

As proteins are digested and metabolized or broken down into amino acids in the intestine, ammonia is produced as a by-product. The ammonia enters and circulates in the bloodstream until the liver removes it from the portal circulation. Liver cells then convert the ammonia to urea. Ultimately, the kidneys remove the urea from the circulation and excrete it in urine.

The two most common causes of an elevated ammonia level are the failure of the hepatic cells to function in the conversion of ammonia to urea and the impairment of the portal vein circulation, which prevents the ammonia from reaching the liver tissue.

REFERENCE VALUES   Neonate: 90-150 µg /dL *or* SI: 64-107 µmol/L
Child >1 mo: 29-70 µg/dL *or* SI: 21-50 µmol/L
Adult: 15-45 µg/dL *or* SI: 11-32 µmol/L

HOW THE TEST IS DONE

An arterial puncture or a venipuncture is performed to collect a sample of arterial or venous blood.

SIGNIFICANCE OF TEST RESULTS

Elevated Values

Liver failure (hepatic necrosis or terminal cirrhosis)
Hepatic encephalopathy
Portal hypertension
Portacaval shunting of the blood
Inborn errors of metabolism that affect the urea synthesis cycle
Reye's syndrome

INTERFERING FACTORS

- Tobacco smoke
- High protein intake
- Gastrointestinal hemorrhage
- Hyperalimentation (total parenteral nutrition)
- Ureterosigmoidostomy
- Hemolysis

NURSING CARE

Nursing actions are similar to those used in other arterial puncture or venipuncture procedures (see Chapter 2), with the following additional measures.

Pretest

○ *Patient Teaching.* Instruct the patient not to smoke before the test. The smoke itself will elevate the results falsely. If venipuncture will be used to collect the specimen, instruct the patient not to clench the fist.

Posttest

- Ensure that the specimen is placed in a bed of ice and sent to the laboratory immediately.
- If the specimen is allowed to warm, it will produce falsely elevated results.

Amniocentesis and Amniotic Fluid Analysis

SPECIMEN OR TYPE OF TEST: Amniotic fluid

PURPOSE OF THE TEST

Amniocentesis is the procedure to obtain a sample of amniotic fluid and fetal cells. The analysis of the fetal epithelial cells in amniotic fluid is used to detect genetic or chromosomal abnormalities of the fetus. The analysis of the amniotic fluid is used to assess fetal maturity or fetal distress in the management of a problem pregnancy.

BASICS THE NURSE NEEDS TO KNOW

Amniocentesis

When the purpose of the amniocentesis is to screen for fetal abnormality, it is performed early in the second trimester. Usually, the procedure is performed in the 15th to 17th weeks of gestation, when the risk to the fetus is lower and sufficient time is available to provide the appropriate counseling and discuss treatment alternatives. When the purpose of the amniocentesis is to evaluate a problem pregnancy or to identify a change in the health status of the fetus, the procedure is performed in the late part of the second trimester or during the third trimester. In a high-risk pregnancy, it may be advisable to terminate the pregnancy by delivery of the preterm infant. Severe maternal illness can adversely affect the fetus. The analysis of the amniotic fluid provides information about the health and development of the fetus.

Amniotic Fluid Analysis

Chromosomal analysis identifies genetic abnormalities that are present in the fetal cells of the amniotic fluid. A *karyotype* is the complement of chromosomes. In humans, the normal karyotype consists of 46 chromosomes aligned in a standard sequence, with defined location, size, structure, and banding patterns.

Trisomy 21 (Down syndrome) and other trisomy conditions caused by the translocation of genes have an identifiable incidence in women older than age 35. Chromosomal analysis also can detect genetic abnormalities that cause many different types of inborn errors of metabolism. They include disorders of lipid, carbohydrate, glycoprotein, mucopolysaccharide, amino acid, and organic acid metabolism. The use of gene probe technology can also identify other autosomal recessive genetic mutations and sex-linked autosomal recessive genetic disorders.

Alpha-fetoprotein (AFP) testing of the amniotic fluid is the more accurate follow-up test when the maternal serum test is positive (see Alpha-Fetoprotein, Serum, p. 62). When the amniotic fluid value of the AFP is >2.1 multiple of median value (MoM), the result is considered abnormal. A value of 7 MoM is considered positive for spina bifida and a value of 20 MoM is considered positive for anencephaly. The calculation of the test value is based on the ultrasound measurement of the gestational age of the fetus.

Acetylcholinesterase is an enzyme present in cerebrospinal fluid. If the fetus has an open neural defect, this enzyme enters the amniotic fluid and the test result is positive.

Bilirubin causes the amniotic fluid to change to a dark yellow or amber color. When the maternal blood is Rh negative or contains atypical antibodies, there is potential for the fetus to develop hemolytic disease of the newborn (erythroblastosis fetalis). In this disorder, the erythrocytes of the fetus undergo hemolysis and the release of bilirubin. An abnormal test result is usually followed up with percutaneous umbilical blood sampling (see p. 483) to obtain a direct sample of the fetal blood.

Lecithin/sphingomyelin (L/S) ratio is an indicator of fetal pulmonary maturity. Lecithin is the primary part of surfactants that line the alveoli and prevent alveolar collapse in the newborn infant. Lecithin increases in production, starting in the 35th week of gestation. Sphingomyelin is a lipid produced at a steady rate by the fetus after the 25th week of gestation. In this test, sphingomyelin serves as a control on which to measure the increase of lecithin. The test is used to help determine the best time for the physician to do the obstetrical delivery of a problem pregnancy that is threatening the health of the mother, the fetus, or both. When the L/S ratio reaches a value of 2.5 or higher, the fetal lungs are mature. An L/S ratio of 1.5 to 2.4 is

A

considered borderline. An L/S ratio of <1.5 indicates fetal lung immaturity, with the increased likelihood that the newborn infant will experience respiratory distress syndrome. If used to measure fetal lung maturity, the L/S ratio is often interpreted in combination with the measurement of phosphatidylglycerol.

The L/S ratio is less precise when the gestational age of the fetus is less than 28 weeks. The L/S ratio is used less commonly today. Fetal lung maturity is more often measured by three newer, cost-effective tests in combination. They are: phosphatidylglycerol immunoassay, fluorescence polarization, and lamellar body density tests.

Phosphatidylglycerol (PG) is a component of pulmonary surfactant that normally appears in the amniotic fluid after the 35th week of gestation. It is a major indicator of fetal lung maturity. Once it is present, there is little risk that the fetus will experience respiratory distress syndrome.

Slide agglutination method (Amniostat-FLM) is a quantitative method to measure the antibody of phosphatidylglycerol. The test result of >2.0 mg/L is a high positive value and correlates with the absence of respiratory distress syndrome. The test result of >0.5 mg/L is a low positive value, but also correlates with fetal lung maturity. However, the negative value of <0.5 mg/L is a poor predictor of fetal lung immaturity.

The foam stability index is one way to measure the amount of pulmonary surfactant in the amniotic fluid. Pulmonary surfactant is a substance produced by the mature epithelial cells of the alveoli and its presence enables the walls of the alveoli to expand and contract in the function of respiration. The surfactant is also in the amniotic fluid in the same concentration as in the lungs. The fetus respirates while in the uterus. A *foam stability index (FSI)* value of SI: 0.47 or more indicates fetal lung maturity.

Fluorescence polarization assay is a new method to measure fetal lung maturity. It measures the amount of surfactant in a ratio with albumin in the amniotic fluid. The test method is very accurate and serves as a screening test. The measure of fetal lung maturity is a value of 55 mg of surfactant per one gram of albumin or greater. The values between 40 mg/g and 54 mg/g indicate neither mature nor immature lung development. A value that is less than 39 mg/g indicates less surfactant and immature lung development.

Lamellar Bodies. This newer test method counts the lamellar body particles in the amniotic fluid specimen as a way to measure fetal lung maturity. The lamellar bodies are phospholipid particles that are the storage form of surfactant. The particles reside in the fetal alveolar spaces to provide surfactant. They are also released into the amniotic fluid during fetal respiration. As the fetus matures, the lungs increase the phospholipids production and the particles can be counted in the amniotic fluid sample. A lamellar body count of 50,000 particles/µL indicates fetal lung maturity. The normal value varies with the different types of analyzers that are available and the laboratory method used.

REFERENCE VALUES

Chromosome analysis: Normal karyotype
Alpha-fetoprotein: <2.0 multiple of median value (MoM)
Acetylcholinesterase: Negative
Bilirubin: 0.01-0.03 mg/dL or SI: 0.02-0.06 µmol/L
Lecithin-to-sphingomyelin ratio: >2.5 mg/L or higher (fetus at 28 weeks gestation)
Phosphatidylglycerol: Present

Slide agglutination method: >2.0 mg/L = high positive value
Pulmonary surfactant: Positive; foam stability index: 0.47
Fluorescence polarization assay: 55 mg surfactant/g albumin or higher
Lamellar bodies: 50,000 particles/μL or more

▽ **Critical Values**   L/S ratio: <1.5

HOW THE TEST IS DONE

For amniocentesis, ultrasound is used to locate the position of the fetus, the placenta, and the pool of amniotic fluid. Using sterile technique, the physician passes a long, sterile needle through the abdominal wall and into amniotic fluid. Syringes are used to aspirate up to 30 mL of amniotic fluid from the uterus (Figure 14). The fluid is placed in sterile brown plastic containers for transport to the laboratory.

SIGNIFICANCE OF TEST RESULTS

Abnormal Findings
Chromosomes
Cystic fibrosis
Sickle cell anemia
Muscular dystrophy

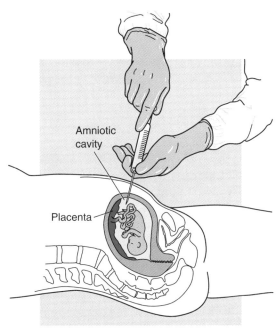

Amniotic
cavity

Placenta

Figure 14. Amniocentesis. Once the needle is inserted through the skin and the uterine wall, a sample of amniotic fluid is aspirated with a syringe.

Hemophilia A, B
Inborn errors of metabolism
Down syndrome
Retinoblastoma
Wilms' tumor
Thalassemias
Phenylketonuria
Enzyme G-6-PD deficiency

Elevated Values
Alpha-Fetoprotein
Neural tube defects: anencephaly, spina bifida, myelocele, hydrocephaly
Acetylcholinesterase
Neural tube defect
Bilirubin
Rh incompatibility
Hemolytic disease of the newborn
L/S Ratio
Maternal diabetes
Pulmonary Surfactant
Maternal diabetes

Decreased Values
L/S Ratio
Fetal lung immaturity
Phosphatidylglycerol
Fetal lung immaturity
Pulmonary Surfactant
Fetal lung immaturity
Polyhydramnios
Fluorescence Polarization Assay
Fetal lung immaturity
Lamellar Body Count
Fetal lung immaturity

INTERFERING FACTORS

- Exposure of specimen to sunlight
- Contamination of specimen (blood, meconium)
- Position of the placenta

NURSING CARE

Pretest

- After the patient receives a complete explanation of the amniocentesis procedure from the physician, obtain the patient's written consent for the procedure and the chromosomal (genetic) analysis. Despite the explanation, the patient may not understand Down syndrome or the amniocentesis procedure, particularly if she recently immigrated from a developing country. A low educational level and language limitations are often the reasons for noncomprehension. Patient comprehension is essential for a valid consent.

○ *Patient Teaching.* Provide instructions regarding pretest preparation. These instructions vary, depending on the gestation of the pregnancy. For a pregnancy that is less than 20 weeks of gestation, instruct the woman to drink extra fluids 1 hour before the test and not to urinate until completion of the test. A full bladder raises the uterus up and out of the pelvis so that the uterine contents can be visualized. For a pregnancy that is greater than 20 weeks of gestation, no requirements exist for fluid intake. Instruct the woman to void before the procedure begins. With the larger size of the uterus, an empty bladder is less likely to be punctured during the procedure.

- The patient will wear a hospital gown and lie supine on the examining table.
- Obtain and record vital signs, including the blood pressure, temperature, pulse, respirations, and fetal heart rate. This establishes the baseline values that are needed for comparison in the posttest period.
- Provide emotional support for the patient. Anxiety is common regarding the procedure, possible abnormal results, and the status of the fetus' health.

During the Test

- Position the patient with her hands behind her head to help prevent contamination of the sterile field.
- After ultrasound images have located the position of the fetus, the placenta, and the pool of amniotic fluid, the nurse washes the abdomen with povidone-iodine solution or other surgical soap and helps drape the sterile field.
- The nurse comforts the patient as the physician administers the local anesthetic into the intended area of the abdomen. The patient will feel some stinging during the injection.
- After the fluid sample is withdrawn by the physician, the nurse assists with its placement in the sterile specimen container. Glass containers cannot be used because the cells would adhere to the surface of the glass. A brown container is used to protect the fluid and bilirubin from sunlight. Exposure to sunlight would reduce the bilirubin amount within 30 minutes. If a brown container is not available, a clear container may be used. Once it has the specimen within, the clear container is closed and immediately wrapped with aluminum foil to prevent bilirubin oxidation by sunlight. Ensure that the specimen is correctly labeled. The laboratory form that is transported with the specimen should state the patient's name, the source of the fluid, the maternal age, and the period of gestation of the pregnancy. Additional information includes the reason for the study and relevant patient history, medication, and transfusion history.
- Once the needle is withdrawn, a small adhesive bandage is placed over the site of the needle puncture.

Continued

A

| **NURSING CARE—cont'd** |

Posttest

- The nurse monitors and records the maternal blood pressure, pulse, respirations, and fetal heart rate every 15 minutes for 30 to 60 minutes. They should remain within normal limits and be comparable to the pretest data.
- If the patient feels faintness, nausea, or cramps, the nurse places the patient on her right side to relieve the uterine pressure.
- After amniocentesis, all nonsensitized patients with an $Rh_o(D)$ negative blood type should receive immunization. The nurse administers the intramuscular injection of $Rh_o(D)$ immune globulin, as prescribed. This helps prevent hemolytic disease of the newborn (erythroblastosis fetalis) in future pregnancy.

○ *Patient Teaching.* At the time of discharge, instruct the patient to rest at home until the cramping subsides. Light activity can then resume. Posttest activity restrictions for the next several days include no bending at the waist, no lifting of anything heavier than 20 lb, and avoidance of strenuous exercise. Provide the patient with written instructions to notify the physician immediately about any symptoms of itching, fever, leakage of fluid, severe abdominal pain, or unusual (increased or decreased) fetal activity.

- Once the test results are known, the patient (or the prospective parents) meets with the physician. In early stage amniocentesis, when a genetic abnormality is encountered, the parents need comprehensive information about the health status of the fetus. They need to make an informed decision about the pregnancy, and the choices are painful. The alternatives include termination of the pregnancy or completion of the pregnancy with preparation for the special health care needs of the newborn. Genetic counseling precedes the amniocentesis and is also provided upon encountering a genetic abnormality. The nurse uses listening skills and a supportive approach in communication and interactions with the patient. The patient may need clarification, time for additional discussion, or to express feelings and concerns. The nurse may need to refer the patient to appropriate health care personnel for in-depth information.

▽ **Nursing Response to Critical Values**

A low L/S ratio indicates fetal lung immaturity. If delivery occurs at this time, the test value is a predictor that the fetus will develop respiratory distress syndrome (RDS). Usually, this value is correlated with a gestation of 34 weeks or less. The nurse informs the physician of the test result. Medical and nursing interventions will be specific to each patient, depending on the physical condition of the mother and fetus. When delivery is anticipated before the fetal lungs are mature, the mother usually receives prescribed antenatal glucocorticoid therapy that will stimulate fetal lung maturity.

◇ **Nursing Response to Complications**

The overall incidence of complications from amniocentesis is less than 0.5%. The complications include spontaneous rupture of the membranes, premature labor, bleeding from a traumatic tap, and infection.

Ruptured membranes, premature labor, bleeding, infection. The patient is asked to describe the symptoms that she is experiencing. Her vital signs are taken, including temperature. The nurse assesses for signs or bleeding or leakage of amniotic fluid from the puncture site or the vagina and asks about any leakage of fluid, blood, or passage of clots that occurred at home. The nurse also questions the patient about cramping or contractions, including the intensity, frequency, and duration. Assessment findings are reported to the physician and entered into the patient's record.

Amylase and Amylase Isoenzymes, Serum

Also called: Amylase, total (AMY), Amylase Isoenzymes: Pancreatic amylase (P-AMY) and salivary amylase (S-AMY)

SPECIMEN OR TYPE OF TEST: Serum

PURPOSE OF THE TESTS

Serum amylase can help diagnose acute pancreatitis, particularly when the specimen is obtained within 6 to 48 hours of the onset of abdominal pain. It is used together with serum lipase to investigate the cause of epigastric pain, nausea, and vomiting.

The serum amylase isoenzymes differentiate between the salivary and pancreatic sources of the enzyme secretions. The total enzyme test is accurate, but not very specific for identifying the cause of hyperamylasemia. The isoenzyme measurements, particularly P-AMY, are more helpful in identifying that the source of excess amylase enzyme in the blood is from the pancreas.

BASICS THE NURSE NEEDS TO KNOW

Amylase enzymes act on dietary starch and convert it to maltose. The salivary source of amylase is produced by the parotid glands and is secreted with saliva to initiate the breakdown of starch. The pancreatic source of amylase is made by the acinar cells of the pancreas and is secreted into the intestine via the pancreatic and common bile ducts. It performs most of the digestive work for the breakdown of starch.

Elevated Values

Inflammation or obstruction in any part of the pancreas or the common bile duct causes obstruction of the flow of amylase and a backup of the enzyme in the pancreatic tissue. The amylase is then absorbed into the bloodstream, with resultant hyperamylasemia (elevated level of amylase in the blood). In acute pancreatitis, the serum amylase value starts to rise within 2 to12 hours of the onset of the inflammation. The total amylase value peaks in 12 to 72 hours and returns to normal in 3 to 5 days. The pancreatic isoenzyme remains elevated in the blood for 1 week.

Other intestinal diseases that cause inflammation of the pancreas or blockage of the common bile duct also cause the serum amylase to rise, as do various pathologies or other organs that also produce some amylase. Acute inflammation of the parotid glands, as in parotitis (mumps) can cause an elevated serum amylase from a salivary source.

Decreased Values

Mucoviscidosis is a congenital pancreatic disease that causes dysfunction of the mucus-secreting glands. Thick mucus obstructs the pancreatic ductal system, causing acinar cell atrophy. In children or adults who have advanced cystic fibrosis, the serum amylase levels may be decreased.

A

REFERENCE VALUES | Adult, total: 24-65 U/L *or* SI: 0.41-1.1/ μKat/L
Adult, Pancreatic amylase isoenzyme: 13-53 U/L
The normal values depend on the method of analysis

▽ Critical Values | An increase of three to five times the upper limit of the normal value

HOW THE TEST IS DONE

Venipuncture is performed to collect a sample of venous blood.

SIGNIFICANCE OF TEST RESULTS

Elevated Values

Acute pancreatitis
Other pancreatic disorders (trauma, abscess, pseudocyst)
Obstruction at the ampulla of Vater
Intestinal obstruction
Perforated peptic ulcer, ruptured appendix, peritonitis
Abdominal trauma
Parotitis (mumps)

Decreased Values

Cystic fibrosis, advanced
Chronic pancreatitis
Pancreatic cancer
Cirrhosis
Hepatitis
Postpancreatectomy
Cancer, ovary, lung

INTERFERING FACTORS

- Drinking alcohol before the test
- Recent administration of morphine or other narcotic analgesic

NURSING CARE

Nursing actions are similar to those used in other venipuncture procedures (see Chapter 2), with the following additional measures.

Pretest

○ *Patient Teaching.* Inquire if the patient has imbibed alcohol in the past 24 hours. Alcohol increases the secretion of salivary amylase. No other fasting measures are required.

- The administration of morphine, codeine, or meperidine (Demerol) to the patient may be omitted in the pretest period. The recent administration of narcotics would close the sphincter of Oddi, with the effect of falsely raising the amylase level.

Posttest
▽ **Nursing Response to Critical Values**
Severe increases in serum amylase are considered significant and the physician must be notified. The sudden rise is usually caused by acute pancreatitis or an acute surgical condition of the abdomen.

When the serum amylase value rises to three to five times the upper limit of normal or more, the nurse should assess the patient for signs of acute abdominal pain, including location and any increase in intensity. Ecchymosis (bruising) may appear in the flank or around the umbilicus. Vital signs must to be taken to help evaluate for shock. Tachycardia, hypotension, and respiratory distress are indicators of severe, acute pancreatitis.

Amylase, Urine

SPECIMEN OR TYPE OF TEST: Urine

PURPOSE OF THE TEST

Urinary amylase is used to help diagnose acute and relapsing pancreatitis, particularly when the serum value is borderline or normal.

BASICS THE NURSE NEEDS TO KNOW

Amylase is cleared from the body in the urine. When the serum amylase level is elevated, the filtration rate by the kidneys increases and a greater rate of amylase clearance occurs. The amount of amylase clearance is measured in units per urine volume in a specific collection period. After the onset of acute pancreatitis, urinary amylase levels remain elevated for up to 2 weeks, as compared with the serum level that declines after 3 to 5 days.

REFERENCE VALUES*   **Adult: 1-17 U/hour**

*The reference range varies with the laboratory and method of analysis.

HOW THE TEST IS DONE

Urine is collected for a specific time period. The most common period is 1 or 2 hours, but 6- , 8- , or 24-hour collection periods are sometimes used.

SIGNIFICANCE OF TEST RESULTS

Elevated Values
Pancreatitis, acute or late stage
Cancer of the head of the pancreas
Pancreatic cyst or pseudocyst
Gall bladder disease
Obstruction (pancreatic ducts, intestine, salivary glands)
Parotitis (mumps)

Decreased Values
Alcoholism
Chronic pancreatitis
Hepatitis
Cirrhosis
Liver cancer or abscess
Pancreatic insufficiency (decreased P-AMY)

INTERFERING FACTORS

- Heavy menstrual flow
- Bacterial contamination of the urine
- Salivary amylase contamination of the specimen
- Omission of any voided specimen in the collection period
- Failure to cool the specimen

NURSING CARE

Nursing actions are similar to those used in other timed urinary collection procedures (see Chapter 2), with the following additional measures.

Pretest

⊙ *Patient Teaching.* Instruct the patient not to drink alcohol for 24 hours before the test. Alcohol stimulates the secretion of salivary amylase. Just before the start of the test, instruct the patient to void and discard the specimen. This urine has been in the bladder for an unknown period.

During the Test

- Write the date and time for the start and finish of the test on the specimen label and the requisition slip.
- During the collection period, refrigerate the urine or place the container in a bed of ice. Amylase is unstable in acidic urine. The patient and personnel must be careful not to cough, sneeze, or talk near the open collection container. Their saliva will add amylase to the content of the specimen.

Posttest

Maintain refrigeration of the specimen until it is sent to the laboratory.

Amyloid, beta

See Lumbar Puncture and Spinal Fluid Analysis on p. 421.

Androstenedione

SPECIMEN OR TYPE OF TEST: Serum, whole blood, amniotic fluid

PURPOSE OF THE TEST

The test is used to evaluate androgen production in the hirsute female and along with other tests it is used to evaluate and manage androgen disorders. It may be used to detect the illegal use of anabolic steroids as performance-enhancing drugs.

BASICS THE NURSE NEEDS TO KNOW

Androstenedione is an androgen precursor hormone that converts to testosterone in the male and to estrogens in the female. It is synthesized by the adrenal cortex in males and females and is also synthesized by the ovaries of the female. In normal physiology, the level of this hormone rises sharply after puberty and peaks in the young adult. After menopause, the level decreases abruptly in women. The hormone has a diurnal pattern and peaks in the blood level at about 7 AM, with the lowest level at about 4 PM each day.

The hirsute female experiences excessive growth of body hair, similar to the hair distribution of the male. An elevated level of androstenedione may be the cause of the hirsutism.

Congenital adrenal hyperplasia can be detected by measuring the elevated androstenedione level in the amniotic fluid sample, the cord blood, or the circulating blood of the neonate. In at least one state, androstenedione is part of the panel of state-mandated tests for newborn screening. Most cases of this disorder are diagnosed in infancy or early childhood.

REFERENCE VALUES

Amniotic fluid (midpregnancy)
Male fetus: 1.0 ng/dL *or* SI: 34.9 pmol/L
Female fetus: 0.7 ng/dL *or* SI: 24.4 pmol/L

Blood
Cord: 30-150 ng/dL *or* 1.0-5.2 nmol/L
Neonate (1-7 days): 20-290 ng/dL *or* SI: 0.7-10.1 nmol/L
Children (1-10 years): 8-50 ng/dL *or* SI 0.3-1.7 nmol/L
Adult: 75-205 ng/dL *or* SI 2.6-72 nmol/L
Postmenopausal female: 82-275 ng/dL *or* SI 3.0-9.6 nmol/L

HOW THE TEST IS DONE

Venipuncture is used to collect a sample of venous blood.
For fingerstick or heelstick method, whole blood is placed on filter paper.
Amniotic fluid is collected during amniocentesis.

SIGNIFICANCE OF THE TEST RESULTS

Elevated Values

Hirsutism
Congenital adrenal hyperplasia
Cushing's syndrome
Ovarian tumor
ACTH-producing tumor

INTERFERING FACTORS

- Menstruation
- Radioactive isotopes

A

Nursing actions are similar to those used in other venipuncture procedures (see Chapter 2), with the following additional measures.

Pretest

- For the menstruating female, schedule the test for at least 1 week before or 1 week after menstruation.
- The patient should fast from food and fluids for 8 hours before the test.
- The blood should be drawn early in the morning because of the diurnal rhythm of the hormone level.

Posttest

- Place the specimen on ice and arrange for prompt transport to the laboratory. The laboratory analysis should be done within 1 hour or the serum must be frozen.

Angiography, Abdomen and Extremities

Also called: CT angiography (CTA)

SPECIMEN OR TYPE OF TEST: Radiography

PURPOSE OF THE TEST

Angiography is used to investigate arterial vascular disease, to provide visualization of the arteries during treatment procedures, to evaluate the arterial circulation after traumatic injury, and to evaluate the effectiveness of vascular surgery.

BASICS THE NURSE NEEDS TO KNOW

Computed tomography (CT) angiography can provide visualization of the lumens of arteries from the diaphragm to the symphysis pubis and the extremities. Within the torso, imaging of the vasculature of specific organs is useful to identify arterial stenosis, occlusion, aneurysm, the effect of trauma on the vasculature of the organs, or other abnormal finding that affects the tissue of the liver, spleen, kidneys, pancreas, aorta, and the arterial circulation to the legs. CT arteriography is also used to evaluate the postoperative patency of arterial grafts and hemodialysis grafts. In preoperative planning for a transplant, CT angiography is done on the donor to evaluate the quality of the vasculature of the donor organ, such as a lobe of a liver or a kidney.

Contrast Medium

In computed tomography arteriography, contrast medium is needed to image the lumen of these arteries. Nonionized contrast is used to minimize the risk of a hypersensitivity reaction. The contrast medium is injected into the vasculature via a venous catheter that has been placed in a vein of the antecubital fossa. Oral ingestion of water also may be used as a contrast to distend the stomach and duodenum. This helps to improve the imaging of the nearby target organs. Within 24 hours, the contrast medium will be cleared from the patient's body in the urine.

Contrast medium is somewhat nephrotoxic. To prevent renal damage, the patient will drink extra fluids before and after the imaging procedure. During the procedure, intravenous fluids will be administered continuously. The contrast medium may cause a hypersensitivity reaction in the patient. To minimize the risk, nonionized contrast is used and the patient is given a low or minimum dose. In case of a severe hypersensitivity reaction, a well-equipped emergency cart is available in a nearby location in the radiography unit.

REFERENCE VALUES
No anatomic or functional abnormalities of the arteries are noted. No stenosis, occlusion, aneurysm, or bleeding is visualized.

HOW THE TEST IS DONE

The patient is placed on the movable table that is attached to the scanner. Correct positioning is very important to achieve quality images. The patient is instructed to avoid any movement as the table moves through the gantry and the scanning is done. The gantry is a large ring that has an x-ray tube that continuously rotates around the patient. The x-ray emissions pass through the body. An array of detectors is also located all around the ring of the gantry and receive the x-ray signals as they exit the body. The simultaneous forward movement of the patient and table, combined with the circling x-ray tube and the detectors of the gantry result in a spiral or helix pattern of data.

The contrast is injected into the patient's vasculature at a specific rate and the scanning of a particular area of vasculature in the torso is based on timing and computer coordination. The imaging of the specific location must be done as the contrast reaches its maximum concentration in a particular region. For example, the CT scanning of the upper abdomen will acquire data when the contrast is in the hepatic arteries and pancreas; after a delay of 65 to 70 seconds, it will then acquire data about the portal vein circulation, where the contrast is now concentrated (Perez-Johnson, Lenhart, & Sahani, 2010).

Complex computer operations reconstruct or convert the raw data into images. The data can be presented from many planes or views. It can image various levels, called slices. The data may be presented as two- or three-dimensional images. With such versatility in treatment of the data, specific and pertinent information is obtained.

SIGNIFICANCE OF TEST RESULTS

Abnormal Values
Peripheral vascular disease
Arterial occlusion
Aneurysm
Vascular fistula
Traumatic arterial injury
Thromboangiitis obliterans
Fibromuscular dysplasia
Collagen vascular disease
Arterial spasm
Tumor
Arteriovenous malformation
Inflammatory vasculitis
Giant cell arteritis
Raynaud's disease or phenomenon

A

INTERFERING FACTORS

- Renal failure
- Movement during the scanning process

NURSING CARE

Pretest

○ *Patient Teaching.* To help reduce distress and anxiety, the nurse instructs the patient regarding the procedure. Most patients do not know much about the test and will benefit from the information. The discussion can help with accurate expectations and reduction of the anxiety associated with the unknown. In addition, the patient instruction provides information so that the patient follows the required preparation measures.

○ *Patient Teaching.* The patient is instructed to drink extra fluids on the days before and after the test. No food can be taken after midnight or 8 hours before the test, but clear liquids and medications can be continued during this time.

○ *Patient Teaching.* The patient is informed that he or she will lie on the radiography table and must not move during the test. The patient will hear clicking and whirring sounds during the procedure. As the contrast medium is injected, the patient may feel a burning sensation or heat, pain, or nausea. Although momentary discomfort occurs, the sensations are normal and brief.

- During the assessment interview, the nurse identifies and reports any patient history of a previous reaction to a radiologic procedure that used a contrast medium. Once the physician has explained the procedure, a written consent form must be signed by the patient and entered into the record.
- The nurse ensures that recent laboratory test results are posted in the patient's record. Blood urea nitrogen and creatinine determinations are needed to verify adequate renal function.
- The nurse monitors the vital signs and records the results in the chart.

○ *Patient Teaching.* The patient is instructed to void to empty the bladder before going to the radiology department. The contrast medium acts as a diuretic and can cause the discomfort of a full bladder. The patient receives assistance, as needed, to remove all clothing and put on a hospital gown. All metal objects, such as jewelry, must be removed from the area of the scanning field.

- Place the patient in supine position on the scanning table. The arms are placed up above the head, to keep them away from the torso.

During the Test

- An intravenous line is established before the test begins and intravenous fluids are administered during the test. Remind the patient to remain motionless on the narrow table during the scanning procedure.

Posttest

- Once the venous catheter is removed, a small bandage covers the needle puncture site.
- Extra fluid intake is essential to prevent nephrotoxicity from the contrast medium. The patient should drink extra fluids to achieve a 2000- to 3000-mL intake in the 24-hour posttest period. Because of the high volume of fluids and the diuretic effect of the contrast material, the patient will experience a frequent need to urinate.

◆ **Nursing Response to Complications**

The overall complication rate for the angiography procedure is 1% to 3%. Reaction to the contrast medium consists of an hypersensitive response that may be a mild or severe form of reaction. The nurse monitors and assesses for this complication and notifies the physician should abnormal findings appear.

Nonimmediate hypersensitivity reaction. A nonimmediate reaction to contrast medium can start from 1 hour to 3 days after the contrast is given. It consists of skin that is reddened with a macular or maculopapular rash, itching, and swelling from hives or angioedema. The nurse prepares to counteract this reaction with the administration of diphenhydramine hydrochloride (Benadryl), as prescribed.

Immediate hypersensitivity reaction. The immediate reaction begins with the sudden appearance of a red rash, hives, urticaria, and angioedema, but it quickly progresses to systemic symptoms that are far more serious.

If the reaction to the contrast medium becomes severe, the nurse begins frequent and specific assessment for potential respiratory and cardiac complications. Respirations are monitored for abnormal rate, rhythm, and effort, particularly when the patient demonstrates dyspnea. The lungs are assessed for the presence of wheezes, crackles, or rhonchi. The patient may develop shock with hypotension and tachycardia. If this very serious anaphylactic reaction begins, its progression can be rapid and unrelenting.

Because complete obstruction of the airway can occur, the nurse brings the emergency cart to the patient's bedside. To assist the patient with breathing, the nurse prepares to administer oxygen and places the patient in the full Fowler's position. The nurse also prepares to assist with additional treatments, including epinephrine (adrenaline), steroids, and the possible insertion of an endotracheal tube. It is essential that the physician assess the patient and begin to treat the complication before the airway closes completely and the heart develops severe arrhythmia or cardiac standstill. The nurse monitors the ABCs of cardiopulmonary resuscitation and CPR may become necessary.

Angiography, Cerebral, Carotid

Includes: CT angiography (CTA) and MR Angiography (MRA)

SPECIMEN OR TYPE OF TEST: Radiography

PURPOSE OF THE TEST

Angiography of the carotid and cerebral arteries locates and identifies circulatory abnormality in the neck vessels and brain. The data provides information regarding possible medical or surgical intervention in various neurovascular abnormalities.

BASICS THE NURSE NEEDS TO KNOW

Angiography of the carotids and cerebral arteries provides for imaging of the arterial circulation and can be done by various methods. Because of recent advances in technology, CT angiography with or without contrast medium (radiocontrast) has become the preferred method of initial imaging of these neurovascular arteries in cases of suspected stroke, transient ischemic attack, ischemia, fracture of the skull, aneurysm, and other neurovascular conditions. It is a very rapid imaging process that enables timely and precise treatment in emergency situations. The vascular imaging may also be done by magnetic resonance angiography that is particularly effective in identification of a cerebral tumor. It is sometimes combined with contrast medium to obtain images of an aneurysm, vascular malformation, and obstruction in blood vessels of the brain. Both these methodologies are minimally invasive and have few complications.

Catheter angiography was once the "gold standard" of cerebral vascular imaging, but now has been surpassed by the CT and magnetic resonance (MR) angiography procedures. Catheter angiography requires an arterial puncture to insert a long catheter, which is advanced through the vascular system to the area of concern. Then contrast is injected and images are taken. The procedure is still used to obtain images of the renal arteries, but is not used very much for other vascular imaging studies because of the higher risk of trauma to the arteries, bleeding at the puncture site, and potential to disrupt plaque and cause occurrence of an arterial embolus. This method also has a higher failure rate in trying to image the targeted tissue.

Carotid Artery Examination by Computed Tomography Angiography

When the carotid arteries exhibit signs of blockage, the patient is at risk for a stroke. The CT angiography identifies the presence of plaque and the degree of occlusion. The examination report will state the results as the degree of occlusion or the degree of lumenal opening that is present, as well as the location of the occlusion. When the obstruction has a hairline or somewhat larger opening in the lumen, there is still some blood that is able to pass through and reach the brain. An endarterectomy or stent then can be used to reduce or remove the blockage and reopen the arterial lumen.

CT angiography of the carotid arteries can also identify other abnormalities in the arterial structure, including an aneurysm (Figure 15). If the aneurysmal wall has a tear or leakage, hemorrhage will occur. The imaging identifies the aneurysm, including its location and size.

Cerebral Arteries Examination by Computed Tomography

When the patient experiences signs of a stroke within the past 48 hours, an emergency CT angiography without contrast is performed. No contrast is used initially, until it is certain that there is no vascular bleeding into brain tissue. The CT angiography provides very rapid imaging of the cerebral arteries and can identify a cerebral hemorrhage or thrombus (Figure 16), as well as ischemia to the brain tissue distal to the vascular abnormality. The data from the CT images can predict whether the ischemia can be reversed and the brain tissue salvaged or not. The imaging helps the physician to determine the appropriate method of intervention, including rapid thrombolysis (a dissolving of the clot), or mechanical thrombectomy (removing the clot). The patient with a hemorrhage may be a candidate for rapid endovascular or surgical intervention to stop the bleeding and prevent rebleeding.

In cases of traumatic injury, CT angiography of the carotid and vertebral arteries of the neck, and arteries of the cerebral tissue provide important data about blunt or penetrating tissue injuries. The imaging may be performed for the head and neck or with whole body CT angiography when suspecting multiple areas of trauma.

Speed in imaging is very important to early medical or interventional treatment. The unenhanced CT angiography of the cerebral tissue is completed in 12 to 15 seconds, and the report of results is available within 20 minutes (Delgado, Almandoz, Romero, Pomerantz, & Lev, 2010).

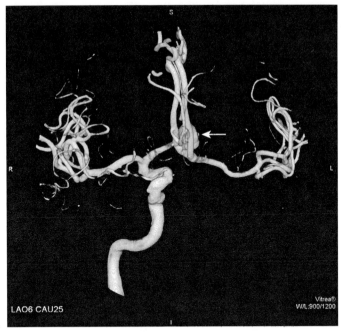

Figure 15. **Computed tomography angiography with contrast.** The three-dimensional reconstruction shows the internal carotid artery and the nearby aneurysm in the anterior communicating artery in the brain. (From Frank ED, Long BW, Smith BJ: *Merrill's atlas of radiographic positioning and procedures,* ed 12, St Louis, 2012, Mosby.)

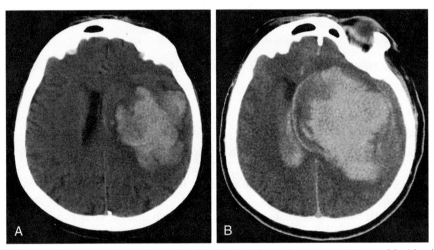

Figure 16. **Computed tomography angiography of the brain.** The patient was an 81-year-old with a history of hypertension. Two to three hours before arrival at the hospital, she had an altered mental status. When the emergency CT angiography without contrast was performed, it demonstrated **(A)** a left basal ganglia cerebral hemorrhage with minimal extension into the ventricle. **B,** Two hours later, the follow-up computed tomography angiography showed a marked increase in size of the cerebral hemorrhage, with greater extension into the ventricle. The patient died shortly after the imaging was completed. (From Delgado Almandoz, JE; Romero, JM; Pomerantz, SR; & Lev, MH (2010) Computed tomography angiography of the carotid and cerebral circulation, *Radiologic Clinics of North America, 48,* (2) 273.)

A

If it is determined that there is no cerebral hemorrhage from a defect in an artery, CT angiography can be done using contrast medium. The radiocontrast provides sharper images of the lumen of the arteries and any abnormality that is present, including aneurysm, arteriovenous malformation, atheromatous plaque, tumor, shift in the position of brain structures, fracture of the skull, or compression of brain tissue from tumor or subdural hematoma.

Carotid and Cerebral Artery Examination with Magnetic Resonance Angiography

This method captures images of the magnetized blood moving through arteries of the carotid and cerebral circulation. It can provide images with and without contrast medium. It is very effective in identifying and sizing benign and malignant cerebral tumors, stroke, thrombus, embolus, and aneurysm. It can locate the source of bleeding from an aneurysm and can identify a cerebral hematoma. In trauma cases, it can locate and image the extent of the injury and edema to the tissue. It is not able to provide images of bone. Sometimes both CT angiography and MR angiography are needed to provide complete information about the patient's condition.

Contrast Media

When radiocontrast is used, the imaging by CT or MRI is very sharp and detailed. There are many types of contrast and the selected choice is specific to the imaging process and the tissue that is to be imaged. Nonionic contrast media has a much lower risk of an adverse reaction and in the United States, it is used almost exclusively. When used for CT or MR angiography, the contrast is injected into a vein. The radiocontrast is cleared from the circulation by the kidneys and is completely eliminated in urine within 24 hours.

There have been many studies to identify what causes a hypersensitivity reaction to contrast medium in some people, but the cause remains unclear. There is no evidence that allergy to the protein in shellfish or iodine in seafood is predictive of a hypersensitivity reaction to the contrast media (Beaty, Liberman, & Stavin, 2008).

REFERENCE VALUES   No abnormalities of the arterial vasculature of the neck or head are visualized.

HOW THE TEST IS DONE

For CT angiography, the patient is placed on the special CT table and is positioned according to the area of tissue being imaged. For head and neck imaging, the patient is in a supine position and a special cradle is placed over the patient's head. The cradle holds the patient's head immobile during the imaging process.

The gantry of the machine consists of a large ring that holds the x-ray tube and many detectors. The tube continuously and rapidly rotates around the ring and x-ray energy passes through the patient's body. The detectors opposite the tube capture the signals from the x-ray energy. At the same time, the table moves the patient through the gantry ring and this provides progressive levels of raw data of the area that are imaged. The combination of rotational direction of the x-rays and the forward movement of the table produce a spiral or helical path of data. Complex computer operations convert the raw data into visual images of the tissues and structures. Other computer operations provide images of particular slices or views to focus on the area of abnormality.

When radiocontrast is used in CT or MR angiography of the head and neck, the contrast is injected intravenously via a vein in the antecubital fossa. The computer software coordinates the timing of the imaging so that images are taken as the contrast material is concentrated in the arterial vasculature of the head and neck.

Complete discussion of the magnetic resonance imaging procedure is found on p. 436.

SIGNIFICANCE OF THE TEST RESULTS

Abnormal Values

Vascular occlusion, stroke
Cerebral aneurysm
Intracranial hemorrhage
Atherosclerotic plaque
Vasospasm, arteritis, stenosis
Arteriovenous malformation
Arteriosclerosis
Brain tumor

INTERFERING FACTORS

- Movement of the head during imaging
- Metal objects in the x-ray field
- Renal insufficiency
- Dehydration

NURSING CARE

Pretest

- If it is possible to obtain blood urea nitrogen (BUN) and creatinine results, the nurse verifies that the results are in the patient's record. These laboratory tests are necessary because the patient must have adequate renal function to filter and remove the contrast at the end of the study. Elevated results indicate that renal function is impaired and the physician is notified.
- Once the physician has informed the patient about the procedure, obtain written consent from the patient and enter the signed document in the patient's record.
- ○ *Patient Teaching.* The nurse instructs the patient regarding the food restrictions to be implemented before the test. Instruct the patient to discontinue food intake for 6 to 8 hours before the test. The contrast medium can cause nausea. If food is in the stomach, vomiting would result in head movement during the imaging process. Most protocols encourage extra intake of clear fluids because adequate hydration will promote renal excretion of the contrast medium.
- Assist the patient in removing all clothing and putting on a hospital gown. For CT angiography of the head and neck, metal objects are removed from the head, mouth, hair, neck, and upper torso. These include hair ornaments or pins, removable metal dental appliances, jewelry, and body-piercing items. For MR angiography, the protocol for removal of metallic items is much more specific (see Magnetic Resonance Imaging on p. 436).
- Take baseline vital signs and enter the results in the patient's record. Many of the patient's are frail and elderly with preexisting diabetes, renal impairment, or a heart condition. Others are severely injured because of trauma. Their medical condition may be unstable.

Continued

A

NURSING CARE—cont'd

During the Test

- Establish an intravenous line for fluid volume and hydration.
- The patient is placed in the supine position. Remind the patient to keep the head and neck absolutely still during the injection of contrast material and the imaging sequence. Inform the patient that he or she may experience a temporary flushing or burning sensation, a salty taste, headache, or nausea as the contrast medium is injected. The unpleasant sensations do not last very long.

Posttest

- Vital signs should be taken and the results recorded. A small bandage is placed over the venous site of injection.
- Instruct the patient to continue drinking extra fluids for the next 24 hours to promote the excretion of the contrast medium.

◆ Nursing Response to Complications

After cerebral angiography, the overall incidence of complication from a hypersensitivity reaction to the nonionic contrast medium is 0.5% to 3%. If any of the nursing assessments demonstrate abnormality associated with complication, the nurse immediately informs the physician. The hypersensitivity reaction may be nonimmediate or immediate. The nonimmediate reaction starts from 1 hour to 3 days after contrast is administered. It is usually a mild and self-limiting reaction. The immediate reaction usually begins within an hour after the contrast is administered, but it progresses rapidly in seriousness. It can be a very severe, life-threatening reaction and may result in death of the patient.

Nonimmediate hypersensitivity reaction to the contrast medium. In this milder form, the nursing assessment findings include urticaria (hives and itching), angioedema (diffuse swelling of the skin), and a macular or maculopapular rash. Vital signs remain stable. Usually diphenhydramine (Benadryl) will be prescribed to relieve the symptoms and reduce the hypersensitive response.

Immediate hypersensitivity reaction to the contrast medium. The adverse reaction usually begins with the cutaneous symptoms of hives, itching of the skin, rash, and the swelling of angioedema. However, additional severe systemic reactions rapidly begin to occur and they affect the respiratory and cardiac functions. The physician is notified immediately.

The nurse assesses the patient's breathing ability, because swelling in the airway and bronchospasm can begin. The patient begins to develop pallor, cyanosis, dyspnea, and respiratory failure. Vital signs are also taken because hypotension and tachycardia may be present and lead to shock. The patient condition has progressed to anaphylaxis. The nurse assists the physician with the treatment to reverse the condition and support the patient's vital functions. Treatment includes subcutaneous injections of epinephrine (adrenalin) and steroids. The emergency cart is kept nearby because an endotracheal tube and oxygen may be required along with the emergency drugs. The nurse continues to monitor for the ABCs of cardiopulmonary resuscitation and CPR may be necessary. If this severe reaction cannot be reversed, the patient will develop seizures, go into a coma, and respiratory and cardiac arrest.

Angiography, Pulmonary

Also called: Pulmonary Arteriography

SPECIMEN OR TYPE OF TEST: Radiography

PURPOSE OF THE TEST

Pulmonary angiography is used primarily to confirm the diagnosis of a pulmonary embolism. It may be performed to diagnose congenital or acquired abnormalities of the pulmonary vasculature.

BASICS THE NURSE NEEDS TO KNOW

Pulmonary angiography is an invasive diagnostic procedure in which radiocontrast medium is injected into the pulmonary artery or its branches to visualize the pulmonary vascular bed. It is usually performed when a pulmonary embolism is suspected and other less invasive procedures cannot exclude or confirm the diagnosis. With the development of multidetector computer tomography (MDCT), which is noninvasive and reliable in diagnosing pulmonary emboli, pulmonary angiography is being done less frequently.

Risks are involved with pulmonary angiography; however, most of the problems are manageable, such as dysrhythmias, an allergic response to the contrast medium, and infection of the venous access site. There is no absolute contraindication for pulmonary angiography, but certain conditions may require adaptations of the technique used. These conditions include systemic anticoagulation, pregnancy, an uncooperative patient, severe hypoxia, pulmonary hypertension, right-sided endocarditis (risk of dislodging vegetation), left bundle branch block (risk of complete heart block), and amiodarone pulmonary toxicity.

REFERENCE VALUES	Pulmonary vessels fill quickly and symmetrically, with no filling defects, narrowing, or obstruction.

HOW THE TEST IS DONE

The procedure is performed in an angiography laboratory in which cardiac monitoring equipment and emergency equipment are available. With the patient supine, a catheter is inserted via the antecubital or femoral vein into the right or left pulmonary artery, or both (the decision is based on previous testing). Multiple films are taken after the dye is administered through the catheter.

Additional imaging techniques are available in some laboratories and may be part of the angiography. These techniques include *high-resolution cineangiography, balloon occlusion angiography,* and *digital subtraction angiography.* Cineangiography has the advantage of delineating flow and motion, and helping to distinguish questionable filling defects and overlapping structures. Balloon occlusion angiography involves occlusion of the pulmonary artery with a balloon catheter. A smaller amount of contrast dye is needed with balloon occlusion angiography, which permits excellent opacification. Digital subtraction angiography allows dye to be inserted into the superior vena cava or right atrium; thus, the procedure is less invasive.

A

SIGNIFICANCE OF TEST RESULTS

Pulmonary embolism
Pulmonary artery stenosis
Pulmonary arteriovenous fistula

INTERFERING FACTORS

- Uncooperative patient
- Noncompliance with dietary restrictions

NURSING CARE

Pretest
- Perform and document baseline assessments.
- Ensure that informed consent has been obtained.
- The nurse checks blood test results for PT, PTT, and platelet determinations. Ensure that a baseline electrocardiogram and electrolyte, blood urea nitrogen, creatinine, and arterial blood gas (ABG) determinations are performed, that the results are in the patient's chart, and that abnormalities are reported.
- The nurse checks with the patient for a history of allergic reactions to contrast dyes or shellfish. The nurse also reports and documents the allergies according to hospital protocol.
- If a femoral vein is to be used as the access site. Shave the area if necessary. If the patient is taking anticoagulants, the angiography procedure is usually performed with the antecubital approach.
- The nurse ensures that the patient maintains adequate hydration. A peripheral intravenous line is usually inserted.

○ *Patient Teaching.* Instruct the patient about the procedure. Warn the patient that a warm, flushed, or nauseated feeling may ensue when the dye is injected but that this feeling passes quickly.

○ *Patient Teaching.* The nurse instructs the patient not to eat or drink, except for sips of water, for 4 to 6 hours before the procedure.

During the Test
- The patient is awake and will need reassurance and explanations by the nurse during the procedure.
- Place the patient on a cardiac monitor and observe cardiac rhythm during the procedure.
- Place the patient in the supine position. The site of venous entry is exposed, and the patient is draped.
- After a local anesthetic is given, right-sided heart catheterization is performed under electrocardiographic monitoring and intermittent fluoroscopy. As the catheter is inserted, the nurse records pressure readings.
- Contrast dye is warmed to body temperature. The nurse again reassures the patient that any discomfort felt when the dye is administered is temporary.
- The nurse continuously monitors the patient for complications related to the dye (sensitivity reaction, anaphylaxis, or bronchospasms) or to catheterization (dysrhythmias, cardiac perforation).

Posttest
- Maintain the patient on bedrest for 2 to 4 hours. Keep the patient warm.
- Apply pressure to the site for a minimum of 5 minutes. The nurse checks the venous access site for hemostasis, and assesses distal pulses.

Angiotensin-Converting Enzyme

Also called: (ACE); Serum Angiotensin-Converting Enzyme (SACE)

SPECIMEN OR TYPE OF TEST: Serum

PURPOSE OF THE TEST

ACE levels are determined to evaluate possible cause of hypertension and to diagnose and treat sarcoidosis.

BASICS THE NURSE NEEDS TO KNOW

Angiotensin-converting enzyme (ACE) is found primarily in the pulmonary epithelial cells. ACE converts angiotensin I to angiotensin II. Angiotensin II stimulates the adrenal cortex to produce and secrete the hormone aldosterone and is also a powerful vasoconstrictor. Because angiotensin II is a vasopressor, ACE levels are determined as part of the diagnostic workup for hypertension.

ACE levels increase with sarcoidosis, a disease that causes widespread granulomatous lesions that may affect any organ, including the lungs. When sarcoidosis is suspected, ACE levels are determined to diagnose the disorder, assess its severity, and evaluate its therapy.

REFERENCE VALUES   Children and adolescents: 15-50 IU/L *or* SI: 15-50 IU/L
Adult male: 12-36 IU/L *or* SI: 12-36 IU/L
Female: 10-30 IU/L *or* SI: 10-30 IU/L

HOW THE TEST IS DONE

A venipuncture is performed; if a delay is expected in sending the specimen to the laboratory, place the specimen on ice.

SIGNIFICANCE OF TEST RESULTS

Elevated Values
Cirrhosis
Gaucher's disease (familial disorder of fat metabolism)
Hansen's disease
Histoplasmosis
Hodgkin's disease
Hyperthyroidism
Myeloma
Pulmonary fibrosis
Rheumatoid arthritis
Sarcoidosis
Scleroderma

Decreased Values
Adult respiratory distress syndrome
Diabetes mellitus
Hypothyroidism
Tuberculosis

INTERFERING FACTORS

• Steroid use

| NURSING CARE

The nursing actions are similar to those for other venipuncture procedures, as presented in Chapter 2.

Anion Gap

Also called: Electrolyte Gap; Ion Gap

SPECIMEN OR TYPE OF TEST: Serum

PURPOSE OF THE TEST

The anion gap is calculated most frequently to determine the cause of metabolic acidosis.

BASICS THE NURSE NEEDS TO KNOW

The anion gap is the sum of unmeasured anions in the serum: phosphates, sulfates, ketones, proteins, and organic acids. It is used to distinguish among causes of metabolic acidosis. The anion gap is used to determine if the metabolic acidosis is a result of the accumulation of hydrogen ions or due to a loss of bicarbonate.

The major determinant of the anion gap is protein. A significant decrease in plasma protein causes a large decrease in the anion gap.

In addition to disease states that cause an increase or decrease in anions or cations, or both, in the blood, fluid volume also affects the anion gap, because it may cause hemoconcentration (higher sodium and potassium concentration) or hemodilution (dilutional hyponatremia).

REFERENCE VALUES	3-11 mEq/L *or* SI: 3-11 mmol/L, *or* 10-15 mEq/L *or* SI: 10-15 mmol/L, depending on laboratory methodology
▼ Critical Value	<3 mEq/L

HOW THE TEST IS DONE

The anion gap is determined by subtracting the sum of measured anions (bicarbonate [HCO_3] and chloride [Cl]) from the measured cations (sodium [Na] and potassium [K]).

SIGNIFICANCE OF TEST RESULTS

Elevated Values

Hypernatremia
Hyperosmolar coma
Hypocalcemia
Hypomagnesemia
Ketoacidosis
Lactic acidosis
Starvation

Decreased Values

Hypercalcemia
Hypermagnesemia
Hypoalbuminemia
Hyponatremia
Multiple myeloma

INTERFERING FACTORS

- Dehydration
- Ingestion of licorice
- Excessive ingestion of antacids, ethylene glycol, methanol, paraldehyde, or salicylates
- Use of medications such as adrenocorticotropic hormones, antihypertensive agents, bicarbonates, chlorpropamide, diuretics, lithium, Na penicillin, phosphates, steroids, sulfates, and vasopressin

❘ NURSING CARE

After the results of blood electrolyte determinations are obtained, calculate the anion gap during the test with the following formula:

$$(Na + K) - (HCO_3 + Cl) = Anion\ gap$$

Antidiuretic Hormone

See Vasopressin on p. 624.

Anti-DNA

Also called: DNA Antibody; Antibody to Double-Stranded DNA (Anti-ds-DNA)

SPECIMEN OR TYPE OF TEST: Serum

PURPOSE OF THE TEST

The anti-DNA test is useful for the diagnosis of systemic lupus erythematosus (SLE). It is also used to monitor the response to treatment of this disorder.

A

BASICS THE NURSE NEEDS TO KNOW

In autoimmune disease, antibodies attach to and destroy nuclear or cytoplasm antigens in one's own body tissue (Figure 17). The autoimmune response causes inflammation, fibrosis, and destruction of a single target organ, or the process is disseminated, meaning that it affects many different organs or tissues.

Elevated Values

Anti-DNA is one of the specific antinuclear antibody (ANA) tests. Antibody to double-stranded DNA is highly elevated in the serum of a majority of patients with systemic lupus erythematosus at some time during an active phase of illness. It is present to a much lesser degree in patients with other collagen vascular or autoimmune diseases. Using the enzyme-linked immunosorbent assay method, a value of 25 to 30 IU/mL is considered to be a borderline result, and a value of 31 to 200 IU/mL or higher is positive. When the value is in the high or very high range, it is specific for SLE. It may take several years before a medical diagnosis of SLE can be made, based on this test, other antibody tests, and clinical symptoms of the illness.

SLE is a disease of exacerbation and remission, meaning there are "flare-ups" of active illness and quiet periods when there is less disease activity. The level of anti-DNA is much higher during exacerbations. To monitor the patient during an active phase, this test may be ordered every 1 to 3 months; during remission, it may be ordered every 6 to 12 months.

REFERENCE VALUES   Enzyme immunoassay method: Negative; <25 IU/mL

HOW THE TEST IS DONE

Venipuncture is used to collect a sample of venous blood.

SIGNIFICANCE OF TEST RESULTS

Active systemic lupus erythematosus
Discoid lupus erythematosus
Rheumatoid arthritis
Chronic active hepatitis (lupoid hepatitis)

INTERFERING FACTORS

- Administration of radioactive isotopes in the preceding 7 days
- Warming of the specimen

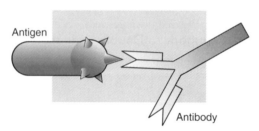

Figure 17. Antigen and antibody.

NURSING CARE

Nursing actions are similar to those used in other venipuncture procedures (see Chapter 2), with the following additional measures.

Pretest

- Schedule this test before any radioactive isotope test.

Posttest

- Arrange for prompt transport of the specimen to the laboratory, because the specimen will require chilling.
- The nurse can assist by obtaining a history of the patient's symptoms. The patient with SLE complains of fatigue, fever, muscle aches, and arthritic pains in small joints, particularly in the hands and wrists. There is a characteristic erythematous rash across the bridge of the nose and on both cheeks. It is called a butterfly rash because of its characteristic shape. The exacerbation of illness often occurs with an emerging rash after exposure to sunlight, stress, infection, and treatment with antibiotic therapy. The nurse also documents the patient's current medications, because some of them can cause drug-induced lupus, a temporary condition. Medications include procainamide hydrochloride (Pronestyl) and hydralazine hydrochloride (Apresoline).

Antiglobulin Tests

Also called: Coombs' tests
Includes: Antiglobulin Test, Direct (DAT); Direct Coombs' Test; Antiglobulin Test, Indirect (IAT); Indirect Coombs' Test

SPECIMEN OR TYPE OF TEST: Blood

PURPOSE OF THE TEST

The *direct antiglobulin test* is part of the posttransfusion workup to detect red blood cell incompatibility between donor and recipient blood. It is also used to help diagnose erythroblastosis fetalis, or hemolytic disease of the newborn, and helps confirm the diagnosis of hemolytic anemia.

The *indirect antiglobulin test* is used as an antibody screen in type and crossmatch testing in preparation for blood transfusion. It detects maternal-fetal blood incompatibility and predicts the hematologic risk to the fetus. It is used to evaluate the need for $RH_o(D)$ immune globulin administration and helps confirm the diagnosis of hemolytic anemia.

BASICS THE NURSE NEEDS TO KNOW

The antiglobulin tests consist of direct and indirect tests. They are used to detect the presence of antibodies in the serum and antigens on erythrocytes. When an antigen-antibody reaction has occurred in the blood, the erythrocytes become coated with antibody globin, and the erythrocytes agglutinate (clump together). In severe conditions, lysis of the coated erythrocytes occurs. The lysis of many erythrocytes results in hemolytic anemia.

A

Direct Antiglobulin Test

The direct antiglobulin test detects antibodies attached to red blood cells. In this antigen-antibody reaction the coated cells are "sensitized" and then clump together in the process called *agglutination*. The severity of the reaction depends on the number of antibodies produced and the number of affected erythrocytes. This test would detect the antigen-antibody reaction during the transfusion of incompatible blood of the donor to the recipient. It also detects the Rh_o incompatibility between the expectant mother and the fetus. Because the blood types of the mother and fetus are incompatible, the maternal antibodies attack the erythrocytes of the fetus. As the erythrocytes of the fetus become coated, agglutinate, and undergo hemolysis, erythroblastosis fetalis or hemolytic anemia of the newborn develops.

Some medications also cause elevation of the direct antiglobulin test. Methyldopa (Aldomet), acetaminophen, and quinidine are the medications often involved, but others are penicillin, cephalosporin, tetracycline, sulfonamides, levodopa, and insulin. Protein in the medication is the antigenic substance, and IgG or complement causes the erythrocytes to become coated. In most of these cases, the direct antiglobulin test result is elevated, but in a few cases, hemolytic anemia results.

Indirect Antiglobulin Test

The indirect antiglobulin test detects the presence of antibodies in the patient's serum.

In the first trimester of pregnancy, this test is used to screen the expectant Rh negative mother for potential blood incompatibility with the fetus. When the test result is negative, the test is repeated in the 28th week of pregnancy and at delivery. Whenever the test becomes positive for the presence of antibodies, it is followed up with antibody identification, a titer reading, and possible amniocentesis. The development of maternal antibodies occurs in the Rh-negative mother who carries an Rh-positive fetus. The antibodies cross the placental barrier, enter the fetal circulation, and result in the coating and agglutination of fetal erythrocytes.

Methyldopa is a common drug cause of elevated indirect antiglobulin test results.

REFERENCE VALUES   Negative

HOW THE TEST IS DONE

Direct Antiglobulin Test
Venipuncture is used to collect a sample of venous blood. Venous cord blood may be collected in the newborn.

Indirect Antiglobulin Test
Venipuncture is used to collect a sample of venous blood.

SIGNIFICANCE OF TEST RESULTS

Positive Values
Direct Antiglobulin
Autoimmune hemolytic anemia
Hemolytic transfusion reaction

Hemolytic disease of the newborn
Sensitivity to particular medications
Indirect Antiglobulin
Maternal-fetal blood incompatibility
Autoimmune hemolytic anemia
Sensitivity to particular medications

INTERFERING FACTORS

- Hemolysis
- Inadequate identification of the specimen

NURSING CARE

Nursing actions are similar to those used in other venipuncture procedures (see Chapter 2), with the following additional measures.

Pretest

- Include the following information on the requisition form: recent history of blood transfusion or plasma expanders, obstetric history, and the pertinent medications taken by the patient.

Posttest

- Ensure that the specimen label and requisition form include the patient's name and identification data, as well as the source of the blood (venous, cord).

Antinuclear Antibody

Also called: (ANA)

SPECIMEN OR TYPE OF TEST: Serum

PURPOSE OF THE TEST

The ANA test is used as a screen to detect connective tissue disorders, particularly systemic lupus erythematosus.

BASICS THE NURSE NEEDS TO KNOW

An autoimmune disease is a disorder caused by an immunologic reaction against one's own tissue antigens. When the antibodies attack one or more antigens in the cell nuclei, the antibodies are called *antinuclear antibodies*, or ANA. Of the many different autoimmune disorders, some affect cell nuclei of a single organ and others cause systemic disease, affecting the cell nuclei of many tissues.

Positive ANA results identify the presence of the antibodies of various systemic rheumatic diseases, but ANA cannot identify a specific disease. As a screening tool, however, ANA is particularly relevant. A titer of 1:160 or higher (SI 3U or higher) is positive for connective tissue disorder, especially systemic lupus erythematosus.

A

Antinuclear Antibody, Specific Autoantibodies

For more specific information, a test panel of specific antibodies may be ordered to follow up on a positive ANA test result. These specific subtypes include anti-ds-DNA, anti-Ro, anti-La, anti-nRNP, anti-Smith autoantibody, and others. When positive, the subtype is an indicator for a specific connective tissue disease. For example, elevated values for anti-Smith and anti-ds-DNA autoantibodies are found only in individuals who have systemic lupus erythematosus.

   The ANA test can produce false-positive results because of medications, including procainamide (Pronestyl) and hydralazine (Apresoline), and a number of other drugs. The test can also produce false-positive results in normal individuals, particularly older women. In these cases, however, the titer elevation is low.

REFERENCE VALUES   Negative: <1:40 dilution *or* SI: <1-3U

HOW THE TEST IS DONE
Venipuncture is used to collect a sample of venous blood.

SIGNIFICANCE OF TEST RESULTS
Elevated Values
Systemic Autoimmune Diseases
Systemic lupus erythematosus
Rheumatoid arthritis
Myositis
Progressive systemic sclerosis (scleroderma)
Mixed connective tissue disease
Sjögren syndrome
Autoimmune Diseases of the Blood and Target Organs
Hashimoto's thyroiditis
Myxedema
Thyrotoxicosis
Hepatic or biliary cirrhosis
Leukemia
Chronic renal failure
Multiple sclerosis
Pernicious anemia
Regional ileitis (Crohn disease)
Ulcerative colitis
Gluten-sensitive enteropathy
Pemphigus vulgaris

INTERFERING FACTORS
• Hemolysis of the specimen of blood

Nursing actions are similar to those used in other venipuncture procedures (see Chapter 2), with the following additional measure.

Pretest

• On the laboratory requisition form, list any medications taken by the patient.

Antithrombin

See Coagulation Inhibitors on p. 199.

Arthrocentesis and Synovial Fluid Analysis

Also called: Joint Fluid Analysis

SPECIMEN OR TYPE OF TEST: Synovial fluid

PURPOSE OF THE TEST

Synovial fluid analysis helps in the diagnosis of rheumatic diseases, infection, inflammation, trauma, or other conditions that result in swelling of the joint, increased production of fluid, and changes in the quality of the fluid.

BASICS THE NURSE NEEDS TO KNOW

Arthrocentesis, a needle aspiration of the joint, is used to obtain a sample of synovial fluid. The procedure can be done on an affected knee, hip, ankle, shoulder, elbow, or wrist.

Joint fluid appearance. Normally, the joint contains a small fluid volume that is clear to pale yellow in color. In infection, inflammation, trauma, or irritation of the joint cartilage or synovial membrane, fluid production increases and fills or distends the joint capsule. Abnormal fluid can be cloudy or milky, indicating crystals in the fluid. Infection or inflammation of the joint produces cloudy, yellow fluid. There should be no red blood cells in the fluid. If blood is present it is usually due to blood leaking into the joint capsule from a bone fracture, trauma, hemophilia, or a traumatic tap.

Synovial fluid analysis of the aspirated specimen provides data regarding the cause of the swelling and the increased fluid production. Cell counts, chemical analysis, microscopic analysis, and culture of the fluid are commonly done.

Leukocytes. An abnormal leukocyte (white blood cell) count can be mildly to severely elevated. In severe infection, the WBC count can rise to 100,000 cells/μL or higher.

WBC differential. The increase in neutrophils in the fluid indicates bacterial sepsis. The increase in the lymphocytes indicates nonseptic inflammation. Additionally, rheumatoid arthritis (RA cells called ragocytes) or lupus erythematosus (LE cells called Reiter cells) may be present, identifying the particular immunologic condition affecting the joint.

Protein. The elevated level of protein (>4.0 g/dL [SI: >40g/L]) indicates pathology, but it is nonspecific as to the cause.

A

Glucose (fasting). The glucose level in the fluid should be equivalent to the level in the blood. A decrease in the glucose level of the synovial fluid is indicative of inflammatory arthritis. For the glucose analysis of the fluid, the patient is usually in a fasting state before the test is performed. This provides a stable baseline value for both the blood and the synovial fluid.

Uric acid. An elevated uric acid level indicates gout.

Mucin clot and mucin string test. In normal viscosity of the fluid, a mucin clot either does not form or it is present and of firm consistency. When a small amount of fluid is poured, it is thick enough to form a long string. Inflammation and excessive synovial fluid lessen the viscosity, resulting in a clot that is friable in texture. When the fluid is poured, only a short string can form.

Microscopic examination. A sample of the fluid is stained and examined microscopically for the presence of crystals, sediment, and particles that do not belong in the joint or its fluid. A culture of the fluid is prepared and the results of any growth of infectious organisms are detected and identified microscopically. Bacterial, viral, fungal, or tubercular organisms can cause joint inflammation. These include the most common bacterial organisms of *Staphylococcus* and *Streptococcus*, but *Haemophilus sp.* or *Neisseria gonorrhea* can also cause the infection of the joint.

REFERENCE VALUES

Synovial Fluid Analysis
Appearance: Crystal clear to pale yellow
Viscosity: High
Volume: <3.5-4mL
Red blood cells: Absent
White blood cells: 0-200 cells/µL *or* SI: 0-200 cells × 10⁹/L
WBC differential
Neutrophil count: <25% of the differential
Leukocyte count: <15% of the differential
Protein: 1.2-3 g/dL *or* SI: 12-30 g/L
Glucose (fasting): <60 mg/dL *or* SI: <3.4 mmol/L
Uric acid: <8 mg/dL *or* SI: 476 µmol/L
Mucin clot: Absent or firm texture
Mucin string test: Formation of a long string (4-6 cm in length)
Culture: No growth

HOW THE TEST IS DONE

Joint

Under sterile conditions, an aspiration needle is inserted into the joint space and 15 mL of fluid is withdrawn.

Blood

Venipuncture is used to obtain a sample of venous blood. The blood is drawn at the same time the joint aspiration is performed.

Culture

If gonococcus is suspected, some synovial fluid is inoculated onto a plate that contains Thayer-Martin culture medium. This is carried out immediately after the completion of arthrocentesis. Other cultures are started in the laboratory.

SIGNIFICANCE OF TEST RESULTS

Abnormal Values

Bacterial sepsis (or viral, fungal infection)
Rheumatoid arthritis
Inflammation of the joint (crystal induced, immunologic, chronic, nonseptic)
Traumatic injury
Synovitis
Osteoarthritis
Gout
Hemophilic arthritis
Systemic lupus erythematosus
Tuberculosis
Lyme disease

INTERFERING FACTORS

• Failure to maintain a nothing-by-mouth status

NURSING CARE

Pretest

• An informed, signed consent is required and is entered in the patient's record.

○ **Patient Teaching.** Instruct the patient to fast for 6 to 8 hours before the test. A fasting blood glucose test will be performed on the blood sample. Also inform the patient that the joint procedure is performed using local anesthesia. Mild discomfort may be felt as the physician injects the anesthetic and as the needle penetrates the joint capsule.

During the Test

• The nurse assists with positioning of the affected extremity. The skin is cleansed with antiseptic, and the area is covered with a sterile drape. The nurse also assists with the preparation of the local anesthetic and the collection of all specimens.

Posttest

• After the physician withdraws the needle, the nurse will use sterile dressing material to apply pressure to the aspiration site for about 5 minutes. This stops the leaking of fluid and blood and helps to prevent a hematoma from forming. An elastic binding may be applied to the joint for 8 to 24 hours to increase the stability of the joint.

○ **Patient Teaching.** Instruct the patient to apply a cold pack intermittently to the joint for 24 to 36 hours to decrease the swelling. The extremity may be elevated on pillows. Instruct the patient to avoid excessive use of the joint for 2 to 3 days. This will help prevent stiffness, pain, and swelling.

◆ **Nursing Response to Complications**

Infection is a possible complication of arthrocentesis or any other procedure that opens the joint capsule. The infection can be introduced from environmental contamination or from aggravation of infection already present in the joint tissues.

Infection. The nurse instructs the patient to notify the physician if the dressing becomes wet with purulent, malodorous secretions. Usually the patient also develops a fever and the joint becomes swollen and painful.

Arthroscopy

SPECIMEN OR TYPE OF TEST: Endoscopy

PURPOSE OF THE TEST

Arthroscopy provides direct visualization of the interior of the joint and tissue surfaces. It is used to detect torn tendon or ligament, injured meniscus, abnormal synovial tissue, pannus formation, and damaged cartilage.

BASICS THE NURSE NEEDS TO KNOW

The arthroscope is a thin, flexible fiberoptic endoscope that provides direct visualization of the joint structures and tissues in the joint space. Special accessory instruments can be used to obtain biopsy specimens or to aspirate synovial fluid.

The joint and its interior ligaments, structures, synovial lining, and bony surfaces can develop infection, inflammation, tumor growth, or injury from trauma. When the pathologic change in the joint is not fully explained by more simple laboratory tests and diagnostic procedures, arthroscopy may be needed to confirm the diagnosis and evaluate the extent of the problem. The knee is the most common joint to be examined by arthroscopy, but the shoulder and other joints also can be examined by this method.

Diagnostic arthroscopy is performed as a same-day surgical procedure. General, spinal, or intraarticular anesthesia may be used. Arthroscopy is an invasive procedure because surgical openings are made into the joint capsule to allow the insertion of the endoscope. After the diagnostic phase, arthroscopic surgical repair of the torn or damaged tissue may be performed.

REFERENCE VALUES   No tissue or structural abnormalities of the joint space are noted.

HOW THE TEST IS DONE

The surgeon makes two incisions in the skin. A trocar is inserted into the joint capsule through one incision, followed by insertion of the arthroscope. A probe or the accessory instruments are inserted through the other incision. Additional incisions may be needed to visualize all aspects of the joint. Tissue and fluid samples may be collected for laboratory analysis. Once the fluid is drained and the instruments removed, sutures or tape strips are used to close the incisions.

SIGNIFICANCE OF TEST RESULTS

Abnormal Values
Torn ligament or meniscus
Degenerative articular cartilage
Synovitis
Loose bodies
Subluxation, fracture, or dislocation of the bone
Chondromalacia
Osteochondritis desiccans

Arthritis
Gout
Ganglion or Baker's cyst

INTERFERING FACTORS

• Failure to maintain nothing-by-mouth status

NURSING CARE

Pretest

• Once the procedure has been explained by the physician, an informed, written consent is signed by the patient and entered into the patient's record. The explanation includes information about the procedure, the anesthetic, the tests that will be done, the incisions, and the postoperative inflammation and any potential risks of complication. Mild postoperative pain will occur, but it will be controlled with analgesics.

○ *Patient Teaching.* The nurse reminds the patient to discontinue all food and fluids for 8 hours before the procedure. In addition, the patient is instructed to have a responsible person available to provide transportation after the procedure. Depending on the medications and anesthetic used, driving is likely to be difficult and hazardous. A review of postoperative instructions is done and the patient has opportunity to ask any additional questions or obtain clarification about information that was given.

• On the day of the test, take baseline vital signs and record the results.

During the Test

• Position the patient, including possible placement of a stabilizing support mechanism. The extremity is prepped and draped. The nurse also sets up the arthroscopy equipment and ensures that it is operational, including the irrigation system and suction unit.

• On completion of the procedure, bulky sterile dressings are applied and covered with an elastic bandage. An immobilizer may also be applied.

Posttest

• If general or spinal anesthetic was administered, monitor vital signs immediately and thereafter every 15 minutes for the first 2 hours, then every 30 minutes for 1 hour, and then every hour for 2 hours or until discharge from the postanesthesia unit.

• The nurse assesses for neurovascular function in the distal extremity every 15 minutes, comparing the findings with assessment of the unaffected side. The distal pulses should be strong, and the skin should be cool to warm with satisfactory color. As the effect of the anesthetic diminishes, movement and sensation should return in the fingers or toes.

• The nurse also assesses for pain and provides the prescribed medication for relief of pain, as needed. The elastic compression dressing is checked for any signs of excessive bleeding, constriction, or excessive swelling of the joint or distal extremity.

• Usually, this procedure is done as an outpatient and that evening, a follow-up phone call may be made by the nurse. The purpose is to evaluate how the patient is feeling and inquire as to any special problems or difficulties that the patient is experiencing. There may be a need to reexplain the postoperative instructions and review the use of the pain medications. The nurse also helps reassure the patient who is worrying about pain, immobility, or other common problems.

Continued

NURSING CARE—cont'd

○ *Patient Teaching.* For discharge instructions, remind the patient to keep the extremity elevated for 24 to 48 hours to reduce the swelling. A cold pack should be applied for 24 hours. The nurse instructs the patient about the prescriptions for medications to be taken at home. Pain is usually minimal and can be relieved by nonsteroidal, antiinflammatory medications and nonnarcotic analgesics.

- With arthroscopy of the knee, remind the patient that walking is permitted, but that no exercise or excessive use of the joint should occur for 24 hours. The patient may be instructed to use crutches to keep all weight off the knee or to walk only with a partial weight-bearing gait. With arthroscopy of the shoulder, the arm is placed in a sling. Activity requirements or restrictions depend on the type of injury and any surgical repair that may have been done after the diagnostic phase of the test. Range-of-motion exercises are usually started on the second to third postoperative day, and physical therapy may be instituted to strengthen the muscles.

◇ **Nursing Response to Complications**

Infection. The complications of diagnostic arthroscopy are rare, but infection can occur. If infection occurs, the patient will develop a fever and experience increased pain in the infected joint. The dressing will become wet with drainage that has a bad odor. The nurse instructs the patient to report any sign of infection to the physician.

Aspartate Aminotransferase

Also called: (AST); Serum Glutamate Oxaloacetate Transaminase (SGOT)

SPECIMEN OR TYPE OF TEST: Serum

PURPOSE OF THE TEST

AST is an indicator of inflammation, injury, or necrosis of the tissues that contain this transaminase enzyme. In liver disease, it is an indicator of liver damage from any cause. The AST test may also be used to monitor liver function in patients who receive medication that potentially is hepatotoxic.

BASICS THE NURSE NEEDS TO KNOW

AST is a transaminase enzyme found in high concentrations in the heart and liver tissues, and to a lesser extent in skeletal muscle, brain, kidney, pancreas, spleen, and lung tissues.

When there is mild or moderate liver inflammation, injury, or necrosis, the liver cells release AST through damaged cell membranes, resulting in rising AST levels in the blood. With severe damage, the liver cells are destroyed and greater amounts of AST are released into the blood stream. For example, in severe, acute hepatitis, the AST level can rise to a value of 20 to 100 times the normal value. The very high values reflect the severity of the disease, the amount of organ damage, and the prognosis for the patient's condition.

Because AST is also present in skeletal muscle tissue and other organs, the serum AST will rise when there is trauma, inflammation, or necrosis in these tissues. Generally these elevations are slight to moderate, although shock, acute pancreatitis, and infectious mononucleosis occasionally cause a severe elevation of the serum value.

Drug-induced liver disease can have a dramatic elevated effect on the AST value and other tests of the liver profile (alanine aminotransferase, alkaline aminotransferase, and bilirubin values). Numerous medications have the potential to cause inflammation and injury to hepatic cells as a result of overdose or by simply taking the medication appropriately, as prescribed. These include antiinflammatory medications, nonsteroidal antiinflammatory drugs (NSAIDs) such as acetaminophen (Tylenol), aspirin, estrogen, oral contraceptives, androgens, anabolic steroids, antimicrobials, antibiotics, antidepressants, antineoplastics, statins, and others. Very high levels of the AST test occur when the damage to the hepatocytes is moderate to severe. The liver inflammation can be temporary and gradually will subside once the particular medication is discontinued. However, acetaminophen (Tylenol, Panadol) in excessive amounts can cause severe, permanent liver damage, liver failure, and the need for a liver transplant.

AST-to-ALT Ratio

A comparison of AST to ALT is sometimes used to differentiate among the causes of damage to liver cells. The results are expressed as a ratio of AST to ALT. Because the amounts of each enzyme are about equal, the ratio is expressed as AST = ALT, or the normal value of AST:ALT = 1.

In alcoholic hepatitis, the AST value is greater than the ALT value, or the ratio is expressed numerically. For example, AST:ALT = 3:1 means that the AST value is three times greater than the ALT value. In viral hepatitis, the ALT value can rise to greater than the AST value, as AST:ALT = 1:3.

REFERENCE VALUES	Newborn: 25-75 U/L *or* SI: 0.43-1.28 µKat/L
	Infant: 15-60 U/L *or* SI: 0.26-1.02 µKat/L
	Adult: 8-20 U/L *or* SI: 0.14-0.34 µKat/L
	Adult >60 years:
	Male: 11-26 U/L *or* SI: 0.19-0.44 µKat/L
	Female: 10-20 U/L *or* SI: 0.17-0.34 µKat/L
	AST:ALT = 1
▽ Critical Values	An AST value that is three times the upper limit of normal.
	An AST:ALT ratio that is greater than 1.

HOW THE TEST IS DONE
Venipuncture is performed to collect a sample of venous blood.

SIGNIFICANCE OF TEST RESULTS
Elevated Values
Hepatitis (viral, toxic, alcoholic, drug-induced)
Cirrhosis
Hemochromatosis
Cancer of the liver

Chronic alcohol abuse
Obstructive jaundice
Myocardial infarction
Heart failure
Severe injury to the skeletal muscle tissues

INTERFERING FACTORS

- Hemolysis
- Failure to maintain a nothing-by-mouth status
- Intensive exercise before the test

NURSING CARE

Nursing actions are similar to those used in other venipuncture procedures (see Chapter 2), with the following additional measures.

Pretest

○ *Patient Teaching.* Instruct the patient to fast for 12 hours before the test. Advise the ambulatory patient to avoid strenuous exercise before the test.

Posttest

▽ **Nursing Response to Critical Values**

If the AST value is greater than three times the upper limit of the normal value or the AST:ALT ratio is greater than 1, notify the physician of this elevated result. Many commonly prescribed medications can cause hepatotoxicity (a toxic effect on liver cells). The rise above the critical value is an indicator to discontinue the particular medication that caused or increased the liver damage. The nurse should review the patient's medication list and ask the physician if any should be withheld or discontinued.

The patient's overall condition may not appear to be changed as a result of the rise in the AST level. Measurement of the vital signs can be done to ensure that shock has not occurred. The nurse also monitors the patient's level of consciousness, observing for increasing somnolence or coma, or the onset of signs of encephalopathy.

Barium Enema

Also called: (BE); Double-Contrast Barium Enema, (DCBE)

SPECIMEN OR TYPE OF TEST: Radiography

PURPOSE OF THE TEST

The barium enema is used to investigate and identify pathologic conditions that change the structure and function of the colon. It may be used as a screening test for early detection of colon cancer.

BASICS THE NURSE NEEDS TO KNOW

The barium enema is a radiographic test that is used to investigate the cause of a change in elimination patterns, melena (blood in the stool), obstruction of the colon, or the presence of an abdominal mass that has a suspected location in the colon. Barium is a contrast medium that is radiopaque, has a different density than body tissue, and can be instilled into hollow organs such as the colon. In the barium enema procedure, the entire colon and the distal portion of the ileum can be visualized on x-ray film (Figure 18). The technique may be done as a single contrast study that takes spot x-ray images of the colon with the barium filling the lumen. Alternatively, a double contrast study may be done. In this method, barium is instilled and then drained out of the colon, leaving a residual coating of contrast on the luminal mucosal surface. Then the colon is slowly filled with air that serves as a second contrast medium and also dilates the lumen of the colon. Spot x-ray images of the colon are taken after the contrasts are instilled completely.

REFERENCE VALUES   No lesions, polyps, tumors, or other abnormalities of the colon are noted. The mucosal lining is intact and the contour of the lumen is normal.

HOW THE TEST IS DONE

After the colon is emptied of feces, the contrast medium enema is administered by the radiology technologist. Barium and possibly additional air contrast are instilled as contrast media. If perforation is suspected or the patient is at risk for intraperitoneal leakage of the contrast, barium is not used and a water-soluble contrast medium is used in substitution. Fluoroscopic images are taken at intervals to monitor the instillation of the contrast. The patient must retain the contrast medium in the colon during the test. The patient's positional changes, (supine, prone, lateral) are used to enhance gravity flow of the contrast medium throughout the entire colon.

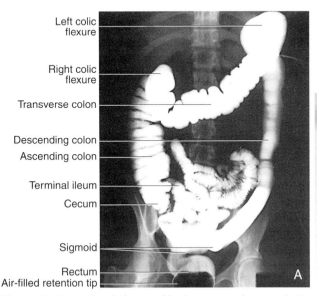
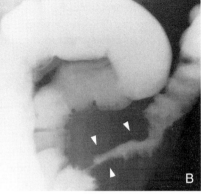

Figure 18. Normal and abnormal barium enema images. **A,** Normal single contrast barium enema image of the colon. **B,** Abnormal single contrast barium enema image of cancer of the colon *(arrowheads)*. (**A,** From Frank ED, Long BW, Smith BJ: *Merrill's atlas of radiographic positioning and procedures,* ed 12, St Louis, 2012, Mosby; **B,** From Major NM: *A practical approach to radiology,* Philadelphia, 2006, Saunders.)

X-rays are taken to image the colon and in particular, the abnormal area(s). The procedure takes 45 minutes to 1 hour to complete.

SIGNIFICANCE OF TEST RESULTS

Adenocarcinoma
Diverticulitis
Sarcoma
Hirschsprung disease
Idiopathic megacolon
Polyps of the colon
Gastroenteritis
Chronic amebic dysentery
Ulcerative colitis
Intussusception

INTERFERING FACTORS

- Upper gastrointestinal series within 3 days before the test
- Inability to retain barium
- Incomplete pretest cleansing of the colon
- Recent myocardial infarction or cerebral vascular accident

NURSING CARE

Health Promotion
The nurse can be very instrumental in health teaching to encourage people to have scheduled colorectal screening tests and not wait until symptoms appear. Early detection leads to early intervention, with a more positive treatment outcome.

Health Promotion
The barium enema is one method of routine screening for colorectal cancer. It has a high level of accuracy and is readily available throughout the nation. Precancerous polyps and cancer of the colon can be detected at a very early stage, before they cause symptoms or become invasive. Most colorectal cancers develop after age 50. If the double contrast barium enema is used as a screening test for asymptomatic adults, the recommended interval for testing is every 5 years, starting at age 50.

Pretest
- Schedule the barium enema before any other barium studies. Residual barium from the upper gastrointestinal tract would obscure the images of the colon.
- The patient receives a complete explanation of the procedure and then signs a consent form that is entered into his or her record.
- For bowel preparation the goal is to eliminate all fecal matter, gas, and mucus so that x-ray imaging is clear. The exact bowel cleansing procedure is defined by the protocol of the radiologist, and variations exist. For children younger than age 4, the bowel preparation is prescribed on an individualized basis. For the adult, a common method of preparation is presented here.

○ *Patient Teaching.* Teach the patient to begin a clear liquid diet 12 to 24 hours before the test to reduce the amount of fecal matter.

- A cathartic such as 300 mL of magnesium citrate is taken on the afternoon before the test and 50 mL of castor oil is taken in the evening before the test. A warm tap water enema (1500 mL for adults) is given at 6:00 AM on the day of the test. When all fecal matter has been removed, the enema returns will be clear.
- Extra oral fluids are taken in the pretest period to prevent dehydration or excess absorption of the barium solution from the colon. Some protocols require extra amounts of oral fluids in the afternoon and evening, but a nothing-by-mouth status is started by midnight before the test.
- It is helpful to provide all pretest and posttest instructions in writing.

During the Test

During the instillation of the barium and air contrast, the radiographer or aide instructs the patient to keep the anal sphincter contracted tightly against the tubing and to relax the abdominal muscles. This limits the leakage or expulsion of the contrast medium. The patient is also instructed to do deep breathing to limit colonic spasm and abdominal cramps. During the imaging process, the patient will be turned and repositioned. This promotes gravity flow of the contrast medium to all parts of the colon. The radiologist takes spot images of the colon as the patient moves through the various positions.

Posttest

- The patient is assisted to the toilet or commode to evacuate the contrast medium.
- A laxative is prescribed to eliminate the residual barium and prevent the constipation caused by the barium. Residual barium changes the color of feces to a gray or whitish color for 24 to 72 hours after the test.
- Encourage the patient to rest for the remainder of the day because this test is tiring.
- Elderly patients are vulnerable to a fall. Since they may also become mentally confused because of dehydration, instruct the patients to increase their fluid intake.

◇ **Nursing Response to Complications**

Complications from the barium enema procedure are not frequent. Perforation can occur when the colon tears and barium spills into the peritoneal cavity. The cause can be excessive intracolonic pressure and distention, or a tear in thin, damaged colon tissue. The instillation of large amounts of fluid into the colon can trigger vagus nerve stimulation, with resultant bradycardia. If a complication occurs, it usually happens during the test. However, complications can progress and cause a very serious illness that becomes apparent in the posttest period. The nurse monitors for complications and notifies the physician of abnormal assessment findings.

Perforation. The nurse assesses for postprocedure complaints of abdominal pain and abdominal distention. With perforation, the patient may develop shock or peritonitis, with changes in vital signs and the onset of fever.

Barium Swallow

See Esophagography on p. 304.

Base Excess/Deficit

See Arterial Blood Gases on p. 139.

ß-Amyloid(1-42)

See Lumbar Puncture and Cerebral Spinal Fluid Analysis on p. 423.

Bilirubin, Serum, Urine

Includes: Total Bilirubin, Direct Bilirubin (Conjugated Bilirubin), Indirect Bilirubin (Unconjugated Bilirubin), Neonatal Bilirubin (Total Bilirubin, Neonatal)

SPECIMEN OR TYPE OF TEST: Serum

PURPOSE OF THE TEST

Total serum bilirubin is the sum total of indirect bilirubin and direct bilirubin. The purposes of the total bilirubin test are to evaluate liver function, diagnose jaundice, and monitor the progression of jaundice.

The purpose of direct and indirect bilirubin tests is to identify the underlying cause of the elevated bilirubin level. In the newborn baby with jaundice, the neonatal bilirubin test is used to determine whether the infant needs treatment to prevent kernicterus (brain damage from high levels of bilirubin).

The purpose of the urinary bilirubin test is to identify the presence or absence of bilirubinuria in the diagnostic workup for liver and biliary diseases.

BASICS THE NURSE NEEDS TO KNOW

Most bilirubin is produced by the liver and spleen as part of the process of hemolysis (breakdown) of senescent (old) or damaged red blood cells. Once created, the bilirubin is transported in the bloodstream as indirect (unconjugated) bilirubin. The liver then converts indirect bilirubin to direct (conjugated) bilirubin. The direct bilirubin mixes with fluid and enters the bile canaliculi and hepatic ducts of the liver in the process that makes bile.

Bile, with its component direct bilirubin, flows from the hepatic ducts of the liver to the biliary ductal system. It is stored in the gallbladder and, on demand, flows through the cystic duct, the common duct, and enters the duodenum to help in the process of digestion of fats.

Jaundice

This is a clinical term that describes the yellow discoloration of the skin and sclera caused by excess bilirubin in the blood and body tissues. The jaundice becomes visible when the total serum bilirubin is elevated to greater than 2 mg/dL. An elevated level of bilirubin in the blood is called hyperbilirubinemia.

Classifications of Jaundice

One way to classify jaundice is based on the physiologic location of bilirubin manufacture, transport, and excretion. As seen in Table 4, pathophysiologic changes will be detected by elevated values of the indirect or direct bilirubin tests. These tests help provide information about the cause of the problem. The prehepatic category refers to bilirubin manufacture and transport before the blood circulation reaches the liver. The hepatic category refers to problems within the liver because of injury to the liver cells or blockage within the intrahepatic bile ducts. The posthepatic category refers to blockage of bile within the liver or in the gallbladder or gallbladder ducts.

Neonatal Jaundice In the first few days of life, newborns experience varying levels of elevated bilirubin. The condition is called physiologic jaundice. It is not clear why this condition occurs, but it is temporary. The indirect bilirubin rises modestly for 3 to 4 days and then declines to a normal value.

Other causes of neonatal jaundice are considered abnormal or pathologic, including ABO and Rh incompatibility. The rapid destruction of red blood cells in hemolytic disease of the newborn causes a great increase in indirect bilirubin. The onset is usually in the first day of life. If the total bilirubin level is greater than 20 mg/dL (SI: 340 µmol/L), potential exists for bilirubin encephalopathy or kernicterus. In kernicterus, bilirubin is deposited in the brain and if untreated, permanent damage can occur.

If the infant is born with biliary atresia, the biliary drainage system is incompletely developed and there is no open passageway for bile to flow into the duodenum. Because of the blockage, a rapid, severe rise in total bilirubin and direct bilirubin will occur. Urinary bilirubin will be positive in biliary atresia and hepatic disease, but not in hemolytic jaundice.

TABLE 4	Classifications of Jaundice	
Category of Jaundice	**Type of Bilirubin Elevation**	**Origin of the Problem**
Prehepatic	Indirect (unconjugated)	Excessive hemolysis of red blood cells Hemolytic jaundice
Hepatic	Indirect (unconjugated)	Defect in transport or conjugation in hepatocytes Physiologic jaundice
	Direct (conjugated)	Injury to, or disease of, hepatocytes Blockage of intrahepatic bile ducts Intrahepatic cholestasis
Posthepatic	Direct (conjugated)	Blockage in the biliary ductal system Extrahepatic cholestasis

There is no specific test for indirect bilirubin. The measurement of indirect bilirubin is a mathematical calculation made by subtracting the value of direct bilirubin from the value of total bilirubin.

REFERENCE VALUES

Total Bilirubin
Cord blood: <2.0 mg/dL *or* SI: <34 µmol/L
0-1 day: 1.4-8.7 mg/dL *or* SI: 24-149 µmol/L
1-2 days: 3.4-11.5 mg/dL *or* SI: 158-197 µmol/L
3-5 days: 1.5-12 mg/dL *or* SI: 26-205 µmol/L
>5 days—adult: 0.3 mg/dL *or* SI: 5-25 µmol/L

Direct Bilirubin
Adult: <0.2 mg/dL *or* SI: <3.4 µmol/L

Indirect Bilirubin
Adult: <1.1 mg/dL *or* SI: 19 µmol/L

▽ Critical Values

Total bilirubin, serum
Term infant: >15 mg/dL *or* SI: >257 µmol/L
Premature infant: 10-15 mg/dL *or* SI: 171-257 µmol/L

HOW THE TEST IS DONE

Adult: Venipuncture is performed to collect a specimen of venous blood.
Infant: Drops of blood are collected from the heel that has been pricked by a sterile lancet.
Urine: A random sample of fresh urine is collected.

SIGNIFICANCE OF TEST RESULTS

Elevated Values
Total Serum Bilirubin
Physiologic jaundice
Hepatocellular damage (toxic, infectious, or malignancy)
Obstruction in the biliary system
Hemolytic diseases
Familial hyperbilirubinemia
Reaction to some medications
Direct Bilirubin
Hepatotoxins that cause liver necrosis
Infection of the liver (hepatitis, bacterial, parasitic)
Cirrhosis
Cystic fibrosis
Cancer (liver, gall bladder, pancreas, ampulla of Vater)
Sclerosing cholangitis

Primary biliary cirrhosis
Biliary atresia
Gallstones
Lymphoma
Acute pancreatitis
Indirect Bilirubin
Inherited defects of red blood cells (sickle cell anemia, spherocytosis)
Inherited enzyme disorders
Reaction to some medications
Malaria
Physiologic jaundice
Rh or ABO incompatibility
Blood transfusion reaction due to incompatibility

INTERFERING FACTORS

- Sunlight
- Hemolysis
- Failure to maintain a nothing-by-mouth status (adults only)

NURSING CARE

Nursing actions are similar to those used in other venipuncture or capillary puncture procedures (see Chapter 2), with the following additional measures.

Pretest

○ *Patient Teaching.* Instruct the patient to fast from food for 8 to 12 hours (overnight) because serum lipids will alter the results.

Posttest

- Ensure that the tube of blood or the microcapillary tube or the urine sample is covered in aluminum foil and sent to the laboratory without delay. Because bilirubin is photosensitive, the specimens must be protected from exposure to light or a prolonged time in a lighted environment.
- The nurse remains vigilant for signs of neonatal jaundice, but observational assessment may not be reliable and is not the best method to detect elevated bilirubin at an early stage. In evidence-based nursing practice, the best approach is to systematically monitor the laboratory results for elevated total serum bilirubin values and identify those neonates who are at risk for hyperbilirubinemia (Watson, 2009).

▽ **Nursing Response to Critical Values**

If the neonatal serum bilirubin rises to a critical value in the newborn or premature infant, notify the physician immediately. If the elevation is considered to be pathologic, rather than physiologic, the baby must be evaluated medically to determine the cause of hyperbilirubinemia. At the level of the critical value, the physician will consider the treatment of phototherapy. If the level goes higher, phototherapy will be performed, and exchange transfusion may also be necessary.

Biopsy, Bone

Also called: Bone Needle Aspiration Cytology

SPECIMEN OR TYPE OF TEST: Biopsy tissue

PURPOSE OF THE TEST

Bone biopsy is performed to examine a specimen of bone tissue for its cell type and to distinguish benign from malignant bone tumor.

BASICS THE NURSE NEEDS TO KNOW

Benign bone tumors are characterized by their uniform density and well-defined margins. The most common benign tumor is the giant cell tumor, often located in the end of a long bone near a joint.

Malignant primary bone tumors are characterized by borders that extend outward into the surrounding fat or muscle tissue or inward into the marrow and medullary cavity, or both (Figure 19). The most common primary bone malignancy is osteogenic sarcoma, which is often located in the region of the knee. Malignant bone tumors may also be metastatic tumors, with the primary site located elsewhere in the body. Most bone metastases are in multiple sites, usually located in the vertebrae, ribs, sternum, or pelvis.

When a bone tumor is suspected, a bone scan or computed tomographic (CT) scan is performed first. These preliminary tests are used to verify the presence of the tumor and identify

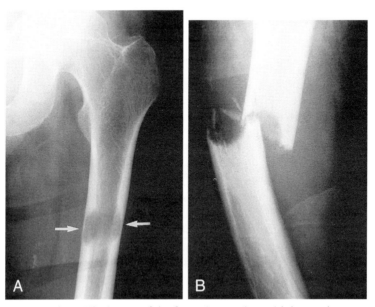

Figure 19. Bone metastasis. **A,** The image of the femur in a patient with known lung cancer shows a destructive lesion expanding from the marrow space and thinning the cortex of the bone *(arrows)*. It is important to locate lesions in weight-bearing bones so that therapy can be undertaken to prevent pathologic fracture. **B,** A view of the femur from the same patient, who returned 2 weeks later with a pathologic fracture. (From Mettler FA: *Essentials of radiology,* ed 2, Philadelphia, 2005, Saunders.)

the site for bone biopsy. They also are used to identify additional metastatic sites and to help assess the extent of growth or invasion of the tumor. Unlike biopsy, the preliminary imaging cannot distinguish benign from malignant disease.

REFERENCE VALUES   Bone tissue is normal, with no tumor cells present.

HOW THE TEST IS DONE

Using local anesthesia, a small incision is made in the skin, and a bone biopsy needle is used to drill or push into the bone. Once it is in place, the biopsy needle is rotated 180 degrees to obtain a core sample of the tissue. The specimen is placed on a slide with fixative or in a specimen jar with 95% alcohol or both. Just before collection of the bone specimen for biopsy, a bone marrow aspiration for biopsy may be done in the same location.

SIGNIFICANCE OF TEST RESULTS

Abnormal Values

Malignant

Osteogenic sarcoma

Ewing sarcoma

Reticulum cell sarcoma

Angiosarcoma

Multiple myeloma

Metastatic tumor

Benign

Giant cell tumor

Osteoma

Osteoid osteoma

Chondroma

INTERFERING FACTORS

- Failure to obtain an adequate sample of tissue
- Failure to send the specimen to the laboratory immediately

NURSING CARE

Pretest

- After the physician has explained the procedure to the patient, obtain an informed, written consent from the patient and enter the document into the patient's record.

○ *Patient Teaching.* The nurse instructs the patient to remove all clothing and put on a hospital gown.

- Baseline vital signs are taken and the results are recorded. The skin at the site of the biopsy location is cleansed with antiseptic. The nurse uses a calm, reassuring approach with the patient. The procedure and potential biopsy results can cause the patient to feel anxious.

Continued

NURSING CARE—cont'd

During the Test

- Provide support to the patient as the local anesthetic is injected into the skin and subcutaneous tissue and the biopsy needle is inserted. Despite the local anesthetic, the patient feels momentary pain as the needle penetrates the periosteum and enters the bone.
- The nurse labels all specimen containers and slides with the patient's name and the tissue source. The requisition form for a tissue cytologic study is completed, including the patient's name, age, history of carcinoma or infection, and the site of biopsy. The slides or specimen, or both, are sent to the laboratory without delay. The final preparation of the slides must be completed within 6 hours to prevent deterioration of the tissue.

Posttest

- The nurse assesses vital signs and monitors them at regular intervals until they are stable.
- Assessment findings should include observation that the pressure dressing remains clean, dry, and intact.

○ *Patient Teaching.* The nurse instructs the patient to rest quietly with an ice pack over the dressing for about 2 hours. In preparation for discharge from the ambulatory setting, instruct the patient to resume routine activity but to avoid strenuous physical activity for a few days. The pressure dressing may be changed to a small adhesive bandage on the day after the procedure, and a shower is permitted. Mild discomfort is common, and the patient can take an analgesic medication as needed.

◇ **Nursing Response to Complications**

Infection. Infection of the bone is a rare, but possible complication. If infection occurs, the patient develops a fever and headache. He or she feels bone pain and pain on movement. The biopsy site becomes red, with purulent drainage or an abscess. The nurse instructs the patient to notify the physician if these symptoms occur.

Biopsy, Bone Marrow

Also called: Bone Marrow Aspiration
Includes: Genetic testing, bone marrow cells

SPECIMEN OR TYPE OF TEST: Bone marrow fluid or tissue.

PURPOSE OF THE TEST

The bone marrow aspiration or biopsy, followed by microscopic examination of the tissue, is used to evaluate hematopoiesis. It diagnoses malignancy of primary and metastatic origin and determines the cause of infection. The examination of the marrow also is used to evaluate the progression of some hematologic diseases or the response of the marrow to chemotherapy treatment, such as in Hodgkin disease and acute myelogenous leukemia.

BASICS THE NURSE NEEDS TO KNOW

The bone marrow is responsible for hematopoiesis—the formation of blood cells. The aspirated cells of the bone marrow are used to investigate hematologic disorders. A small sample of the cells is often representative of the whole marrow. Microscopic examination of the cells provides information about the cause, type, and extent of the abnormality. A peripheral blood smear is performed on the same day to compare and incorporate pertinent findings.

The marrow cells are examined for characteristics of the tissue including *cellularity*, the proportion of aspirate that is hematopoietic cells rather than fat cells; *distribution*, an estimate or count of the number of each type of cell found in the marrow specimen; *maturation,* the balance of cells in stages of development; and abnormal cells, the presence of irregular or *abnormal cells* in the marrow. In addition, the examination provides data about the underlying cause of the abnormality in the cells of the blood.

Leukocytes from the marrow have a number of different proteins attached to the cell surfaces. Many blood disorders have distinctive distributions and patterns of the proteins on these cell surfaces. In the presence of fluorescent antibodies, the different cellular proteins will react and bond with specific antibodies and the analysis of the cell patterns provides for many diagnoses. The proteins serve as markers to help diagnose different diseases, such as leukemia and lymphoma, and can distinguish between different types of each of these cancers (Jenkins, Karunanithi, & Hewamana, 2008).

Genetic Testing of Bone Marrow Cells

Cytogenic studies are performed to identify acquired disorders of chromosomes in malignant cells of the marrow. The alterations provide information about the type of malignancy and prognosis in response to conventional cancer therapy.

Molecular analysis examines the DNA in nuclei of the white blood cells in the marrow specimen, identifying the altered or defective DNA. When molecular defects are identified, they can be used to monitor the response to therapy or identify a relapse at an early stage when additional treatment can still be effective. The cancer patient who is undergoing treatment or who is in remission will need to undergo repeated, planned bone marrow aspirations and biopsies over time. This process of surveillance of bone marrow cells is called *minimal residual disease monitoring.*

REFERENCE VALUES   Normal bone marrow.

HOW THE TEST IS DONE

A local anesthetic is injected in the skin, into subcutaneous tissues, and at the bone site. In bone marrow aspiration, a bone marrow needle is inserted into the medullary cavity of a bone. Fluid and marrow cells are aspirated into several syringes. When a bone marrow biopsy is required, a wider, bone trephine needle with an inner core is inserted. After the inner core is removed, the hollow, outer component of the needle is advanced into the marrow and a core of marrow tissue is removed. Slides are prepared and tissue specimens collected. When indicated, culture specimens are obtained.

The aspiration and biopsy sites include the iliac crest and proximal tibia (Figure 20). In adults, the posterior iliac crest is the best site. In infants and young children, the proximal tibia is used. The sternal site is only used for obese patients.

Conscious sedation may be indicated for bone marrow biopsy, particularly for the children and adults who have undergone treatment for cancer. In the minimal residual disease monitoring process, the bone marrow biopsy sites are often multiple, with multiple specimens obtained.

B

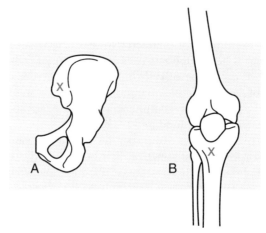

Figure 20. Anatomic sites (X) for bone marrow aspiration and biopsy. **A,** Posterior iliac rim. **B,** The proximal tibia, about 1 to 2 inches below the patella of the infant or small child.

SIGNIFICANCE OF TEST RESULTS

Abnormal Values
Iron deficiency anemia
Infection: histoplasmosis, miliary tuberculosis, infectious mononucleosis
Sideroblastic anemia
Anemia of chronic disease
Megaloblastic anemia
Macroglobulinemia
Agammaglobulinemia
Myelofibrosis
Aplastic anemia
Leukemia
Collagen disease
Multiple myeloma
Parasitic disease: malaria, leishmaniasis
Hodgkin's disease
Lymphoma
Metastatic bone cancer

INTERFERING FACTORS
• Failure to obtain an adequate specimen

NURSING CARE

Pretest

- After the physician explains to the patient the reason for the bone marrow examination and how the procedure will be done, the patient signs the informed consent form. This form is entered into the patient's record.
- The nurse assesses the patient for anxiety and provides a calming, supportive presence. Common sources of anxiety are fear of the procedure and fear of the possible diagnosis.

During the Test

- The nurse positions the patient according to the site that will be biopsied. For a sternal or tibial biopsy, the supine position is used. Biopsy of the iliac crest requires a lateral recumbent position, with the hip flexed. Prepare the skin by cleansing it with an antiseptic solution.
- The nurse provides support and reassurance as the local anesthetic is instilled. The patient feels brief discomfort as the needle and anesthetic solution penetrate the skin and infiltrate the periosteum. Caution the patient to remain immobile as the biopsy needle is inserted into the marrow. Despite the use of the anesthetic, the patient will experience some pain as the periosteum is penetrated and the marrow is aspirated.
- The nurse assists with the preparation and labeling of the slides. The clot and biopsy tissue are placed in a sterile specimen jar that contains fixative (formalin or Zenker's solution). Once the needle is removed, the nurse applies pressure to the site, using small sterile gauze. After bleeding has stopped, a small sterile dressing is placed over the puncture site. The patient with a low platelet count is prone to prolonged bleeding so it may take longer to stop blood from oozing out.

Posttest

- Arrange for prompt transport of the request form and the identified specimens and slides to the laboratory.
- Reassure the patient that for a few days, mild discomfort at the biopsy site is expected. Any signs of persistent bleeding or infection should be reported to the physician.

Biopsy, Breast

Includes: Estrogen receptor (ER), progesterone receptor (PR), HER-2/*neu* receptor

SPECIMEN OR TYPE OF TEST: Tissue biopsy

PURPOSE OF THE TEST

The pathology examination of the biopsy specimen is used to distinguish benign from malignant change in the breast tissue.

BASICS THE NURSE NEEDS TO KNOW

A suspicious, palpable or nonpalpable lesion of the breast requires a biopsy to determine the cause and differentiate between benign and malignant tissue. Imaging by ultrasound, computed tomography (CT), or magnetic resonance imaging (MRI) is done to visualize the size and location of the suspicious tissue. A core needle biopsy, or an open surgical biopsy are commonly used because of their high level of accuracy in obtaining a tissue sample. A fine needle aspiration biopsy may be used, but is not as accurate in obtaining a tissue sample.

When the suspicious tumor or microcalcification is small and nonpalpable, the radiologist uses CT imaging to insert a clip as a tissue marker. This marker is left in place so that malignant tissue can be located for excision. Alternatively, a localizing needle wire can be placed directly into the tissue site or very close to it. The needle is then removed and the wire is left in place, held firm by a hook in the tip of the wire (Figure 21). The wire will provide additional guidance for the surgeon to locate the specific tissue to take a biopsy. Shortly after the wire is in place, the biopsy is performed.

Estrogen receptor (ER), progesterone receptor (PR), and HER-2/*neu* receptor

These tests are all tumor markers for breast cancer. These tests are done on the biopsy tissue when the biopsy result is invasive cancer of the breast. Estrogen receptor and progesterone receptor assay results provide information about prognosis and responsiveness to hormonal therapy, such as tamoxifen or aromatase therapy. Positive results for each of these tests can indicate that the tumor is highly likely to respond to hormonal therapy and a negative result means that the tumor is not likely to respond to this therapy. In recent testing advances, the

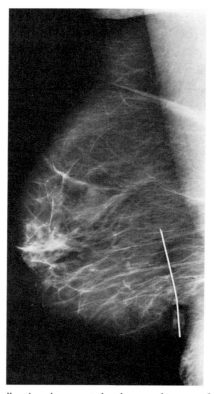

Figure 21. Successful breast needle wire placement that locates the area of suspicious tissue. After breast biopsy, the lesion was diagnosed as a 9-mm infiltrating ductal carcinoma. (From Frank ED, Long BW, Smith BJ: *Merrill's atlas of radiographic positioning and procedures,* ed 12, St Louis, 2012, Mosby.)

patient with a positive ER-PR assay also can have genetic testing to identify a genetic variant that would prevent tamoxifen from being effective. If the patient is genetically resistant to tamoxifen, an alternative treatment with an aromatase inhibitor (anastrozole) would also act to inhibit the effect of estrogen on breast cancer.

The HER-2*neu* receptor is an oncogene for breast cancer and other cancers. An oncogene is a gene that can mutate and cause normal cells to become cancer cells. From the biopsy specimen, the positive result correlates with the extent of the tumor and is the best indicator of long-term survival. The HER-2*neu* can also be measured in the serum and has a high correlation with the biopsy results.

REFERENCE VALUES   Normal breast tissue.

HOW THE TEST IS DONE

For the core needle biopsy, the patient is placed in prone position on the biopsy table, with the affected breast hanging down through a special opening in the table. The table is then elevated and the surgeon works beneath the table. Under local anesthesia and using ultrasound for imaging, the wire is removed and a sample of tissue from the breast lesion is obtained from the designated area. With the core needle method, multiple core tissue samples are obtained. Special vacuum suction equipment may be used to help extract the tissue samples.

For an open biopsy, the patient is in a supine position on the operating room table. Conscious sedation or general anesthesia is administered. Conscious sedation consists of the combination of the sedative hypnotic midazolam hydrochloride (Versed) and a narcotic analgesic fentanyl citrate (Sublimaze) or meperidine hydrochloride (Demerol). An incision is made and the identified section of breast tissue is excised.

The tissue is sent to the pathology laboratory for frozen section for immediate analysis; a follow-up with permanent slides will be made of the fluid and tissue samples. Using a microscope, the pathologist examines and identifies, classifies, and stages the abnormal tissue. If the surgeon excises the small tumor at the time of the biopsy, the pathologist also examines the margins (edges of the tissue samples) to determine that the entire tumor has been removed and the margins are clear of malignant cells, or not. When the tissue is highly suspicious or confirmed as malignant, a sentinal node biopsy will be done immediately after the breast biopsy (See Biopsy, Sentinel Node on, p. 132).

SIGNIFICANCE OF TEST RESULTS

Abnormal Values
Fibroadenoma
Carcinoma
Duct papilloma
Calcification
Fat necrosis
Cystosarcoma
Granular cell tumor

INTERFERING FACTORS

• Inadequate tissue sample

NURSING CARE

Pretest

- After the doctor informs the patient of the procedure, the reason for the biopsy, and possible complications, the nurse obtains a signed consent from the patient. This consent is entered into the patient's record.
- The patient who must undergo a breast biopsy experiences varying degrees of distress, depression, anxiety, and heightened emotion. The anxiety can be very high, particularly in those women who have limited social support or increased stress from other causes. The emotions may be due to fears of a possible malignancy, uncertainty, the biopsy procedure, or pain from the procedure. In a personalized approach, the nurse provides emotional and educational support. Assist the patient in reducing stress by listening, providing explanations, affirming feelings, or using diversions, as indicated. The nursing interactions with the patient need to be culturally sensitive and communication must be in language that the patient can understand (Laio, Chen, Chen, et al, 2009).
- If general anesthesia is planned, instruct the patient to fast from food and fluids for 12 hours before the surgery.
- On the morning of the biopsy, the patient should bathe, but not apply deodorant, lotion, perfume, or powder to the breasts and underarms.
- The nurse also assesses and records the patient's vital signs, including temperature, blood pressure, pulse, and respirations. If the patient is very anxious before the core biopsy is done, diazepam (Valium) will be given.

During the Test

Assist the patient in proper positioning. For the core needle biopsy procedure, pillows may be used to help with comfort because the patient will not be allowed to move during the procedure.

- Clean the breast tissue with povidone-iodine or other surgical antiseptic preparation. Assist with the preparation of the local anesthetic.
- When the procedure is to be done with a local anesthetic, the nurse provides support to the patient. The patient can feel the injection of the anesthetic. Some patients can feel the push and pull of the needle, some pain, and other sensations such as stinging. Assess the patient for early signs of fainting, such as lightheadedness, dizziness, pallor, and diaphoresis.
- Once the tissue is obtained, place the fresh tissue specimen in a sterile jar for a frozen section, or in fixative solution for permanent slides. The container is labeled with the patient's name, medical record number, date of the biopsy, and the exact location of the biopsy site. When a fresh tissue specimen is to be analyzed immediately, the laboratory physician comes to the location where the biopsy is performed and receives the specimen personally. The pathology requisition form has the identical written information that is on the specimen label.
- Apply a dry, sterile dressing to the incision or puncture site.

Posttest

- The nurse takes vital signs and records the results. When a general anesthetic is used, vital signs must be monitored every 15 to 30 minutes until the patient is reactive, alert, and stable.
- Until the biopsy results are known, it is common for the patient to continue to experience anxiety and uncertainty in the posttest period. To help the patient cope, encourage her to return to normal activity as soon as possible. After an open biopsy, however, vigorous exercise must be avoided for 2 weeks.

⦿ *Patient Teaching.* To relieve surgical pain, the nurse instructs the patient to use warm, moist compresses or a heating pad. Female patients should wear a supportive bra. The patient may shower or bathe as usual, using unscented soap at the needle puncture site. The method of cleansing of the surgical incision is prescribed by the surgeon. The patient will change the surgical dressing once a day. Inform the patient that the core needle method does cause bruising, particularly when multiple needle insertions and aspirations occur during the procedure.

- Advise the patient to inform the surgeon of inflammation, infection, or excessive pain in the incision.

◇ **Nursing Response to Complications**

Hematoma. The assessment findings for hematoma include swelling, pain, and ecchymosis in the breast. The nurse assesses the breast, and abnormal findings include extensive bruising, asymmetrical swelling, and leakage of fluid from the incision.

Cellulitis or infection. The nursing assessment findings of cellulitis or infection include pain, swelling, and redness in the breast tissue. In addition, the patient feels ill (malaise) and complains of a headache and elevated temperature.

Biopsy, Endomyocardial

SPECIMEN OR TYPE OF TEST: Pathology

PURPOSE OF THE TEST

An endomyocardial biopsy is usually performed to determine if a transplanted heart is being rejected. Other purposes for the biopsy are to diagnose myocarditis or doxorubicin (Adriamycin)-induced cardiomyopathy and to determine the cause of restrictive heart disease.

Studies are currently being done to develop blood tests to identify rejection of transplanted hearts. They center on measuring the immune status of the transplant recipient. If these molecular expression tests are successful, endomyocardial biopsy will no longer be necessary.

BASICS THE NURSE NEEDS TO KNOW

Endomyocardial biopsy is an invasive procedure requiring cardiac catheterization. It permits sampling of right or left ventricular tissue.

REFERENCE VALUE   No pathology.

HOW THE TEST IS DONE

The procedure involves a cardiac catheterization (see p. 221). A catheter with a jawlike tip is inserted under fluoroscopy or echocardiography, and several small tissue samples are obtained. Echocardiography is considered superior to fluoroscopy because of improved visualization of the tricuspid value. A right or left ventricular sample may be taken. For patients at high risk, such as those with a history of left ventricular thrombus or infarction, a right ventricular biopsy may be preferred.

SIGNIFICANCE OF TEST RESULTS

Abnormal Values

Doxorubicin-induced cardiomyopathy

Cardiac amyloidosis

Cardiac fibrosis (especially radiation injury)

Chagas' cardiomyopathy

Myocarditis

Rejection of transplanted heart

Scleroderma

Toxoplasmosis

Tumor infiltrates

Vasculitis

INTERFERING FACTORS

* Bleeding disorders
* Severe thrombocytopenia
* Systemic anticoagulation
* Uncooperative patient

NURSING CARE

See section on Cardiac Catheterization.

◆ **Nursing Response to Complications**

Although complications of endomyocardial biopsy are rare, they include accidental biopsy of papillary muscle or chordae tendineae, cardiac perforation, and hemopericardium. Other complications can occur but are related to the catheterization rather than to the biopsy.

   Accidental biopsy of papillary muscle or chordae tendineae. The nurse assesses the heart sounds of patients after an endomyocardial biopsy for new onset of a murmur. Report the existence of a new murmur to the physician, who may want to order an echocardiogram.

   Hemopericardium. Bleeding into the pericardial sac will interfere with cardiac movement. The nurse will observe signs of cardiac tamponade: decrease in cardiac output, muffled heart sounds, increase in right atrial pressure, and pulsus paradoxus.

   Notify the physician immediately. If cardiac output is significantly compromised, anticipate need for pericardiocentesis.

   Cardiac perforation. See above, plus the nurse will assess for shock, as evidenced by hypotension, tachycardia, and dyspnea.

Biopsy, Liver

Also called: Percutaneous Liver Biopsy

SPECIMEN OR TYPE OF TEST: Tissue biopsy

PURPOSE OF THE TEST

The biopsy sample is used to diagnose pathologic changes in the liver and to help evaluate the extent of the disease process.

BASICS THE NURSE NEEDS TO KNOW

The indicators for liver biopsy are unexplained, abnormal liver function tests, jaundice, and an enlarged liver or a history of cancer that commonly metastasizes to the liver. The tissue sample is obtained by fine needle biopsy, using needle aspiration or a needlelike instrument that shaves a very small core tissue sample. If the disease is diffuse and affects all parts of liver tissue, the biopsy sample may be aspirated without direct visualization of the organ. When a small and specific area of tissue is located more deeply into the liver tissue, ultrasound or CT provides visualization for placement of the tip of the needle directly into the affected area.

REFERENCE VALUES   The liver cells are normal, with no evidence of inflammation, scarring, degeneration, infection, tumor, malignancy, or other pathologic change.

HOW THE TEST IS DONE

After administration of local anesthetic, the physician places the needle between the anterior and midaxillary lines, usually at the level of the sixth or seventh intercostal space (Figure 22). While the patient holds his or her breath on expiration, the needle is inserted into the liver. Aspiration is performed with a 10 mL syringe that is connected to the needle; cutting is done by rotating the needle apparatus so the cutting edge shaves off small bits of tissue. Once the needle

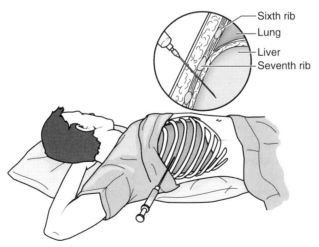

Sixth rib
Lung
Liver
Seventh rib

Figure 22. Liver biopsy procedure. The patient is positioned in supine or left lateral position with the arm raised and hand under the head. The biopsy needle is inserted below the seventh rib. Ultrasound is usually used to image the precise location for the biopsy of the liver tissue. (Adapted from Burden N: *Ambulatory surgical nursing*, ed 2, Philadelphia, 2000, Saunders.)

is removed, the patient resumes breathing. The aspiration must be coordinated with breathing because during expiration, the liver and diaphragm are at their highest positions and while the patient holds his or her breath, the liver tissue is immobile. Both these factors help prevent laceration of the liver or diaphragm.

Once the tissue sample is collected, the physician prepares some slides immediately. The remainder of the tissue is placed in a sterile container filled with formalin or saline. The slides are labeled with the patient's identification. Additionally, the specimen container and the pathology request form have the patient's identification, the date, type of tissue, and the procedure used. The slides, tissue sample, and request form are all sent to the laboratory for pathology examination.

SIGNIFICANCE OF TEST RESULTS

Cirrhosis
Cancer of the liver, primary or metastatic
Cyst of the liver
Chronic hepatitis B or C
Sarcoidosis
Amyloidosis
Wilson's disease
Miliary tuberculosis

INTERFERING FACTORS

- Obesity
- Infection in the right pleural cavity or right upper quadrant of the abdomen
- Uncooperative patient behavior
- Abnormal clotting ability

NURSING CARE

Pretest

- Once the physician has explained the procedure to the patient, the nurse obtains the patient's written consent. The form is entered into the patient's record.

○ *Patient Teaching.* Provide pretest teaching about positioning, breathing instructions, and posttest instructions. Patients tend to feel anxious about this test, so the nurse provides reassurance and support, as needed. The patient must discontinue all food and fluids for 8 hours before the test. If the procedure is to be done in an outpatient setting, instruct the patient to arrange for transportation home, accompanied by a competent adult. Because of the medications given at the start of the procedure, the patient will not be competent to drive for some hours afterward.

- Before the biopsy is done, the patient's clotting ability is evaluated because liver disorders can cause impaired clotting ability. The prothrombin time should not be more than 3 seconds longer than the control time, and the platelet count should be greater than 100,000 cells/mm³. The nurse reviews the test results and ensures that they are in the patient's record. If the results are abnormal, the nurse informs the physician.

- Baseline vital signs are taken and the results are recorded. About 1 hour before the biopsy procedure, the nurse administers the prescribed pretest medication. Commonly, meperidine (Demerol) or diazepam (Valium) is injected intramuscularly to promote relaxation and analgesia.

During the Test

- The patient is positioned on the left side or supine, with the arm under the head. The skin is cleansed and draped with a sterile cloth.
- The nurse stands beside the patient to provide reassurance and help keep the patient immobile. Despite the use of local anesthesia, the patient feels some pain in the side and top of the shoulder as the needle passes through the phrenic nerves and into the liver.
- The nurse assists with the placement of the tissue in a specimen container and labels all slides and the container appropriately.
- The skin at the biopsy site is covered with a sterile bandage. The nurse takes and records vital signs, and places the patient on his or her right side.

Posttest

The specific routine for monitoring by the nurse is usually based on hospital or physician protocol and varies somewhat from one institution to another.

- For 1 to 2 hours, the patient remains positioned on the right side with a pillow pressing on the waist and rib area. This helps the liver remain somewhat compressed against the rib cage to promote clotting.
- Take vital signs regularly and frequently because of the risk of hemorrhage or hypotension. Generally, the pattern is every 15 minutes for 1 hour, every hour for 4 hours and every 4 hours thereafter, until the patient is stable. The nurse observes the lower right side of the rib cage for signs of bleeding. This may appear as oozing at the needle insertion site or as ecchymosis in a nearby area.
- The patient may resume food and fluid intake soon as desired. Bed rest is maintained for 12 to 24 hours. If the patient is to be discharged to the home, he or she remains on bed rest in the recovery area for up to 6 hours before discharge.

○ *Patient Teaching.* The nurse provides discharge instructions for the patient who is going home. The patient must avoid aspirin for 2 weeks. There must be no heavy lifting efforts until healing is complete. In 24 hours, the patient may remove the bandage and bathing can be resumed. Finally, the patient is instructed to notify the physician of any malaise, fever, pain, shortness of breath, or signs of bleeding.

◆ **Nursing Response to Complications**

Usually, complications do not occur, but bleeding is possible. A blood vessel may have been punctured during the procedure, or impaired clotting ability may contribute to some blood loss. If excess bleeding or other abnormal assessment findings occur, the nurse takes vital signs and notifies the physician immediately.

Bleeding. The nurse assesses for blood on or under the skin. Localized ecchymosis (bruising) would appear on the lower right lateral ribs or on the side of the abdomen just below the ribs. Signs of shock include restlessness, hypotension, tachycardia, dyspnea, pallor, and diaphoresis (cold, sweaty skin). The abdomen may be distended and painful. If bleeding occurs after discharge from the outpatient setting, the patient should know how to recognize the problem and how to contact his physician for immediate assistance.

Biopsy, Lung, Open

Also called: Pulmonary Biopsy, Open Lung Biopsy

SPECIMEN OR TYPE OF TEST: Pathology

PURPOSE OF THE TEST

A lung biopsy is performed to diagnose pulmonary disorders such as cancer and sarcoidosis. Lung biopsy can confirm the diagnosis of fibrosis and degenerative or inflammatory diseases of the lung.

BASICS THE NURSE NEEDS TO KNOW

A lung biopsy is performed to remove lung tissue so that the cells may be examined microscopically for pathologic features. A variety of methods are used to obtain these lung cells. Tissue samples may be obtained by bronchoscopy (see p. 153), by percutaneous or fine-needle biopsy (see p. 127), or by open biopsy.

With an open biopsy, surgery is required, with its potential risks. It involves the resection of a small portion of tissue, which is sent to the laboratory for histology examination.

REFERENCE VALUES   Normal tissue.

HOW THE TEST IS DONE

For an open biopsy of the lung, a thoracotomy is required, which is a surgical procedure. After a small incision is made in the chest wall, the lung is exposed and tissue is excised. A chest tube or tubes are inserted to restore negative pleural pressure.

SIGNIFICANCE OF TEST RESULTS

Carcinoma
Diffuse alveolar damage (DAD)
Granuloma
Infection
Interstitial lung disease
Sarcoidosis

INTERFERING FACTORS

• Noncompliance with dietary restrictions
• Smoking
• Obesity

NURSING CARE

Follow hospital protocol for the preoperative and postoperative care of a patient requiring open chest surgery.

◆ **Nursing Response to Complications**

Potential complications of an open lung biopsy are bleeding, pneumothorax, and empyema.

Bleeding. The nurse assesses for indications of bleeding: tachycardia, restlessness, hypotension, and tension pneumothorax. The nurse reports indications of bleeding immediately. Depending on the size of the hemothorax, the nurse would anticipate the need for chest tube(s) and thoracotomy tray.

Pneumothorax. Anxiety, restlessness, dyspnea, tachypnea, pallor, and decreased breath sounds are indications of pneumothorax. If a tension pneumothorax has occurred, there will be a mediastinal shift to the unaffected side. Notify the physician immediately and anticipate an order for chest x-ray to evaluate the size of the pneumothorax. Depending on the size of the pneumothorax, the nurse would anticipate the need for chest tubes and a thoracotomy tray.

Empyema. Empyema is an infection in the pleural cavity with an accumulation of pus. The patient usually presents with fever, chills, and sweating. The patient will complain of malaise, dyspnea, pain, and cough. The nurse should anticipate that the physician will order a white blood cell count and antibiotics and may want to insert chest tubes to drain the pleural cavity.

Biopsy, Lung, Percutaneous, Needle

Also called: PNB of the Lung; Fine-Needle Biopsy of the Lung; FNB of the Lung; Transthoracic Needle Biopsy

SPECIMEN OR TYPE OF TEST: Pathology

PURPOSE OF THE TEST

A percutaneous needle biopsy of the lung is performed to determine the pathology of a lung lesion such as cancer, granuloma, infection, and sarcoidosis. It is used for staging of malignant tumors. Percutaneous needle biopsy is also indicated for diagnosis of mediastinal masses.

BASICS THE NURSE NEEDS TO KNOW

Percutaneous needle biopsy of the lung has been made possible by the use of fluoroscopy and CT guidance. Intrathoracic lesions, especially of the lung parenchyma, can usually be visualized by biplane or C-arm fluoroscopy technique. For small intrathoracic tumors or those located in the hilar or mediastinal area, a CT scan is used to guide the biopsy.

REFERENCE VALUES   No pathology.

HOW THE TEST IS DONE

Under the guidance of CT scanning or fluoroscopy, a biopsy needle is inserted into a lesion and a specimen is aspirated for histology examination.

SIGNIFICANCE OF TEST RESULTS

Carcinoma

Granuloma

Infection

Sarcoidosis

NURSING CARE

Pretest

- The patient is kept on nothing-by-mouth status for 4 hours before the procedure, but may take medications (except aspirin and anticoagulants).
- The nurse takes and records baseline vital signs and ensures that an informed consent form is signed.
- The nurse assesses the patient for bleeding disorders because the needle path may be close to major vessels. The nurse also assesses the patient's history for contraindications to percutaneous needle biopsy: pulmonary hypertension, severe chronic obstructive lung disease, or arteriovenous malformation.

○ *Patient Teaching.* Instruct the patient about the procedure and the need to remain still and not cough when instructed not to move. Practice with the patient holding breath on command.

○ *Patient Teaching.* The nurse warns the patient that minor discomfort may be experienced during the biopsy and that multiple biopsies may be necessary.

- Transport the patient to the CT laboratory; if fluoroscopy is planned, bring the patient to the radiology department.

During the Test

- The patient is positioned according to the location of the lesion.
- The skin is marked as a guide for needle insertion.
- The pulse oximeter is applied and baseline readings are taken and recorded. The nurse also checks vital signs. Have oxygen available in case a pneumothorax occurs during the procedure.
- Remind the patient not to cough or take deep breaths.
- Skin preparation is carried out, and the area is draped. A local anesthetic is given before the skin is nicked with a scalpel. The physician inserts the biopsy needle and tissue samples are taken. During insertion of the needle and any needle manipulation and biopsy, the patient is instructed to hold his or her breath and not move.
- A pathologist may be present to prepare slides from the aspirated specimen. If a pathologist is not present, the nurse places the tissue specimen in a sterile container, usually with a fixative. Special techniques may be required depending on studies being done. Check with the physician for desired media to use in the container. The tissue container and the requisition slip contain the appropriate patient information, the date, time, and the source of the tissue. The specimen is then sent to the laboratory.

Posttest

- The nurse records vital signs every 15 minutes during the first hour.
- Position the patient with the biopsy side down.

B

- Observe the patient for a minimum of 2 hours.
- Instruct the patient to avoid coughing and limit talking for 2 hours.
- A chest x-ray study is usually ordered immediately after the procedure and again 2 hours later to identify any pneumothoraces. Patients with small pneumothoraces (10% or less) are usually discharged. If a significant pneumothorax occurs, the patient is admitted to the hospital.

○ *Patient Teaching.* The nurse instructs the patient being discharged to rest at home, to limit activities for the rest of the day, and return to the hospital if chest pain, discomfort, or shortness of breath is experienced.

◆ **Nursing Response to Complications**

The nurse needs to observe for indication of the complications of percutaneous needle biopsy, which are pneumothorax, hemorrhage, bile leak, and infection.

Pneumothorax. Anxiety, restlessness, dyspnea, tachypnea, pallor, and decreased breath sounds are indications of pneumothorax. If a tension pneumothorax has occurred, there will be a mediastinal shift to the unaffected side. Notify the physician immediately and anticipate an order for chest x-ray to evaluate the size of the pneumothorax.

Hemorrhage. Observe for overt or covert bleeding. Bleeding into the pleural space will cause a tension pneumothorax. The nurse will assess for tachycardia, restlessness, pallor, and hypotension. Response to bleeding will depend on the site and amount. Exert pressure if bleeding is at site of needle insertion. If large amount of bleeding has occurred into the pleural space, prepare for chest tube(s) insertion.

Bile leak. Bile is very alkaline; if it leaks into the peritoneal space, the patient will complain of abdominal pain. Notify the physician. The nurse also positions the patient to maximize comfort.

Infection. Since the procedure is done under sterile technique, infection is rare. However, if indications of infection occur; such as fever, malaise, tachycardia, or elevated WBCs, the nurse informs the doctor. The nurse should anticipate that the physician will order cultures, so appropriate antibiotics may be ordered.

Biopsy, Lung, Transbronchoscopy

See Bronchoscopy on p. 153.

Biopsy, Pleural

See Thoracentesis, Pleural Fluid Analysis, and Pleural Biopsy on p. 567.

Biopsy, Renal

Also called: Kidney Biopsy; Fine-Needle Aspiration Biopsy of the Kidney; FNB of the Kidney

SPECIMEN OR TYPE OF TEST: Tissue biopsy

PURPOSE OF THE TEST

Renal biopsy is used to determine the exact pathologic state and diagnosis of a renal disorder, monitor the progression of the renal disease, evaluate the response to treatment, and assess for rejection of a renal transplant.

BASICS THE NURSE NEEDS TO KNOW

Biopsy of the kidney provides specific information regarding the pathophysiologic changes in the tissue. Other laboratory tests and noninvasive procedures are performed first to obtain as much diagnostic information as possible. The broad categories of pathophysiologic conditions that require renal biopsy include acute renal failure, renal tumor, renal transplant rejection, asymptomatic hematuria, proteinuria of unknown origin, or questions regarding drug toxicity and untoward reaction to medication.

A renal biopsy may be done as a surgical procedure or more frequently by fine needle biopsy. Needle biopsy may be performed to diagnose renal cancer. It is used when CT or magnetic resonance imaging (MRI) findings are inconclusive to investigate metastatic disease or recurrence of cancer, and to diagnose the type of renal tumor in the patient who is a poor surgical risk.

In renal transplant patients, the donor kidney can show signs of transplant rejection. Without biopsy, early accurate diagnosis of rejection is difficult because of other possible causes of renal dysfunction that produce the same symptoms. Fine needle aspiration biopsy is minimally invasive and can be used repeatedly on the same patient.

REFERENCE VALUES   No pathology.

HOW THE TEST IS DONE

After administration of local anesthesia, the physician inserts a biopsy needle percutaneously (through the skin) or through a small incision. Ultrasound or x-ray films are used to guide the exact placement and location of the biopsy needle. A syringe is used to aspirate a small core of tissue from the renal cortex. The total time needed to obtain the specimen is about 15 minutes.

SIGNIFICANCE OF TEST RESULTS

Abnormal Values
Acute or chronic glomerulonephritis
Goodpasture's syndrome
Amyloid infiltration of the kidney
Systemic lupus erythematosus
Renal transplant rejection or failure
Renal cell carcinoma
Wilms' tumor

INTERFERING FACTORS

- Failure to maintain nothing-by-mouth status
- Coagulation disorder
- Urinary tract infection
- Nonfunction or presence of only one kidney

NURSING CARE

Pretest
- Ensure that written informed consent has been obtained and is entered in the patient's record.
- The nurse checks that all screening tests are completed and that the results are posted in the patient's chart. Coagulation studies, including prothrombin time, activated partial thromboplastin time, platelet level determination, and hematocrit are performed to verify clotting ability. Urinalysis identifies the presence of any infection.
- Check for a history of contraindications: allergies to dye, renal cyst, one kidney, acute or chronic perirenal infection and hydronephrosis.
- The nurse takes baseline vital signs and records the results. Report *uncontrolled* severe hypertension, which is a contraindication for the procedure.
- The nurse administers sedation as ordered.

During the Test
- Cleanse the skin over the site with antiseptic.
- Provide reassurance to the patient to help alleviate anxiety. When the physician is about to insert the biopsy needle, instruct the patient to take a deep breath and hold it. Assist the patient in remaining still. A brief sensation of pain may occur.
- After the needle is removed, apply pressure to the puncture site for 20 minutes to help promote hemostasis. Then apply a sterile dressing and adhesive bandage to the puncture site.
- The nurse places the biopsy specimen in a sterile container with normal saline and ensures that the container is labeled with the patient's name and the tissue source of the specimen.
- Arrange for immediate transport of the specimen to the laboratory.

Posttest
- The nurse monitors vital signs every 15 minutes for 1 hour, every 30 minutes for the next hour, and at regular intervals thereafter. At frequent intervals, the nurse observes the dressing and surrounding tissue for signs of bleeding.
- For 8 hours, the nurse checks each voided specimen for hematuria. Initially, a small amount of blood may be present, but it should disappear within the 8-hour period. In some institutions, the protocol is to collect every urine specimen separately, with a notation of the time and date of voiding written on the container. Over time, progressively less blood should be present, and the urine should return to its normal color.
- If not contraindicated, the nurse encourages the patient to drink extra fluids to help promote urination.
- Eight hours after the test, the nurse obtains a blood specimen for hemoglobin and hematocrit determination. When bleeding is excessive, different time intervals and repeat testing may be necessary.

○ *Patient Teaching.* Instruct the patient to lie flat for 12 to 24 hours. A sandbag may be used to help promote compression of the tissue. After this period of immobility, bed rest or limited activity is maintained for 24 hours to prevent the onset of fresh bleeding. The nurse also instructs the patient to avoid physical exertion, heavy lifting, and trauma to the lower back for several days.

◇ **Nursing Response to Complications**

Although renal biopsy is considered safe, with a low complication rate, the procedure has some risks. These complications include retroperitoneal and urinary tract hemorrhage, pneumothorax, biopsy of other abdominal viscera, and infection.

Continued

B

Bleeding. The nurse observes for overt and covert bleeding. Vital signs may indicate tachycardia and hypotension. The nurse should also observe for restlessness, confusion, pallor, cool skin, and decreased urinary output. The patient may complain of dorsal, flank, or shoulder pain. The nurse immediately notifies the physician and anticipates an order for hemoglobin and hematocrit. A blood typing and cross-matching may also be ordered.

Infection. The nurse assesses site for inflammation (redness, warmth) and patient complaint of discomfort or tenderness at the site. The nurse notifies the physician and anticipates an order for a WBC.

Pneumothorax. Anxiety, restlessness, dyspnea, tachypnea, pallor, and decreased breath sounds are indications of pneumothorax. Notify the physician immediately and anticipate an order for chest x-ray to evaluate the size of the pneumothorax.

Biopsy, Sentinel Lymph Node

Also called: SNLB; Sentinel Node Biopsy; SNB

SPECIMEN OR TYPE OF TEST: Tissue Biopsy

PURPOSE OF THE TEST

This tissue biopsy is used to investigate a particular regional lymphatic basin to detect metastasis in patients who have cancer of the breast or cutaneous melanoma. It is also used to help with staging of these cancers and provides part of the information needed to determine the most effective methods of treatment for these patients.

BASICS THE NURSE NEEDS TO KNOW

The sentinel node is the first lymph node in the regional chain of nodes that drains lymphatic fluid from the tissue where the primary cancer is located. It is the most likely node to be affected by invading cancer cells that have traveled from the primary site via the lymphatic system. The sentinel lymph node biopsy procedure is widely accepted for use in cases of breast cancer and melanoma. Of all the diagnostic tests and procedures that will be done on patients with cancer of the breast or cutaneous melanoma, the sentinel lymph node biopsy is the best predictor of the patient's long-term survival (Weidner, Cote, Suster, & Weiss, 2009; Stebbins, Garibyan, & Sober, 2010).

When the biopsy specimen is positive for cancer cells, metastasis is already in the sentinel node. The whole lymphatic chain of nodes will be removed surgically at the same time that the primary tumor is excised. If the biopsy specimen is negative for metastasis, the patient will have a surgical removal of the primary site of the cancer, but is spared having a lymphadenectomy and the subsequent problem of poor lymphatic drainage from distal tissues.

There is a small percentage of "false negative" results that can occur. This means that the pathology report is negative, but undetected cancer cells actually are present in the sentinel node.

REFERENCE VALUES   Normal lymphatic cells and fluid within the sentinel node.

HOW THE TEST IS DONE

There are two methods that are used together to locate the sentinel node. One way is by lymphatic scintigraphy. A radioactive colloid is injected into tissue near the primary cancer site, 2 to 6 hours before the biopsy. The radioactive colloid will drain out of the tissue and move to the regional nodal basin via specific lymphatic channels. A gamma probe will detect the radioactive material as it pools in the regional lymphatic bed and forms a "hot spot" in the sentinel node. The other way is to use a blue dye that is injected into tissue that is very near the primary cancer site 5 to 10 minutes before the biopsy. The dye moves through the lymphatic channels to the regional nodal basin and into the sentinel node, staining the tissue with blue color as it moves with the lymphatic fluid. The surgeon dissects the tissue along the blue-stained pathway and then uses the gamma probe to identify which node is the sentinel node to be removed in an open biopsy procedure. Sometimes the second node in the lymphatic chain is also removed for pathology analysis.

SIGNIFICANCE OF THE TEST RESULTS

Abnormal Values

Metastasis of cancer of the breast
Metastasis of melanoma

INTERFERING FACTORS

- Previous extensive excision of the malignant tumor at the primary site
- Previous flap reconstruction after excision of the cancer at the primary site

NURSING CARE

Pretest
- Once the physician has explained the procedure to the patient, the nurse obtains the patient's written consent. The form is then placed in the patient's record.
- Because general anesthesia will be used for this biopsy, the patient is told to discontinue food for 12 hours and discontinue drinking fluids for 8 hours before the surgery.
- The nurse provides emotional support to the patient who experiences anxiety and fear about the diagnosis and outcome of the surgery (see also Biopsy, Breast on p. 117).

During the Test
- Once the node is removed, it is submitted fresh, or is placed in fixative solution and sent immediately to the pathology laboratory for analysis. The tissue container is labeled with the patient's name and identification number, the time and date, the physician's name, the location of the node, and the method of detection. The container has a label stating that the contents are radioactive. The accompanying pathology request contains the same information as is written on the specimen container.

Continued

The amount of radioactivity varies with the procedure that is used. Overall, the amount is small and when handling the specimen, there is no significant risk of radioactivity exposure (Weidner, et al, 2009). For precautionary measures, the specimen container should be handled as little as possible, while wearing gloves. The gloved hands should be washed after handling the specimen container and then hands should be washed after removing the gloves.

Posttest

- Surgery to excise the cancerous tumor, with or without lymphadenectomy is usually done immediately after the results of the breast biopsy and sentinel node biopsy are known.
- If instead, no further surgery is to be done immediately after the biopsy procedure, the incision is sutured closed and a sterile dressing is applied. Aftercare of the incision is per the surgeon's instructions. For discharge, the patient is taught to observe the bandage and the skin for signs of infection or bleeding, such as redness, swelling, ecchymosis, purulent drainage, fever, malaise, or incisional pain that is not relieved by the prescribed medications.

Biopsy, Skin

Also called: Gross and Microscopic Pathology, Skin

SPECIMEN OR TYPE OF TEST: Tissue biopsy

PURPOSE OF THE TEST

Skin biopsy is performed to make an exact diagnosis and exclude alternative diagnoses. It may be used to evaluate and monitor a disease or response to treatment. Microscopic analysis of the biopsy tissue provides evidence of the clinical diagnosis. It is used to identify malignancy or premalignancy and to investigate any lesion that increases in size, bleeds easily, or ulcerates spontaneously.

BASICS THE NURSE NEEDS TO KNOW

When a skin lesion is present and the clinical diagnosis is uncertain or must be verified, a skin biopsy is carried out to determine the cellular composition of the lesion, the presence of infection, or inflammation. Skin biopsy can be performed by several different types of technique, all of which cause minimal amounts of discomfort, scarring, and bleeding. Common biopsy methods are shave biopsy, punch biopsy, and excision biopsy (Figure 23).

Shave Biopsy

This procedure is used when a small, raised growth or lesion is present. The physician places the scalpel parallel to the surface of the growth, and a shallow cut is used to remove some of the superficial tissue layers.

Punch Biopsy

This technique is used when the lesion extends into the middle to lower portion of the dermis. The physician places a circular cutting tool against the desired tissue and rotates with downward pressure to cut and remove a core sample of the skin. The small hole may be closed with a suture or allowed to heal by granulation.

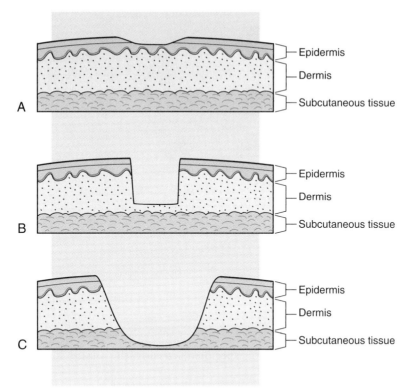

Figure 23. Skin biopsy. The depth of tissue removal for **(A)** shave biopsy, **(B)** punch biopsy, and **(C),** elliptical excision biopsy.

Excision Biopsy

This method is used when the lesion or growth is greater than 4.5 mm in diameter or is thought to extend deeper than the middermis. The solitary lesion is removed in its entirety and the tissue is excised to a depth that includes some subcutaneous fat. The tissue defect is closed with sutures.

REFERENCE VALUES   **Benign; no malignant cells are present. No infectious organisms are present.**

HOW THE TEST IS DONE

After local anesthetic is administered, the skin tissue is removed surgically for histology (determination of cell types) and microbiologic examination. If an inflammatory disease is suspected, a sample of venous blood is also obtained. Both the blood and the tissue sample will be analyzed for the presence of autoantibodies.

SIGNIFICANCE OF TEST RESULTS

Abnormal Values

Malignant melanoma
Seborrheic dermatitis
Basal cell carcinoma
Squamous cell carcinoma
Keratosis
Cyst
Neurofibroma
Bacterial infection
Dermatofibroma
Lupus erythematosus
Discoid lupus
Pemphigus
Fungal infection
Nevus

INTERFERING FACTORS

- Failure to identify the specimen
- Inaccurate identification of the specimen
- Improper preservation of the tissue specimen, causing the tissue specimen to become "dried out"
- Culture specimen was fixed in a preservative, such as formalin

NURSING CARE

Pretest

- After the physician has explained the procedure, the nurse obtains a written consent from the patient and enters it into the patient's record.
- The nurse instructs the patient to remove the necessary clothing to expose the biopsy site. A hospital gown may be worn as needed. Vital signs are taken and the results are recorded. Depending on the site of the lesion, the nurse instructs the patient to sit or lie on the examining table.

During the Test

- The nurse cleanses the skin site with alcohol. The nurse also assists with the application of the surgical drape and the preparation of the local anesthetic.
- Once the tissue sample has been removed by the physician, it is placed in a sterile, covered container with formalin or some other preservative. If a tissue sample is needed for culture, place a small amount of the tissue in a separate sterile container *without a preservative*.
- The nurse closes and labels each container accurately, including the patient's name, the date, and the tissue source. Place the same information on the laboratory requisition form.
- After the bleeding ceases, the nurse places a small sterile dressing over the biopsy site.

Posttest
- After the biopsy is completed, the nurse takes the patient's vital signs and records the results.
- The dressing is assessed for signs of bleeding. It should be clean, dry, and intact.
- ○ *Patient Teaching-Wound Care.* The nurse instructs the patient to change the dressing three to four times a day, washing the skin with soap and water and applying an antibiotic ointment to the wound to keep it moist. The wound will heal best in a moist environment. Cover the biopsy site to keep it protected from trauma or the rubbing of clothes.
- If sutures are in place, the patient will return to the physician for their removal. Facial sutures are removed in 3 to 5 days. For other sites, the time of suture removal is 7 to 14 days.
- The nurse ensures that the specimens are transported to the laboratory promptly. Microbiologic specimens must be sent immediately because they can dry out. The specimens in preservative are sent on a routine basis.

Biopsy, Thyroid

SPECIMEN OR TYPE OF TEST: Pathology

PURPOSE OF THE TEST

A biopsy is performed to differentiate the cause of thyroid nodules or lumps. Thyroid nodules are more common in women and occur at any age. Thyroid cancer is rare; most nodules are benign. The biopsy will identify malignant thyroid nodules, follicular neoplasms, and benign lesions.

BASICS THE NURSE NEEDS TO KNOW

A thyroid biopsy is usually performed by fine needle aspiration (FNA). FNA has replaced surgical removal as a diagnostic technique because it avoids surgical risk and is less traumatic for the patient.

REFERENCE VALUES   No pathology.

HOW THE TEST IS DONE

FNA is usually carried out in the operating room or in the interventional radiology department to maintain sterile technique. It usually requires a local anesthetic only, which permits it to be performed on an outpatient basis. A 23- or 25-gauge biopsy needle is used to aspirate tissue from the nodule. Another method is called the capillary method, in which the needle is inserted into the nodule; with an up-and-down motion, tissue accumulates in the needle until blood is seen in the hub of the needle. The tissue is assessed by cytologic examination.

SIGNIFICANCE OF TEST RESULTS

Benign thyroid nodules
Cancer of the thyroid gland
Follicular neoplasm (cancerous or benign)

INTERFERING FACTORS

- Noncompliance with dietary restrictions
- Failure to place specimen in preservative immediately after aspiration
- Inadequate amount of tissue obtained

NURSING CARE

Pretest
- The nurse assesses the patient's level of anxiety because fear of cancer may be significant or may interfere with the patient's ability to understand explanations.
- ○ *Patient Teaching.* The nurse instructs the patient not to eat or drink for 12 hours before the test.
- Prepare the patient for the operating room according to hospital protocol.
- Ensure that a signed informed consent has been obtained.
- Administer preprocedure medication as prescribed.

During the Test
- The patient is positioned supine with a small pillow under the shoulders.
- A local anesthetic may or may not be given by the physician. General anesthesia may be required in some cases.
- The nurse instructs the patient not to move or swallow as the local anesthetic is given.
- The nurse supports the patient, who will feel pressure as the procedure is performed.
- After the needle is removed, the nurse maintains direct pressure on the site for 10 to 15 minutes.

Posttest
- The nurse reassures the patient that tenderness is expected at the biopsy site.
- Position the patient in a semi-Fowler position with a small pillow under the head to remove stress from the site. The nurse provides an ice pack if it is ordered.
- ○ *Patient Teaching.* Instruct the patient to support the head when changing position to prevent stress on the site.
- ○ *Patient Teaching.* The patient should keep the site clean and dry.
- ◇ Nursing Response to Complications

Complications from a thyroid biopsy are rare. Most patients complain only of some tenderness, but the nurse should observe for possible overt bleeding, hematoma, edema, or infection. If abnormal findings are present, the nurse notifies the physician immediately.

Bleeding. The nurse assesses for indications of bleeding: tachycardia, restlessness, hypotension, and overt bleeding at the site or at the back of the neck. The nurse reports indications of bleeding immediately.

Hematoma. Hematoma at the site of the biopsy may cause swelling, dyspnea, or stridor.

Infection. The nurse assesses site for inflammation (redness, warmth) and the patient's complaint of discomfort or tenderness at the biopsy site. The nurse anticipates an order for a WBC.

Blood Gases, Arterial

Also called: ABGs

SPECIMEN OR TYPE OF TEST: Arterial blood

PURPOSE OF THE TEST

ABG determinations are obtained for a variety of reasons, including the diagnosis of chronic and restrictive pulmonary disease, adult respiratory failure, acid-base disturbances, pulmonary emboli, sleep disorders, central nervous system dysfunctions, and cardiovascular disorders, such as congestive heart failure, shunts, and intracardiac atrial or ventricular shunts, or both.

ABG determinations also are used in the management of patients on mechanical ventilators and during the weaning process from the ventilators.

BASICS THE NURSE NEEDS TO KNOW

ABGs provide valuable information about the acid-base balance, ventilatory ability, and oxygenation status of the individual. The data derived from blood gas determination support clinical assessments and are invaluable in evaluating medical treatment and nursing interventions. ABG determinations provide the pH, partial pressure of carbon dioxide (pCO_2), partial pressure of oxygen (pO_2), bicarbonate (HCO_3), O_2 saturation (SaO_2), and base excess/deficit levels.

The pH (the partial pressure of hydrogen [H^+] ions in the blood) reflects the acid-base balance of the blood. A narrow normal range of pH reflects the body's need to maintain a relatively constant internal environment. An inverse relationship exists on the pH scale between H^+ concentration and pH. As the H^+ ion concentration goes up, the pH goes down. As the H^+ ion concentration increases in solution, H^+ ions can be given up. This is *acidosis*. As the H^+ ion concentration decreases in solution, H^+ ions may be taken on (H^+ ion receiver). This is *alkalosis*.

The pH of human blood is normally 7.35 to 7.45, which on the pH scale of 1 to 14 is above the neutral point of 7 and therefore slightly alkaline. In the clinical setting, however, a pH of 7.35 to 7.45 is used as the neutral state. A pH below 7.35 is acidotic, and a pH above 7.45 is alkalotic. One must remember that other body fluids have a different normal pH.

To maintain a normal pH, the body has evolved several mechanisms, including buffering systems and the respiratory and renal systems. Within seconds, the body buffers respond to changes in pH. Within minutes, the respiratory system adapts to changes in H^+ ion concentration, and in days, the kidneys respond to the acid-base needs of the body. These changes reflect the body's ability to compensate for deviations in the acid-base balance and the need to maintain that balance within a narrow range.

The pCO_2 value reflects the ventilatory ability of the body to maintain a normal pH. Carbon dioxide (CO_2) in blood travels as an acid (carbonic acid) until it dissociates in the lungs to be exhaled as CO_2. If the blood becomes acidotic, the respiratory system increases its rate and depth of ventilation to blow off CO_2 and thus reduce the acid load in the blood. If the blood becomes alkalotic, the respiratory system hypoventilates to retain CO_2 and thus moves the pH toward normal. Pathologic conditions of the pulmonary system may interfere with this normal compensatory action. When an individual cannot adequately ventilate, CO_2 is retained, and acidosis occurs. Because this acidosis results from a pulmonary cause, it is called respiratory acidosis. If the lungs blow off too much CO_2, respiratory alkalosis occurs. Table 5 presents causes of respiratory acid-base imbalances and the nursing assessments for the imbalances.

TABLE 5	Causes and Assessments of Acid-Base Imbalances
Cause	**Clinical Assessment**
Respiratory Acidosis	
Respiratory center dysfunction	Dyspnea
Opiates, anesthetics, sedatives	Tachycardia
Oxygen-induced hypoventilation	Headache
Central nervous system lesions	Confusion
Disorders of the respiratory muscles	Pallor
or chest wall	Diaphoresis
Myasthenia gravis, amyotrophic lateral sclerosis	Apprehension
Kyphoscoliosis	Restlessness
Pickwickian syndrome	Lethargy
Splinting caused by pain	Drowsiness
Disorders of gas exchange	Coma
Chronic obstructive pulmonary disease	Hypertension
Acute pulmonary edema	Papilledema
Asphyxia	
Hypoventilation while on a mechanical ventilator	
Respiratory Alkalosis	
Hyperventilation	Restlessness
Atelectasis	Dizziness
Severe anemia	Agitation
Pulmonary emboli	Tetany
Anxiety	Numbness
Central nervous system disorders	Tingling
Brain stem dysfunction	Muscle cramps
Subarachnoid hemorrhage	Seizures
Salicylate poisoning	Increased deep tendon reflexes
Hypermetabolic states	
Fever	
Thyrotoxicosis	
Sepsis	
Hyperventilation while on mechanical ventilation	
Metabolic Acidosis	
Diabetic ketoacidosis	Lethargy
Lactic acidosis	Nausea
Cardiac arrest	Vomiting
Anaerobic metabolism	Dysrhythmias

TABLE 5 Causes and Assessments of Acid-Base Imbalances—cont'd	
Cause	**Clinical Assessment**
Ingestion of acid	Coma
Salicylates	Hypotension
Ethylene	Hyperventilation
Methanol	
Paraldehyde	
Loss of bicarbonate	
Diarrhea	
Fistulas	
Renal failure	
Metabolic Alkalosis	
Loss of acid	Dullness
Vomiting	Weakness
Excessive gastric suction	Dysrhythmias
Urine loss	Tetany
Diuretics	Hypokalemia
Excessive corticosteroids	Hyperactive reflexes
Exogenous	
Endogenous	
Hypokalemia	
HCO_3 overload	
Excessive ingestion of $NaHCO_3$*	
Massive blood transfusions	
Excessive ingestion of licorice	
Nonparathyroid hypercalcemia	

*$NaHCO_3$, sodium bicarbonate.

    The bicarbonate ion concentration in the blood (HCO_3) reflects the renal system's response to the acid-base balance. HCO_3 is made by the kidneys, and its production is increased whenever acidosis is present. However, it takes several days for the kidneys to respond fully to changes in pH. If the kidneys are unable to make HCO_3 to buffer the acid in the blood, the patient will be in a state of metabolic acidosis. If the patient has too much HCO_3 or has lost acid from the gastrointestinal or genitourinary tract, a state of metabolic alkalosis occurs. Table 5 presents causes of metabolic acid-base imbalances and the nursing assessments for the imbalances.

    The pulmonary and renal systems are constantly balancing and adapting to maintain a normal pH. An abnormality in pH initiates a compensatory mechanism to restore the pH to normal or to achieve at least a partial compensation. For example, a patient with chronic obstructive pulmonary disease retains CO_2 and thus experiences respiratory acidosis. The kidneys respond to the decrease in pH and increase their production of HCO_3. This response results in a normal pH and high pCO_2 and HCO_3 levels (Figure 24). For the process used to assess acid-base balance. A serious clinical problem occurs with mixed acid-base imbalances, in which the patient has

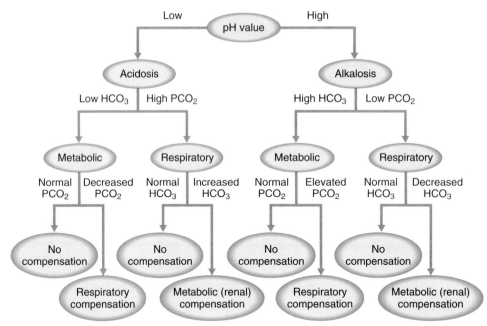

Figure 24. Analysis of arterial blood gas results. (Adapted from Lehmann CA, ed: *Saunders manual of clinical science*, St Louis, 1998, Saunders.)

either respiratory and metabolic acidosis or both respiratory and metabolic alkalosis because compensation cannot take place.

The partial pressure of oxygen in the blood (pO_2) is the amount of O_2 dissolved in the plasma. SaO_2 is the percentage of hemoglobin saturated with O_2. Together, the pO_2 and the SaO_2 form the O_2 *content*, the total amount of O_2 in the blood.

When interpreting the O_2 levels in the blood, barometric pressure must be considered. At sea level, barometric pressure is 760 mm Hg; at 5000 feet above sea level, barometric pressure is 630 mm Hg; thus the norms for pO_2, SaO_2, and O_2 content must be adjusted. Use the normal values of the laboratory doing the testing to interpret oxygen levels.

The base excess or base deficit on the ABG determinations reflects the metabolic nonrespiratory contribution to the maintenance of normal pH. With a base excess, a positive balance greater than 2 correlates with metabolic alkalosis, and with a base deficit, a negative balance less than −2 correlates with metabolic acidosis.

REFERENCE VALUES

pH: 7.35-7.45 *or* SI: 7.35-7.45
PCO_2: 35-45 mm Hg *or* SI: 4.7-5.3 kPa
HCO_3: 21-28 mEq/L *or* SI: 21-28 mmol/L
pO_2: Newborn: 60-70 mm Hg *or* SI: 8.0-10.33 kPa
Adult: 80-100 mm Hg *or* SI: 10.6-13.3 kPa
SaO_2: Newborn: 40%-90% *or* SI fraction saturated 0.40-0.90
Adult: >95% *or* SI fraction saturated >0.95
Base excess/deficit: ±2 mEq/L *or* SI: ±2 mmol/L

▽ **Critical Values**

pH: < 7.26 *or* >7.55
pCO_2: <20 mm Hg *or* >75 mm Hg
HCO_3: <15 mEq *or* >40 mEq
pO_2: <60 mm Hg

HOW THE TEST IS DONE

An arterial blood sample of approximately 0.6 to 1.0 mL is obtained via an arterial puncture or arterial line. The radial or femoral artery is usually used in adults, whereas the temporal artery is used in infants.

Intraarterial blood gas monitoring provides continuous pO_2, pCO_2, and pH levels to be displayed. In addition, derived parameters of O_2 saturation, bicarbonate, base excess, and total CO_2 content are calculated and displayed every 20 to 30 seconds. With continuous intraarterial blood gas monitoring, a sensor is inserted into a radial or femoral artery via an arterial catheter. The tip of the sensor is advanced 1 to 2 inches beyond the tip of the catheter, so it is exposed to nonheparinized arterial blood. This method decreases the number of blood samples needed, thus conserving the patient's blood.

SIGNIFICANCE OF TEST RESULTS

Acid-base imbalances (see Table 5)
Hypercapnia
Hypocapnia
Hypoxia

INTERFERING FACTORS

- Noncompliance with proper collection procedure, including air bubbles in syringe and hemolysis of sample
- Low hemoglobin level
- With continuous intraarterial blood gas monitoring, clot formation at sensor tip, sensor lying against arterial wall, and transition periods, when a change in FiO_2 occurs

NURSING CARE

Nursing actions are similar to those used in other arterial puncture procedures (see Chapter 2), with the following additional measures.

Pretest

- Before a radial artery puncture is executed or a radial arterial line is inserted, perform an Allen test to ensure adequate collateral circulation to the hand. With the Allen test, occlude the radial and ulnar arteries with the fingertips while instructing the patient to tighten the fist (Figure 25). Ask the patient to open the fist and remove pressure from the ulnar artery while maintaining pressure on the radial artery. If color returns to the palm and fingers within 5 seconds, adequate ulnar circulation exists.
- Prepare ice and a heparinized syringe.

Continued

NURSING CARE—cont'd

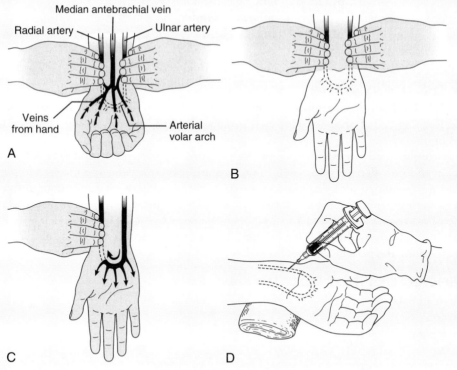

Figure 25. The Allen test.

- The patient's temperature affects results because the ABG machines are calibrated using gases at 37° C. The nurse writes on the requisition slip the patient's temperature at the time the blood is drawn.
- The nurse reassures the anxious patient, since arterial punctures are painful and hyperventilation may occur, giving false readings because CO_2 is blown off.
- Do not obtain an ABG reading for 20 to 30 minutes after a procedure or event that does not reflect the patient's current status (e.g., suctioning).

During the Test

- The procedure is usually performed by a physician or a respiratory therapist, but nurses in specialized units may perform arterial punctures. In critical care units, nurses usually obtain samples from arterial lines. If a femoral puncture is needed, a physician performs the procedure.
- If a radial artery is used, the wrist is hyperextended and the arm is externally rotated.
- Palpate the artery for the point of maximal impulse. Cleanse the site according to hospital policy.
- The needle is inserted at a 45- to 90-degree angle at the point of maximal pulsation.
- Observe the syringe; the plunger will move upward under arterial pressure.
- Withdraw the needle and cap the syringe with the airtight rubber stopper.
- Roll the syringe between your palms.

- Label the syringe and place it on ice.
- Send the specimen to the laboratory immediately with a requisition slip marked with the patient's temperature, the FiO_2 value, and the time.
- Care of the continuous intraarterial blood gas line is similar to care of any arterial line.

Posttest

- Immediately after the needle is withdrawn, exert pressure on the arterial site for a minimum of 5 minutes or according to hospital protocol. If the patient is taking anticoagulants, pressure on the site should be maintained for at least 10 minutes.

◆ **Nursing Response to Complications**

Complications from ABG determination result from the trauma of arterial puncture. They include arterial occlusion from hematoma formation or thrombosis, bleeding, and infection.

Arterial occlusion. The nurse needs to check sites distal to arterial puncture for pulse, skin color, and temperature. If distal site is cold, pale, or if patient reports numbness, report findings immediately to the physician.

Bleeding. Bleeding may be overt or a hematoma may occur at the site of the arterial puncture. Keep site visible, except if using the femoral artery. Check site frequently. Palpate around site for hematoma formation. A hematoma may press on the artery, so assess for arterial occlusion. If bleeding occurs, apply pressure; notify the physician immediately if bleeding does not stop or significant blood has been lost. If a hematoma is causing a decrease in perfusion to distal parts, notify the physician immediately.

Infection. The nurse assesses the site for inflammation (redness, warmth) and patient complaint of discomfort or pain at the arterial site.

Blood Gases, Mixed Venous

SPECIMEN OR TYPE OF TEST: Venous blood

PURPOSE OF THE TEST

Mixed venous blood gases are obtained to assess the O_2 supply and tissue O_2 consumption. Changes in SvO_2 (venous oxygen saturation) indicate a need to determine which factor in O_2 supply and delivery is abnormal: cardiac output, hemoglobin level, tissue O_2 consumption, or SaO_2 (arterial oxygen saturation).

BASICS THE NURSE NEEDS TO KNOW

Mixed venous blood gases provide a method for evaluating the dynamic balance between O_2 supply and O_2 consumption of the body. Because the organs of the body use various amounts of O_2, mixed venous blood gases measure the blood in the pulmonary artery, which contains the venous return from all the body systems. Arterial blood gases (ABGs) reflect what is available for body use (supply), whereas venous blood gases tell how well the body uses this supply.

With ABGs, the nurse can assess the oxygen supply available to the body tissues and determine oxygen delivery (see Blood Gases, Arterial on p. 139). With mixed venous oxygen saturation (SvO_2), the nurse can assess oxygen consumption and whether the person has adequate venous reserves of oxygen.

Venous reserve is that amount of oxygen in the blood that returns to the right side of the heart after systemic circulation. If oxygen demand is greater than oxygen supply, the amount of oxygen in the returning blood decreases. This is assessed by a low SvO_2.

Mixed venous blood gases may be obtained periodically, or the mixed venous oxygen saturation (SvO_2) may be monitored continuously.

SvO_2 monitoring has been made possible by the development of fiberoptic pulmonary catheters. It is measured by light emitted from the catheter and reflected onto red blood cells within the pulmonary artery. The wavelength of reflected light is interpreted by the SvO_2 computer and continuous readings of the SvO_2 in the blood after systemic circulation is provided. Because the hemoglobin normally unloads about 25% of its O_2 during systemic circulation, the normal SvO_2 is 75%, with a range of 60% to 80%.

Continuous SvO_2 monitoring is used to evaluate the response to nursing care. For an unstable patient, changes in position, bathing, suctioning, and so forth can increase O_2 consumption, resulting in a corresponding lowering of the SvO_2.

REFERENCE VALUES

pH: 7.33-7.43 *or* SI: 7.33-7.43
pCO_2: 41-51 mm Hg *or* SI: 5.3-6.0 kPa
HCO_3^-: 24-28 mm Hg *or* SI: 24-28 mmol/L
pvO_2: 35-49 mm Hg
SvO_2: 60%-80%

▽ Critical Values

No specific value for SvO_2 is correlated with anaerobic metabolism. A pvO_2 of 28 mm Hg does correlate with lactic acidosis; however, and this pvO_2 corresponds to a SvO_2 of 53%, which seems to be a critical value.

HOW THE TEST IS DONE

A mixed venous sample may be obtained in a heparinized syringe from the distal port of the pulmonary artery catheter, or continuous SvO_2 may be assessed from a fiberoptic pulmonary artery catheter attached to an oximeter.

SIGNIFICANCE OF TEST RESULTS

Elevated Values (SvO_2 greater than 80%)
Anesthesia
Cyanide toxicity
High fractional concentration of oxygen in inspired gas (FiO_2)
Hypothermia
Left-to-right shunt
Neuromuscular blockade
Relaxation
Sepsis, early stages
Sleep
Vasodilation

Decreased Values (SvO$_2$ less than 60%)

Anemia
Anxiety
Bleeding
Cardiogenic shock
Congestive heart failure
Fever
Hyperthermia
Hypovolemia
Inadequate FiO$_2$
Large burns
Pain
Pulmonary disease
Multiple traumas
Position changes
Seizures
Severe pain
Shivering
Stress
Strenuous exercise
Suctioning

INTERFERING FACTORS

- Inadequate perfusion
- Poorly positioned pulmonary artery catheter

NURSING CARE

Care is based on the technique used. With a random mixed venous blood gas determination, use the procedures that follow:

Pretest
- Explain the procedure to the patient.
- Check the hemodynamic monitoring system. Ensure proper position of the catheter.
- Gather the following equipment: a heparinized syringe, two 10-mL syringes, a syringe cap, and ice.

During the Test
- Wear gloves.
- Attach an empty 10-mL syringe to the sampling stopcock at the distal port of the pulmonary artery catheter.
- Turn the stopcock to close off the flow of the infusion solution.
- Aspirate 5 mL into the syringe to clear the distal line of blood mixed with infusion solution. Turn the stopcock to close off both the infusion line and the portal accessed for blood sampling.

Continued

| NURSING CARE—cont'd

- Remove the syringe and discard. In special situations, such as in neonates, the blood is saved and returned to the patient after the sample is drawn. Check hospital protocol.
- Attach the 3-mL heparinized syringe to the stopcock.
- Open the stopcock to the syringe and aspirate the blood slowly.
- Close the stopcock, remove the 3-mL syringe, and expel any air bubbles. Cap the syringe.
- Gently roll the syringe in your hand. Place on ice.
- Attach a 10-mL syringe to the stopcock. Open the stopcock to the solution and flush to clear the stopcock of blood.
- Turn solution off to the stopcock port used to obtain the sample and cap the sampling port.
- Flush the line and ensure the patency of the distal port. Check the monitor for pulmonary artery waveform.
- Obtain and send an ABG sample, if ordered.

Posttest

- Send blood to the laboratory immediately; clearly indicate on the slip that the blood is a mixed venous sample.
- Compare ABG and mixed venous blood gas samples.

▽ **Nursing Response to Critical Values**

If the SvO_2 falls to less than 60% or varies by 10% from the patient's baseline for longer than 3 minutes (10 minutes after suctioning), a full assessment of the patient is needed, including a cardiac output determination.

Blood Urea Nitrogen

See Urea Nitrogen, Blood on p. 604.

Bone Mineral Density

See Dual Energy X-Ray Absorptiometry on p. 264

Bone Scan

Also called: Bone Scintigraphy

SPECIMEN OR TYPE OF TEST: Nuclear scan

PURPOSE OF THE TEST

The bone scan is used to detect the presence and extent of metastatic disease of the bones. In addition, it is used to monitor degenerative bone diseases, detect osteomyelitis, determine bone viability, identify bone biopsy sites, and evaluate difficult fractures or fractures in battered children.

BASICS THE NURSE NEEDS TO KNOW

Radionuclide bone studies produce sensitive, high-resolution images of the skeleton and joints. Because of the effectiveness of bone-seeking radiopharmaceuticals, the bone scan is sensitive to changes in bone. The bone scan procedure uses the physiology of bone turnover to ensure uptake of the radiopharmaceutical into the bone where it can be detected by the scintillation camera or scanner.

Bone Imaging

The normal scan demonstrates symmetrical activity throughout the skeleton. In children, greater uptake occurs in the growth regions of the epiphyses, cranial sutures, and joints of the pelvic bones. The abnormal scan presents "hot" or "cold" spots and an asymmetrical uptake of the radiopharmaceutical. A *hot spot* is an area of increased uptake of the radiopharmaceutical that indicates increased blood flow or increased osteogenic activity (Figure 26). The cause of increased activity can be a primary or metastatic malignancy, Paget's disease, infection, healing activity in the repair of a fracture, or other conditions. A *cold spot* indicates decreased uptake because of an absence of osteogenic activity or destruction of an area of the bone. Causes of

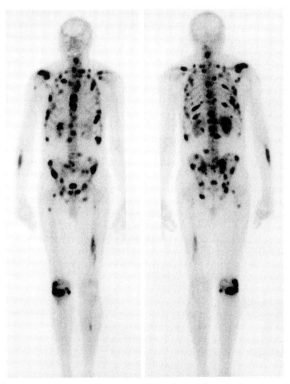

Figure 26. Bone scan of metastatic prostate cancer. Anterior and posterior views of the whole body show many metastatic deposits in the bones. The metastatic deposits are seen as dark areas, or "hot spots" of increased activity. (From Mettler FA, Guiberteau MJ: *Essentials of nuclear medicine imaging*, ed 5, Philadelphia, 2006, Saunders.)

decreased or absent activity include a lack of blood supply (infarction) to the bony area or destruction of bone tissue by such conditions as multiple myeloma, metastatic cancer, an inflammatory mass, or irradiation.

Joint Imaging

Because joints can be imaged, the bone scan can evaluate inflammatory joint disease. The radionuclide collects in tissues with increased blood flow, such as in the increased vascularity of synovitis or degenerative arthritis. Often, early joint inflammation is detected by radionuclide scan before it can be seen on x-ray film.

REFERENCE VALUES	Symmetry of uptake of the radionuclide, with no bone abnormalities noted

HOW THE TEST IS DONE

An intravenous injection of a technetium radiopharmaceutical is followed 1 to 4 hours later by scanning with a gamma camera. The time variable depends on the type of radiopharmaceutical used. Scans are done of anterior and posterior views. The images can be seen on the monitor and photographed for further study.

SIGNIFICANCE OF TEST RESULTS

Abnormal Values

Primary malignant bone tumor
Metastatic tumors
Osteomyelitis
Paget's disease
Fractures
Arthritis
Loose prosthesis
Soft tissue activity
Aseptic necrosis
Postradiation therapy

INTERFERING FACTORS

- Metallic objects
- Full or enlarged bladder
- Pregnancy

NURSING CARE

Pretest

- The procedure requires a signed consent from the patient that is entered into the patient's record. Ensure that the patient is not pregnant because the radioactivity presents a potential danger to the fetus.

○ *Patient Teaching.* Teach the patient that the radiopharmaceutical is a radioactive substance, but it is of low dosage and has a short half-life. After the test, it will be excreted rapidly in the urine so that radiation exposure is minimal. Also instruct the patient to remove all clothing and jewelry and put on a hospital gown. The bladder must be emptied before the start of the procedure because retained urine will contain the radiopharmaceutical and prevent a clear view of the pelvis.

During the Test

- In the radiology department, the radiopharmaceutical is injected intravenously, usually in an arm vein. After the injection but before the scanning process begins, the patient will be asked to drink several glasses of water. These extra fluids will help the patient void at the end of the procedure.

Posttest

- When disposing of the patient's urine, the nurse should wear gloves and wash his or her hands afterward. The radionuclide is excreted over 1 to 2 days, although the radioactivity level is minimal after a few hours. The urine can be disposed of in the toilet.

○ *Patient Teaching.* Instruct the patient to wash his or her hands after voiding. Reassure the patient that the amount of radioactivity in the urine is minimal, but it will remain on the hands unless they are washed.

Brain Natriuretic Peptide

Also called: BNP, B-type Natriuretic Peptide

SPECIMEN OR TYPE OF TEST: Plasma

PURPOSE OF THE TEST

BNP levels are most frequently used to assess for heart failure. It may be used as a biomarker for prognosis. The higher the BNP, the poorer the outcome for patients with congestive heart failure.

BASICS THE NURSE NEEDS TO KNOW

BNP is a neurohumoral hormone produced primarily by the myocardial myocytes in the ventricles of the heart and to a lesser degree within the atria. BNP is secreted in response to ventricular stretching and increasing ventricular pressures. BNP causes a decrease in sodium retention by the kidneys, an increase in diuresis by improving glomerular filtration, and a decrease in renin and aldosterone secretion.

Similar to BNP is *atrial natriuretic hormone* (ANH). ANH is secreted by the atria in response to increased cardiac filling pressures. It may also be used to monitor heart failure. Like BNP, ANH causes sodium and therefore fluid excretion by inhibiting aldosterone and renin secretion.

REFERENCE VALUES*	BNP <80 pg/mL or SI <80 ng/L

▽ Critical Values

Because values vary widely among laboratories, specific critical values will also vary. However, a value greater than 100 pg/mL or SI: 100 ng/L is highly suggestive of congestive heart failure, except for patients with kidney failure.

*Values vary among laboratories.

HOW THE TEST IS DONE
A venipuncture is done and the sample placed on ice and sent to the laboratory immediately.

SIGNIFICANCE OF TEST RESULTS
Increased Values
Acute myocardial infarction
Advanced liver disease
Congestive heart failure
Diastolic dysfunction
Excessive cortisol levels
Kidney failure
Hypervolemic states (e.g., renal failure)
Left ventricular hypertrophy
Pulmonary hypertension

Decreased Values
Medications: ACE inhibitors, beta-blockers, diuretics
Obesity

INTERFERING FACTORS
- Kidney failure/dialysis
- Medications: cardiac glycoside, diuretics
- Not placing the sample on ice

NURSING CARE

Pretest
○ *Patient Teaching.* Instruct patient to fast except for water for 8 to 12 hours before blood is drawn. Check that the patient is not receiving nesiritide (Natrecor), which is an exogenous BNP.
▽ Nursing Response to Critical Values
Assess for indications of acute pulmonary edema and notify physician immediately of test result and clinical findings.

Bronchial Provocation Test

See Pulmonary Function Studies on p. 528.

Bronchoalveolar Lavage

See Bronchoscopy on p. 153.

Bronchoscopy

SPECIMEN OR TYPE OF TEST: Endoscopy

PURPOSE OF THE TEST

Bronchoscopy may be performed for therapeutic or diagnostic purposes. Bronchoscopy is used diagnostically to visualize possible tumors, obstructions, secretions, bleeding sites, or foreign objects in the tracheobronchial system. It permits the collection of secretions for cytologic and bacteriologic study, as well as for assessing tumors for potential resection. Tissue for lung biopsy may be obtained through the bronchoscope.

Bronchoscopy is used therapeutically to remove foreign objects from the tracheobronchial tree and to remove secretions that are obstructing the air passages. A bronchoscope may be used to fulgurate (electrodesiccate) and excise lesions.

BASICS THE NURSE NEEDS TO KNOW

Bronchoscopy is an endoscopic diagnostic procedure involving the inspection and observation of the trachea, larynx, and bronchi. Bronchoscopy is ordered when patients have unexplained pulmonary signs and symptoms or when nonspecific radiographic abnormalities exist.

A bronchoscope permits direct visualization of the tracheobronchial tree down to the subsegmental bronchi. Newer developments in bronchoscopy include ultrathin bronchoscopes and *virtual bronchoscopic navigation* (VBN). VBN permits the advancement of the scope beyond what is visible through the scope by creating digital images. VBN images are created using software attached to a CT system, endobronchial ultrasonography, or even fluoroscopy. These images are used to guide the placement of the scope into the peripheral bronchi and obtain tumor samples for cytology.

A biopsy of lung tissue may be performed via the bronchoscope (*transbronchial lung biopsy*). A transcatheter bronchial brushing may also be carried out to obtain a biopsy. A small brush is inserted through the bronchoscope, which is moved back and forth until cells adhere to the brush. Once the brush is removed, the cells are brushed onto slides. Most bronchoscopies are performed with a fiberoptic bronchoscope, which is flexible. To remove foreign objects lodged in the larger airways, a rigid bronchoscope is usually used.

Bronchoalveolar lavage (BAL) is an additional technique, which can be performed with a fiberoptic bronchoscope. It is used to diagnose and manage interstitial lung disease. It is also used in the diagnosis of lung cancer and pulmonary infections.

REFERENCE VALUES   No abnormalities visualized.
No growth in culture specimen.

HOW THE TEST IS DONE

A rigid (metal) or flexible fiberoptic bronchoscope (FFB) may be used. The rigid bronchoscope uses a hollow metallic tube with a light at its distal end. It is useful in removing secretions, in evaluating future surgical interventions, and in dilating endobronchial strictures. The rigid bronchoscope has almost been replaced by the FFB. However, the physician may prefer the metal scope under certain circumstances, such as in the case of endobronchial tumor resection, massive hemorrhage, foreign body removal, and treatment of small children.

The bronchoscope is inserted through the nose or mouth. The tube is inserted as the physician observes the condition of the upper airways through the eyepiece and guides the tube to the area of the lung to be evaluated (Figure 27).

If BAL is desired, the tip of the fiberoptic catheter is inserted until it wedges in the respiratory tract. Several boluses of 20 mL of normal saline at body temperature are injected distal to the wedge

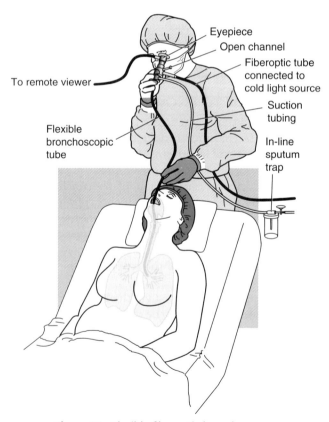

Figure 27. Flexible fiberoptic bronchoscopy.

catheter. After each bolus, the BAL fluid is aspirated. Usually, approximately 50% of the fluid is aspirated. Total bolus fluid should not exceed 300 mL or 3 mL/kg of patient's body weight.

SIGNIFICANCE OF TEST RESULTS

Atelectasis
Bleeding
Bronchial adenomas
Diffuse alveolar damage
Fibrosis
Foreign objects
Infection
Lung cancer
Sarcoidosis
Secretions
Tuberculosis
Tumors

INTERFERING FACTORS

- Patient distress (may require general anesthesia)
- Patient who is hemodynamically unstable or with poor oxygenation
- For BAL: Less than 25 mL specimen volume

NURSING CARE

Pretest
- The nurse ensures that a signed consent form has been obtained.
- Follow hospital policy regarding use of two patient identifiers.
- The nurse assesses for and reports indications of hypoxia or history of asthma or chronic obstructive pulmonary disease
- Obtain a medication history to determine whether the patient is receiving anticoagulant therapy or aspirin preparations. If a prothrombin time (PT), a partial thromboplastin time (PTT), and a platelet count were ordered, the nurse checks the results and reports any bleeding problems to the physician.
- ○ *Patient Teaching.* The nurse instructs the patient not to eat or drink for 6 to 8 hours before the test and explains the purpose of and procedure for the test. Explain the need to maintain NPO status until the gag reflex returns.
- ○ *Patient Teaching.* Warn the patient that the local anesthetic may taste bitter.
- ○ *Patient Teaching.* Inform the patient that as the tube is inserted, it may feel like something is caught in the throat; provide reassurance that the airway is not blocked.
- The nurse evaluates and records baseline vital signs. The nurse administers atropine if prescribed to reduce tracheobronchial secretions and inhibit vagal stimulation. Choice of sedation during the procedure varies based on the preference of the person doing the procedure and hospital policies. Common medications used are the benzodiazepines, opioids, propofol, and fos propofol. Some practitioners do not order any medication to prevent the complications associated with them.
- Have a code cart and suctioning available.

Continued

NURSING CARE—cont'd

During the Test

- The patient is positioned in the semi-Fowler or Fowler position and the pulse oximeter is attached to the patient. The physician sprays a local anesthetic onto the pharynx, and the solution is dropped onto the vocal cords, epiglottis, and trachea to abolish the gag reflex.
- The nurse provides the patient with continuous emotional support during the procedure.
- ○ *Patient Teaching.* Instruct patient about the need for and rationale for the intravenous infusion, pulse oximetry, and electrocardiac monitoring.
- Ensure suctioning equipment is available.
- Encourage the patient to breathe through the nose or to pant.
- The nurse maintains supplemental O_2 for nonintubated patients and continuously monitors the patient's response, electrocardiogram, vital signs, and SaO_2.
- Nurse reports any indication of hypoxia, hypercapnia, or bradycardia.
- Nurse observes for vasovagal response and has atropine on hand, if needed.
- In the elderly, the nurse assesses for indication of dehydration due to the patient being NPO.
- The nurse ensures that the staff wears gowns, gloves, masks or a visor.
- If tuberculosis is a concern, the staff should wear N95 masks.

Posttest

- The nurse continues to assess the patient's vital signs.
- Food and fluids are withheld until the gag reflex returns. The nurse reassures the patient that hoarseness, sore throat, and blood-streaked sputum are common. Provide throat lozenges or throat sprays as comfort measures. The nurse instructs the patient to expectorate rather than swallow saliva, because it may contain the local anesthetic.
- If a biopsy or bronchoalveolar lavage has been performed, the nurse sends the specimen to the histology laboratory and the microbiology laboratory.
- If done as an out-patient procedure, be certain the patient has transportation home and arrange for a follow-up appointment.

◆ **Nursing Response to Complications**

Complications are rare but include bleeding, drug reactions, hypotension, laryngospasm, bronchospasm, hypoxia, dysrhythmia, pneumothorax, and cardiopulmonary arrest.

Bleeding. Bleeding after a bronchoscopy may vary from slight pink-tinged sputum to frank bleeding. The bleeding may also be overt or covert. The nurse assesses vital signs for tachycardia, tachypnea, and hypotension. The nurse observes for restlessness and hemoptysis. Because bleeding may occur into the pleural cavity, the nurse checks for tension pneumothorax. The nurse reports evidence of bleeding to the physician. If a tension pneumothorax is suspected, anticipate the physician need for chest tube(s) and a thoracotomy tray.

Hypoxia. A patient presenting with hypoxia after a bronchoscopy may complain of dyspnea, appear short of breath, will be restless or confused, and his or her skin will be pale or cyanotic. If pulse oximetry is available, a low SaO_2 will be noted. If the patient is on a cardiac monitor, assess for dysrhythmias associated with hypoxia. Notify the physician and anticipate an order for oxygen therapy. Hypoxia may also occur during the procedure. The goal is to maintain oxygen saturation above 90%. If this is not possible, the procedure may need to be cancelled.

Bronchospasm. The nurse assesses for bronchospasm by listening for breath sounds and checking for indications of hypoxia. If wheezing is heard, notify the physician. Anticipate need for respiratory therapy.

Laryngospasm. If there was difficulty in inserting the bronchoscope, the trachea may have been traumatized. If the trachea swells, there may be partial occlusion of the trachea or it may go into spasms. Partial occlusion of the upper airway will cause a high-pitched sound on inspiration, which is called stridor. The nurse notifies the physician because this may interfere with the patient's oxygenation.

Pneumothorax. Nursing assessment consistent with a pneumothorax is dependent on its size. The nurse listens for decreased or absent breath sounds and observes for indications of hypoxia. Patients may complain of tightness of the chest. If a tension pneumothorax has occurred, there will be a mediastinal shift to the unaffected side. The nurse will note the trachea shifting to the unaffected side. Depending on the size of the tension pneumothorax, a thoracotomy may be needed. Anticipate the physician need for chest tube(s) and thoracotomy tray. Some institutions have a policy of having a radiogragh taken 1 hour after the procedure to exclude the presence of a pneumothorax.

Dysrhythmias. During the procedure the nurse observes the cardiac monitor for dysrhythmias. Atrial and/or ventricular dysrhythmias may occur. A code cart with emergency medications should be available.

Calcitonin

Also called: (CT); Thyrocalcitonin

SPECIMEN OR TYPE OF TEST: Serum

PURPOSE OF THE TEST

A calcitonin determination is usually performed to diagnose medullary carcinoma of the thyroid gland.

BASICS THE NURSE NEEDS TO KNOW

Calcitonin is a hormone produced and secreted by the parafollicular cells (C cells) of the thyroid gland. It may also be produced and secreted by ectopic sites such as the lungs, intestines, pituitary gland, and bladder. The action of calcitonin is to inhibit bone reabsorption, inhibit calcium absorption in the gastrointestinal tract, and increase calcium and phosphate excretion from the kidneys. It is believed that calcitonin is not secreted until plasma calcium levels reach 9.3 ng/dL.

To assess familial medullary cancer in relatives of patients with the cancer, a provocation test (also called a stimulation test) may be performed. Calcium chloride is given intravenously over 10 minutes, or pentagastrin is given intravenously over 5 to 10 minutes. Patients with medullary cancer will respond to these stimulants with excessive secretion of calcitonin.

C

REFERENCE VALUES*

Infant (cord blood): 25-150 pg/mL *or* SI: 25-150 ng/L
Infant (7 days old): 77-293 pg/mL *or* SI: 77-293 ng/L
Adult: <150 pg/mL *or* SI: <150 ng/L

Calcitonin stimulation test
Male: <190 pg/mL *or* SI: <190 ng/L
Female: <130 pg/mL *or* SI: <130 ng/L

*Reference values vary among laboratories

HOW THE TEST IS DONE

A venipuncture is performed. Calcitonin is measured using radioimmunoassay (RIA).

SIGNIFICANCE OF TEST RESULTS

Elevated Values

Cancer of the thyroid
Chronic renal failure
Ectopic secretion by malignant tumors
Endocrine tumors of the pancreas
Pernicious anemia
Subacute Hashimoto's thyroiditis
Parathyroid adenoma or hyperplasia
Pregnancy

INTERFERING FACTORS

• Noncompliance with fasting requirement

NURSING CARE

Nursing actions are similar to those used in other venipuncture procedures (see Chapter 2), with the following additional measures.

Pretest

• Schedule isotope scans or other exposure to radioactivity after blood is drawn for this test.

◉ *Patient Teaching.* The nurse instructs the patient not to eat or drink anything except for sips of water for 8 hours before the blood is drawn.

Posttest

• Inform the laboratory personnel that a calcitonin level is being obtained, because the blood sample must be separated immediately. The blood sample must be sent to the laboratory on ice immediately after it is drawn.

• The patient may resume a normal diet.

Calcium, Total and Ionized, Serum

Also called: Total calcium (CA); Ionized calcium (Ca1)

SPECIMEN OR TYPE OF TEST: Blood

C

PURPOSE OF THE TEST

The total serum calcium or ionized (free) calcium levels are used to assist in the diagnosis of acid-base imbalance, coagulation disorders, pathologic bone disorders, endocrine disorders, cardiac arrhythmia, and muscle disorders.

BASICS THE NURSE NEEDS TO KNOW

Calcium is one of the essential mineral elements of the body and is needed for bone structure and for the process of bone formation. Almost all of it is concentrated in bone, with the remainder of the body's calcium present in the cells or extracellular fluids, including the serum. Most of the serum calcium is either physiologically active in a free or ionized state or it is bonded to albumin and other plasma proteins. In the serum and other extracellular fluids, the normal level of ionized calcium is maintained in homeostatic balance by the actions of the small intestine, bones, and kidneys.

Serum calcium is needed for many physiologic functions, including coagulation of the blood, excitation of cardiac and skeletal muscle, maintenance of muscle tone, conduction of neuromuscular impulses, and synthesis and regulation of the endocrine and exocrine glands. On the cellular level, calcium preserves the integrity and permeability of the cell membrane, particularly for sodium and potassium exchange.

Elevated Values

An elevated level of calcium in the blood is called *hypercalcemia*. It causes neuromuscular hypoactivity and alters the function of most body organs. Hypercalcemia can be a life-threatening complication. Hyperparathyroidism and malignancy are the most common causes of hypercalcemia.

Decreased Values

A decreased level of calcium in the serum is called *hypocalcemia*. It causes neuromuscular hyperactivity, affecting many organs and functions. Very low calcium levels also can be life threatening. Total serum calcium is lowered in conditions that decrease plasma proteins, impair intestinal absorption, alter renal filtration and resorption functions, or decrease the amount of parathyroid hormone.

REFERENCE VALUES

Total Calcium
Premature: 6.2-11.2 mg/dL *or* SI: 1.55-2.75 mmol/L
Infant (0-10 days): 7.6-10.4 mg/dL *or* SI: 1.90-2.60 mmol/L
(10 days to 24 months): 9.0-11.0 mg/dL *or* SI: 2.25-2.75 mmol/L
Child (24 mo-12 yr): 8.8-10.8 mg/dL *or* SI: 2.20-2.70 mmol/L
(12 - 18 yr): 8.4-10.2 mg/dL *or* SI: 2.10-2.55 mmol/L
Adult (18-60 yr): 8.6-10.0 mg/dL *or* SI: 2.15-2.50 mmol/L
(60-90 yr): 8.8-10.2 mg/dL *or* SI: 2.20-2.55 mmol/L

Continued

Ionized (Free) Calcium
Whole blood Adult (18-60 yr): 4.6-5.08 mg/dL *or*
    SI: 1.15-1.27 mmol/L
(60-90 yr): 4.64-5.16 mg/dL *or* SI: 1.12-1.32 mmol/L
Serum neonate, 24 hr: 4.40-5.44 mg/dL *or* SI: 1.10-1.36 mmol/L
Youth: 4.80-5.52 mg/dL *or* SI: 1.20-1.38 mmol/L
Adult: 4.64 mg/dL *or* SI: 1.16-1.32 mmol/L
Urine neonate, 24 hr: 4.20-5.48 mg/dL *or* SI: 1.05-1.37 mmol/L

▽ **Critical Values**

Total: <6.0 mg/dL (SI: 1.50 mmol/L) *or* >13 mg/dL
    (SI: >3.25 mmol/L)
Ionized (free): 3.2 mg/dL (SI: <0.80 mmol/L) *or* >6.0 mg/dL
    (SI: >1.5 mmol/L

HOW THE TEST IS DONE

Adult: Venipuncture is performed to collect venous blood.
Infant: A capillary pipette is used to collect capillary blood via the heelstick method.

SIGNIFICANCE OF TEST RESULTS

Elevated Values

Hyperparathyroidism
Metastatic cancer
Multiple myeloma
Vitamin D intoxication
Milk-alkali syndrome
Overuse of calcium antacids
Paget's disease
Idiopathic hypercalcemia of infancy
Polycythemia vera
Pheochromocytoma
Sarcoidosis
Adrenal insufficiency
Thyrotoxicosis
Bacteremia
Dehydration

Decreased Values

Hypoparathyroidism
Vitamin D deficiency
Alcoholism
Chronic renal failure
Hypoalbuminemia

Massive blood transfusions
Prolonged intravenous fluid therapy
Acute pancreatitis
Anterior pituitary hypofunction
Renal tubular disease
Cirrhosis of the liver
Malnutrition
Neonatal prematurity

INTERFERING FACTORS

- Upright position or prolonged activity before the test
- Prolonged storage of the blood specimen

NURSING CARE

Nursing actions are similar to those used in other capillary puncture or venipuncture procedures (see Chapter 2), with the following additional measures.

Pretest

○ *Patient Teaching.* Instruct the patient to fast from food and fluids for 8 hours.

- Some medications (e.g., thiazides and other diuretics, lithium, calcium salts) cause a rise in serum value and should be withheld during the period in which the patient fasts.
- Arrange to have the blood drawn in the morning. This is because the calcium level normally fluctuates in a diurnal rhythm, with the lowest serum calcium levels in the very early morning (2 to 4 AM) and the highest values in the early evening (8 PM).

Posttest

- Arrange for prompt transport of the specimen to the laboratory. The analysis must be performed on a fresh sample to prevent a false elevation of the calcium value.

▽ **Nursing Response to Critical Values**

The nurse must notify the physician of any test result in the abnormal, critical value range. The nurse should also take the patient's vital signs and assess for specific manifestations that occur with calcium imbalance.

Hypocalcemia. The very low serum calcium can induce depression or psychosis, laryngeal stridor, tetany, convulsions, hypotension, and a weak, thready pulse. The patient will have hyperactive reflexes and positive Trousseau's and Chvostek's signs (Table 6). A severe decrease to 6 mg/dL (SI: 1.5 mmol/L) or less can be life threatening.

Hypercalcemia. The very high serum calcium level can induce polyuria, anorexia, nausea, tachycardia in an early stage or bradycardia in a later stage, muscle weakness, lethargy, and absent deep tendon reflexes. A severe elevation of 14 mg/dL (SI: 3.5 mmol/L) or more is likely to induce coma and can cause death from a cardiac arrest.

TABLE 6	Nursing Assessment for Hypocalcemia	
Test	**Method**	**Positive result**
Trousseau's sign	Apply a blood pressure cuff to the arm. Inflate the cuff to 10 mm above the patient's systolic pressure for 3 minutes. Observe the hand. Then deflate the cuff.	When the serum calcium level is low, the patient's hand will develop a carpal spasm. The first three fingers extend rigidly. The fourth and fifth fingers flex and curl toward the palm of the hand.
Chvostek's sign	Use the tip of the index or middle finger to tap just beneath the cheekbone (zygoma) and towards the ear.	When the serum calcium level is low, the same side of the face will demonstrate repeated tics or involuntary spasms of the facial muscles.

Calculus Analysis

Also called: Kidney Stone Analysis; Renal Calculus Analysis

SPECIMEN OR TYPE OF TEST: Kidney stone

PURPOSE OF THE TEST

The analysis of urinary calculi is used in the workup for nephrolithiasis. It determines the chemical composition of the stone and the metabolic factors that result in stone formation.

BASICS THE NURSE NEEDS TO KNOW

A renal *calculus* is commonly called a stone. It forms in the renal pelvis; descends through the ureter, bladder, and urethra; and exits from the body in urine. Calculi are of various sizes, textures, colors, and chemical compositions. Common chemical compositions are: calcium, struvite, uric acid, and cystine. The composition of the stone will affect treatment to prevent reoccurrence.

Calcium stones are the most common type of renal calculi. These calculi are caused by excess calcium in the urine and consist of calcium phosphate, calcium oxalate, or a combination of the two chemical salts. These dark-colored stones are usually hard and have a rough surface. The underlying causes of calcium stone formation are thought to be increased intestinal absorption of dietary calcium, poor renal tubular resorption of calcium, a loss of calcium from bone, or any combination of these factors. The pH of the urine is often >6.0.

Struvite stones are sometimes called infection stones because of their association with chronic urinary tract infection. It is not known whether the stone causes the infection to occur or the infection causes the stone to form. These pale stones are usually large and soft. They are also called a staghorn calculus because of their characteristic shape. The chemical composition of struvite stones is magnesium ammonium phosphate and carbonate apatite. Struvite stones are sometimes called phosphate stones based on their chemical composition. The pH of the urine is often >6.0.

Uric acid stones consist of uric acid and urate crystals. They are yellow-brown and moderately hard. They form in the presence of excess uric acid and concentrated acidic urine. Underlying causes include high intake of food that is high in purine, primary gout, dehydration, and some medications, including thiazide diuretics and salicylates. The pH of the urine is acidic.

Cystine stones occur rarely. They are dark yellow-brown and greasy. Their formation is caused by an autosomal recessive inborn error in metabolism that impairs the absorption of amino acids. Because of this deficit in metabolism, cystine and other amino acids are excreted in urine. The precipitate forms both crystals and stones.

C

REFERENCE VALUES   **No kidney stones are present in the urine.**

HOW THE TEST IS DONE

All urine is strained through a gauze strainer or a fine mesh sieve. Any stones that are recovered are placed in a glass bottle or plastic container, and are sent to the laboratory for qualitative analysis.

SIGNIFICANCE OF TEST RESULTS

Abnormal Values
Urolithiasis
Hypercalciuria
Hyperparathyroidism
Gout
Primary cystinuria
Dehydration
Urinary tract infection
Other infection

NURSING CARE

Pretest
○ *Patient Teaching.* The nurse teaches the patient to use a clean container to collect the urine every time he or she voids. The first voided specimen of the morning is particularly important because the stone may pass during the night.
- Each collected specimen is then poured through a strainer or sieve. The gauze or mesh is examined to see if a stone is present. Teach the patient to look carefully because the stone can be extremely small. When a stone is recovered, it is washed of blood and tissue and placed in a clean, lidded container.

○ *Patient Teaching.* The nurse instructs the patient not to wrap or place the stone on adhesive tape to secure it. The adhesive interferes with the x-ray crystallography that is used to analyze the stone.

Posttest
- The nurse sends the stone to the laboratory in the labeled container. If the stone is enmeshed in the gauze, place both the stone and the gauze in the container.
- Specify on the requisition form that the source of the stone is urinary. Include patient's identification and the date and time that the stone was passed. The same identifying information is placed on the specimen container.

Cancer Antigen 125

Also called: CA 125

SPECIMEN OR TYPE OF TEST: Serum, body fluids

PURPOSE OF THE TEST

In patients with cancer of the ovary, this test is used to monitor the response to treatment or the progression of the disease.

BASICS THE NURSE NEEDS TO KNOW

Cancer antigen 125 (CA 125) is a tumor marker for ovarian cancer. Normally, this antigen is present in small amounts in the serum of healthy women. It will be present or rise slightly with menstruation, the first trimester of pregnancy, and with endometriosis. If ovarian or endometrial cells are destroyed by cancer or the cancer begins to grow, the persistently increasing level of the antigen can be detected in the blood. Because of the lack of specificity and sensitivity, this test cannot be used as a screening test for the general population. It is, however, a very helpful and reliable test to monitor the activity of known cancer of the ovary. A serum value greater than 35 U/mL (SI: >35 kU/L) is positive and correlates with malignancy.

Elevated Values

In a patient with known cancer of the ovary, a persistently rising value of cancer antigen 125 is associated with advancing or recurrent malignancy and possible intraperitoneal tumor. When the value rises after cancer treatment, the test gives an early warning that the treatment response is poor.

Decreased Values

In the patient with known ovarian cancer, a decline in the cancer antigen 125 value indicates a good response to treatment.

REFERENCE VALUES   <35 U/mL *or* SI: <35 kU/L

HOW THE TEST IS DONE

Venipuncture is performed to collect a sample of venous blood.

SIGNIFICANCE OF TEST RESULTS

Elevated Values

Ovarian cancer
Adenocarcinoma of the cervix, endometrium, or fallopian tubes
Adenocarcinoma of the lung, colon, pancreas, or breast
Acute pelvic inflammatory disease
Endometriosis
Pregnancy

INTERFERING FACTORS

- Pregnancy
- Menstruation
- Recent radioisotope scan or abdominal surgery

NURSING CARE

Nursing actions are similar to those used in other capillary puncture or venipuncture procedures (see Chapter 2), with the following additional measures.

Pretest

- This test should be scheduled no sooner than 3 weeks after abdominal surgery to avoid a false positive result. The test should also be scheduled before or at least 7 days after any radioisotope scan so that the radioisotopes of the scan will not interfere with the test methodology. The test should not be done during the woman's menstruation because the value will be much higher at that time.
- For the patient with a history of cancer, provide empathetic support. Her anxiety level is likely to be high because of the implications of a potentially elevated test result.

Posttest

- When the patient with a known history of ovarian cancer has a persistently rising level of cancer antigen 125, a high probability exists that the cause is progression or recurrence of the malignancy. Before new treatment is instituted, additional diagnostic testing is indicated to locate metastasis. Provide continuing emotional support to help the patient cope during the stress of additional testing and in the decision making that is part of the overall treatment plan.

Capillary Glucose/Sugar Monitoring

See Glucose, Capillary on p. 336.

Capnogram

Also called: Exhaled Carbon Dioxide; Capnography; End-Tidal Carbon Dioxide; $ETCO_2$; ($PETCO_2$) Partial Pressure End Tidal CO_2

SPECIMEN OR TYPE OF TEST: Spectrometry

PURPOSE OF THE TEST

Monitoring exhaled carbon dioxide (CO_2) permits continuous evaluation of alveolar ventilation, reducing the number of ABG determinations needed. $ETCO_2$ may be used to evaluate ventilator changes and weaning parameters from mechanical ventilation. It will confirm endotracheal intubation because no capnographic waveform will occur if the tube is in the esophagus.

Capnography may be used to monitor the patient during an *apnea test*. An apnea test is done to diagnosis brain death. This test requires the observation of spontaneous respiration when the arterial CO_2 is above 60 mm Hg.

BASICS THE NURSE NEEDS TO KNOW

Capnography provides a CO_2 waveform, which visualizes CO_2 elimination patterns during exhalation and a total percentage of CO_2 exhaled per breath. CO_2 is measured at the end of exhalation because at this point the exhaled CO_2 approximates arterial CO_2 levels. With normal perfusion of the lungs, arterial CO_2 will be a few millimeters higher (5 mm Hg) than end-tidal CO_2 ($ETCO_2$). When perfusion is not adequate, this assumption cannot be made. Figure 28 shows a typical tracing of a capnogram.

Elevated Values

The $ETCO_2$ increases in hypermetabolic states because of increased production of CO_2, and during hypoventilation because CO_2 is retained and not excreted.

Decreased Values

The $ETCO_2$ decreases when the metabolic rate is reduced, as production of CO_2 decreases, and when there is reduced perfusion, causing a decrease in pulmonary blood flow.

REFERENCE VALUES   35 to 45 mm Hg.

HOW THE TEST IS DONE

Exhaled CO_2 is measured with exhaled gas analyzers. These analyzers measure the CO_2 by mass spectrometry or infrared analysis. Mass spectrometry requires aspiration of exhaled gas, whereas the infrared gas analyzer is usually attached to the exhalation tubing on a ventilator. The recorded value refers to the amount of infrared light absorbed by the exhaled breath. The higher the CO_2 level, the more infrared light is absorbed and the higher the reading.

For endotracheal tube placement, disposable colorimetric devices are available for single use.

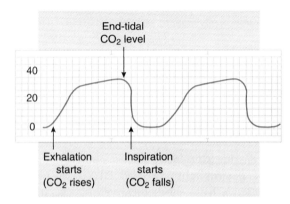

Figure 28. Capnographic tracing. On exhalation, the capnographic tracing shows a rapid rise in carbon dioxide followed by a plateau. At the end of exhalation, the end-tidal carbon dioxide level is obtained. As inspiration begins, there is a dramatic decrease in carbon dioxide.

C

SIGNIFICANCE OF TEST RESULTS

Elevated Values

Burns
Hypermetabolic states
Hypoventilation
Malignant hyperthermia
Multiple trauma

Decreased Values

Acute cardiac failure
Anesthesia
Aspiration
Bronchial spasms
Cardiac and pulmonary arrest
Dislodgment of the endotracheal tube
Hypothermia
Hypothyroidism
Hypovolemia
Mucous plug
Pulmonary edema
Pulmonary embolism

INTERFERING FACTORS

- Cardiopulmonary abnormalities
- Leak in system
- Metabolic disorders

▮ NURSING CARE

During the Test

- Check the capnographic waveform. It should return to zero baseline on inspiration. If it does not, check the seal of the expiratory demand valve on the ventilator and the fresh gas flow in the tube.
- If the waveform disappears or drops to zero, it may indicate accidental extubation, obstruction, esophageal intubation, or cardiac and/or pulmonary arrest.

Carbohydrate Antigen 19-9

Also called: CA 19-9; Cancer Antigen CA19-9

SPECIMEN OR TYPE OF TEST: Serum

C

PURPOSE OF THE TEST

Carbohydrate antigen 19-9 (CA 19-9) is a tumor marker that is used in preoperative staging for cancer of the pancreas. It is also used to monitor the course of pancreatic cancer, the response to treatment, and to predict recurrence.

BASICS THE NURSE NEEDS TO KNOW

CA 19-9 is an antigen made by the pancreas, liver, colon, and other tissues. The antigen appears in the serum when these source tissues undergo healing or when there is a tumor growing in that organ or tissue. This tumor marker is most accurate in cases of pancreatic cancer. The serum level does not rise in an early stage of disease, but is most accurate in the late stages of cancer or during recurrence.

Malignancy causes this test result to rise dramatically. Tumors of the pancreas can cause the serum level to rise to >1000 units/mL (SI: >1000 kU/L). Any result greater than 300 units/L (SI: 300 kU/L) is an indicator that the pancreatic cancer may be too advanced for surgical removal.

After treatment of the cancer of the pancreas, CA 19-9 is used to monitor the patient's condition. A renewed elevation of CA 19-9 indicates that the cancer has returned. The serum level will rise before clinical symptoms appear.

Benign conditions of the pancreas, liver, and gall bladder also can cause an elevation of CA 19-9. In benign disease, the elevation is much lower than the dramatically high elevations associated with cancer. This test has a lack of specificity because it cannot distinguish between benign and malignant causes of hepatobiliary and pancreatic disease and various other diseases. Thus, because of false-positive results in benign conditions, this tumor marker does not have a clear role in the management of cancer patients (Marrelli, Caruso & Pedrazzani, 2009).

REFERENCE VALUES   Adult: <37 U/mL *or* SI: <37 kU/L

HOW THE TEST IS DONE

Venipuncture is used to collect a sample of venous blood.

SIGNIFICANCE OF TEST RESULTS

Elevated Values

Malignant Conditions

Cancer of the pancreas
Cancer of the stomach
Cancer of the colon
Hepatobiliary cancer
Cancer of the lung
Cancer of the head and neck
Gynecologic cancer

Benign Conditions

Hepatobiliary disease
Acute and chronic pancreatitis

INTERFERING FACTORS

- None

NURSING CARE

Nursing actions are similar to those used in other venipuncture procedures (see Chapter 2), with the following additional measures.

Pretest

- Provide emotional support for the patient. Ongoing testing for cancer and tumor markers can create anxiety because of the implications of an elevated result.

Posttest

- When the elevated test result indicates recurrence of cancer, the patient will need emotional support. In some cases, there may be additional treatment options, but in cases of recurrent cancer of the pancreas, the prognosis is bleak. The nurse can use listening skills and empathy to allow the patient to verbalize or express emotion. As the patient becomes aware of declining health, he or she may express denial or anger, or may become depressed. Some will express hope and others will begin to make decisions regarding their future. Listening to the patient can provide the cues as to what the patient believes and how he or she wants to use the time that remains.

Carbon Dioxide, Total

Also called: tCO_2; TCO_2; CO_2 Content

SPECIMEN OR TYPE OF TEST: Whole blood, serum, plasma

PURPOSE OF THE TEST

The total carbon dioxide (TCO_2) determination is used to help evaluate acid-base balance and the bicarbonate buffer system.

BASICS THE NURSE NEEDS TO KNOW

Total CO_2 measures the combined forms of CO_2 in the blood. The largest component is bicarbonate ion, composing 90% of the total CO_2 content in the blood. The total CO_2 content provides the principal extracellular buffer system, which is called the bicarbonate carbonic acid buffer. Buffer systems are needed in the regulation of acid-base balance. The concentration of carbon dioxide is controlled by the lungs, and the concentration of bicarbonate is controlled by the kidneys.

Elevated Values

An elevated serum level of TCO_2 is called *hypercapnia*. It often is caused by poor CO_2 excretion by the lungs or an inadequate respiratory drive.

Hypercapnia is associated with respiratory acidosis, CO_2 retention, and metabolic alkalosis.

C

Decreased Values

A low serum level of TCO_2 is called *hypocapnia*. It is caused by excess elimination of CO_2, excess elimination of bicarbonate, excess accumulation of hydrogen ions in the blood, or a combination of these conditions. Hypocapnia is associated with respiratory alkalosis or metabolic acidosis.

REFERENCE VALUES	Whole blood (venous), adult: 22-26 mEq/L *or* SI: 22-26 mmol/L Whole blood (arterial), adult: 19-24 mEq/L *or* SI: 19-24 mmol/L Serum, adult: 23-29 mEq/L *or* SI: 23-29 mmol/L >60 yr: 23-31 mEq/L *or* SI: 23-31 mmol/L Capillary (plasma), Newborn: 13-22 mEq/L *or* SI: 13-22 mmol/L Infant: 20-28 mEq/L *or* SI: 20-28 mmol/L Child: 20-28 mEq/L *or* SI: 20-28 mmol/L Adult: 22-28 mEq/L *or* SI: 22-28 mmol/L
▽ Critical Values	<10 mEq/L (SI: <10 mmol/L) *or* >40-45 mEq/L (SI: >40-45 mmol/L)

HOW THE TEST IS DONE

Venipuncture or arterial puncture is done to collect a sample of venous or arterial blood. A capillary pipette is used to collect capillary blood.

SIGNIFICANCE OF TEST RESULTS

Elevated Values

Respiratory acidosis
Emphysema
Pneumonia
Cystic fibrosis
Congestive heart failure
Pulmonary edema
Metabolic alkalosis
Hypokalemia
Excessive intake of antacids
Severe, prolonged vomiting
Cushing's syndrome
Primary aldosteronism

Decreased Values

Respiratory alkalosis
Hyperventilation
Metabolic acidosis
Diabetes mellitus
Severe diarrhea
Renal tubular acidosis

Renal failure
Dehydration
Hypovolemia

INTERFERING FACTORS

• Exposure of the specimen to air

NURSING CARE

Nursing actions are similar to those used in other arterial, venipuncture, or capillary blood collection procedures (see Chapter 2), with no additional measures.

▽ **Nursing Response to Critical Values**

The physician must be notified immediately if the total or ionized carbon dioxide reaches a critical value (either very low or very high). The blood pH and serum electrolytes also are likely to be in serious imbalance. The patient requires an immediate nursing assessment of all vital signs, with particular attention to abnormal changes in the rate and quality of respirations.

Carboxyhemoglobin

Also called: COHb

SPECIMEN OR TYPE OF TEST: Whole blood

PURPOSE OF THE TEST

Carboxyhemoglobin measures the amount of carbon monoxide that is in the blood, bound to hemoglobin molecules.

BASICS THE NURSE NEEDS TO KNOW

Carbon monoxide enters the body by inhalation of exhaust from the burning of fossil fuels, including gasoline, kerosene, coal, charcoal, wood, and oil. The exhaust enters the air from a defective heater, furnace, stove, or generator, exhaust from an automotive vehicle, or by burning fuel in an area with poor ventilation. The exposure can be accidental or a suicide attempt. The person who is in fire may also breathe a substantial amount of carbon monoxide in the smoky air. Carbon monoxide is present in tobacco smoke and may also come from industrial sources. Depending on the amount of exposure, carbon monoxide poisoning can kill in minutes or hours.

The hemoglobin molecule of a red blood cell has four receptor sites that will bind with oxygen molecules for transport of the oxygen to cells. When carbon monoxide is present in the blood, the hemoglobin has a powerful affinity to quickly attach the carbon monoxide instead of oxygen. The combination of carbon monoxide and hemoglobin form a compound called carboxyhemoglobin that cannot transport oxygen. As carboxyhemoglobin accumulates in the blood, tissue hypoxia begins to develop. In addition, the increasing accumulations of carboxyhemoglobin cause a shift of the hemoglobin-oxygen dissociation curve to the left, adding to the anoxia.

C

In laboratory measurements, the amount of carboxyhemoglobin in the blood is expressed as the percentage of hemoglobin that is saturated with carbon monoxide or the fraction of the whole that is saturated. As the amount of carboxyhemoglobin increases to 20% to 30% of hemoglobin saturation, symptoms of carbon monoxide poisoning appear. In children, lower concentrations may be toxic (McPherson & Pincus, 2007).

REFERENCE VALUES	Nonsmokers: 0.5%-1.5% Hb saturation *or* 0.005-0.015 Fraction of Hb saturation Smokers (1-2 packs per day): 4%-5% Hb saturation *or* 0.04-0.05 Fraction of Hb saturation Toxic: >20% Hb saturation *or* >0.20 Fraction of Hb saturation Lethal: >50% Hb saturation *or* >0.50 Fraction of Hb saturation
▽ Critical Values	>20% Hb saturation *or* >0.20 Fraction of Hb saturation

HOW THE TEST IS DONE

Venipuncture is performed to collect a sample of venous blood.

SIGNIFICANCE OF THE TEST RESULTS

Evaluated Values

Carbon monoxide poisoning
Hemolytic disease

INTERFERING FACTORS

- Oxygen

NURSING CARE

Nursing actions are similar to those used in other venipuncture procedures (see Chapter 2), with the following additional measures.

Pretest

- If the blood specimen can be drawn before oxygen therapy is started, an accurate carboxyhemoglobin value will be identified. Oxygen administration accelerates the elimination of carbon monoxide from the body and the carboxyhemoglobin value will begin to decline.

Posttest

◉ *Patient Teaching.* At the time of discharge after a low level of accidental exposure in the home, instruct the patient to get plenty of fresh air in the next few hours. In addition, instruct the patient not to return home until the furnace and all gas appliances are checked by a professional. Keep all windows opened to eliminate any residual carbon monoxide that is present.

▽ **Nursing Responses to Critical Values**

The patient may already have a toxic level of carbon monoxide poisoning at the time of admission for emergency treatment. The nurse assesses for symptoms including headache, nausea, dizziness, mental confusion, and elevations of the pulse, blood pressure, and respiratory rate.

Late signs are the presence of the characteristic cherry red skin, loss of consciousness, hypotension, coma, seizures, and cardiac arrest (Goldstein, 2008). The nurse prepares to administer prescribed 100% pure oxygen via a tight-fitting, nonrebreather mask. Other emergency measures may be needed, such as intubation and cardiac/respiratory support.

Carcinoembryonic Antigen

Also called: CEA

SPECIMEN OR TYPE OF TEST: Serum, body fluid

PURPOSE OF THE TEST

Carcinoembryonic antigen (CEA) is a tumor marker used to monitor for and detect recurrence of colorectal, breast, and gastric cancer. It also may be used to measure the extent of malignant disease and help in the staging of the cancer.

BASICS THE NURSE NEEDS TO KNOW

In cancer, the necrosis of malignant tissue permits large amounts of this antigen to leak out of the tumor and enter the blood and body (effusion) fluids. An elevated value of serum CEA indicates that there is extension or recurrence of cancer at the primary site or metastases to a distant site (often liver, lung, or bone). The CEA value often rises many months before other laboratory tests become abnormal and before the patient experiences symptoms.

Elevated levels can occur in benign disease, but the test values are in a lower range than those of malignancy. Smokers have a normal value that is higher than nonsmokers, but do not necessarily have benign or malignant disease. A CEA value of >20 ng/mL (SI: >20 mcg/L) usually indicates cancer at a primary or metastatic site.

Interpretation of the test results is made with consideration of when the test is done. If the CEA value is normal after surgical removal of the cancer, the information means that no new cancer is growing. If the CEA value rises in the weeks, months, or years after surgical removal, it provides very early warning that cancer has recurred in the primary or metastatic site. Additional testing to locate the site of the cancer and additional cancer treatment are likely. In colorectal cancer, a preoperative elevation of CEA indicates a poorer long-term prognosis.

REFERENCE VALUES	Adult, nonsmoker: <3.0 ng/mL *or* SI: <3.0 mcg/L
	Adult, smoker: <5.0 ng/mL *or* SI: <5 mcg/L

HOW THE TEST IS DONE

Blood: Venipuncture is used to obtain a sample of venous blood. Blood specimens are generally done before surgery, 4 weeks postoperatively, and at regular intervals thereafter for 5 years.

Body fluid: A sample of the body fluid is collected by the physician during a diagnostic procedure, such as a thoracentesis, or paracentesis.

C

SIGNIFICANCE OF TEST RESULTS

Elevated Values
Malignant Conditions
Colorectal cancer
Stomach cancer
Pancreatic cancer
Breast cancer
Lung cancer
Thyroid cancer
Ovarian cancer
Cancer metastases (liver, bone, lung)
Benign Conditions
Ulcerative colitis
Crohn's disease
Hepatitis
Cirrhosis
Pulmonary infection
Radiation therapy

INTERFERING FACTORS

- Recent administration of radioisotopes
- Smoking
- Heparin
- Hemolysis

NURSING CARE

Nursing actions are similar to those used in other venipuncture procedures (see Chapter 2), with the following additional measures.

Pretest
- Schedule any nuclear scan after this test is completed. The radioisotopes of the nuclear scan would interfere with the laboratory method of analysis for CEA.

Posttest
- When colorectal cancer has been diagnosed and has been treated with surgical removal of the tumor, the nurse should emphasize the importance of follow-up medical care. This includes follow-up CEA testing, abdominal imaging, and a repeat colonoscopy at scheduled intervals for the next 5 years. Most patients are aware of the possibility of recurrence of colorectal cancer and the benefit of early identification and treatment. Improved patient compliance with follow-up testing would occur if the patient receives clear guidance about follow-up medical care, including laboratory and diagnostic testing (Cardella, Coburn & Gagliardi, 2008)
- The postsurgical patient with colorectal cancer may experience anxiety regarding follow-up testing because of the potential for recurrence. A negative or normal CEA value is "good news" because it means there is no evidence of the recurrence of cancer. If the CEA test becomes elevated at any time after the initial treatment, the patient's anxiety level will rise. The elevated CEA may occur up to 36 months before cancer symptoms are present.

Cardiac Markers

Also called: Biochemical Cardiac Markers; Biomarkers; Cardiac Enzymes; Cardiac Isoenzymes

SPECIMEN OR TYPE OF TEST: Serum

PURPOSE OF THE TEST

Cardiac markers are used with clinical presentation and electrocardiographic studies to diagnose acute myocardial infarction (AMI). Accurate and rapid diagnosis of an MI will lead to early intervention, which will decrease mortality and infarction size. Based on clinical presentation, to rule out an acute MI, CK-MB (creatine kinase-MB) and troponin levels are usually ordered. These tests may be done at the point of care, usually in the Emergency Department. This permits early intervention, which can save myocardial tissue. It also helps to prevent unnecessary admissions to the coronary care units.

BASICS THE NURSE NEEDS TO KNOW

Currently, no single test can absolutely rule out an AMI. Based on timing (when the infarction actually occurs), there are cardiac markers with a high degree of sensitivity and specificity. The nurse needs to be aware that whereas the AMI is assumed to occur when chest pain is experienced, this is not always so. Patients may have severe chest pain from angina before the infarction. Also, patients may experience atypical chest pain or no chest pain with an AMI.

The following is a brief discussion of the varied laboratory tests that may be ordered.

Enzymes are complex compounds found in all tissues that speed up the biochemical reactions of the body. Damage to body tissue causes release of the enzymes from the injured cells into the serum. Enzymes may be common to more than one type of tissue. Elevated serum levels of the enzymes reflect tissue damage, but because the enzymes are not specific, patterns of enzyme elevations are used to determine myocardial tissue damage.

Creatine kinase (CK) is an enzyme found in the heart, brain, and skeletal muscle. The individual with greater muscle mass has a higher CK level than does the average person. CK levels may be higher in African Americans. CK may be separated into three isoenzymes. Isoenzymes refer to the various forms of an enzyme, which can differ chemically, physically, or immunologically, but catalyze the same reaction. The CK isoenzymes include CK-MM, CK-MB, and CK-BB. With myocardial damage, the elevated fraction that rises is CK-MB. CKMB isoforms, a new cardiac marker, have even greater specificity.

Troponin is a protein found in skeletal and cardiac muscle fibers. Troponins are considered the gold standard biomarker for assessing myocardial tissue damage. Three forms of troponin exist, two of which are used in diagnosing cardiac disorders (cardiac troponin T [cT_nT] and cardiac troponin I [cT_nI]). Normally, cardiac troponin levels are very low, but the level increases rapidly with an MI. Troponin I is found only in the cardiac muscle complex; therefore, it is very specific to cardiac injury. This is especially important if the person being evaluated for a cardiac problem has renal disease or a musculoskeletal disorder, which would make interpretation of the CK-MB difficult. Troponin levels increase earlier than CK-MB levels; thus their evaluation may be helpful in diagnosing MI earlier than the enzyme studies. Earlier diagnosis may lead to earlier treatment and salvaging more myocardium. Under investigation at this time is *hs-cTnT*, which may permit the identification of people at risk for a cardiac event.

C

Myoglobin (Mb, S-Mgb) is an oxygen-binding protein found in striated muscle. It releases oxygen at very low tensions. Any injury to skeletal muscle will cause a release of myoglobin into the blood. Because myoglobin rises and falls so rapidly, its use in diagnosing AMI is limited.

Lactate dehydrogenase (LDH) is present in almost all metabolizing cells but is especially high in the heart, kidneys, brain, red blood cells, liver, and skeletal muscles. Because LDH is present in so many tissues of the body, the origin of its release cannot be determined without the use of electrophoresis, which separates out its five isoenzymes. The LDH isoenzymes, LDH_1 and LDH_2, are used to assess myocardial damage.

C-reactive protein (CRP) is a marker for inflammation. It is produced by the liver and increases in response to tissue inflammation or injury. It lacks specificity in identifying myocardial injury. Currently, some studies have shown CRP as a better predictor for an MI than cholesterol. It is believed inflammation in the arterial walls and the body's response to inflammation may trigger a "cardiac event." (See C-Reactive Protein, p. 229.) *High-sensitivity C-reactive protein* (hs-CRP) is being investigated to assess "healthy" people, who may be at risk for cardiovascular disease. Its reference value is less than 2 mg/L.

REFERENCE VALUES

CK
Newborn: 50-525 U/L *or* SI: 0.85-8.93 µKat/L
Adult male: 38-174 U/L *or* SI: 0.65-29.6 µKat/L
Adult female: 26-140 U/L *or* SI: 0.44-2.38 µKat/L

CK-MB
0%-6% of total CK *or* SI: 0.00%-0.06% (fraction of total CK)

Cardiac Troponin T
<0.2 µg/L

Cardiac Troponin I
<0.35 µg/L

Myoglobin
<90 µg/L

LDH
Adult: 200-400 U/L
Neonate: 400-700 U/L

LDH Isoenzymes
LDH_1 14%-26% *or* SI: 0.14-0.26 (fraction of total LDH)
LDH_2 29%-39% *or* SI: 0.29-0.39 (fraction of total LDH)

HOW THE TEST IS DONE

A venipuncture is necessary.

SIGNIFICANCE OF TEST RESULTS

In diagnosing MI, a pattern of test changes supports the diagnosis. CK levels begin to rise 6 hours after the infarction; they peak in 18 hours, and return to normal in 2 to 3 days. CK-MB levels rise within 3 to 6 hours after an infarction, peak in 12 to 24 hours, and return to normal in 12 to 48 hours. An increase in CK-MB, expressed as a percentage of the total CK, supports the diagnosis of myocardial damage. The percentage accepted as diagnostic of an infarction varies from laboratory to laboratory. If the CK-MB level rises quickly and then drops quickly, myocardial contusion may be suspected. CK-MB levels will also drop quickly if thrombolytic therapy for an AMI has been successful.

Cardiac troponin is cardiac specific. It rises 2 to 6 hours after the onset of an AMI, peaks in 16 hours, and returns to normal in 5 to 9 days.

Myoglobin rises and falls within 2 to 6 hours of the onset of MI; therefore, timing of the specimen is crucial. If the patient delayed seeking treatment, myoglobin is not helpful in diagnosing an MI.

LDH elevations do not occur until 24 to 48 hours after an infarction. They peak in 3 to 4 days and do not return to normal levels for 10 to 14 days after an infarction. LDH_2 levels are normally greater than LDH_1 levels. A "flipped" LDH, which occurs when LDH_1 levels become greater than those of LDH_2, is indicative of an MI. The flipped LDH is especially helpful if the person delayed seeking help when chest pain occurred. Figure 29 shows a schematic of the cardiac biomarker patterns after an acute MI.

The rise of cardiac markers correlates positively with the size of the infarction after 7 days and negatively correlates with the person's ejection fraction.

Because of their nonspecificity, other clinical problems may create changes in the cardiac markers. Common causes of these changes are as follows:

CK

Elevated Values
Amyotrophic lateral sclerosis
Biliary atresia
Burns

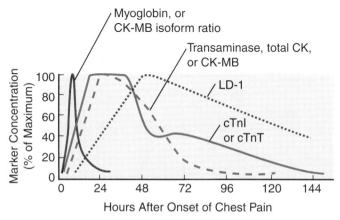

Figure 29. Pattern of cardiac markers increases following an acute myocardial infarction. (From McPherson RA, Pincus MR: *Henry's clinical diagnosis and management by laboratory methods,* ed 21, Philadelphia, 2007, Saunders.)

Some cancers
Cardiomyopathy
Central nervous system trauma, including cerebrovascular accident
Hypokalemia, severe
Hypothermia
Hypothyroidism
Infarction: cerebral, bowel, myocardial
Intramuscular injections
Muscular dystrophy
Myocarditis
Organ rejection
Pulmonary edema
Pulmonary embolism
Renal insufficiency or failure
Surgery

Decreased Values
Addison's disease
Anterior pituitary hyposecretion
Connective tissue disease
Cirrhosis, alcoholic
Metastatic cancer
Steroid administration

Troponin I
Elevated Values
Acute myocardial infarction

Troponin T
Elevated Values
Acute myocardial infarction
Angina
Renal failure
Muscle trauma
Rhabdomyolysis
Polymyositis
Dermatomyositis

Myoglobin
Elevated Values
MI
Muscle injury or breakdown
Polymyositis
Renal failure

Rhabdomyolysis
Open heart surgery
Exhaustive exercise

LDH
Elevated Values
Alcoholism
Anemia
Burns
Cancer
Cardiomyopathy
Cerebrovascular accident
Cirrhosis
Convulsions
Delirium tremens
Hepatitis
Hypothyroidism
Infectious mononucleosis
Codeine
Lithium carbonate
Meperidine
Morphine
Niacin
Pneumonia
Pulmonary infarction
Procainamide
Propranolol
Shock
Thyroid hormones
Ulcerative colitis

Decreased Values
Radiation therapy
Oxalates

INTERFERING FACTORS
- CK: Cardioversion, drugs (alcohol, aspirin, halothane, lithium, succinylcholine), gross hemolysis of specimen, muscle trauma, recent vigorous exercise or massage, surgery
- Troponin: Hemolysis of specimen
- LDH: Pregnancy, prosthetic heart valves, recent surgery, hemolysis of specimen
- Myoglobin: Any trauma to skeletal muscle. Recent administration of radioactive material, if radioimmunoassay (RIA) is used for analysis.

NURSING CARE

Nursing actions are similar to those used in other venipuncture procedures (see Chapter 2), with the following additional measures.

Pretest
- The nurse reassures the patient, who is usually frightened and having chest pain, and may also be in denial.
- Do not give intramuscular injections or perform repeated venipunctures, if possible, until all the initial enzyme studies are completed.
- Instruct the patient about the need for repeat blood sampling.
- The nurse determines if alcohol or drugs that affect results have been ingested.

During the Test
- Serial specimens are taken according to hospital protocol.
- If the tourniquet is in place too long, inaccurate results may occur.

Posttest
- Nursing actions are similar to those for any venipuncture.

Catecholamines, Plasma

Also called: Catecholamine Fractionalization, Plasma

SPECIMEN OR TYPE OF TEST: Plasma

PURPOSE OF THE TEST

Plasma catecholamines are usually assessed to diagnose pheochromocytoma or to identify extraadrenal tumors after abdominal surgery. Pheochromocytomas are tumors developing in the sympathetic nervous system. These tumors usually secrete epinephrine, norepinephrine, or both, and sometimes dopamine.

A *clonidine suppression* test may be performed to differentiate between pheochromocytoma and essential hypertension. With this test, clonidine is given 2 to 3 hours before a venous blood sample is taken. Clonidine suppresses neurogenic catecholamine release. If suppression occurs, the test result is consistent with the diagnosis of essential hypertension. If the catecholamines remain elevated, the diagnosis of pheochromocytoma is supported.

BASICS THE NURSE NEEDS TO KNOW

The catecholamines are three hormones produced and secreted by the adrenal medulla. This structure is the inner core of the adrenal glands, which lie at the superior pole of each kidney. The catecholamines are epinephrine, norepinephrine, and dopamine (a precursor of norepinephrine). The adrenal medulla secretes the catecholamines when stimulated by preganglionic neurons. The result mimics the effect of a mass discharge of the sympathetic nervous system. Their secretion is part of the "fight or flight" response. The catecholamines help maintain serum glucose levels by promoting liver glycogenolysis, by stimulating the secretion of insulin and glucagon, and by lipolysis. The catecholamines stimulate the reticular activating system, making the person more alert.

REFERENCE VALUES*   Epinephrine (supine): <110 pg/mL *or* SI: <650 pmol/L
Epinephrine (standing): <140 pg/mL *or* SI: <900 pmol/L
Norepinephrine (supine): <750 pg/mL *or* SI: <4431 pmol/L
Dopamine (supine): <30 pg/mL *or* SI: <178 pmol/L

*Values vary among laboratories.

HOW THE TEST IS DONE

Plasma catecholamines are measured using a radioenzyme technique. A venous sampling of 10 mL of blood is drawn once while the patient is lying down and then once with the patient standing. The normal values vary among laboratories. Results may not reveal a tumor that secretes intermittently, so the test may be ordered for when the patient is symptomatic. To localize small tumors, percutaneous venous catheterization may be needed.

SIGNIFICANCE OF TEST RESULTS

Elevated Values

Pheochromocytoma
Ganglioneuroma
Neuroblastoma

INTERFERING FACTORS

- Noncompliance with diet and relaxation requirements
- Amine-rich food and drink
- Anger
- Cold environment
- Medications such as amphetamines, barbiturates, decongestants, epinephrine, levodopa, phenothiazines, reserpine, sympathomimetics, and tricyclic antidepressants
- Sample not sent to the lab immediately
- Severe anxiety

▌ NURSING CARE

Nursing actions are similar to those used in other venipuncture procedures (see Chapter 2), with the following additional measures.

Pretest

- Since many drugs interfere with test results, the nurse should check with the physician if any medications are to be withheld.

○ *Patient Teaching.* The nurse instructs the patient to avoid amine-rich food and drink (e.g., avocados, bananas, beer, cheese, Chianti wine, cocoa, coffee, and tea) for 48 hours before the test.

○ *Patient Teaching.* Instruct the patient not to smoke for 4 hours before the test.

○ *Patient Teaching.* The nurse explains to the patient that a venous catheter (heparin lock) is inserted 24 hours before the blood sample is drawn, because venipuncture may increase catecholamine levels.

Continued

C

| NURSING CARE—cont'd

○ *Patient Teaching.* Instruct the patient to lie down and relax for an hour before the blood is drawn.

During the Test

- The nurse carries out duties similar to those of other venipuncture procedures, except that blood is drawn through the heparin lock. If the heparin lock has been flushed with heparin, withdraw 3 mL of blood and discard it before drawing the sample.
- After the first sample is drawn, the patient may be asked to stand for 10 minutes, and a second sample is drawn.
- Include the position of the patient when the blood was drawn on the requisition slip.
- The nurse flushes the heparin lock according to hospital protocol.

Posttest

- The patient may resume pretest diet and activity. Notify the laboratory that the specimen is coming, because it must be frozen immediately.

Catecholamines, Urinary

Also called: Catecholamines; Fractionation; Free Catecholamine Fractionation

SPECIMEN OR TYPE OF TEST: Urine

PURPOSE OF THE TEST

Urinary catecholamine determinations are usually obtained as a part of the workup to identify the cause of hypertension and to diagnose pheochromocytoma.

BASICS THE NURSE NEEDS TO KNOW

Catecholamines are excreted in the urine in conjugated and unconjugated (free) forms. Together these forms make up the total urinary catecholamines. As serum catecholamines are metabolized, several end-product metabolites are created, which are excreted in the urine (Figure 30). The primary metabolite is vanillylmandelic acid (VMA). Other major metabolites of epinephrine and norepinephrine are metanephrine and normetanephrine. Dopamine's metabolites are 3-methoxy-4-hydroxyphenylacetic acid (*homovanillic acid,* or HVA) and 3,4-dehydroxyphenylacetic acid (DOPA$_c$).

REFERENCE VALUES*

Norepinephrine: 15-56 μg/24 hr *or* SI: 88.6-331 nmol/24 hr
Epinephrine: <20 μg/mL *or* SI: <109 nmol/24 hr
Dopamine: 100-400 pg/mL *or* SI: 625-2750 nmol/24 hr
Vanillylmandelic acid: 2-7 mg/24 hr *or* SI: 10-35 μmol/24 hr
Metanephrine: <1.4 mg/day *or* SI: <7.0 μmol/day
Normetanephrine: <0.4 mg/day *or* SI: <2.0 μmol/day
Homovanillic acid: <0.8 mg/day *or* SI: <44.0 μmol/day

*Values vary among laboratories.

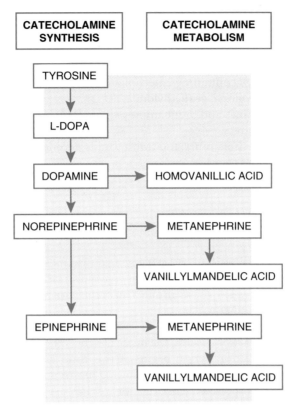

Figure 30. Catecholamine synthesis and metabolism.

HOW THE TEST IS DONE

A 24-hour urine specimen is collected, with a boric or acetic acid or potassium bisulfate preservative added to the container. A random sample may be done, but does not reflect the diurnal changes that occur.

SIGNIFICANCE OF TEST RESULTS

Elevated Values

Catecholamines and Vanillylmandelic Acid

Pheochromocytoma

Neuroblastoma

Ganglioneuroma

Homovanillic Acid

Pheochromocytoma ruled out

Tumors of the autonomic nervous system

Ganglioblastoma

INTERFERING FACTORS

- Epinephrine: Stress
- Norepinephrine: Exercise
- Dopamine: Food and drugs containing catecholamines, high-fluorescent compounds (e.g., tetracycline, quinidine), levodopa, or methyldopa
- Metanephrine: Catecholamines and monoamine oxidase (MAO) inhibitors
- Normetanephrine: Severe stress
- Vanillylmandelic acid: Catecholamines; food with vanilla, levodopa, and MAO inhibitors

■ NURSING CARE

Nursing actions are similar to those used in other 24-hour collections of urine procedures (see Chapter 2), with the following additional measures.

Pretest
- The nurse checks with the physician to see if any medications are to be held.
- ○ *Patient Teaching.* The nurse instructs the patient to avoid stress, exercise, smoking, and pain before and during the testing. The nurse also instructs the patient to avoid chocolate, coffee, bananas, food with vanilla, and citrus fruit.

During the Test
- ○ *Patient Teaching.* At the start of the test, the nurse instructs the patient to void at 8 am and discard this urine. The collection period begins at this time, and all urine is collected for 24 hours, including the 8 am specimen of the following morning.
- On the requisition slip and specimen label, the nurse writes the patient's name, and the time and date of the start and finish of the test period.
- Keep the urine specimen refrigerated or on ice throughout the collection period.

Posttest
- Arrange for prompt transport of the cooled specimen to the laboratory.

Ceruloplasmin

SPECIMEN OR TYPE OF TEST: Serum

PURPOSE OF THE TEST

Ceruloplasmin is one of the tests used to diagnose Wilson's disease, a genetic disorder of copper metabolism that causes liver degeneration and in later life, unexplained central nervous system disorders that affect coordination, motor control, and mental stability.

BASICS THE NURSE NEEDS TO KNOW

Ceruloplasmin is a plasma protein made by the liver. The exact function is unknown, but in the liver, ceruloplasmin molecules bind to copper atoms and the molecules are then released into the circulation. Ceruloplasmin contains most of the total plasma copper. In Wilson's disease, the liver cannot release copper into the bile and the copper then is deposited in all tissues of the body. The accumulated copper is toxic to the tissues of the liver, brain, parathyroid glands, kidneys, corneas, and bones.

Elevated Values

Ceruloplasmin is one of the serum proteins that are part of the body's acute phase response in conditions of extensive physical insult or trauma. The serum value rises in conditions of inflammation, infection, surgery, trauma, and malignancy.

Decreased Values

A low level of ceruloplasmin is associated with malabsorption, protein loss, and advanced liver disease that results in inadequate manufacture of all serum proteins. A low serum value of ceruloplasmin is specifically associated with Wilson's disease, an autosomal recessive disease. A ceruloplasmin value of <10 mg/dL (SI: <100 mg/L) is an indicator of Wilson's disease.

REFERENCE VALUES   Adult: 20-35 mg/dL *or* SI: 200-350 mg/L

HOW THE TEST IS DONE

Venipuncture is performed to obtain a sample of venous blood.

SIGNIFICANCE OF TEST RESULTS

Elevated Values

Leukemia
Hodgkin's disease
Cancer
Tissue necrosis
Trauma
Primary biliary cirrhosis
Systemic lupus erythematosus
Rheumatoid arthritis
Inflammation

Decreased Values

Wilson's disease
Hepatocellular disease
Malabsorption syndrome
Nephrotic syndrome

INTERFERING FACTORS

- Pregnancy
- Hemolysis
- Failure to maintain a nothing-by-mouth status

C

⏐ NURSING CARE

Nursing actions are similar to those used in other venipuncture procedures (see Chapter 2), with the following additional measures.

Pretest

○ *Patient Teaching.* Instruct the patient to fast from food for 8 to 12 hours before the test. High levels of serum lipids will alter the test results.

- Inform the laboratory if the patient is pregnant or taking oral contraceptives because high levels of estrogen will elevate the test results.

Posttest

- Ensure that the vial of blood is placed on ice and sent to the laboratory immediately. Warming of the specimen by prolonged exposure to room temperature will result in a false lowering of the test value.

Chlamydia trachomatis Tests

Includes: Genital culture, Antigen/antibody tests, DNA testing

SPECIMEN OR TYPE OF TEST: Urine, vaginal, or urethral swab

PURPOSE OF THE TEST

The various test methods help detect infection with *Chlamydia trachomatis,* a sexually transmitted disease. These tests are used for screening, diagnosis, and posttreatment evaluation.

BASICS THE NURSE NEEDS TO KNOW

Chlamydia trachomatis is a bacterium that causes genital infection that is often asymptomatic. Untreated, it can ultimately result in pelvic inflammatory disease, ectopic pregnancy, and infertility in women. In pregnancy, the infected mother can transmit the infection to the newborn during vaginal delivery, resulting in severe conjunctivitis or chlamydial pneumonia in the newborn infant.

Recommendations for Testing

Because chlamydial infection is the most common bacterial sexually transmitted disease (STD) in the United States, screening tests are recommended for all sexually active, adolescent females. Other women who are at risk include pregnant women, unmarried females, and those who have sex with multiple partners. At risk men who have sex with men are recommended to have screening for anal, urethral, and pharyngeal chlamydia infection at least annually.

Diagnostic Methods

Genital culture is considered the "reference standard" for diagnosis, but it is time consuming and costly to do. It is used when there are medicolegal implications such as suspected sexual assault or child sexual abuse.

   Direct fluorescent antibody (DFA) testing may be used for women, using a cervical swab and for men, using a urine specimen or urethral swab. The test provides for microscopic visualization of the antibody-stained elementary bodies of the bacterium. *Enzyme-linked immunoabsorbent*

assay (ELISA) detects *C. trachomatis* by use of an antibody that is specific to detect the chlamydial antigen. For women, the test is performed on a cervical swab specimen and for men, a urine specimen or urethral swab. Point of Care testing or "Rapid Tests" use the ELISA method of analysis. There is a higher rate of false positives with the DFA and ELISA methods, so additional testing is recommended to verify the results.

DNA Testing

The newest methodologies identify the DNA of *Chlamydia trachomatis*. The *Nucleic Acid Hybridization* test uses a DNA probe to identify the ribosomal RNA (rRNA) in the chlamydial genome. The specimen is a cervical swab of the female or urethral swab from the male. For either gender, urine specimens are also acceptable. The *Nucleic Acid Amplification testing-Polymerase Chain Reaction (PCR)* identifies single-stranded DNA or RNA of *Chlamydia trachomatis*. The test is performed on cells in the urine of men and women, or on the cervical swab of women or the urethral swab of men. The DNA methods are highly specific and sensitive (more than 95%) in the accurate detection of chlamydia (Mahon, Lehman & Manuselis, 2011).

REFERENCE VALUES   Negative for *Chlamydia trachomatis*

HOW THE TEST IS DONE

Cervical or Urethral Swabs: Dacron swabs are used to obtain mucosal cells from the urethral meatus of the male or the cervix of the female (see also Culture, Genital, p. 239). For a genital culture, a specific culture test kit for *Chlamydia trachomatis* is used.

The swabs are placed in a sterile tube with transport medium. Depending on the patient's sexual history, the individual also may need a cell culture sample from the anus, conjunctiva, nasopharynx, or throat.

Urine Specimen: A urine specimen container is used to collect a sample of a first morning specimen of urine.

SIGNIFICANCE OF TEST RESULTS

Positive Values

Chlamydia trachomatis infection

INTERFERING FACTORS

• Inadequate swab sample

NURSING CARE

Nursing actions are similar to those used for the collection of the first morning urine specimen (see Chapter 2), with the following additional measures.

Pretest

• The patient's history includes a sexual history, particularly for the high-risk populations of adolescents and young adults, ages 15 to 25, who are sexually active. Low-risk factors include a history of sexual activity that is monogamous, with a previous negative result for

Continued

NURSING CARE—cont'd

Chlamydia trachomatis. High-risk factors include unprotected sexual activity, inconsistent use of condoms, sexual intercourse with more than one partner, and a change in partners.

Posttest

- When the test result is positive for *Chlamydia trachomatis*, it is a reportable disease in every state in the United States. The nurse or physician advises the patient that the sexual partner(s) should also be tested or treated for presumptive disease.

Health Promotion.

Routine screening for *Chlamydia trachomatis* is recommended for sexually active females, ages 25 and younger. It is also recommended for those individuals who engage in high-risk sexual activity. One goal is to detect and treat this infection in females before it progresses to a complicated gynecologic problem or it infects the newborn child. The other is to reduce the overall number of infections caused by this organism.

- When working in a community or with population groups that have a high incidence of this infection, the nurse can participate with the health care team to develop a screening protocol. Communication with the local public health authorities would provide the data regarding the incidence of this infection in the local or regional area.

Chloride, Serum

Also called: Cl^-

SPECIMEN OR TYPE OF TEST: Blood

PURPOSE OF THE TEST

Serum chloride measurements are obtained in the evaluation of electrolyte levels, water balance, and acid-base balance and in the measurement of the cation-anion balance (anion gap).

BASICS THE NURSE NEEDS TO KNOW

Sodium (Na^+), potassium (K^+), bicarbonate (HCO_3^-), and chloride (Cl^-) are electrolytes with positive or negative charges. In combination, the electrolytes determine the osmolarity, pH, and hydration status in intracellular and extracellular fluids. In addition, the concentration differences between intracellular and extracellular electrolytes regulate the functions of the nervous system, cardiac, respiratory, and muscle tissues. Chloride is a major electrolyte in extracellular fluid and it generally increases or decreases with the sodium level. Chloride also increases or decreases inversely with bicarbonate, meaning as the bicarbonate level increases, chloride decreases, or as bicarbonate decreases, the chloride level increases. There are also a number of medications that can increase or decrease chloride values.

Elevated Values

An elevated level of chloride in the blood and extracellular fluid is called *hyperchloridemia*. It occurs during dehydration, metabolic acidosis, resulting from excessive loss of bicarbonate fluids and electrolytes from the lower intestine, from renal tubular acidosis, and from mineralocorticoid deficiency.

Decreased Values

A decreased level of chloride in the blood and extracellular fluid is called *hypochloridemia*. It occurs during prolonged vomiting from any cause, a loss of hydrochloric acid during nasogastric suction, from mineralocorticoid excess, salt-losing renal disease, or diabetic acidosis. The low level of chloride may also occur in conditions that cause a rise in bicarbonate or a decreased sodium concentration.

REFERENCE VALUES	Premature infant: 95-110 mEq/L *or* SI: 95-110 mmol/L
	Newborn: 98-110 mEq/L *or* SI: 98-110 mmol/L
	Child and Adult: 98-107 mEq/L *or* SI: 98-107 mmol/L
▽ Critical Values	<80 mEq/L (SI: <80 mmol/L) *or* >115 mEq/L (SI: >115 mmol/L

HOW THE TEST IS DONE

Venipuncture is performed to collect a specimen of venous blood; in infants, a heelstick puncture and a capillary tube may be used to collect capillary blood.

SIGNIFICANCE OF TEST RESULTS

Elevated Values

Dehydration
Renal tubular acidosis
Prolonged diarrhea
Acute renal failure
Diabetes insipidus
Respiratory alkalosis
Hyperparathyroidism
Adrenocortical hyperfunction

Decreased Values

Prolonged vomiting
Nasogastric drainage
Salt-losing nephritis
Chronic renal failure
Chronic respiratory acidosis
Metabolic alkalosis
Addison's disease
Congestive heart failure
Intestinal fistula
Overhydration
Diuretic therapy

INTERFERING FACTORS

• Hemolysis

NURSING CARE

Nursing actions are similar to those used in other venipuncture procedures (see Chapter 2), with the following additional measures.

Pretest

○ *Patient Teaching.* For a routine test, instruct the patient to discontinue all food for 8 hours before the test. This prevents the normal drop in chloride value after eating. For tests performed on an urgent or emergency basis, fasting is omitted.

Posttest

• If the patient receives intravenous fluids, the nurse monitors the flow of fluids and electrolyte replacement, as prescribed. The goal is to control the amount of fluid and the rate of flow correctly, so that the replacement is received in the prescribed time period.

• The nurse also monitors the laboratory results for alterations of other electrolytes because changes in the chloride level are usually accompanied by changes in carbon dioxide and sodium levels. Because of the patient's disease process, changes in the potassium level and the pH also may be in the abnormal range. The chloride measurement is not used as an independent test, but is interpreted together with the other electrolyte tests.

• The monitoring and recording of intake and output are important nursing assessments. Outputs include measurement of drainage (fistula, vomitus, gastric suction, urine) and inputs, include recording oral and intravenous intake.

▽ **Nursing Response to Critical Values**

A severe elevation or loss of chloride indicates serious fluid and electrolyte imbalance. The physician must be notified immediately. Specific medical treatment and nursing intervention depend on the cause of the problem, but immediate action will be taken to restore the electrolyte balance.

Cholangiography, CT

See Computed Tomography on p. 215

Cholangiography, MR

See Magnetic Resonance Imaging on p. 436

Cholangiography, Percutaneous Transhepatic

Also called: (PTC); Transhepatic Cholangiography

SPECIMEN OR TYPE OF TEST: Radiography

PURPOSE OF THE TEST

Percutaneous transhepatic cholangiography is used to demonstrate biliary anatomy in conditions of biliary tract obstruction. It may also be the first step in procedures to insert a drainage catheter to remove infected bile and treat obstructive jaundice.

BASICS THE NURSE NEEDS TO KNOW

When obstructive jaundice is present and ultrasound has demonstrated dilated biliary ducts, the site of the obstruction may be in the intrahepatic or extrahepatic ducts. The usual causes of obstruction are gallstones, tumor, or parasites. If endoscopic cholangiography is incomplete or cannot be performed, this procedure can be used to visualize the biliary tract and the location of the obstruction. Contrast medium is instilled into the biliary tree via the needle that has been inserted into a hepatic duct of the liver. Fluoroscopy is used to assist the physician in the placement of the needle and imaging of obstruction in the biliary ductal system.

REFERENCE VALUES   **The biliary ducts are patent and demonstrate normal anatomic structure.**

HOW THE TEST IS DONE

Percutaneous transhepatic cholangiography is performed in a radiology room equipped with fluoroscopy. The patient is placed on the fluoroscopy table and sedated with heavy conscious sedation or general anesthesia. The skin is prepared, draped, and anesthetized locally. The site of the needle insertion is at the lower right aspect of the rib cage at or near the mid axillary line. A special "skinny" needle is used.

The physician inserts the needle through the skin and into the liver until the tip is well into one of the larger hepatic ducts (Figure 31). When excess bile has dilated the ducts, the bile is removed and a specimen is sent to the laboratory for culture and cytologic analysis. Contrast medium is injected slowly into the ducts until the entire biliary tree is filled with the contrast medium. Using fluoroscopy, the physician is able to visualize the needle placement, the gradual aspiration of bile, and injection of contrast medium.

The tilt table used to move the patient into various positions to promote gravitational flow of the contrast medium. Multiple x-ray images are taken until the total biliary tree is visualized.

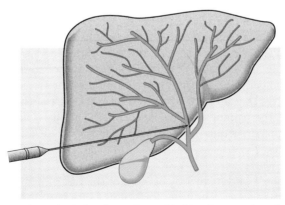

Figure 31. Percutaneous transhepatic cholangiography. Guided by ultrasound on fluoroscopy, the aspirating needle is passed through the patient's skin and liver tissue until the tip penetrates one of the hepatic bile ducts. Radiopaque medium is then instilled into the biliary tree to enhance radiographic imaging.

At the end of the procedure, contrast medium is aspirated from the biliary ducts and the dilated ducts are decompressed. At this time, a biliary catheter may be inserted to establish biliary drainage for a prolonged period.

SIGNIFICANCE OF TEST RESULTS

Abnormal Values

Biliary stone
Malignancy
Hilar cyst
Sclerosing cholangitis

INTERFERING FACTORS

- Uncooperative patient
- Massive ascites
- Gas in the intestinal tract
- Failure to maintain a nothing-by-mouth status
- Bleeding abnormalities
- Sepsis, peritonitis
- Allergy to contrast medium

NURSING CARE

Pretest

- Question the patient about any hypersensitivity reaction during a previous radiology procedure that used contrast medium.
- An informed consent form must be signed and entered in the patient's record.
- To prevent sepsis, intravenous antibiotics are started 1 hour before the procedure and continued into the posttest period.

○ *Patient Teaching.* Instruct the patient to take a prescribed laxative on the night before the test. A cleansing enema is done on the morning of the test. The patient discontinues all food and oral fluids for 12 hours before the test. Additional pretest instructions relate to the procedure itself. This procedure is quite painful. The patient is reassured that pain control will be provided. Either intravenous sedation or a general anesthetic will be used.

- The nurse assesses and records baseline vital signs, including blood pressure, pulse, and respirations and temperature. Any elevation of temperature is reported to the physician and radiologist because sepsis and peritonitis are absolute contraindications to performing the procedure.
- The nurse also ensures that a recent prothrombin time, partial thromboplastin time, and platelet count are in the patient's record. Poor clotting ability is an absolute contraindication to performing this procedure. The nurse notifies the physician and radiologist of these abnormal test values.

Posttest

- Take vital signs regularly and frequently because of the risk of hemorrhage or hypotension. Generally, the pattern is every 15 minutes for 1 hour, every hour for 4 hours thereafter, until the patient is stable. Take the temperature initially and every 4 hours thereafter because of the risk of sepsis and cholangitis.

- Place the patient on his or her right side, with a pillow or sandbag pressed against the lower ribs and abdomen. The gentle pressure and immobility help to promote clotting. Bed rest is maintained for 6 hours after the procedure. Because hemorrhage or biliary leakage could require surgery, nothing-by-mouth status is maintained until the patient is stable.
- The nurse observes the lower right side of the rib cage for signs of bleeding, hematoma formation, ecchymosis, or leakage of bile onto the skin. Some small leakage of blood is expected.

◆ **Nursing Response to Complications**

Bleeding complications can begin during or after the procedure is completed and may require emergency surgery to correct or control. The complications of bleeding, sepsis, cholangitis, and peritonitis tend to appear within hours after completion of the procedure.

Bleeding. In the assessment for bleeding, the nurse assesses for signs of shock, including hypotension, tachycardia, dyspnea, pallor, and *diaphoresis* (cold, sweaty skin). The abdomen may be distended and painful. Localized ecchymosis (bruising) would appear on the lower right lateral ribs or on the side of the abdomen just below the ribs.

Cholangitis and sepsis. Cholangitis (infection in the biliary tree) and *sepsis* (infection in the blood and other tissues) can cause a rapid rise of temperature, with shaking chills. In addition to monitoring the temperature and vital signs, the nurse should also review posttest laboratory reports for an abnormally elevated white blood count and abnormal liver function studies (particularly, elevations of the ALT and AST values).

Peritonitis. Infected bile can leak into the peritoneal cavity and cause acute peritonitis. The nurse takes vital signs, noting pertinent changes associated with shock and infection. These include hypotension, tachycardia, dyspnea, and fever. Using the technique of light palpation, assessment reveals that the abdomen is distended and boardlike. The patient also experiences acute abdominal pain.

Cholesterol, Serum

See Lipid Profile on p. 417.

Chorionic Gonadotropin, Human

Also called: Human Chorionic Gonadotrophin (hCG); ß Human Chorionic Gonadotrophin (ß-hCG)

SPECIMEN OR TYPE OF TEST: Serum, urine

PURPOSE OF THE TEST

The serum and urine tests are used to detect pregnancy and, as part of multiple marker testing, are used to identify Down syndrome in the first and second trimesters of pregnancy. The serum test (ß-hCG) is also used to help confirm the diagnosis of a trophoblastic or germ cell tumor and is a tumor marker for monitoring the patient after treatment by surgical removal of the tumor or chemotherapy.

C

BASICS THE NURSE NEEDS TO KNOW

Human chorionic gonadotropin (hCG) is a hormone normally produced by the developing placenta. In the normal, nonpregnant person, only a trace amount of this hormone is found in the blood. In abnormal conditions, the hormone is produced by some germ cell malignancies and malignancy of other organs.

Pregnancy

The measurement of the serum value detects a normal pregnancy within 2 to 3 weeks after fertilization or 4 to 5 weeks after the last menstrual period. During the early part of a normal pregnancy, the amount of hCG in the blood rises dramatically. The level generally peaks in the seventh to 10th week of gestation. Very high values suggest a multiple pregnancy. In ectopic pregnancy, however, the secretion of hCG is much lower and does not progress in the same pattern.

If urine is used to identify pregnancy, the test result is positive in 10 to 14 weeks after the first missed period. The urine test may be used when a teratogenic medication or treatment such as x-ray, chemotherapy, or radiotherapy must be given to a young, sexually active female patient. The test can screen for an unknown pregnancy before treatment begins or to help determine the cause of pelvic pain. Home pregnancy tests analyze the hCG level in the urine, but use a different method of analysis. Pregnancy is detected at an earlier stage—1 week after implantation or 4 to 5 days before the first missed period.

Screening for Down Syndrome

Pregnant women can now be tested for fetal Down syndrome in the first trimester (11th to 14th week). The recommended tests are interpreted in combination to provide more accurate assessment of the condition of the fetus. This combined first-trimester screen includes human chorionic gonadotrophin, pregnancy-associated plasma protein-A (see p. 514), and nuchal translucency imaging by ultrasound (see Genetic Sonogram, p. 328).

The screening for Down syndrome can also be done early in the second trimester (15th to 22nd week), using the recommended quadruple-marker screening test (Quad test). This combination of serum tests consist of alpha-fetoprotein, human chorionic gonadotrophin, unconjugated estriol, and inhibin A. When Down syndrome affects the fetus, the quadruple-marker screening test demonstrates characteristic changes. The alpha-fetoprotein result is 25% lower than normal, and the unconjugated estriol result is 30% lower than normal. Both hCG and inhibin A rise to twice the normal value. The quadruple-marker screening test detects 81% of fetal Down syndrome pregnancies, with a 7% false-positive rate of error (Peterson, 2006). Because they are screening tests, they are not considered diagnostic of Down syndrome. Further diagnostic testing with ultrasound and possible chorionic villus sampling or amniocentesis is needed to confirm the diagnosis. The recommended screening tests for Down syndrome are now offered routinely to pregnant women of all ages.

Tumor Marker

Benign or malignant trophoblastic disease and germ cell tumors are usually associated with very high levels of ß-hCG. After surgical removal of the tumor, the serum level recedes and returns to normal within 8 to 12 weeks. Because the ß subunit hCG is a tumor marker, the serum level continues to be monitored monthly for 1 year. A persistent or recurrent elevation of the serum value indicates an invasive malignancy with the need for additional diagnostic testing and treatment.

REFERENCE VALUES	Serum: Negative

Male and nonpregnant female: <5 mU/mL *or* SI: <5 IU/L
Pregnant female:
2 weeks of gestation or 4 weeks after the last menstrual period:
  5-50 mU/mL *or* SI: 5-50 IU/L
4 weeks of gestation or 6 weeks after the last menstrual period:
  10,000-80,000 mU/mL *or* SI: 10,000-80,000 IU/L
13-24 weeks of gestation *or* 15-26 weeks after the last menstrual
  period: 5,000-80,000 mU/mL *or* SI: 5000-80,000 IU/L
ß subunit hCG (ß-hCG) <5 ng/mL *or* SI: 5 IU/L
Urine: Negative

HOW THE TEST IS DONE

Serum: Venipuncture is performed to obtain a sample of venous blood.
Urine: A clean plastic container is used to collect a first voided morning specimen of urine.

SIGNIFICANCE OF TEST RESULTS

Elevated Values
Pregnancy
Down syndrome in the fetus
Hydatidiform mole
Choriocarcinoma
Ovarian-testicular cancer
Metastatic cancer

Decreased Values
Threatened abortion
Ectopic pregnancy

INTERFERING FACTORS
• Recent radioactive isotope scan

NURSING CARE

Nursing actions are similar to those used in other venipuncture procedures (see Chapter 2), with the following additional measures.
Pretest
Serum
• It is preferable to schedule this test for before or at least 7 days after a nuclear scan, because the radioisotopes of the scan would interfere with the laboratory method of analysis.
Urine
○ *Patient Teaching.* Instruct the patient to collect a single specimen of urine in the laboratory collection container. The urine should be from the first voided morning specimen, collected on arising from sleep. This urine sample is more concentrated and produces the most accurate result.

Continued

C

Posttest

- On the laboratory requisition, the nurse includes the date of the female patient's last menstrual period. This information is used to help determine whether the results are within normal limits.

Chorionic Villus Sampling and Prenatal Genetic Testing

Also called: CVS

SPECIMEN OR TYPE OF TEST: Placental Tissue

PURPOSE OF THE TEST

The procedure is used to obtain a small sample of chorionic villus tissue of the placenta. The analysis of the tissue identifies genetic abnormalities of the fetus.

BASICS THE NURSE NEEDS TO KNOW

The genetic material of the placenta is exactly the same as the genetic makeup of the fetus. The genetic analysis of the placental tissue reveals genetic fetal abnormality at a very early stage of the pregnancy. When it is needed, the chorionic villus sampling is done in the 10th to 12th week of gestation, approximately 4 to 6 weeks earlier than the more traditional procedure of amniocentesis. When information of genetic abnormality in the fetus becomes known at an early date, termination of the pregnancy in the first trimester is possible. A first-trimester abortion is safer and less traumatic emotionally for the woman.

There are several reasons why chorionic villus sampling may be helpful. The abnormal triple marker screening tests of nuchal translucency (p. 328), chorionic gonadotrophin (p. 193), and pregnancy-associated plasma protein A (p. 514), can indicate an abnormal fetus, Down syndrome, and other abnormalities. Chorionic villus sampling can confirm or exclude the fetal diagnosis. In addition, the procedure is used when both reproductive partners are known carriers of genetic mutations that can produce offspring with the inherited disease. Chorionic villus sampling is also useful for the couple who already had a child with an inherited genetic disorder or multiple congenital abnormalities.

REFERENCE VALUES   There is no evidence of genetic mutations of the fetal trophoblast tissue; the molecular DNA of the fetus is normal.

HOW THE TEST IS DONE

Guided by ultrasound, the physician uses a catheter (transcervical approach) or spinal needle (transabdominal approach) to penetrate the placenta (Figure 32). Either the needle and syringe or a biopsy forceps is used to obtain a sample of placental tissue. The tissue is placed in a sterile tube or container with transport medium for delivery to the laboratory. DNA analysis using gene probes is available to detect various prenatal genetic disorders.

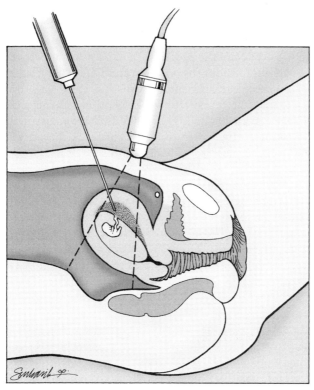

Figure 32. **Chorionic villus sampling, transabdominal approach.** With ultrasound guidance for visualization, the abdomen, uterus, and placenta are penetrated by a needle. Aspiration of a small sample of placental tissue is obtained. (From Gabbe SG, Niebyl JR, Simpson JL: *Obstetrics: Normal and problem pregnancies,* ed 5, Philadelphia, 2007, Churchill Livingstone.)

SIGNIFICANCE OF TEST RESULTS

Abnormal Findings

Genetic mutations of the fetus:
  Down syndrome
  Hemoglobinopathies
  Hemophilia A and B
  Duchenne's muscular dystrophy
  Cystic fibrosis
  Skeletal disorders
  Various metabolic disorders

INTERFERING FACTORS

- Failure to aspirate placental cells
- Contamination of the specimen

C

NURSING CARE

Pretest

- After the physician has explained the procedure and all other appropriate information, the patient must sign a consent form for the procedure and the genetic analysis of the specimen. The consent form is entered in the patient's record.
- The nurse provides emotional support to the patient. Often the patient is apprehensive about the results of the genetic analysis. There may be a strong desire for a good pregnancy outcome, but it is tempered by anxiety or fear. The fetus may have a serious inherited disorder that would negatively affect its life or health.

During the Test

- Depending on the approach that is used, the nurse assists the physician with the antimicrobial cleansing of the abdomen or vaginal canal and surface of the cervix. This helps reduce bacteria that could contaminate the specimen or infect the uterine cavity.
- The specimen and the laboratory requisition form must have the appropriate patient identification and the source of the tissue. The request form should also include the maternal age, gestational age (as determined by ultrasound), and relevant patient history (number of pregnancies, miscarriages). In addition, a history of recent maternal medications, viral infections, or blood transfusions is included.

Posttest

- If bleeding from the vagina or at the abdominal puncture site happens, it is likely to occur very soon after the procedure is completed. The nurse observes for this complication and notifies the physician immediately.
- If the mother has an Rh negative blood type, she is given an injection of immune globulin (RhoGAM). The CVS procedure can cause some mixing of the fetal and maternal blood. If the fetus is Rh positive and the mother Rh negative, a mixing of the two blood types would result in an antigen-antibody response that affects the fetal red blood cells. The maternal injection of immune globulin prevents isoimmunization (the production of the antibodies).
- The patient or the couple will return to the physician for the results of the genetic analysis of the fetus and discussion of the findings.

○ *Patient Teaching.* In discharge teaching, the nurse instructs the patient to notify the physician of any unusual bleeding or cramping sensations, leakage of amniotic fluid, or fever.

◆ **Nursing Response to Complications**

For this procedure, the complication rate of fetal loss is approximately 1%. The complications that can occur include bleeding, rupture of the membranes, chorioamnionitis (infection), and miscarriage.

   Bleeding, ruptured membranes, infection or onset of labor. If the patient returns to the physician or specialized center with procedure-related health concerns, the nurse interviews the patient quickly and carefully to determine the nature of the problem. The nurse asks the patient to describe bleeding, spotting, or leakage of fluid, including duration and amount. If the patient has cramping or pelvic pain, the nurse asks the patient to describe the sensation, including the intensity, frequency, and duration. Vital signs, including temperature, are also taken and the physician is notified immediately of the assessment findings.

Clonidine Suppression Test

See Catecholamines, Plasma on p. 180.

Coagulation Inhibitors

Includes: Antithrombin; Protein C; Protein S

SPECIMEN OR TYPE OF TEST: Plasma

PURPOSE OF THE TEST

The three tests are used to investigate the underlying cause of a thrombus, particularly in young adults or in patients who have a family history of thrombus formation. These tests also are used to assess the cause of a hypercoagulable state and a fibrinolytic state. Antithrombin is used to evaluate the response to heparin or to investigate the cause of heparin failure.

BASICS THE NURSE NEEDS TO KNOW

The regulation of the coagulation cascade consists of a balance between the activation and the inhibition of coagulation factors. Antithrombin, protein C, and protein S all are natural inhibitors of coagulation and they promote thrombolysis. With deficiencies of one or more of these coagulation inhibitors, thrombus formation will occur. The reference values vary according to the method of analysis that is used.

Antithrombin

Antithrombin is a primary inhibitor of thrombin and several factors in the coagulation cascade. The deficiency of antithrombin can result in the formation of recurrent or extensive thrombus formation or a thromboembolic disorder. The disorder can be hereditary or caused by illness, as disseminated intravascular coagulation (DIC) or liver disease. When the amount of antithrombin is adequate, the anticoagulant action of heparin is increased. With low or inadequate levels of antithrombin, patients can experience a resistance to heparin, but they respond to anticoagulant therapy with warfarin sodium (Coumadin).

Protein C

Protein C is synthesized by the liver and is a natural inhibitor of coagulation. Its actions delay or reduce thrombus formation and help to dissolve the thrombus that has already formed. Extensive or recurrent thrombus formation occurs with decreased levels of protein C. When the cause is hereditary, homozygous protein C deficiency usually results in death from massive clot formation in infancy. Heterozygous protein C deficiency is less severe. These patients often experience thrombus formation in adulthood in the form of a deep vein thrombosis, thrombophlebitis, pulmonary embolus, or a hypercoagulable state. Acquired deficiency is associated with the decreased synthesis of protein C in liver disease.

Protein S

Like protein C, protein S is a vitamin K-dependent coagulation protein that is synthesized by the liver. It is a cofactor of protein C, accelerating and enhancing the effect of protein C. In combination, proteins C and S inhibit the formation of a thrombus. The patient who has a deficiency of protein S also has the tendency to form recurrent thrombi in the form of a deep vein thrombosis, thrombus, embolus, or hypercoagulable state. The condition may be of hereditary or acquired origin.

REFERENCE VALUES

Antithrombin
21-30 mg/dL *or* SI: 210-300 mg/L
80%-120% of normal activity *or* SI: 0.80-1.20 (fraction of normal activity)

Protein C
70%-140% of normal activity *or* SI: 0.70-1.40 (fraction of normal activity)

Protein S
65%-140% of normal concentration *or* SI: 0.65-1.40 (fraction of normal concentration)

HOW THE TEST IS DONE

Venipuncture is performed to collect samples of venous blood. Alternatively, a heelstick puncture may be used to collect capillary blood.

SIGNIFICANCE OF TEST RESULTS

Decreased Values
Antithrombin
Congenital deficiency
DIC
Nephrotic syndrome
Pregnancy or postpartum condition
Liver transplant
Hepatectomy
Cirrhosis
Chronic liver failure
Proteins C and S
Congenital deficiency
DIC
Cirrhosis

INTERFERING FACTORS

- Hemolysis
- Coagulation of the specimen
- Warming of the specimen
- Heparin
- Time delay in analysis of the specimen

NURSING CARE

Nursing actions are similar to those used in other venipuncture procedures (see Chapter 2), with the following additional measures.

Pretest

- The nurse schedules the test 2 to 4 weeks after anticoagulation therapy has been discontinued. This is because warfarin (Coumadin) therapy lowers the patient's protein C value and may increase the antithrombin value. Heparin can cause erroneous results for the antithrombin and protein C tests.
- If the patient is currently receiving anticoagulant therapy, the nurse includes the name and dosage of the drug on the requisition form.

During the Test

- The blood is not collected from the arm with an intravenous line or a saline lock device. The heparin flush procedure that is used to keep a venous catheter patent would contaminate the specimen and cause erroneous test results.

Posttest

- The antithrombin tube is placed on ice immediately and all specimens are transported to the laboratory promptly.

Colonoscopy

Includes: Endoscopic Ultrasound (EUS), Lower Panendoscopy, CT Colonography

SPECIMEN OR TYPE OF TEST: Endoscopy or computed tomography

PURPOSE OF THE TEST

The purposes of a colonoscopy by endoscopic method are to perform a routine screening of the colon for detection of polyps and cancer and to investigate the cause of chronic diarrhea and other gastrointestinal complaints related to the colon. Colonoscopy may be done to further investigate an abnormal result of a fecal occult blood test, barium enema, or sigmoidoscopy. It may be used to locate and evaluate the colon pathology before surgical intervention. The purpose of lower panendoscopy is to examine the terminal ileum, particularly for sources of inflammation and bleeding. The purpose of the CT colonography is to image the colon, examining for polyps or tumor.

BASICS THE NURSE NEEDS TO KNOW

Colorectal cancer is the second leading cause of cancer death in the United States. There is evidence that polyps grow slowly and some eventually become malignant. Colorectal cancer also may be present in the colon or rectal area, and it grows slowly. Early detection and removal of a precancerous or cancerous growth provides for a high rate of survival. Late detection and late-stage cancer is associated with a much lower cure rate and lower survival rate. Many major health organizations now recommend routine screening for colorectal cancer. Colonoscopy is the most thorough and accurate method for colorectal screening.

C

Colonoscopy

Colonoscopy is performed with a flexible fiberoptic endoscope. This instrument enables the physician to insert the endoscope through the entire length of the colon, and view the walls of the lumen. The flexibility of the instrument allows it to curve around the flexed areas of the colon (sigmoid, splenic, and hepatic flexures) without interrupting the viewing or damaging the tissue of the colon walls (Figure 33). The instrument provides light, focus, flexibility for positioning, and special channels for instillation of gas or air, cautery, suctioning, removal of polyps, and the taking of biopsy specimens. The colon must be completely clean, without fecal material that would obstruct the view. Almost all patients require conscious sedation and narcotic medications to tolerate the procedure comfortably.

Endoscopic Ultrasound

An ultrasound probe is placed on the tip of the endoscope. During the examination, the ultrasound can provide sonograph images of the tissue layers beneath the mucosal lining of the lumen and beyond the colon into the surrounding tissues and lymph nodes. Images of hidden tumor can be detected to a depth of 3 to 4 inches beyond the mucosal surface. This imaging ability is very useful in presurgical evaluation, in staging of the colorectal malignancy, and in determining the depth of a rectal fistula.

Lower Panendoscopy

This procedure is the same as an endoscopic colonoscopy, but proceeds farther to enter and explore the terminal ileum. It is used primarily to explore the cause and extent of inflammatory illness of the colon and ileum. It is possible to pass the instrument tip of the colonoscope through the ileocecal valve and into the distal ileum for a distance of 8 to 10 inches (20 to 30 cm).

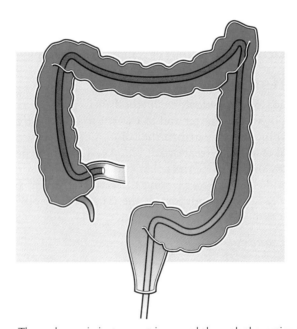

Figure 33. Colonoscopy. The endoscopic instrument is passed through the entire colon. As needed, the tip of the endoscope can be passed into the distal segment of the ileum. Examination is performed as the endoscope is slowly withdrawn. The examination is used to identify sites of bleeding, inflammation, and abnormal tissue, including polyps and tumors. Biopsy samples are taken as needed.

CT-Colonography

This is the newest method of examining the lumen of the colon. It is sometimes called virtual colonoscopy because it uses an abdominal CT scan to image the colon, searching for polyps and bowel cancer. With the advances in CT, contrast medium, and the use of carbon dioxide to insufflate the colon, the imaging of the lumen is quite clear (Poulios & Beaulieu, 2010).

CT colonography is noninvasive, so it has the advantage of not requiring conscious sedation of the patient. There is no risk of a complication of perforation of the bowel, a potential problem with colonoscopy. CT colonography can image the colon when an obstruction prevents the passage of an endoscope. Compared with the colonoscopy, CT-colonography is faster, painless, noninvasive, and easily tolerated. The patient does not lose a day of work recovering from a lengthy procedure and the sedation that is used with colonoscopy.

The disadvantages of CT colonography is that small-sized polyps are difficult to detect. Additionally, when abnormality of colon tissue is encountered, specimens or removal of polyps cannot be done. Although this test is noninvasive, computed tomography does increase the individual's lifetime cumulative radiation risk (US Preventive Services Task Force, 2008).

REFERENCE VALUES   No abnormalities of colon tissue are observed.

HOW THE TEST IS DONE

Colonoscopy and Lower Panendoscopy

A complete bowel preparation is done by the patient to empty the colon of all feces. Almost all patients have the procedure done after receiving conscious sedation. Infants and small children generally require general anesthesia. Once sedated or anesthetized, the physician passes the endoscope into the rectum and advances the instrument on through the sigmoid, descending, transverse, and ascending colon. The colonoscopy procedure reaches the cecum; the lower panendoscopy procedure continues the advance of the endoscope into the terminal part of the ileum. As the instrument is withdrawn slowly, the physician examines all parts of the lumen of the colon and biopsy samples are taken, as needed.

CT Colonoscopy

A complete bowel preparation is done by the patient to empty the colon of all feces. At the beginning of the procedure, the colon is insufflated with carbon dioxide or room air. This distends the walls of the colon and enhances the imaging results. A CT scan of the abdomen is used for imaging of the colon, without any need for pain medication or sedation of the patient.

SIGNIFICANCE OF TEST RESULTS

Polyps in the colon
Colorectal cancer
Ulcerative colitis
Colitis (radiation, ischemia, infection)
Lower intestinal bleeding
Diverticulitis
Crohn's disease

INTERFERING FACTORS

- Poor bowel preparation
- Uncooperative patient behavior
- Retained barium
- Failure to maintain pretest dietary restrictions
- Pregnancy
- Acute medical conditions such as a recent heart attack, toxic colitis, peritonitis, and others

NURSING CARE

Health Promotion.
The nurse can teach people to begin routine health screening for colorectal cancer. After age 50, the healthy individual is at an increased risk to develop colon cancer. Colonoscopy is one of the available methods to detect colon abnormalities. Screening offers prevention by removing polyps before they become cancerous and detecting tumors before symptoms occur. Early detection of abnormality leads to early intervention, when a cure is still possible.

Screening Recommendations.
The US Preventive Task Force (2008) recommends that colorectal screening can be done by fecal occult blood test, flexible sigmoidoscopy, or colonoscopy. For the average-risk individual, the recommended routine screening schedule for adults should begin at age 50 and continue to age 75. They also recommend against routine screening for colorectal cancer for asymptomatic people aged 76 to 85 because the net benefits are small, and against routine colorectal screening of asymptomatic adults older than 85 because the benefits of screening do not outweigh the harm. The American Cancer Society recommends that asymptomatic adults have a colorectal cancer screening starting at age 50. The screening options are flexible sigmoidoscopy, double contrast barium enema, or computed tomography colonography every 5 years or colonoscopy every 10 years (Wilkins & Reynolds, 2008).

Health Promotion.
There is a need for education of the public as to the benefits of regular screening tests. For many years, people were taught to observe for symptoms of disease and then seek medical advice and a diagnosis. Today, the emphasis is on screening to detect abnormality before the problem is advanced enough to cause symptoms. The educational focus should include "unlearning" old information and learning the new and greatly improved methods of detection, as well as the recommended schedule to perform the diagnostic procedure.

Pretest
- Schedule the colonoscopy before performing any barium studies.
- After the physician has explained the procedure, a consent form must be signed by the patient and the form is entered in the patient's record.

○ *Patient Teaching.* Provide written instructions about bowel cleansing. The nurse emphasizes the importance of performing a complete colon cleansing so that the colonoscopy can be performed completely, safely, and accurately. Because there are several possible bowel cleansing protocols that can be used, the nurse follows the endoscopist's requirements. General guidelines are presented here.

- The patient is instructed to modify his or her food intake before the test. On the evening before the test, this can include no intake of solid food or a light diet for supper. Generally, clear fluids are permitted. The process to evacuate all fecal matter from the colon begins in the late afternoon on the day before the procedure. The patient accomplishes this by completing the prescribed regimen of drinking a large volume of PEG-ELS solution (polyethylene glycol-electrolyte lavage solution) or taking the prescribed amount of magnesium citrate solution, or multiple sodium phosphate tablets. The specific cathartic regimen instructions will be provided to the patient. The bowel begins to empty of feces and watery diarrhea soon after the regimen begins. The bowel is considered to be clear of feces when the patient expels clear, watery fluid. On the morning of the test, some procedures involve taking the remaining amount of cathartic preparation to completely empty the colon of any residual feces and liquids.

- The nurse takes the patient's vital signs and enters the results in the patient's record.
- The nurse and physician provide emotional support to the patient before, during, and after the colonoscopy procedure.

During the Test

- For the colonoscopy, conscious sedation is used. The patient is premedicated with intravenous meperidine (Demerol) or fentanyl (Sublimaze) for analgesia and relaxation. This may be followed by intravenous diazepam (Valium) or intravenous midazolam (Versed). Because these drugs can cause apnea, respiratory depression, or cardiac arrest, the medications are administered very slowly, over a period of 5 minutes. Naloxone (Narcan) must be kept on hand to reverse the respiratory depression of meperidine or fentanyl, but it is ineffective against diazepam.
- Oxygen by nasal cannula increases the patient's oxygen reserves and helps prevent hypoxia from the effects of intravenous sedation. The nurse monitors the vital signs at frequent intervals throughout the procedure. Automated blood pressure, pulse oximetry, and cardiac monitoring may be used for all endoscopy patients or for selected patients who are more vulnerable, including the elderly or those with a history of cardiac disease.
- The nurse and physician also monitor for the vasovagal reflex that can occur during the procedure. Atropine sulfate is kept on hand to reverse sudden bradycardia.
- The nurse provides comfort and emotional support to help promote relaxation. As the physician insufflates and manipulates the endoscope, the patient may become uncomfortable and restless, requiring more medication.
- When a biopsy is done, the nurse assists with the collection of tissue specimen. The tissue is placed in a sterile container with fixative solution. The container label has the patient's name, the procedure and type of tissue, and the time and date of collection. The laboratory request form contains this same information and also includes the patient's identification number and the name of the physician. The specimen is sent to the laboratory as soon as the procedure is completed.

Posttest

- Vital signs are monitored every 15 minutes or the automated monitoring is continued until the patient is stable. The nurse checks the rectal area for signs of blood. As soon as the patient is more responsive, food and fluid intake can resume. On discharge from the ambulatory care setting, the patient must be accompanied by a responsible person who will take the patient home. Because of the effects of the intravenous sedation, the patient cannot drive the car for 8 to 12 hours, until thinking is clear and memory is restored.
- Infection control measures regarding the manual cleaning and disinfecting of the endoscope after every procedure are absolutely essential to prevent transmission of infection

Continued

NURSING CARE—cont'd

from one patient to another. Standardized guidelines from various gastroenterology professional organizations provide current protocols for infection control. Because of trained personnel who follow the protocol carefully and consistently, endoscopic transmission of infection is extremely rare (Greenwald, 2007).

◆ **Nursing Response to Complications**

The overall risk of complication from colonoscopy is very low. The two complications are bleeding and perforation of the colon. If complications occur, the nurse must notify the physician of abnormal assessment findings.

Bleeding. The nurse observes the rectal area for signs of bleeding. The amount of visible blood loss is estimated and vital signs are taken. The physician is notified of the bleeding.

Perforation. If the colon is perforated, the patient would complain of malaise and persistent abdominal pain. On palpation of the abdomen, the nurse's findings would include distention and tenderness. An elevated temperature and elevated white blood count are early signs of infection in the peritoneal cavity.

Colposcopy

SPECIMEN OR TYPE OF TEST: Endoscopy, Biopsy

PURPOSE OF THE TEST

Colposcopy is performed to further evaluate an abnormal Pap smear, to monitor for precancerous abnormalities, or to evaluate a lesion of the vagina, cervix, and genitalia.

BASICS THE NURSE NEEDS TO KNOW

The colposcope is a microscope that provides magnification when examining the cervix, vagina, and genitalia for cellular and vascular changes. The procedure is usually indicated to follow-up investigation of an abnormal result of a Papanicolaou (Pap) smear, but also used to investigate unexplained vaginal discharge, pelvic pain, postcoital bleeding, or cervicitis.

When informed of the need for further investigation because of an abnormal result of the Pap smear test, many women experience psychologic reactions of shock, fear, sleep disturbance, disruption of self-image, increased vulnerability, loss of interest in sexual activity, and crying episodes. They may fear the procedure and/or worry about a diagnosis that could be cancer. As many as 45% will be noncompliant in making or keeping their appointment for colposcopic examination. Most of the reported noncompliance occurs with low-income, minority women. (Apgar, Brotzman & Spitzer, 2008).

REFERENCE VALUES   No abnormalities of the vaginal or cervical tissue are noted.

HOW THE TEST IS DONE

A colposcope is inserted into the vagina to provide magnification and illumination of vaginal and cervical tissue. Endocervical curettage is used to scrape the tissue and obtain cell samples of the endocervical canal, and a biopsy forceps is used to obtain samples of abnormal tissue from the cervix. The cell and tissue samples will be sent to the laboratory for histological examination.

SIGNIFICANCE OF TEST RESULTS

Abnormal Values

Atrophic cellular changes
Cervical intraepithelial neoplasia
Papilloma
Condyloma
Infection, inflammation
Cervical erosion
Invasive carcinoma

INTERFERING FACTORS

- Vaginal creams
- Menstruation
- Uncooperative patient
- Acute pelvic inflammatory disease
- Acute inflammatory cervicitis

NURSING CARE

Pretest

- After the physician informs the patient about the procedure, obtain written consent from the patient and enter it into the patient's record.
- Telephone counseling is particularly helpful for those patients who did not keep their appointment for the examination. The counseling approach should include informational needs, the patient's psychological feelings, and any logistical barriers that prevented the patient from keeping the appointment. Addressing these factors can help reduce the patient's anxieties and increase the patient's participation.
- Schedule the procedure for the early part of the menstrual cycle, preferably between days 8 and 12. In this period, the cervical mucus is clear and thin and allows maximum visibility.

○ *Patient Teaching.* The nurse instructs the patient to refrain from the application of any creams or vaginal medications before the test because they obscure the view of the cervix.

During the Test

- The patient changes into a hospital gown. The nurse then assists the patient into a lithotomy position on the examination table, with the patient's legs placed in stirrups.
- As the physician inserts the speculum and colposcope, the nurse instructs the patient to breathe through the mouth to help relax the muscles. As the physician performs endocervical

Continued

| NURSING CARE—cont'd

curettage of the specimen, the patient can feel a "pinch" or a brief cramping sensation. Also, she can hear the snipping sound when the clamp closes and a small piece of biopsy tissue is obtained.

Once the glass slides are prepared with cell scrapings, the nurse can apply the fixative to prevent drying of the cells. If biopsy specimens are taken, place the tissue on hard brown paper or on nonstick gauze (Telfa). Each sample is placed in a separate specimen jar that contains fixative. The nurse ensures that all specimens are labeled appropriately with the patient's name and that the requisition slip also identifies the name, source of the tissue, and date of the procedure.

Posttest

◯ *Patient Teaching.* The patient can resume normal activities and return home or to work after the procedure is completed. It is normal to experience some discomfort for a few hours.

After a biopsy, vaginal discharge and some spotting of blood is expected for 1 to 2 days. Instruct the patient to wear feminine hygiene pads but not to use tampons for the temporary discharge. Sexual intercourse is avoided for 48 hours. Arrange for a follow-up appointment so that the physician can evaluate the healing process and discuss the results of the test.

◆ **Nursing Response to Complications**

Infection can occur 3 to 4 days after the biopsy is done. Instruct the patient to return to the physician if she has a fever, foul-smelling vaginal discharge, and pelvic pain.

Complete Blood Cell Count

Also called: (CBC)

SPECIMEN OR TYPE OF TEST: Whole blood

PURPOSE OF THE TEST

The CBC is used to assess the patient for anemia, infection, inflammation, polycythemia, hemolytic disease, and the effects of ABO incompatibility, leukemia, and dehydration. It is also used to identify the cellular characteristics of the peripheral blood and help manage the side effects of chemotherapy or radiation treatment for cancer.

BASICS THE NURSE NEEDS TO KNOW

The complete blood count (CBC) is a series of different tests used to evaluate the blood and the cellular components of red blood cells, white blood cells, and platelets. Abnormal values require follow-up testing to investigate the underlying cause.

Hemoglobin (Hgb) is the primary component of the red blood cell. An elevated hemoglobin value often is the result of excess production of red blood cells, but it also may be the result of dehydration, which causes a higher concentration of red blood cells in a smaller volume of plasma. A decreased value of hemoglobin is the major indicator of anemia. The decreased value can be caused by a low red blood cell count, by a lack of hemoglobin in the erythrocytes, or by fluid retention, which dilutes a normal number of red cells within a larger than normal volume of plasma. The adult is considered anemic when the hemoglobin for the male is less than 13 g/dL (SI: <130 g/L) and for the female is less than 11 g/dL (SI: <110 g/L).

Hematocrit (Hct) is the ratio of the volume of erythrocytes to that of whole blood and is usually expressed as a percentage value. It used to evaluate blood loss, anemia, polycythemia, and dehydration. The Hct value is elevated when the number of red blood cells increases or when the volume of plasma is reduced. The Hct value falls when there is excessive loss of red blood cells, such as in anemia or after a large blood loss. It can also decrease because of fluid overload that dilutes the concentration of red blood cells. In hemorrhage, the Hct value drops several hours after the bleeding episode. The severity of the drop in value correlates directly with the amount of blood lost.

Red blood cell count, or erythrocyte count, is used to evaluate polycythemia and anemia. An increased red cell count may be the result of hyperactivity of the bone marrow in the manufacture of the erythrocytes or an increase of erythropoietin from renal disease. In dehydration, there is a relative increase of red blood cells, meaning that there are a normal number of erythrocytes, but they are concentrated in decreased plasma volume. A decreased red cell count can occur from excessive loss of the cells, as in hemorrhage, or excessive destruction of red cells, as in hemolytic anemia. The decreased count also may be caused by impaired bone marrow production of the blood cells, such as in bone marrow damage from radiation therapy or chemotherapy in the treatment of cancer.

Red cell indices are used to help diagnose, classify, and evaluate the different types of anemia. The tests measure the size and weight of the average erythrocyte, the amount of hemoglobin in the average erythrocyte, and the average hemoglobin concentration. The tests include the mean corpuscular volume (MCV), mean corpuscular hemoglobin (MCH), the mean corpuscular hemoglobin concentration (MCHC), and the red cell distribution width (RDW). Additional information related to changes in the characteristics of red blood cells can be done by laboratory examination of the peripheral blood smear (see Red Blood Cell Morphology, p. 535).

Mean corpuscular volume calculates the average erythrocyte size. If the MCV value is elevated, the erythrocytes are large, or macrocytic. *Macrocytosis* is defined by a mean corpuscular volume >100 fL (Kaferle & Strzoda, 2009). If the MCV value is decreased, the erythrocytes are small, or microcytic.

Mean corpuscular hemoglobin calculates the weight of the hemoglobin in the average erythrocyte. The MCH value is elevated when the erythrocyte is macrocytic and decreased when the erythrocyte is microcytic.

Mean corpuscular hemoglobin concentration measures the average concentration or percentage of hemoglobin in the average erythrocyte. When the MCHC value is elevated, a high concentration of hemoglobin exists in the erythrocyte, and the cell is hyperchromic. When the value is in a normal range, the red cell is normochromic. When the MCHC value is decreased, a lower concentration of hemoglobin exists, and the erythrocyte is hypochromic.

Red cell distribution width is a numeric calculation of the widths of the erythrocytes. When the RDW value is elevated, the peripheral blood smear is reviewed for *anisocytosis*, a variation in the size of erythrocytes. The presence and amount of anisocytosis is used to estimate the severity of anemia and to differentiate among the microcytic anemias.

White blood cell, or leukocyte, count is the total number of the five types of leukocytes present in the blood. The leukocyte count is a general indicator of infection, tissue necrosis, inflammation, or bone marrow activity.

Leukocytosis is an elevated number of white blood cells. The elevated value occurs in response to infection and is usually directly proportionate to the degree of bacterial invasion. The elevated value also may be caused by necrosis of tissue or malignancy of the bone marrow. A white blood cell count of 11,000 to 17,000 cells (11 to 17 $\times$ 10^3/μL or SI: 11 to 17 $\times$ 10^9/L) is considered to be a mild to moderate leukocytosis. When the white blood cell count falls to less than normal limits, it is called *leukopenia*. Mild leukopenia is indicated by a white blood cell count of 3000 to 5000 cells (3 to 5 $\times$ 10^3/μL or SI: 3 to 5 $\times$ 10^9/L). Decreases in the leukocyte count usually are a result of bone marrow depression or a particular infection that has exhausted the supply of neutrophils and bone marrow reserves. Specific diagnostic information is obtained by the WBC differential count that identifies the numbers of each type of white blood cell (see White Blood Cell Differential Count, p. 640).

Platelet count is used to assess the ability of the bone marrow to produce platelets and to identify the destruction or loss of platelets in the circulation. It also is used to evaluate the untoward effects of chemotherapy or radiation treatment. Platelets function to initiate the process of coagulation. When there is a nick or opening in a blood vessel, platelets quickly aggregate, adhere to the endothelial surface of the blood vessel, and plug the opening. As additional platelets and clotting factors arrive, the clot becomes firm and seals off the opening effectively.

Thrombocytosis is an excess number of platelets (>400,000 cells/μL or SI: >400 $\times$ 10^9/L) in the blood. The condition may occur when platelets are produced at a fast rate in response to injury. This condition rarely causes symptoms and is self-limiting. Thrombocytosis also may be a symptom of myeloproliferative disease, such as chronic myelocytic leukemia. The platelet count rises severely, and potential exists for hemorrhage or thrombosis. *Thrombocytopenia* is a decreased number of platelets (<100,000 cells/μL or SI: <100 $\times$ 10^9/L) in the blood. The patient's clotting ability is seriously compromised and the patient is vulnerable to bleeding, particularly into the skin. The decrease in platelets is often caused by rapid platelet destruction.

Reticulocyte count is used to evaluate erythropoiesis, distinguish among different types of anemia, assess the severity of blood loss, and evaluate the bone marrow response to treatment of anemia. Reticulocytes are immature erythrocytes. Normally, few reticulocytes exist in the circulation in proportion to the number of erythrocytes.

An increase in reticulocytes indicates the ability of the bone marrow to produce erythrocytes. The elevated value is considered a healthy response after a loss of erythrocytes from hemorrhage or hemolysis. It also is a healthy response to anemia or to a reduced amount of hemoglobin in the red blood cells. The reticulocyte count may also rise after treatment for anemia. A decreased reticulocyte count indicates that erythropoiesis is diminished in the bone marrow. The cause may be a lack of stimulation by erythropoietin, a disease that affects the bone marrow function, or a faulty maturation process in the bone marrow.

REFERENCE VALUES

Hemoglobin
Fetal Values: see Percutaneous umblical blood sampling, p. 483.
Cord blood 12.5-20.5 g/dL *or* SI: 125-205 g/L

Neonate
2 weeks 113.4-19.8 g/dL *or* SI: 134-198 g/L
1 month 10.7-17.1 g/dL *or* SI: 107-171 g/L

Infant
2 months 9.4-13 g/dL *or* SI: 94-130 g/L
6 months 11.1-14.1 g/dL *or* SI: 111-141 g/L
1 year 11.3-14.1 g/dL *or* SI: 113-141 g/L

Child
2-5 years 11-14 g/dL *or* SI: 110-140 g/L
9-12 years 12-15 g/dL *or* SI: 120-150 g/L

Adult
Adult Male: 14-18 g/dL *or* SI: 140-180 g/L
Adult Female: 12-15g/dL *or* SI: 120-150g/L

Hematocrit
Fetal Values: see Percutaneous umblical blood sampling, p. 483.
Cord blood: 42-60% *or* SI: 0.42- 0.60 (volume fraction)

Neonate
1 day 61% $\pm$ 7.41% *or* SI: 0.61 $\pm$ 0.07 (volume fraction)
1-2 weeks 54% $\pm$ 8.3% *or* SI: 0.54 $\pm$ 0.08 (volume fraction)

Infant (capillary whole blood values)
5-6 weeks 36% $\pm$ 6.2% *or* SI: 0.36 $\pm$ 0.06 (volume fraction)
10-12 weeks 33% $\pm$ 3.3% *or* SI: 0.33 $\pm$ 0.03 (volume fraction)

Child
1-3 years 34%-48% *or* SI: 0.34-48 (volume fraction)
4-7 years 36%-46% *or* SI: 0.36-46 (volume fraction)
8-13 years 35%-49% *or* SI: 0.35-49 (volume fraction)

Adult
Adult Male: 40%-54% *or* SI: 0.40-0.54 (volume fraction)
Adult Female: 35%-49% *or* SI: 0.35-0.49 (volume fraction)

Red Blood Cell Count
Male: 4.6-6.0 $\times$ 10^6/μL *or* SI: 4.6-6.0 $\times$ 10^{12}/L
Female: 4.0-5.4 $\times$ 10^6 /μ /L *or* SI: 4.0-5.4 $\times$ 10^{12} /L

Red Cell Indices
MCV: 80-100 fL *or* SI: 80-100 fL
MCH: 26-32 pg *or* SI: 26-32 pg
MCHC: 32%-36% *or* SI: 0.32-0.36 (concentration fraction)
RDW-CV: 11.5%-14.5% *or* SI: 0.115-0.145 (number fraction)

Continued

White Blood Cell Count
4.5-11.5 × 10³/μL *or* SI: 4.5-11.5 × 10⁹/L

Platelet Count
150,000-450,000 cells/μL *or* SI: 150-450 × 10⁹/L

Reticulocyte Count
Manual count, Adult: 24,000-84,000 cells/μL *or* SI: 24-84 × 10⁹/L
Manual count, Adult: 0.5-1.5 % (percentage of reticulocytes)
Automated count, 12 yr-Adult: 58,600-146,200 *or* SI: 56.8-146.2 × 10⁹/L
Automated count, 12 yr-Adult: 1.32-4.91 % (percentage of reticulocytes)

▽**Critical Values**

Hemoglobin: <6.0 g/dL *or* >20.0 g/dL *or* SI: <60 g/L *or* >200 g/L
Hematocrit: <18% *or* >54% *or* SI: <0.18 *or* >0.54 (number fraction)
WBC: <2.5 × 10³/μL *or* >50 × 10³/μL *or* SI: 2.5 ×10⁹/L *or* >50 × 10⁹/L
Platelets: <40,000 cells/μL *or* >1,000,000 cells/μL *or* SI: <40 cells × 10⁹/L *or* >1000 cells × 10⁹/L

HOW THE TEST IS DONE

Venipuncture is performed to obtain a sample of venous blood. For infants, the heelstick method and capillary tubes are used. In children, capillary puncture and capillary tubes or special filter paper are used for collection of the blood sample.

SIGNIFICANCE OF TEST RESULTS

Elevated Values
Hemoglobin
Polycythemia
Dehydration
Hematocrit
Polycythemia
Dehydration
Red Blood Cell Count
Polycythemia
Renal tumor
Dehydration
Red Blood Cell Indices
MCV: Alcoholism, pernicious anemia, deficiency of vitamin B_{12} and/or folate, hypothyroidism
MCH: Hereditary spherocytosis
MCHC: Hereditary spherocytosis
RDW: Iron deficiency anemia, pernicious anemia, deficiency of vitamin B_{12}, folate, β-thalassemia major

White Blood Cell Count
Infection
Inflammation
Leukemia
Platelets
Myeloproliferative diseases
Multiple myeloma
Iron deficiency anemia
Hodgkin's disease
Lymphomas
Renal disease
Infection or inflammation
Reticulocytes
Treatment for iron deficiency anemia and pernicious anemia
Hemolytic anemia
Hemorrhage
Chronic blood loss

Decreased Values
Hemoglobin and Hematocrit
Hemorrhage
Anemia
Hemolysis of erythrocytes
Fluid overload
Red Blood Cells
Hemorrhage
Fluid overload
Anemia
Aplastic anemia
Bone marrow depression
Hemolysis of erythrocytes
Red Blood Cell Indices
MCV: Iron deficiency anemia, chronic inflammation, lead poisoning, thalassemia
MCH: Iron deficiency anemia
MCHC: Iron deficiency anemia
White Blood Cells
Aplastic anemia
Bone marrow depression
Pernicious anemia
Some infectious or parasitic diseases
Platelets
Idiopathic thrombocytopenic purpura
Aplastic anemia
Anemias
Disseminated intravascular coagulation
Bone marrow depression

Systemic lupus erythematosus
Uremia
Liver disease
Reticulocytes
Anemias (aplastic, iron deficiency, chronic disease, sideroblastic, pernicious)
Renal disease
Endocrine disease

INTERFERING FACTORS

- Hemolysis or coagulation of the specimen
- Hemodilution

NURSING CARE

Nursing actions are similar to those used in other venipuncture procedures (see Chapter 2), with the following additional measures.

Pretest

- No special measures are needed.

During the Test

- Ensure that the blood is not taken from the hand or arm that has an intravenous line. Hemodilution with intravenous fluids causes a false decrease in the values of some tests.

Posttest

- Assess the puncture site for signs of bleeding or bruising (ecchymosis) of the skin. If the platelet count is decreased, clotting will occur slowly. To promote clotting, the nurse can use sterile gauze to apply pressure to the site or raise the arm above the head while maintaining pressure on the site.

▽ **Nursing Response to Critical Values**

If the test result is in the range of the critical values, the nurse notifies the physician immediately. When the change develops slowly or gradually, the patient may not have immediate abnormal assessment findings. When the result occurs rapidly or is severely decreased, assessment findings are more likely to be abnormal. Further medical investigation is needed to determine the cause of the abnormal value.

Hemoglobin, hematocrit, and red blood cell count. When the hemoglobin, hematocrit, and red blood cell count are severely decreased, nursing assessment findings may include fatigue, pallor, tachycardia, rapid respirations, dyspnea on exertion, and a low blood pressure.

White blood count. For a severely low white blood count (leukopenia), the patient is at risk to develop an infection that can become life threatening. The patient has too few white blood cells to protect against infection or combat one that occurs. The nurse prepares to implement measures that will help protect the patient from acquiring an infection. A severely elevated white blood count (hyperleukocytosis) is a potential emergency situation. Hyperleukocytosis is usually the result of leukemia in the crisis stage. The patient may have a fatal hemorrhage in the lung or brain as leukocytes clump or aggregate in small blood vessels. The nurse assesses for any change in vital signs, dyspnea, or levels of consciousness and for other signs of a stroke.

Platelets. When the platelet value shows a severe depletion, the patient is at risk to develop a spontaneous hemorrhage. The nurse assesses for bruising or bleeding in the skin, as evidenced by petechiae or ecchymosis, or bleeding from the nose or gums of the mouth (gingivae). More seriously, a hemorrhage in the brain can occur, causing a stroke. The nurse assesses for any change in the patient's level of consciousness or loss of speech, motor, or sensory function. When the platelet count rises severely, the patient is at risk of developing a thrombosis (clot) that can form anywhere, including in the blood vessels of the heart, brain, fingers, toes, or abdominal organs. The nurse assesses for change in vital signs and levels of consciousness, changes in the circulation to the extremities, or the patient's complaint of pain.

Computed Tomography

Also called: CT Scan, Computerized Axial Tomography, CAT Scan

SPECIMEN OR TYPE OF TEST: Radiography

PURPOSE OF THE TEST

The CT scan provides precise visualization of the structure, size, shape, and density of soft tissue, bone, major blood vessels, and organs of the head and torso. It distinguishes between benign and malignant tissue and is used in the staging of cancerous tumors. In cases of blunt trauma, it provides images of the bones and also the fluid collection at the site of the injury. It can be used to analyze the bone mineral content of the vertebrae and proximal femur in the assessment of osteoporosis. It provides visual guidance in procedures as draining an abscess or performing a biopsy.

BASICS THE NURSE NEEDS TO KNOW

The Imaging Process

CT uses x-rays, a scanner with a gantry ring, and specialized computer software to produce detailed images of the internal organs and tissues. The views are cross-sectional images of the anatomic structures and each individual image is called a *tomographic slice or axial slice*. In the CT scanning process, the patient is on the moving table that advances through the ring of the gantry. At the same time that the patient is moving forward, the x-ray tube rotates around the gantry ring continuously. The photons pass through the body and are received and measured by multiple detectors on the opposite side of the ring (Figure 34). After computerized treatment of the data, the CT scan provides clear and very detailed digital images of the desired slices. The CT images are reviewed for pathologic changes, identifying the size, shape, and structure of the organs, including the positions and spatial relationships to the other nearby tissues.

The newest generation of CT scanners has 64 stationary detectors in the gantry ring; for the future generations of scanners that are already in development, greater numbers of detectors will be used (Frank, Long & Smith, 2007). The imaging is accomplished quickly because of the increased numbers and fixed position of the detectors, thinner axial slices, and other factors. The images are sharp and the patient has less exposure to radiation.

The CT images are usually two-dimensional cross-sections of particular slices. The viewer is facing the patient's image, so the left side of the CT image is the actual right side of the patient. For cross-sectional images, the view is anterior-posterior and the upper portion of the image is anterior unless otherwise stated. The computer also can rotate the image to present different views from various planes. Using the same data of the scan, the computer can create a three-dimensional reconstruction to provide clear detail of a specific tissue abnormality (Figure 35).

C

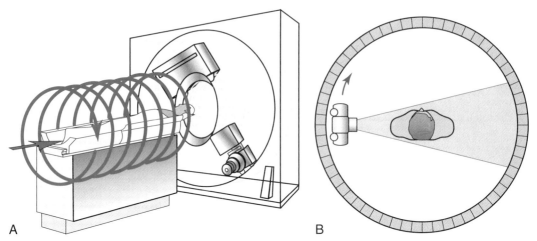

A

B

Figure 34. The scanning process in computed tomography. **A,** As the patient is moved forward into the gantry and the x-ray detector system rotates continuously around the patient, a spiral path of data is obtained. **B,** Inside the gantry, as the x-ray tube circles the patient, the radiation passes through the patient's body and is received by the stationary detectors that surround the patient. (From Frank ED, Long BW, Smith BJ: *Merrill's atlas of radiographic positioning and procedures*, ed 12, St Louis, 2012, Mosby.)

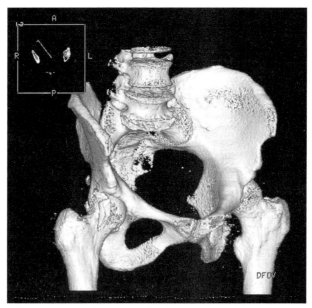

Figure 35. Three-dimensional computed tomography image of a pelvic and acetabular fracture, with displacement. The three-dimensional view enhances accuracy in diagnosis and is useful in surgical planning for the repair of the injury. (From Major NM: *A practical approach to radiology*, Philadelphia, 2006, Saunders.)

Contrast Medium

CT may be done with or without contrast. The contrast medium provides greater clarity and detail in the vasculature, organs, and tissues. Gastrointestinal contrast may be barium, air, or carbon dioxide. The injectable contrast is an iodine-based medium. It is usually a low-osmolarity preparation because that type causes many fewer allergic reactions. The injectable contrast will be excreted from the body by the kidneys.

CT Scan of the Head

The imaging of the head can be done with or without contrast medium. When contrast is used, the brain tissue is imaged more clearly. The CT of the head is often needed in cases of trauma or head injury. A fracture of the skull can be identified and the CT can demonstrate hematoma, swelling, or bleeding within the brain or space between the brain and skull. Because the helical CT examination is so rapid, treatment of life-threatening injury can begin at a much earlier time.

CT of the Brain and Spinal Cord

The CT scan can investigate intracerebral, extracerebral, and spinal lesions. The abnormalities may be congenital, degenerative, inflammatory, vascular, or tumor in origin. In CT of the brain, the initial scanning is done without contrast because a hemorrhage or bleeding may exist. If there is no bleeding, contrast can then be used (see also, Angiography, Cerebral, Carotid, p. 81).

Intracranial lesions that are identified by CT are hydrocephalus and aqueduct stenosis, cerebral atrophy, hemorrhage, hematoma, infarction, and edema of the brain. Tumors within the cranium may be (1) intracerebral and often malignant or (2) extracerebral and probably benign. Extracerebral tumors include meningiomas, acoustic neuromas, epidermoid tumors, dermoid tumors, craniopharyngiomas, and pituitary tumors.

In imaging the spinal cord, the CT scan demonstrates the bony and soft tissue abnormalities that compress the cord and nerve roots. It images a bulge in a disc, a degenerative change, the alignment and structure of the vertebrae, spinal infection, and hypertrophy of the ligaments. Also the diameter of the spinal cord can be measured. CT is often used to confirm spinal stenosis as a cause of spinal cord disorder.

CT of the Chest

The CT scan can be used to diagnose benign or cancerous pulmonary lesions (Figure 36). With some bronchogenic cancers, the CT scan can be used to determine the invasive extent of the cancer into the chest wall, diaphragm, and mediastinum, as well as extrathoracic metastasis.

The CT scan is used to plan surgery or radiation therapy for the patient with cancer of the lung. It may also be useful in the diagnosis of silicosis, asbestosis, lung abscess, and empyema. (See also Angiography, Pulmonary, p. 87.)

CT of the Coronary Arteries

See Coronary Angiography, Computed Tomography, p. 226.

CT of the Abdomen

This procedure provides a view of the bowel wall, mesentery, peritoneum, and organs adjacent to the gastrointestinal tract (Figure 37). CT is used to detect intraabdominal masses, including abscess, tumor, infarct, perforation, obstruction, inflammation, and diverticulitis. It is also useful

C

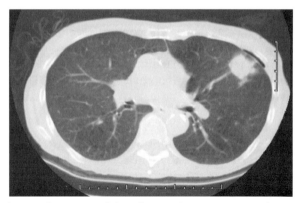

Figure 36. Malignant solitary pulmonary nodule (adenocarcinoma). CT scan demonstrates a mass with ill-defined contour. (From Eisenberg RL, Johnson NM: *Comprehensive radiographic pathology*, ed 4, St Louis, 2007, Mosby.)

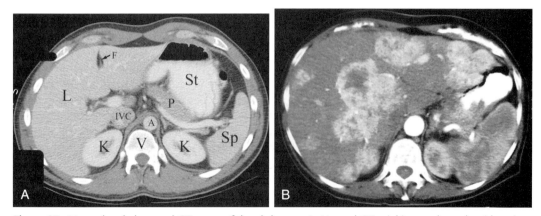

Figure 37. Normal and abnormal CT scans of the abdomen. **A,** Normal CT axial image through midportion of the abdomen, with the anatomical structures identified. A, aorta; F, falciform ligament; IVC, inferior vena cava; K, kidney; L, liver; P, pancreas; Sp, Spleen; St, stomach; V, vertebral body. **B,** Abnormal CT axial image showing an enlarged liver and liver metastases. Intravenous contrast was used in both images. (From Major NM: *A practical approach to radiology*, Philadelphia, 2006, Saunders.)

in detection of metastases and in the staging of abdominal malignancy. CT cholangiography is the preferred method to assess for biliary obstruction when ultrasound results are not effective.

With or without intravenous iodinated contrast, CT of the abdomen can be useful in identifying changes in the pancreas. The CT scan is useful to visualize benign or malignant tumors of the pancreas, diagnose acute or chronic pancreatitis, and locate a pancreatic abscess.

CT of the Kidneys, Ureters, and Bladder

This imaging procedure is known as **intravenous urography** and it replaces the older test called intravenous pyelogram (IVP). Using intravenous contrast medium, the contrast flows through the vascular system and enters the kidneys by the physiologic function of renal filtration. Initially, the glomeruli, renal pelvis of each kidney, and the calyces fill with contrast. Then the contrast flows through the excretory system so that all parts of the urinary system can be imaged by computed tomography. The CT provides images of the renal cancer, cyst, polycystic disease, pyelonephritis, trauma to the kidneys or renal artery, obstruction of the ureter, and hydronephrosis. The bladder also reveals abnormalities, including bladder outlet obstruction, cancer, and bladder rupture. CT without contrast will provide imaging of kidney stones.

Retrograde urography is the procedure that instills contrast medium into the bladder via a catheter. The procedure is done with the assistance of a cystoscope. Contrast medium can be instilled into the ureters, to detect constriction, tumor or cyst, bladder cancer, and cystitis.

CT of the Pelvis

In the evaluation of the female pelvis, CT with intravenous contrast material produces clear, cross-sectional images of the pelvic tissues and organs. The pelvic CT scan is used to observe for pelvic fracture or other damage from trauma. It is often used to determine the extent of malignancy or the source of infection. For these purposes, the scan usually includes the abdomen and the pelvis so that nearby organs, structures, and blood vessels are visualized. Oral and rectal barium contrast material may be administered to opacify the bowel loops. If a pelvic tumor or abscess is located, the CT scan is used to guide the placement of a needle in a percutaneous aspiration biopsy or in percutaneous needle drainage of the purulence.

CT of Bones and Joints

In orthopedics, the CT scan is particularly useful because the bone tissue is dense and absorbs many of the x-ray photons. Thus the image of the bones appears white or bright on the film. The scan gives accurate definition of the structure of the bones and demonstrates subtle pathologic changes, such as the small linear fracture, stenosis of a bony canal, erosion of the bone, or degenerative changes from osteoporosis. It also images problems of subluxation, dislocation, calcification, and cancer of the bone.

Traditional CT also may be used to assess the spinal column, confirming the presence of bony or soft tissue changes that affect the vertebrae or spinal canal. CT detects congenital malformation, bony overgrowth, bone spurs, lumbar stenosis, cervical spondylosis, scoliosis, degenerative changes, a bulging disk, and ligament hypertrophy.

The CT scan is particularly useful in cases of cervical spine trauma with a suspected fracture, subluxation, or dislocation that could result in compression of the spinal cord. It also is very useful in cases of massive or multiple fractures, such as trauma to the pelvis involving the pelvic and hip bones. CT also is used to identify abnormality in the bone due to neoplasm, infection, degenerative disease of the spine, and postsurgical difficulty with a spinal repair.

REFERENCE VALUES   No structural or anatomic abnormalities are noted.

HOW THE TEST IS DONE

The patient is placed on the gantry table and positioned carefully. If intravenous contrast is to be administered, a vein in the antecubital fossa is commonly used. The advancement of the gantry table, the infusion of the contrast, and the timing of the imaging are all computer coordinated so that the imaging occurs when the patient is at the correct location within the gantry ring and the contrast has circulated to the target location.

SIGNIFICANCE OF TEST RESULTS

Abnormal Values
Tumor
Malignancy
Cyst
Stenosis
Thrombus
Embolus
Arteriosclerotic plaque
Calcification
Congenital malformation
Abscess
Inflammation
Fluid collection
Bleeding or hemorrhage
Organ atrophy
Bone fracture

INTERFERING FACTORS
- Jewelry or metal in the CT field
- Patient movement during the imaging
- Pregnancy
- Failure to maintain nothing-by-mouth status (as indicated)
- Previous reaction to contrast medium (with the use of intravenous contrast medium)
- Severe kidney disease (with the use of intravenous contrast medium)

▌NURSING CARE

Pretest
- When iodinated contrast is planned, a blood urea nitrogen (BUN) and creatinine should be done and the results posted in the patient's record. These laboratory tests are needed because the patient must have adequate renal function to eliminate the contrast at the end of the study. Elevated results of these tests indicate that renal function is impaired and the physician must be notified.

○ *Patient Teaching.* If intravenous contrast medium is used, instruct the patient to discontinue all food and fluids for 4 to 8 hours before the test. In gastrointestinal CT imaging, instruct the patient to drink prescribed amounts of liquid contrast on the night before the test and again at timed intervals in the hours before the scan. If the colon is imaged by a CT scan, pretest bowel preparation will be required to cleanse the organ and remove the feces. Just before the scan, a barium enema, and air or carbon dioxide will be instilled in the colon.

- The nurse or technologist explains that the patient will be positioned on a movable table and restrained to prevent movement. The table will move the patient into the scanner, which has a small, air-conditioned chamber, equipped with a microphone. The patient can communicate with the technologist at all times. To help the patient remain motionless during scans of the abdomen or chest, the technologist will instruct the patient to hold his or her breath at intervals. While the scanning is performed, the patient will hear the quiet whirring of the machine and feel the table move further into the chamber, or tilt to achieve different angles of imaging. When no contrast is used, the scanning procedure is painless.

- To help the patient control anxiety or a mild feeling of claustrophobia, the nurse can suggest various diversionary or relaxation techniques. The patient may already have a preferred way to help control anxiety or remain calm. Suggestions can include visual imagery, muscle relaxation, meditation, and prayer.
- After the physician informs the patient about the procedure, obtain written consent from the patient and enter it into the patient's record.

○ *Patient Teaching.* The nurse inquires if the patient has any history of a hypersensitivity reaction during a previous radiograph study. If affirmative, the radiologist is informed. When the contrast is administered, the patient may feel a sensation of warmth, a salty taste, headache, or nausea. These are temporary sensations that will disappear in a few minutes.

- Instruct the patient to remove all clothes, jewelry, and other metal objects. For the procedure, a hospital gown is worn. The patient's blood pressure is taken and the results are entered in the record.
- Sedatives are usually used for the infant or young child, particularly when the scan requires an extended period of immobility.

During the Test

- Instruct the patient to remain motionless while in the scanner and to hold his or her breath when instructed to do so. Keep an emesis basin in a nearby area in case the patient vomits after receiving the contrast medium.

Posttest

- If sedatives were administered, the nurse monitors the vital signs on a regular basis until the patient is responsive and awake.
- If barium was used in a gastrointestinal scan, the nurse explains that the barium will appear as gray material in the feces. It will be eliminated from the body within a day or two. Intravenous contrast medium is excreted in the urine within 24 hours, with no noticeable impact on the patient.

Coombs' Tests, Direct, Indirect

See Antiglobulin Tests, direct, indirect on pages 93-95.

Coronary Angiography; Catheterization, Cardiac

Also called: Angiocardiography; Coronary Arteriography

SPECIMEN OR TYPE OF TEST: Radiography

C

PURPOSE OF THE TEST

A cardiac catheterization is performed to (1) evaluate coronary artery disease with unstable, progressive, or new-onset angina or angina that is not responsive to medical therapy; (2) diagnose atypical chest pain; (3) diagnose complications of myocardial infarction, such as septal rupture and refractory dysrhythmias; (4) diagnose aortic dissection; (5) evaluate the need for coronary artery surgery or angioplasty; (6) assess valvular function; and (7) determine the efficacy of a heart transplant. Rarely, a cardiac catheterization may be carried out to obtain a biopsy specimen.

BASICS THE NURSE NEEDS TO KNOW

Cardiac catheterization is an invasive procedure that permits the assessment of anatomic abnormalities of the heart, as well as the state of the coronary arteries. Cardiac catheterization may assess (1) pressures, oxygen content, and oxygen saturation in the various heart chambers; (2) cardiac output and index; (3) patency of the coronary arteries; and (4) pressure gradients across the valves.

Cardiac catheterization may be a right-sided catheterization, a left-sided catheterization, or both. A right-sided catheterization is performed today in specialized units under the category of hemodynamic monitoring; therefore, this section will focus on left-sided catheterization.

Left-heart cardiac catheterization, because it is invasive, has significant risk. Increasingly, *impedance cardiography* (ICG) is being used to obtain noninvasively many of the parameters obtained by cardiac catheterization. These measurements include cardiac output, left ventricular ejection fraction, stroke volume, left cardiac work indexes, and systemic vascular resistance. ICG obtains hemodynamic data with application of electrodes on the neck and thorax. It measures cardiac flow, not pressure. Very-low-grade electrical stimuli are emitted from electrodes on one side of the body and sensed by the electrodes on the opposite side. The wave form created is interpreted and cardiac values are displayed.

While cardiac catheterization is still the gold standard in diagnosing coronary artery disease, it is invasive. Increasingly, a noninvasive procedure, coronary CT angiography is being used. See Coronary Angiography, Computed Technology on pp. 226-227.

REFERENCE VALUES	**Pressures**
	Right atrium: 2-6 mm Hg
	Neonate: 0-3 mm Hg
	Child: 1-5 mm Hg
	Right ventricle: 20-30/2-8 mm Hg
	Neonate: 30-60/2-5 mm Hg
	Child: 15-30/2-5 mm Hg
	Pulmonary artery pressure: 20-30/8-15 mm Hg
	Neonate: 30-60/2-10 mm Hg
	Child: 15-30/5-10 mm Hg
	Pulmonary artery wedge pressure: 4-12 mm Hg
	Left atrium: 4-12 mm Hg
	Neonate: 1-4 mm Hg
	Child: 5-10 mm Hg
	Left ventricle: 90-140/4-12 mm Hg
	Neonate: 60-100/5-10 mm Hg
	Child: 80-130/10-20 mm Hg

C

Cardiac Output
4-8 L/min

Cardiac Index
2.5-4 L/min
Neonate and child: 3.5-4 L/min

Stroke Index
30-60 mL/beat/min

Ejection Fraction
55%-75%

Oxygen Saturation
75% (right side of heart); 95% (left side of heart)

Oxygen Content
14-15 volume % (right side of heart)
19 volume % (left side of heart)

Oxygen Consumption
250 mL/min

Volume
Left ventricular end-diastolic: 50-90 mL
Left ventricular end-systolic: 14-34 mL
Right ventricular end-diastolic: 70-90 mL
Left atrium: 57-79 mL

Mass
Left ventricular thickness
Male: 12 mm
Female: 9 mm
Left ventricular wall mass
Male: 99 g
Female: 76 g

Wall Motion
Normal

Valve Gradient
None

Valve Orifice Areas
Aortic valve: 0.7 cm^2
Mitral valve: 1 cm^2

HOW THE TEST IS DONE

A left-sided catheterization is performed in a cardiac catheterization laboratory. This laboratory is designed with fluoroscopy, electrocardiographic equipment, and emergency equipment and drugs (code cart). For a left-sided catheterization, the physician must thread a catheter through an artery into the left side of the heart; therefore, arterial access is necessary (usually, the brachial or femoral artery is used). Pressure measurements are obtained in the aorta and left atrium and ventricle. Samples of blood are obtained for oxygen analysis. Cardiac output, stroke volume, and ejection fractions are measured.

When a *coronary angiogram* is included in the catheterization, dye is instilled into the heart to visualize the size of the ventricles, wall motion, and contractility and to identify valvular dysfunction. Pregnancy is a contraindication for the use of a dye.

A *coronary arteriogram* also may be obtained. The catheter is withdrawn from the left ventricle and positioned at the coronary ostia, where small boluses of dye are injected into the coronary arteries while a series of x-ray films are taken.

SIGNIFICANCE OF TEST RESULTS

Cardiac catheterization provides a significant amount of data for analysis, which may support the following diagnoses:

Coronary artery disease (CAD)
Coronary occlusions and degree of blockage
Congenital abnormalities
Septal defects
Shunting
Aneurysms
Valvular defects

INTERFERING FACTORS

- Allergic reactions to contrast medium
- Uncontrolled congestive heart failure
- Dysrhythmias
- Renal insufficiency
- Electrolyte imbalances
- Infection
- Drug toxicity

NURSING CARE

Pretest

○ *Patient Teaching.* The nurse instructs the patient and family about the purpose and procedure for the study. Explain to the patient that the table rotates and that the physician may ask the patient to change positions or cough. Unless instructed tell patient to lie still during the procedure. Explain to the patient that when the dye is given, a feeling of warmth, or flushing, or a metallic taste may be sensed.

- The nurse verifies that an informed consent has been obtained.
- Assist with the precatheterization evaluation: blood tests, including a prothrombin time test and a partial thromboplastin time test; an electrocardiogram (ECG); and chest x-ray film if the procedure will be performed on an outpatient basis.

- Question patient about possible pregnancy.
- Obtain baseline vital signs.
- Mark distal pulse sites for evaluation of pulses after the test.
- Obtain patient weight and height.
- If contrast dye is used, the nurse checks for allergies. Report elevated blood urea nitrogen (BUN) or creatinine levels, because these patients are at risk for renal failure.
- The nurse assesses the patient's fears and anxieties. Correct any misperceptions and reassure the patient that the nurse, physician, and technicians are there to assist during the procedure and will be continuously present.
- The patient is to have nothing by mouth after midnight, except if the catheterization is planned for late in the afternoon. In that case, a clear liquid breakfast may be taken.
- The nurse checks with the physician(s) if they want cardiac drugs withheld.
- The nurse prepares the catheter site according to laboratory protocol. The femoral artery is commonly used for the percutaneous insertion of the catheter. Usually both sides of the groin are prepared.
- The nurse gives the premedication as ordered to reduce the patient's anxiety. In some catheterization laboratories, the patient also is medicated routinely to decrease the risk of allergic reaction to the contrast dye.
- Encourage the patient to wear his or her glasses to the catheterization laboratory.
- The patient is instructed to void before going to the catheterization laboratory.

During the Test
- The patient is awake. The nurse provides emotional support and reinforces explanations given about the procedure.
- Baseline vital signs are obtained and documented.
- Continuous cardiac monitoring is maintained. The nurse observes constantly for complications, especially dysrhythmia from catheter irritation or sensitivity to the contrast dye.
- The physician uses a local anesthetic after the insertion site is prepared and draped.
- The physician inserts the cardiac catheter under fluoroscopy.
- The patient may be asked to change position or cough during the procedure.

Posttest
- The nurse observes the insertion site for signs of bleeding. Palpation around the puncture site will help detect bleeding into tissue. If bleeding is present, the nurse exerts pressure just proximal to the puncture site with a gloved hand for a minimum of 15 minutes.
- The nurse checks distal pulses for arterial patency and then documents the findings.
- The nurse monitors vital signs and cardiac rhythm according to hospital protocol.
- Report any significant changes in vital signs, rhythm, and circulation or the occurrence of chest pain.
- Bed rest is maintained for 4 to 6 hours depending on the type of hemostasis used.
- Evaluate the patient's psychologic response to the procedure and its findings.
- ○ *Patient Teaching.* If cardiac catheterization is performed as an outpatient procedure, instruct the patient (1) not to drive or climb stairs for 24 hours; (2) to avoid heavy lifting, sports, and strenuous housework for 3 days; and (3) to take no baths until the wound is healed. Instruct outpatients that they may shower and change the dressing after 24 hours.

◆ **Nursing Response to Complications**
The nurse needs to assess for and report any observations indicating complications that may occur during or after the cardiac catheterization. Complications include dysrhythmias, asystole, vasovagal reaction, retroperitoneal bleeding, air embolism, contrast media reaction,

Continued

NURSING CARE—cont'd

thrombus, or hematoma formation at the insertion site, cardiac tamponade, myocardial infarction, pulmonary edema, cerebral vascular accident, and infection.

Dysrhythmias. During and after the procedure, the patient is kept on a cardiac monitor. The nurse needs to monitor for dysrhythmias and respond to possible lethal dysrhythmias. Supraventricular and ventricular tachycardia and fibrillation may occur. Cardiac arrest, especially in patients with preexisting heart blocks, may also occur. Dysrhythmias may also occur because of a vasovagal response. Notify the physician and anticipate treatment based on established protocols.

Bleeding. Bleeding may occur at the access site of the catheterization. It may be overt bleeding, or a thrombus or hematoma may occur. The nurse checks the arterial puncture site frequently for overt bleeding. Assess pulses, skin temperature, and color distal to the insertion site. If retroperitoneal bleeding has occurred, there will be tachycardia, tachypnea, restlessness, hypotension, and a drop in hematocrit. The patient may also complain of lower abdominal pain or flank pain. The nurse notifies the physician immediately if bleeding is suspected. If bleeding is significant, the nurse checks to see if the patient has been typed and cross-matched for blood.

Cardiac tamponade. A feared complication of cardiac catheterization is cardiac tamponade, which occurs from bleeding into the pericardial sac. As blood accumulates into the pericardial sac, the heart is restricted. The nurse will observe a decrease in cardiac output, muffled heart sounds, increase in right atrial pressure, and pulsus paradoxus. Notify the physician immediately. If the size of the pericardial effusion is significant, emergency surgery may be necessary.

Coronary Angiography, Computed Tomography

Also called: (CTCA); Coronary CT Angiography (CCTA)

SPECIMEN OR TYPE OF TEST: Radiology

PURPOSE OF THE TEST

Because of its high specificity and sensitivity, CTCA is assuming an increasing importance in the evaluation of chest pain. It is used to confirm or exclude the presence of coronary artery disease and to distinguish between cardiac and noncardiac causes of chest pain.

BASICS THE NURSE NEEDS TO KNOW

With the advent of multidetector computed tomography (MDCT), it is possible to assess noninvasively the presence and severity of coronary atherosclerosis. It can be used to triage patients who present in the Emergency Department with chest pain, preventing unnecessary admissions. However, it is only part of the patient's evaluation. A medical history, physical examination, ECG, and cardiac markers are necessary.

With the introduction of the 64-slice system to CT scanners, the test takes seconds. Radiation dosage is significant, so concern for its use in younger persons must be considered.

REFERENCE VALUES | Patent coronary arteries
No structural *or* anatomic abnormalities

HOW THE TEST IS DONE

See Computed Tomography on pp. 219-220.

INTERFERING FACTORS

- Rapid heart rate (frequently controlled with β-blockers)
- Dysrhythmias
- Obesity

NURSING CARE

See Computed Tomography on pp. 220-221.

Corticotropin, Plasma

See Adrenocorticotropic Hormone, Plasma on p. 44.

Cortisol, Total

Also called: Hydrocortisone, Serum

SPECIMEN OR TYPE OF TEST: Plasma, serum

PURPOSE OF THE TEST

Cortisol levels are used to diagnose Cushing's syndrome, Cushing's disease, and primary and secondary adrenal insufficiency. Primary adrenal insufficiency is called Addison's disease.

BASICS THE NURSE NEEDS TO KNOW

The adrenal cortex produces a group of hormones called glucocorticoids. The primary glucocorticoid is cortisol. Secretion of cortisol is regulated by ACTH, which is secreted by the anterior pituitary gland. It is secreted in a diurnal pattern; highest in the morning and lowest in the evening. When secreted, most of the cortisol in the plasma binds with corticosteroid-binding globulin (CBG) and 10% to 20% binds with albumin. The free cortisol is the biologically active form, whereas the bound hormone acts as a storehouse to replace the free cortisol.

The actions of cortisol and the other glucocorticoids are multiple and relate to their plasma concentrations. At normal plasma levels, glucocorticoids, as the name implies, maintain glucose levels by promoting hepatic gluconeogenesis and glycogenolysis, prevent fatigue by making tissues more responsive to glucagon and catecholamines, reduce the secretion of antidiuretic hormone (ADH), increase glomerular filtration rates, and make the distal tubules of the kidneys more permeable to water reabsorption.

Elevated Values

At elevated levels, for example in times of stress or in pharmacologic doses, the glucocorticoids have an immunosuppressive and an antiinflammatory effect.

Cushing's syndrome includes excessive secretion of the adrenal cortex hormones resulting from a primary adrenal dysfunction. When a pituitary or hypothalamic disorder causes an increase in the production of glucocorticoids, including cortisol, it is called Cushing's disease. The high cortisol levels may be dangerous for the individual because the inflammatory response is suppressed. The inflammatory response is necessary to destroy invading microorganisms, to wall off infected areas, and to initiate normal wound healing.

REFERENCE VALUES	Newborn: 8-10 AM: 0.1-3.4 μg/dL *or* SI: 28-938 nmol/L
	4-6 PM: 0.1-8.0 μg/dL *or* SI: 28-288 nmol/L
	Adult: 8-10 AM: 5-23 μg/dL *or* SI: 138-635 nmol/L
	4-6 PM: 3-16 μg/dL *or* SI: 83-441 nmol/L

HOW THE TEST IS DONE

Venipuncture is performed. Varied methods are used to measure cortisol, including radioimmunoassay (RIA), competitive protein-binding assay, fluorometric assay, and high-performance liquid chromatography.

For newborns, instead of performing a heelstick or venipuncture when doing cortisol levels, saliva may be used to test for cortisol. If a saliva specimen is used, no milk should be present in the infant's mouth.

SIGNIFICANCE OF TEST RESULTS

Elevated Values

Cushing's syndrome
Cushing's disease
Stress
Acute illness
Surgery
Trauma
Excessive exogenous glucocorticoids
Exogenous estrogen
Anxiety
Starvation
Anorexia nervosa
Alcoholism
Chronic renal failure
Adrenal hyperfunction
Excessive ACTH (pituitary or ectopic production)

Decreased Values

Addison's disease
Pituitary destruction or failure
Hypophysectomy

Postpartum pituitary necrosis
Pregnancy
Hepatitis
Cirrhosis of the liver

INTERFERING FACTORS

- Noncompliance with dietary or activity restrictions
- With RIA: Androgens, estrogens, phenytoin, hepatic dysfunction, and renal failure
- With competitive protein-binding assay: Prednisolone and 6-alpha-methylprednisolone
- With fluorometric assays: Jaundice, renal failure, and medications (niacin, quinacrine, quinidine, spironolactone)
- With high-performance liquid chromatography: Prednisone, prednisolone

NURSING CARE

Nursing actions are similar to those used in other venipuncture procedures (see Chapter 2), with the following additional measures.

Pretest

- The nurse obtains a medication history and asks the physician if any interfering drugs should be withheld. The nurse also inquires and notes on the requisition slip if the patient is pregnant, because this may affect test results.

○ *Patient Teaching.* The nurse explains to the patient the need to obtain two specimens of blood, one in the early morning and one in the evening to obtain the peak and low secretion times. Instruct the patient to ingest nothing by mouth for 12 hours before the test. Some physicians recommend a low-carbohydrate diet for 2 days before the test. The nurse also instructs the patient to limit physical activity for 12 hours before the test and to lie down for 30 minutes before the blood is drawn.

Cortrosyn Stimulation Test

See Adrenocorticotropic Hormone Stimulation Test on p. 44.

Cosyntropin Test

See Adrenocorticotropic Hormone Stimulation Test on p. 44.

C-Reactive Protein

Also called: (CRP)
Includes: High Sensitivity C-Reactive Protein (hs-CRP)

SPECIMEN OR TYPE OF TEST: Serum

PURPOSE OF THE TEST

C-reactive protein is used as a nonspecific indicator of infection or inflammation and also is used to monitor the response to antibiotic or antiinflammatory medication. It is commonly used to help with the diagnosis of rheumatoid arthritis and rheumatic fever, particularly when the erythrocyte sedimentation rate and other test results are inconclusive. It is also being investigated by research as a possible risk factor or cause of cardiovascular disease.

BASICS THE NURSE NEEDS TO KNOW

C-reactive protein is a serum protein that is normally absent from the blood, except when tissue necrosis, trauma, inflammation, or infection exists. The older test method, called standard CRP, is not sensitive at the lower range of positive serum values. The new method, called high sensitivity CRP (hs-CRP), is more accurate in measurement of CRP values.

The serum level of C-reactive protein rises rapidly and dramatically higher in response to bacterial infection and acute inflammation. The progressive rise in value reflects increasing infection, inflammation, or tissue damage. Equally, the progressive fall in the serum value indicates healing or the effectiveness of antibiotic or antiinflammatory medication. In detecting sepsis and estimating its severity, CRP monitoring is more accurate than the leukocyte (WBC) count and the body temperature. Because the protein level does not rise in the presence of viral infection, the test may be used to differentiate between viral and bacterial sources of infection.

High-Sensitivity C-Reactive Protein (hs-CRP)

If an acute myocardial infarction occurs, the hs-CRP level will rise modestly above the normal value. Research has identified that a high normal value of hs-CRP is a possible cardiovascular risk factor, but the relationship of hs-CRP to coronary artery disease remains unclear. More research is needed to clarify the role of CRP as a possible risk factor and investigate whether it is a possible cause or consequence of atherosclerosis formation (Boekholdt & Kastelein, 2010; McPherson & Pinkus, 2007). Ultimately, the goal is to determine the best use of the hs-CRP results in the clinical treatment to reduce the risk of a heart attack.

REFERENCE VALUES   Standard CRP: <1 mg/dL *or* SI: <10 mg/L
High-sensitivity CRP: <1-10 mg/dL *or* SI: <1-10 mg/L

HOW THE TEST IS DONE

Venipuncture is performed to collect a sample of venous blood.

SIGNIFICANCE OF TEST RESULTS

Elevated Values
Rheumatoid arthritis
Rheumatic fever
Systemic lupus erythematosus
Bacterial sepsis
Tuberculosis
Pneumococcal pneumonia

Crohn's disease
Myocardial infarction

INTERFERING FACTORS

- Oral contraceptives
- Serum lipidemia
- Hemolysis

NURSING CARE

Nursing actions are similar to those used in other venipuncture procedures (see Chapter 2), with the following additional measures.

Pretest

○ *Patient Teaching.* Instruct the patient to fast from food for 4 to 8 hours before the test. Fluids are permitted. Fasting is necessary because it is desirable to have the level of serum lipids as low as possible. Serum lipids cause a false-positive result.

Posttest

- The nurse monitors the CRP results of the patient as one of the indicators that infection or inflammation is increasing or decreasing, particularly in response to medication. Inflammatory disorders may be arthritic, affecting joints or involving specific organs. If, however, the heart tissue is inflamed, the nurse monitors the pulse for an elevated rate and altered rhythm. If CRP is used as a predictor of coronary artery disease, the nurse monitors for a sudden onset of chest pain and altered vital signs.

Creatine Kinase

See Cardiac Markers on p. 175.

Creatine Kinase Isoenzymes

See Cardiac Markers on p. 175.

Creatinine Clearance

Also called: (Ccre)

SPECIMEN OR TYPE OF TEST: Urine, blood

PURPOSE OF THE TEST

A creatinine clearance is performed to measure glomerular filtration rates. Almost all the creatinine produced by protein metabolism is filtered by the glomeruli. Creatinine clearance is often done to evaluate the progression of renal insufficiency. It is sometimes done to ensure adequate filtration and removal of medications from the blood.

BASICS THE NURSE NEEDS TO KNOW

Creatinine clearance is the total amount of creatinine excreted in the urine within a designated time period. Creatinine is an amino acid waste product that is derived from muscle creatinine, a product of protein metabolism. It is distributed throughout body fluids and is excreted by the kidneys. In the process of urinary elimination, creatinine is almost totally filtered by the glomeruli. Age affects the creatinine clearance value. After age 40, creatinine clearance decreases every 10 years by almost 10%.

Elevated Values

Creatinine clearance increases after intense exercise, with infection, diabetes mellitus, and after eating a meat meal.

Decreased Values

Urinary creatinine decreases with acute and advanced chronic renal failure because the glomeruli are impaired or unable to remove the creatinine from the blood. In these conditions, the serum creatinine level rises, but the urinary creatinine and creatinine clearance rate decreases.

REFERENCE VALUES | Children: 70-140 mL/min/1.73 m² *or* SI: 1.17-2.33 mL/s/1.73m²
Adults: 75-125 mL/min/1.73 m² *or* SI: 1.25-2.08 mL/s/1.73 m²

▼Critical Values | <30 mL/min/1.73 m² *or* SI: <0.02 mL/s/1.73 m²

HOW THE TEST IS DONE

Blood: A venipuncture is done. For infants and small children, a heelstick puncture is used to fill a capillary pipette. The blood is collected at the midpoint of the time of the urine collection period.

Urine: Urine is collected for a 4-, 12-, or 24-hour period.

Creatinine clearance is a calculated value obtained by using the urine and plasma creatinine levels, urinary volume, and the patient's body surface area.

SIGNIFICANCE OF TEST RESULTS

Increased Values

Pregnancy
Burns
High-protein diet
Hypothyroidism
Diabetes mellitus

Decreased Values

Renal insufficiency or failure
Glomerulonephritis
Nephrotic syndrome

Dehydration
Pyelonephritis
Shock
Congestive heart failure
Hyperthyroidism

INTERFERING FACTORS

- Exercise
- Ingestion of meat
- Ketosis
- Many medications: androgens, ascorbic acid, anabolic steroids, barbiturates, many antibiotics, thiazides

NURSING CARE

Nursing actions are similar to those used in other venipuncture and timed urine collection procedures (see Chapter 2), with the following additional measures.

Pretest

- The nurse asks the physician if any medications are to be withheld during the test. Generally, medications including cephalosporins are withheld because they alter the test result.
- The patient's height, weight, and age are recorded in the patient's record and on the laboratory requisition slip. The data are used in the calculation of the creatinine clearance.

○ *Patient Teaching.* The nurse instructs the patient to discard the first urine of the morning at 8 AM and then begin the urine collection. All urine for the timed period is to be placed in a special collection container, including the last voided specimen at the end of the collection period. The container with the urine is kept on ice. The patient is instructed to maintain fluid intake before and throughout the collection period.

During the Test

- The nurse writes the date and time of the start and finish of the collection period on the collection container and the requisition slip.

Posttest

- The nurse arranges to send the urine to the laboratory promptly.

▽ **Nursing Response to Critical Values**

A creatinine clearance value at the critical value level or worse occurs in advanced renal failure. The nurse assesses the patient's intake and output of fluids, vital signs, and mental status. In advanced renal failure, the patient has decreased urinary output, or *oliguria*; that is, a urine output of 100 to 400 mL per day, or *anuria*, a urine output of 100 mL or less per day. When the kidneys cannot filter and remove water, the patient develops edema in body tissues. The patient develops hypertension and tachypnea and may be somnolent (excessively drowsy). The nurse notifies the physician of the creatinine clearance result and the assessment findings, including the patient's intake and output.

Creatinine, Serum, Plasma

Also called: (pCR); Plasma Creatinine

SPECIMEN OR TYPE OF TEST: Serum, plasma

PURPOSE OF THE TEST

Serum creatinine determination is the most common laboratory test used to evaluate renal function and to estimate the effectiveness of glomerular filtration.

BASICS THE NURSE NEEDS TO KNOW

Creatinine is an amino acid and waste product of protein metabolism. It is derived from creatine, which is synthesized in the liver, kidneys, and pancreas, and stored in muscle tissue. As creatine is metabolized in the muscle, creatinine is produced. Creatinine is released into the extracellular fluid and excreted through the kidneys.

In the kidneys, creatinine is filtered by the glomeruli and is usually not resorbed. Additional creatinine is secreted by the renal tubules. When the kidneys are functional, they maintain the serum creatinine level at a minimal, low level.

Elevated Values

When renal function is impaired, the creatinine level increases.

Decreased Values

The serum levels of creatinine decrease in conditions that cause a decrease in muscle mass, including old age and muscle-wasting diseases. In these conditions, there is less creatine synthesis and storage, and therefore less creatinine production.

REFERENCE VALUES	
	Newborn: 0.3-1 mg/dL *or* SI: 27-88 μmol/L
	Infant: 0.2-0.4 mg/mL *or* SI: 18-35 μmol/L
	Child: 0.3-0.7 mg/dL *or* SI: 27-62 μmol/L
	Adolescent: 0.5-1 mg/dL *or* SI: 44-88 μmol/L
	Adult male: 0.7-1.3 mg/dL *or* SI: 62-115 μmol/L
	Adult female: 0.6-1.1 mg/dL *or* SI: 53-97 μmol/L

▽ Critical Values	
	Renal insufficiency: 1.5-3.0 mg/mL
	Renal failure: >3.0 mg/mL

HOW THE TEST IS DONE

A venipuncture is done to obtain a specimen of blood. For infants and small children, a heelstick puncture is used to fill a capillary pipette.

SIGNIFICANCE OF TEST RESULTS

Elevated Values

Acute or chronic renal insufficiency/failure
Contrast-induced nephropathy
Uremia or azotemia
Renal artery stenosis
Congestive heart failure
Shock
Dehydration
Rhabdomyolysis
Acromegaly

Decreased Values

Advanced liver disease
Long-term corticosteroid therapy
Hyperthyroidism
Muscular dystrophy
Paralysis
Dermatomyositis
Polymyositis

INTERFERING FACTORS

- Hemolysis
- Warming of the specimen
- Lipemia
- Recent ingestion of meat

NURSING CARE

Nursing actions are similar to those used in other venipuncture procedures (see Chapter 2), with the following additional measures.

Pretest

○ *Patient Teaching.* When indicated by the laboratory protocol, the nurse instructs the patient to fast from food and fluids for 8 hours before the test.

Posttest

- Arrange for prompt transport of the specimen to the laboratory. Prolonged delay causes ammonia to form in the specimen. Warming will cause a falsely elevated test result.

▽ **Nursing Response to Critical Values**

When the serum creatinine elevates to the critical value level or higher, the finding indicates acute or severe chronic renal insufficiency or renal failure. The glomeruli are unable to filter the blood and remove the accumulating creatinine. The nurse assesses the patient for signs of renal failure, including hypertension, tachypnea, edema, and somnolence (drowsiness). The urine output may be *oliguric*, with an output of 100 to 400 mL per day, or *anuric*, with a volume of 100 mL per day, or less. The nurse notifies the physician of the elevated serum creatinine level and of the assessment findings.

Creatinine, Urine

Also called: Urinary Cre

SPECIMEN OR TYPE OF TEST: 12- or 24-hour urine

PURPOSE OF THE TEST

The urine creatinine test is performed to assess renal function. It usually is not assessed alone, but is done as part of the Creatinine Clearance Test (see p. 231).

BASICS THE NURSE NEEDS TO KNOW

Creatinine is an amino acid waste product that is derived from muscle creatine, a product of protein metabolism. It is distributed throughout body fluids and is excreted by the kidneys. In the process of urinary elimination, creatinine is almost totally filtered by the glomeruli. After age 60, there is a progressive decrease in the amount of creatinine excreted by the kidneys.

REFERENCE VALUES

Child: 6-30 mg/kg/day *or* SI: 53-264 μmol/kg/day
Adult male: 1-2 g/day *or* SI: 8.8-17.7 mmol/day
Adult female: 0.8-1.8 g/day *or* SI: 7.1-15.9 mmol/day

HOW THE TEST IS DONE

The test usually requires urine collection for 24 hours, but collection periods of 12 hours are sometimes prescribed.

SIGNIFICANCE OF TEST RESULTS

Elevated Values
Muscular dystrophy
Polymyositis
Paralysis
Muscular inflammatory disease
Hyperthyroidism
Anemia
Leukemia

Decreased Values
Glomerulonephritis
Congestive heart failure
Acute tubular necrosis
Advanced pyelonephritis
Shock
Polycystic kidney disease
Renal malignancy
Dehydration
Bilateral ureteral obstruction
Nephrosclerosis

INTERFERING FACTORS

- Excessive exercise during the test period
- Failure to collect all the urine
- Failure to time the test accurately
- Warming of the urine specimen
- High protein intake before the test

NURSING CARE

Nursing actions are similar to those used in other timed urine collection procedures (see Chapter 2), with the following additional measures.

Pretest

○ *Patient Teaching.* The nurse instructs the patient to avoid excessive intake of meat on the day before the test. The patient is taught to collect all urine for the 24-hour period of the test, storing the container in the refrigerator or on ice. The nurse encourages the patient to maintain adequate hydration before and during the test and to omit coffee and tea during the test.

During the Test

○ *Patient Teaching.* At 8 AM, instruct the patient to void and discard the urine. The test begins at this time, and all subsequent urine specimens are collected for 24 hours, including the 8 AM specimen of the next morning. Advise the patient to avoid vigorous exercise during the test period.

○ *Patient Teaching.* The nurse ensures that the patient's name and the time and date of the start and finish of the test are written on the label and requisition slip.

Posttest

- Arrange for prompt transportation of the refrigerated specimen to the laboratory.

Culture, Blood

SPECIMEN OR TYPE OF TEST: Blood

PURPOSE OF THE TEST

The blood culture identifies the organism that is causing *bacteremia* (an infection in the bloodstream). Susceptibility testing determines which antibiotics will be effective in elimination of the pathogen.

BASICS THE NURSE NEEDS TO KNOW

Septicemia, an infection of the blood, can be caused by almost any bacterial organism. In sepsis, some bacteria are present in the circulation continuously and others are present in the blood on an intermittent or transient basis only. The timing of the specimen collection depends on when the bacteria are likely to be present in the blood. When the suspected organism is one that is intermittent or transient, the best time to collect the blood and obtain a positive culture is just before or during a chill or temperature spike in the patient. If the suspected organism is in the blood continuously, the blood culture specimen can be obtained at anytime.

In the past, blood collections were repeated multiple times within a few hours or daily for several days, in efforts to capture the microbes in the circulation. Today, however, research shows that the volume of blood drawn at a single time is more important than multiple specimens obtained at different intervals. Best practice methods today are to draw blood one time only, obtaining at least 30 mL of blood (for adults) from 2 different venipuncture sites. Antibiotic therapy is initiated or maintained until 3 days later when the culture and susceptibility results are known (Mahon, Lehman & Manuselis, 2011).

Susceptibility Testing

When bacteria are identified, susceptibility testing will be done, if requested. In the presence of antibiotic or antimicrobial medication, bacteria are described as susceptible, intermediate, or resistant. Susceptible means that the bacteria can be treated effectively with a specific antibiotic or antimicrobial. Intermediate means that the bacteria can be treated effectively with a higher dosage of the medication or with medication that concentrates in a particular body site where the bacteria are located. Resistance means that the bacteria will not be killed or eliminated by particular medications.

REFERENCE VALUES	Negative; no growth of organisms
▽ Critical Values	Positive culture *or* a first time positive culture

HOW THE TEST IS DONE

For the adult, needles and syringes, culture bottles, a blood culture system, or a special set of blood tubes with culture media are used to collect at least a total of 30 mL of venous blood, divided in two separate samples. Two different venipuncture sites are used to obtain the two samples of the blood. At each venipuncture site, the skin is first disinfected with alcohol and then povidone iodine to kill most surface bacteria.

For infants and small children, the procedure is the same, but the volume of blood is much less. For children younger than 10 years, the specimen's blood volume is 1 mL for each year of life. For children older than 10 years, the amount of blood is 20 mL. For the neonate, 4% of their total blood volume is sufficient.

SIGNIFICANCE OF TEST RESULTS

Positive Values
Bacterial endocarditis
Bacterial meningitis
Septic arthritis
Typhoid fever
Brucellosis
Sepsis or septicemia
Osteomyelitis
Bacterial pneumonia
Toxic shock syndrome

INTERFERING FACTORS

- Contamination of the specimen
- Clotted blood specimen

NURSING CARE

Nursing actions are similar to those used in other venipuncture procedures (see Chapter 2), with the following additional measures.

Pretest

- If possible, schedule the tests before antibiotic therapy is administered.
- The nurse informs the patient about the procedure, including blood specimens and the skin asepsis. The patient is asked about any history of skin sensitivity to iodine.
- To assist with the timing of the blood sampling, the nurse monitors the patient's temperature, pulse, respiration, and blood pressure at frequent and regular intervals. The results are recorded in the patient's chart.

During the Test

- The nurse assists the physician or lab technician as needed. The skin of the venipuncture site is scrubbed in concentric circles in an outward direction with 80% to 95% alcohol and then allowed to dry. The second scrub is done in the same pattern, using povidone-iodine (Betadine). This solution remains on the skin for at least 1 minute. If the patient is sensitive to iodine, green soap may be substituted or the alcohol preparation alone can be used. If an intravenous catheter is in place, the specimen is obtained from a venous site distal to the catheter or from the opposite extremity. This prevents hemodilution with intravenous fluids. Blood is never drawn from the intravenous line, central line, or the heparin-lock device because of the risk of external contamination.

Posttest

- Ensure that each requisition slip and all collection containers or tubes are correctly identified. The patient's name, identification number, room number, physician, the time, date, and culture site are included. In the patient's record, the nurse documents the blood culture specimen collection, the time, date, and venous sites that were used.

▽ **Nursing Response to Critical Values**

Institutions vary in their critical value identification of blood culture findings. In many places, the physician must be notified immediately of a positive blood culture or of a first time positive blood culture result. Septicemia is very serious, and effective antibiotic treatment should be started as quickly as possible.

Culture, Genital

Also called: Genitourinary Culture, Cervical Culture, Endocervical Culture, Prostatic Fluid Culture, Vaginal Culture

SPECIMEN OR TYPE OF TEST: Secretions

C

PURPOSE OF THE TEST

The genital culture is used to identify the pathogenic organism that causes abnormal discharge and inflammation of the vagina or urethra.

BASICS THE NURSE NEEDS TO KNOW

A genital infection in the female is indicated by inflammation of the vagina and vulva, with the presence of vaginal secretions. In the male, it is indicated by inflammation of the urethra and urethral discharge. The infection may be caused by a sexually transmitted disease, or it may be the result of other causes that are not related to sexual contact. Numerous pathogens may be responsible for a sexually transmitted disease. The culture of the secretions or tissue scrapings is used to identify the causative organism.

Susceptibility Testing

When bacteria are identified, susceptibility testing may be done. In the presence of antibiotic or antimicrobial medication, bacteria are described as susceptible, intermediate, or resistant. Susceptible means that the bacteria can be treated effectively with a particular antibiotic or antimicrobial medication. Intermediate means that the bacteria can be treated effectively with a higher dosage of the medication or with medication that concentrates in a particular body site where the bacteria are located. Resistance means that the bacteria will not be killed or eliminated by the particular medication.

REFERENCE VALUES   Negative; normal flora present

HOW THE TEST IS DONE

For any of the following procedures, a sterile culture tube is used to receive the specimen of cell scrapings or fluid aspirate,

Male

A sterile cotton swab is used to collect secretions from the penile discharge. The physician may insert a wire loop into the urethra to obtain cell scrapings or a swab to obtain urethral secretions (Figure 38, *A*).

Female

Using a speculum, a sterile swab or wire loop is inserted into the cervical canal to obtain secretions or endocervical cell scrapings (Figure 38, *B*).

For chancroid, the base of the genital ulcer is irrigated with saline. The fluid is aspirated with a sterile pipette or a moist, sterile cotton swab.

For herpes simplex, a sterile cotton swab is used to remove epithelial cells from the base of fresh lesions. Fluid from vesicles may also be obtained by aspiration with a sterile pipette.

SIGNIFICANCE OF TEST RESULTS

Positive Values

Neisseria gonorrhoeae
Candida albicans
Staphylococcus aureus
Group B streptococcus

C

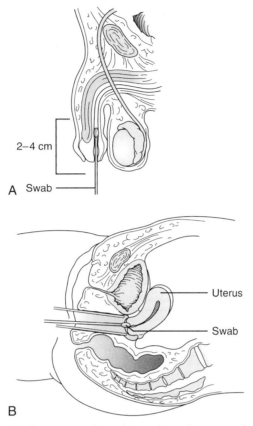

Figure 38. Specimen for genital culture. **A,** Sterile swab in male urethra. **B,** Sterile swab in female endocervical canal. (From Steppe CA, Woods MA: *Laboratory procedures for medical office personnel*, Philadelphia, 1998, Saunders.)

Gardnerella vaginalis
Giardia lamblia
Herpes simplex virus
Trichomonas vaginalis
Chlamydia trachomatis
Human papillomavirus
Haemophilus ducreyi

INTERFERING FACTORS

- Recent urination
- Recent douching
- Improper collection technique
- Contamination of the specimen
- Antibiotic administration

NURSING CARE

Pretest

○ *Patient Teaching.* Instruct the patient about pretest conditions as follows:

Male: Do not urinate within 1 hour of the test, because there will be fewer organisms available for culture.

Female: Do not douche for 24 hours before the test, because douching results in fewer organisms available for culture.

- The nurse inquires about any current use of antibiotics. The culture should be performed before starting any antibiotic therapy.

During the Test

- Place the male in the supine position. The female is placed in the lithotomy position, as for gynecologic examination.
- The nurse provides emotional support to the patient during the collection of the specimen. For the female, the procedure may produce mild apprehension or discomfort, but it is not painful. The male may experience nausea, sweating, fainting, or weakness as the wire loop or swab is inserted into the urethra. These discomforts are temporary.
- The requisition form and the specimen sample should include information regarding the source of the specimen, the patient's name and age, the clinical diagnosis, the time and date of the specimen collection, and any current antibiotic therapy.

Posttest

○ *Patient Teaching.* Instruct the patient to abstain from sexual contact until any infection is identified, treated, and cured. With gonorrheal infection, instruct the patient to have the culture repeated 1 week after the completion of antibiotic therapy.

○ *Patient Teaching.* When the culture is positive for a sexually transmitted disease, counsel the patient to inform all sexual partners of the test results. Sexual contacts are advised to undergo testing.

○ *Patient Teaching.* As part of follow-up nursing care for a sexually transmitted disease, the nurse discusses ways to reduce risk for a repeat infection. From the patient's sexual history, the nurse can identify the individual's high-risk practices that resulted in infection and make suggestions for the future. The best protection from sexually transmitted disease is achieved through abstinence, a long-term monogamous relationship, or the use of condoms.

Culture, Nasopharyngeal

SPECIMEN OR TYPE OF TEST: Secretions

PURPOSE OF THE TEST

The nasopharyngeal and throat cultures are performed to identify the bacteria that cause upper respiratory tract infection.

C

BASICS THE NURSE NEEDS TO KNOW

A variety of normal flora exists in the nose and nasopharynx. These normal organisms may multiply and cause illness, particularly in children, the elderly, immunocompromised individuals, or individuals in a weakened condition. A nose culture positive for one of these organisms may indicate infection in the nasopharynx, sinuses, oropharynx, or tonsils. Infection can also occur elsewhere in the body, with the source of the infection being in the nose or throat.

Staphylococcus aureus

The anterior nasal cavity is a major reservoir of *S. aureus*. In drug addicts with bacterial endocarditis, or in renal dialysis patients with septicemia, the nasal passageway may be the source of infection. This bacterium is also implicated in postoperative wound infection and in *furunculosis,* a bacterial infection of the skin. As asymptomatic carriers, individuals may harbor *S. aureus* and the incidence is higher in hospital personnel and hospitalized patients. When an outbreak of this infection occurs, the nasopharyngeal culture may be performed as a screening test to identify asymptomatic carriers.

Bordetella pertussis

Bordetella pertussis and *Bordetella parapertussis* are the organisms that cause pertussis or whooping cough. This respiratory tract infection usually occurs in infants who are not vaccinated or who are incompletely vaccinated and are in close contact with an infected individual. The nasopharyngeal culture is a very important test when this infection is suspected.

Susceptibility Testing

When bacteria are identified, susceptibility testing may be done. In the presence of antibiotic or antimicrobial medication, bacteria are described as susceptible, intermediate, or resistant. Susceptible means that the bacteria can be treated effectively with the particular medication. Intermediate means that the bacteria can be treated effectively with a higher dosage of the medication or with medication that concentrates in a particular body site where the bacteria are located. Resistance means that the bacteria will not be killed or eliminated by the particular medication.

Severe Acute Respiratory Syndrome (SARS)

SARS is a respiratory infection that causes severe pneumonia from a newly recognized corona virus. The RNA of the virus may be detected in the respiratory tract within a period of 72 hours after symptoms begin. When SARS is suspected, the patient must be placed in isolation. Contact and respiratory droplet precautions are maintained.

The nasopharyngeal swab or aspirate is an early part of the diagnostic testing that is done when this lung infection is suspected. Each swab or aspirate sample of the secretions is placed in separate culturette tubes with a viral transport medium. The specimens of mucus and cells are tested by polymerase chain reaction (PCR) technology to identify the RNA of the virus. If the nurse assists the physician with collection of diagnostic samples from the suspected SARS patient, the nurse, physician, and all other personnel must use protective equipment and adhere to the procedures of droplet precautions. This includes gown, a respirator mask, and goggles and double gloves. Before specimen collection begins, the departments of epidemiology and the laboratory should be consulted.

REFERENCE VALUES	Normal flora are present.

▽ Critical Values	Positive culture or a first time positive culture

HOW THE TEST IS DONE

A special sterile, flexible nasopharyngeal wire swab or Dacron swab is used to collect a specimen from the posterior nasopharynx. The wire swab should be in contact with the mucosa for 5 seconds. For the pertussis culture, the swab is placed near the septum and floor of the nose and is rotated against the mucosal surfaces. For the nasal culture, a sterile Dacron swab is premoistened with saline and then inserted 1 inch into the nares. It is rotated against the nasal mucosa. Once collected, the swab is placed in the swab transport system and sent to the laboratory.

SIGNIFICANCE OF TEST RESULTS

Positive Values
Pharyngitis
Scarlet fever
Diphtheria
Thrush
Pertussis
Staphylococcus aureus
Severe acute respiratory syndrome (SARS)

INTERFERING FACTORS

- Antibiotic therapy
- Improper technique in specimen collection

▎ NURSING CARE

Pretest
- If possible, the nurse ensures that the specimen is obtained before antibiotics are started.
- ○ *Patient Teaching.* Inform the patient that the sterile wire swab will be put into the back of the nose and throat or a soft-tipped swab will be inserted a short distance into the nose. The swab will collect samples of cells and secretions from the tissue lining. Any mild discomfort disappears after the swab is removed. Instruct the patient to cough before the swab is inserted.

During the Test
- For the nasopharyngeal culture, help the patient sit up and tilt the head back. Use a light or sterile nasal speculum to visualize the nasal passage and nasopharynx. The wire swab in the posterior nasopharynx may stimulate the patient's gag reflex.

Posttest
- Place the swab or wire in the sterile culture tube.
- On the laboratory form, and the culture tube, write the time, date, source of the specimen, the patient's name, identification number, and physician's name. Include the suspected clinical diagnosis and any current antibiotic therapy.

▽ **Nursing Response to Critical Values**
Institutions vary in their critical value notification policy regarding culture results. In many places, the physician must be notified immediately of a positive culture result. Some infections are very serious; effective antibiotic treatment should be started as quickly as possible.

Culture, Sputum

SPECIMEN OR TYPE OF TEST: Sputum

PURPOSE OF THE TEST

Sputum culture is performed to identify the pathogenic organism responsible for the lower respiratory tract infection, particularly pneumonia. Susceptibility testing determines the selection of appropriate antibiotic therapy.

BASICS THE NURSE NEEDS TO KNOW

Sputum is a product of the lower respiratory tract, not a product of the oropharynx, such as saliva. Sputum cultures are obtained to identify pathogenic organisms in patients with suspected pulmonary infection. If bacteria are present, microscopic examination of a *Gram stain* of the specimen identifies the bacteria as gram positive or gram negative. This knowledge may be used to initiate appropriate antibiotic therapy until the bacterial culture and susceptibility testing is completed. A stat (immediate) Gram stain result is available in 15 to 30 minutes. Identification of the specific organism growing in the culture medium requires about 48 hours.

Susceptibility Testing

When bacteria are grown in the culture and identified, susceptibility testing is usually done. In the presence of antibiotic or antimicrobial medication, bacteria are described as susceptible, intermediate, or resistant. Susceptible means that the bacteria can be treated effectively with the particular medication. Intermediate means that the bacteria can be treated effectively with higher dosage of the medication or with medication that concentrates in a particular body site where the bacteria are located. Resistance means that the bacteria will not be killed or eliminated by the particular medication.

Severe Acute Respiratory Syndrome (SARS)

Severe acute respiratory syndrome (SARS) is a respiratory infection that causes severe pneumonia from a newly recognized corona virus. The virus may be detected in the respiratory tract within a period of 72 hours after symptoms begin. When SARS is suspected, the patient must be placed in isolation. Contact and respiratory droplet precautions are maintained.

The sputum specimen or bronchial aspirates are part of the diagnostic testing that is done when this lung infection is suspected. Collected by the patient's ability to cough productively or by aspiration or bronchial suction methods, each sputum sample is placed in separate culturette tubes with a viral transport medium. The specimens of mucus and cells are tested by PCR technology to identify the DNA of the virus.

If the nurse assists the physician with collection of diagnostic samples from the suspected SARS patient, the nurse, physician, and all other personnel must use protective equipment and adhere to the procedures of droplet precautions. This includes wearing a gown, a respirator mask, and goggles or face mask. The departments of epidemiology and the laboratory should be consulted before specimen collection begins (see also Severe Acute Respiratory Syndrome Tests on p. 546).

REFERENCE VALUE   No growth

HOW THE TEST IS DONE

Expectoration Method

A sputum specimen may be obtained by the patient coughing up the sputum into a wide-mouthed sterile container with a cap.

Aspiration Method

A bronchial sputum specimen may be obtained by aspiration. If a bronchial specimen is needed, suctioning equipment and a sterile sputum trap are used.

Bronchoscopy or Transtracheal Method

A sputum specimen may also be obtained during a bronchoscopy or via transtracheal aspiration. The nurse may assist with these procedures but does not perform them.

SIGNIFICANCE OF TEST RESULTS

Positive Values
Pneumonia
Influenza
Gonorrhea
Diphtheria
Tuberculosis
Parasitic infection of the lungs
SARS

INTERFERING FACTORS

- Contamination of the specimen
- Antibiotic therapy

▌ NURSING CARE

Pretest
- The nurse has the patient complete this test before starting antibiotic therapy. This timing helps prevent a false-negative result. The nurse also assesses the patient's ability to follow instructions in coughing up the sputum, as well as his or her ability to expectorate.
- Provide a sterile container with a cap.

○ *Patient Teaching.* Instruct the patient to do the following:

1. Collect the specimen on arising in the morning before eating or drinking. Dentures should be removed. Rinsing the mouth with water is done before collecting the sputum.
2. Take several deep breaths.
3. Cough up the sputum from deep within the lungs.
4. Instruct patient not to spit or salivate into the container.
5. Expectorate into the sterile container.

The nurse teaches the procedure to help the patient avoid contamination of the container and lid during the collection procedure. A major problem with the expectoration method is contamination of the specimen by the normal flora, the microorganisms found in the mouth and throat.

During the Test

Expectoration Method

- Support and encourage the patient's attempts to produce sputum. If it is not contraindicated, postural drainage, clapping, and vibration of the back may assist in raising the sputum. If the sputum is very tenacious, aerosol therapy may be necessary.
- Approximately 1 tsp of sputum is necessary for a sputum culture and sensitivity test. When the patient is unable to produce this amount in one attempt, the container should be capped between attempts to expectorate.
- If the patient is intubated, a sputum trap is used to obtain the specimen (Figure 39). In this case, suctioning is performed as usual, except that the sputum trap is inserted between the sterile suction catheter and the suction tubing attached to the wall suction regulator.

Aspiration Method

- Use the sputum trap as follows:
  1. Tighten the cap to obtain an airtight seal.
  2. Attach the wall suction tubing to the plastic "chimney" on the cap.
  3. Connect the distal end of the sterile container to the latex tubing.
  4. Suction as usual, but do not flush the catheter while the trap is in place.
  5. After suctioning, disconnect the suction tubing and catheter.
  6. Connect the latex tubing to the chimney of the cap.

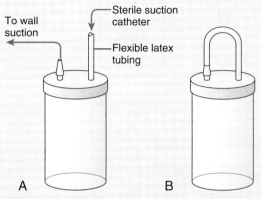

Figure 39. Sputum aspiration. **A,** Sputum trap. **B,** Closed sputum trap.

Continued

NURSING CARE—cont'd

Posttest
- Ensure that the lid is tightly sealed and that the container is labeled correctly.
- Send the specimen to the laboratory as soon as possible. Do not refrigerate the specimen.
- No complications result from the sputum collection procedure. The nurse should be aware, however, of the complications that can result from endotracheal suctioning, if that method is used to obtain the specimen.

Culture, Stool

Also called: Stool Culture for Enteric Pathogens

SPECIMEN OR TYPE OF TEST: Feces

PURPOSE OF THE TEST

The stool culture is used to identify the bacterial organism that caused intestinal infection and determine susceptibility to antibiotics.

BASICS THE NURSE NEEDS TO KNOW

Stool culture may be used when the patient experiences severe, persistent, or recurrent bloody diarrhea with fever and tenesmus, a painful, ineffectual straining at stool. The patient may have a history of travel to a developing country, a recent dietary intake of seafood, or exposure to a known bacterial agent. Routine stool culture will include testing for *Shigella, Salmonella, Campylobacter, Vibrio* sp., *Aeromonas, Plesiomonas, Yersinia, and Escherichia coli* Testing for *Clostridium difficile* may be indicated for patients with diarrhea who have been hospitalized for more than 3 days but were not originally admitted with the diarrhea.

Susceptibility Testing

When bacteria are identified, susceptibility testing may be done. In the presence of antibiotic or antimicrobial medication, bacteria are described as susceptible, intermediate, or resistant. Susceptible means that the bacteria can be treated effectively with a particular antibiotic. Intermediate means that the bacteria can be treated effectively with a higher dosage of the medication or with medication that concentrates in a particular body site where the bacteria are located. Resistance means that the bacteria will not be killed or eliminated by the particular antibiotic.

REFERENCE VALUES	Negative; no growth
▽ Critical Values	Positive for enteric pathogens

HOW THE TEST IS DONE
Random Stool Method

A small amount of freshly passed feces is evacuated directly into a clean, dry container. The specimen can have no contact with urine or the water and cleansers of the toilet bowl. If bacterial infection is suspected, the patient should have one specimen collection each day for 3 days. (See also, Chapter 2) .

Rectal Swab Method

The swab is inserted past the anal sphincter and into the rectum. The swab is gently rotated around the canal. To attain maximum absorption, the swab is kept in place for 15 to 20 seconds before it is withdrawn. It must have visible feces on it. The swab is placed in the special culture tube with media.

SIGNIFICANCE OF TEST RESULTS
Positive Values

Shigellosis
Salmonella infection
E. coli infection
Cholera
Bacillary dysentery
Botulism
Enteric fever
Acute gastroenteritis
Typhoid fever
Food poisoning
Legionnaire's disease

INTERFERING FACTORS

- Contamination of the specimen with urine, detergent, or soap
- Improper technique of specimen collection
- Antibiotic therapy

NURSING CARE

Pretest

○ *Patient Teaching.* The nurse instructs the patient to evacuate a small amount of feces directly into the container or collection device. If a bedpan is used, it must be rinsed with water and dried thoroughly before use. The nurse obtains the specimen before any antibiotic therapy is started.

- The specimen in a clean container must be delivered to the laboratory within 30 minutes. If delivery will be delayed, the specimen is placed in a transport container with medium to prevent drying.

Continued

| NURSING CARE—cont'd

Posttest

- The nurse uses gloves to handle the open container or culturette until it is sealed. Hands are washed thoroughly after the gloves are removed. These bacteria are highly transmissible via a fecal-oral route.
- The specimen and lab request form are labeled with the patient's name, identification number, the time, date of the collection, the source of the specimen, and the physician's name.

▼ **Nursing Response to Critical Values**

- Institutions vary in their critical value notification policy regarding the results of a stool culture. Some include all positive cultures in their critical value list. Some identify only certain organisms in the stool and some do not include stool culture on their critical value list. The nurse follows the institutional decision regarding rapid notification of the physician.
- The department of epidemiology of the institution must be notified because the patient with a positive stool culture result needs to be placed on isolation precautions.

Culture, Throat

Also called: Oropharyngeal Culture
Includes: Rapid Antigen Detection Test

SPECIMEN OR TYPE OF TEST: Secretions

PURPOSE OF THE TEST

The throat culture identifies the bacteria that cause infection of the oropharynx, pharynx, and tonsils. It is also used to screen for an asymptomatic carrier of the infection.

BASICS THE NURSE NEEDS TO KNOW

When acute pharyngitis occurs, or when a clinical illness indicates an oropharyngeal source of infection, a throat culture may be indicated. Untreated for 9 days or more, a throat infection caused by group A β-hemolytic streptococcal infection could develop complications of rheumatic fever, scarlet fever, glomerulonephritis, wound infection, and sepsis.

Other serious organisms that produce a positive throat culture include *Corynebacterium diphtheriae,* the cause of diphtheria, and *Neisseria gonorrhoeae,* the gonorrheal cause of an infected oropharynx. Diphtheria infects the tonsils, oropharynx, nasopharynx, larynx, and trachea. Generally, a routine throat culture and a nasopharyngeal culture are performed simultaneously. When gonorrhea infection is in the throat, the infection may be asymptomatic or may cause tonsillitis and acute pharyngitis. The throat is a primary site of sexually transmitted infection in men who have sex with men. Often, cultures of the genitalia and anal canal are performed at the same time. In children, a throat culture positive for gonorrhea is indicative of child sexual abuse.

Rapid Antigen Detection Test (RADT) and Other Test Methods

In the case of the sore throat, the rapid antigen detection test is often used instead of the throat culture to confirm the presence of group A β-hemolytic streptococcus antigen. (Alcaide & Bisno, 2007). Within minutes it can identify the bacteria, whereas 18 to 48 hours are needed to obtain the results of a throat culture. If the RADT is negative, a throat culture is often done to verify the results. Other detection methods to identify group A β-hemolytic streptococcus include antigen-antibody tests and a chemiluminescent DNA probe to identify this organism (Choby, 2009).

REFERENCE VALUES   Negative; no growth of pathogens

HOW THE TEST IS DONE

For the throat culture, two sterile Dacron swabs are used to obtain a specimen of exudates from the throat (Figure 40). The swab is then placed in a culture tube with media and is capped tightly.

SIGNIFICANCE OF TEST RESULTS

Abnormal Values

Group A β-hemolytic streptococcus throat infection
Scarlet fever
Pertussis
Pharyngitis
Thrush
Diphtheria
Gonococcal infection

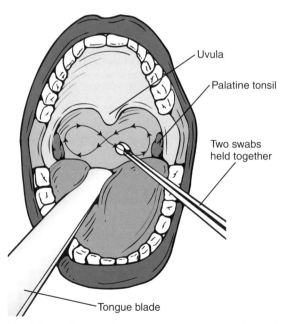

Figure 40. Technique for obtaining a throat culture. (From Steppe CA, Woods MA: *Laboratory procedures for medical office personnel*, Philadelphia, 1998, Saunders.)

C

INTERFERING FACTORS
- Antibiotic therapy
- Contamination of the specimen

NURSING CARE

Pretest
- Obtain the culture specimen before antibiotic therapy is started. Inform the patient that the test involves swabbing the throat. The swabbing may cause a brief gagging sensation. The discomfort disappears as soon as the procedure is finished.
- In cases of acute epiglottitis or suspected diphtheria, the nurse does not perform the throat culture, but would assist the physician. The test should not be performed until preparation has been made to establish an alternate airway, as needed. If diphtheria is suspected, the nurse notifies the laboratory in advance so that a special isolation medium can be prepared.

During the Test
- Instruct the patient to tip the head back. Use a tongue blade to depress the tongue.
- The two sterile swabs are used together to rub the inflamed sites and areas of exudate in the oropharynx and tonsils. These tissues commonly have many organisms present and poor technique will cause a false-positive result. During the swabbing of the throat, ensure that the tongue, cheeks, and uvula are not touched.
- The swabs of routine culture are placed in a regular culture tube with medium. A throat culture for suspected diphtheria or gonococcal infection requires a special swab and culture-transport medium.

Posttest
- Ensure that the specimen is placed in the sterile culture tube or transport medium as appropriate for the specific test.
- On the requisition request and the specimen container, identify the source of the specimen, the name and identifying number of the patient, the clinical diagnosis, the physician, and any antibiotic therapy that the patient is currently undergoing.

◆ **Nursing Response to Complications**
There are no complications from a routine throat culture. In cases of acute epiglottitis or suspected diphtheria, however, the patient may experience a laryngospasm immediately after the specimen is obtained.

Laryngospasm. The nurse assesses for signs of respiratory obstruction, including dyspnea and stridor (a high-pitched, crowing sound) and increased respiratory effort. The nurse records the results of the respiratory assessment in the patient's chart. If laryngospasm and respiratory obstruction begins, the nurse prepares to support oxygenation and assist the physician with the establishment of an airway, as needed.

Culture, Urine

Also called: Midstream Urine Culture Midvoid Specimen; Urine Culture, Clean Catch

SPECIMEN OR TYPE OF TEST: Urine

PURPOSE OF THE TEST

Culture of the urine is used to diagnose a urinary tract infection and to monitor the number of microorganisms in the urine. Sensitivity testing identifies the appropriate antibiotics and antimicrobials that are effective.

BASICS THE NURSE NEEDS TO KNOW

Bacteriuria is the presence of bacteria in urine. A lower urinary tract infection consists of an infection in the bladder or urethra, or both. An upper urinary tract infection involves the renal pelvis or renal interstitial tissues, or both. Any bacterial or fungal organism can cause a urinary tract infection, but the most common pathogens are those that are present in normal feces.

A bacterial count of 10,000 colony-forming units per milliliter (CFU/mL) or more is considered positive and indicates significant bacteriuria. The count of the organism is evaluated together with the patient's symptoms, predisposing factors, and the type of organism(s) isolated. In the female patient, the test may be repeated once or twice to ensure the accuracy of the diagnosis, because contamination of the specimen could cause a false-positive result. In the male patient, only one specimen is needed for a correct diagnosis.

Susceptibility Testing

When bacteria are identified, susceptibility testing may be done. In the presence of antibiotic or antimicrobial medication, bacteria are described as susceptible, intermediate, or resistant. Susceptible means that the bacteria can be treated effectively with a particular medication. Intermediate means that the bacteria can be treated effectively with a higher dosage of the medication or with medication that concentrates in a particular body site where the bacteria are located. Resistance means that the bacteria will not be killed or eliminated by the particular medication.

REFERENCE VALUES   No growth

HOW THE TEST IS DONE

Midstream catch: A clean-voided midstream technique is used to obtain 15 mL or more of urine in a sterile container. A first voided specimen of the day is used because it has the highest colony count after an overnight incubation period.

Indwelling catheter: The top of the collection port of the Foley catheter is disinfected with alcohol. A sterile needle and syringe are used to obtain 4 mL or more of urine from the urine sample port of the catheter. The urine is then placed in a sterile container.

Suprapubic puncture: Occasionally, suprapubic puncture is used to obtain the specimen. Using sterile technique, a needle is inserted into a full bladder and the urine is aspirated with a syringe. The nurse may assist with this procedure but does not perform a suprapubic aspiration.

SIGNIFICANCE OF TEST RESULTS

Abnormal Values

Escherichia coli
Enterobacter spp.
Klebsiella spp.

Staphylococcus aureus
Mycobacterium spp.
Proteus spp.
Pseudomonas
Streptococcus faecalis
Candida albicans

INTERFERING FACTORS

- Contamination of the specimen
- Antimicrobial therapy
- Inadequate volume of urine

NURSING CARE

Pretest
◎ *Patient Teaching.* The nurse instructs the patient regarding the proper procedure for collection of a clean-catch midstream urine sample (see also, Chapter 2). The patient must wash his or her hands with soap before the specimen is collected. The perineum and urinary meatus must be cleansed carefully. The procedure for cleansing is very important because contamination of the specimen from the external genitalia, hair, vagina, or rectum would introduce microbes into the urine sample and cause a false-positive result.

During the Test
Midstream or Clean-Catch Method
◎ *Patient Teaching.* Instruct the patient to begin the urinary stream and void about 1 oz; then, as the urine flow continues, collect the urine by catching it midstream into the container. The first and last parts of the urinary stream are not used for the collection of the specimen. During the collection process, the container must not touch the perineal skin or hair. Once the specimen is obtained, the patient screws the lid onto the container without touching the inner surfaces.

Indwelling Catheter Method
- When the urinary catheter is already in place, the nurse obtains the specimen from the collection port. Disinfect the port with an alcohol sponge. A sterile needle and syringe are used to collect the urine sample through this port. The urine is then placed in a sterile container.
- Urine must not be collected from the drainage bag because bacteria can be present on the outside of the bag. Additionally, the urine is not fresh, and bacteria have had an opportunity to colonize while the specimen remained at room temperature. Lastly, the Foley catheter must not be separated from the collecting tube to obtain the specimen. If the closed drainage system is opened, bacteria will enter the tubing and cause infection in the bladder.

Posttest
- The specimen and requisition request are labeled, including the patient's name, identification number, identification of the specimen, the time of collection, the date, and the physician's name. On the requisition request, also include the method of collection and any antibiotic therapy that may have been initiated already.

Culture, Wound

Also called: Bacterial Culture, Wound

SPECIMEN OR TYPE OF TEST: Secretions, cell scrapings

PURPOSE OF THE TEST

The wound culture is used to determine the presence of infection and to identify the causative organism.

BASICS THE NURSE NEEDS TO KNOW

Soft tissue infections affect various depths of tissue layers, including the epidermis, dermis, subdermis, fascial planes, and muscle tissue. The infectious organism may be enclosed, such as in an abscess. The pathogens also may be in an open, ulcerated, or necrotic wound or fistulous tract that is exposed to the external environment.

One of the problems in culturing the infected wound is that many normal flora grow in an open, draining wound, fistula, or opened abscess. In the case of an ulcerated or necrotic infection, the wound must be cleansed and débrided to remove dead tissue and many of the surface bacterial flora. Then the culture is performed on the underlying tissue or sinus tract at the base of the wound.

Susceptibility Testing

When bacteria are identified, susceptibility testing may be done. In the presence of antibiotic or antimicrobial medication, bacteria are described as susceptible, intermediate, or resistant. Susceptible means that the bacteria can be treated effectively with a particular medication. Intermediate means that the bacteria can be treated effectively with a higher dosage of the medication or with medication that concentrates in a particular body site where the bacteria are located. Resistance means that the bacteria will not be killed or eliminated by the particular medication.

REFERENCE VALUES   **No growth**

HOW THE TEST IS DONE

The physician may use a syringe and needle to aspirate purulent material from a wound. The liquid can be placed in a sterile tube. Tissue samples from a biopsy or scraping of the wound may also be obtained. For transport, the tissue sample is protected from drying by the addition of a small amount of sterile saline.

Swabs and a culture tube can be used. Two swabs are needed, one for culture and one for a smear. The ends of the swabs are twirled around the outer rim of the infected area where bacteria are growing. The swabs cover approximately ½ inch of tissue for 5 seconds, applying enough pressure to cause minimal bleeding and expression of fluid from the tissue. (Bonham, 2009). The swabs are then placed in culture tubes with transport medium.

SIGNIFICANCE OF TEST RESULTS

Positive Values

Staphylococcus aureus
Streptococcus pyogenes
Staphylococcus epidermidis
Escherichia coli
Proteus spp.
Pseudomonas spp.
Bacteroides spp.
Clostridium spp.
Group D streptococci
Klebsiella spp.

INTERFERING FACTORS

• Antibiotic therapy
• Contamination of the specimen

NURSING CARE

Pretest
• If possible, schedule this procedure before antibiotic therapy is started.
• Explain that only minor discomfort occurs as an open wound is swabbed. If the physician must open an abscessed area surgically or perform a tissue biopsy, débridement, or scraping, a local anesthetic may be used. A written consent is needed for these surgical procedures.

During the Test
• Before obtaining the specimen from an open wound, the wound must be thoroughly cleansed with surgical soap and then alcohol. The goal is to culture the infecting organism and avoid contamination by flora and colonizing organisms in pus, old exudate, and dead or necrotic tissue. The contamination of the specimen with surface organisms produces invalid results.

Posttest
• The culture tube must be labeled with the patient's identifying information, date, and time. Ensure that the requisition request indicates the patient's name, identification number, age, specific culture site, time, date, clinical diagnosis, reason for the culture, and any current antibiotic therapy. The specimen is sent to the laboratory promptly.

Cystourethroscopy

SPECIMEN OR TYPE OF TEST: Endoscopy

PURPOSE OF THE TEST

Cystourethroscopy is used to investigate the cause of painless hematuria, particularly when cancer of the epithelial lining of the bladder is suspected. It also is part of the investigation into recurring urinary infection, or the cause of urinary incontinence or retention, related to a problem in the bladder or urethra.

BASICS THE NURSE NEEDS TO KNOW

Cystoscopy provides direct visualization of the urinary bladder. When the urethra also is examined, the procedure is called cystourethroscopy. The examination is performed with a cystoscope—a thin, lighted tube with a telescopic lens. The procedure may be performed in the urologist's office or in the operating room with local, spinal, or general anesthetic. Following the diagnostic component, treatment may include dilation of stricture, surgical removal of some tissue of the prostate gland, cauterization of bleeding spots, implantation of radium seeds, or placement of a ureteral stent or catheter.

REFERENCE VALUES   **The bladder wall is smooth. The bladder is normal in size, shape, and position. There are no obstructions, growths, or stones.**

HOW THE TEST IS DONE

Once the patient is anesthetized, the cystoscope is inserted through the urethra into the urinary bladder. Once the bladder is filled with sterile saline or water for irrigation, all aspects of the bladder walls are examined. The cystoscope has video-camera device that fits over the eyepiece and special lighting, so that the interior surface of the bladder can be imaged. The imaging appears on the monitor and a videotape copy is made for later review. Biopsy samples for tissue examination and cell washings for cytologic analysis may be carried out. Urine samples may be collected from the bladder or from each ureter. The procedure takes approximately 30 to 45 minutes.

SIGNIFICANCE OF TEST RESULTS

Abnormal Values

Tumor
Polyps
Cyst
Cancer of the bladder
Diverticulum of the bladder
Bladder fistula
Bladder stones (calculi)
Urethral stricture
Chronic urethritis
Congenital anomaly
Abnormal prostate (bleeding, enlargement, obstruction)
Traumatic injury (bladder, urethra)

INTERFERING FACTORS

- Failure to maintain nothing-by-mouth status
- Acute infection of the bladder, urethra, or prostate gland

NURSING CARE

Pretest

- After the physician has explained the procedure, the purpose, benefits, and risks, the nurse ensures that written informed consent is obtained from the patient and that the signature is witnessed. The nurse ensures that the consent is entered in the patient's record.

○ *Patient Teaching.* When bowel emptying is part of the protocol, instruct the patient to administer a cathartic or enema, as ordered, the night before or the morning of the test.

○ *Patient Teaching.* For general or spinal anesthesia preparation, the nurse instructs the patient to fast from food and fluids for 8 hours before the procedure. For local anesthesia, fasting from food is required, but clear liquids on the morning of the test are permitted.

- On the morning of the procedure, the nurse obtains baseline vital signs and records the results. The nurse also administers preoperative sedatives or antispasmodics as prescribed.

During the Test

- The nurse provides reassurance to the patient who may be awake during the procedure. The instillation of the local anesthetic into the urethra is mildly painful until the tissue becomes numb. When the bladder is filled with saline, discomfort and the urge to void are normal sensations.
- The biopsy tissue is placed in a sterile glass container with formalin preservative. For the cytologic study, 50 to 75 mL of bladder irrigation fluid is placed in a sterile jar with 50% alcohol as a preservative.
- The nurse assists with the collection of urine specimens. On the container and requisition form, the nurse writes the patient's name, identification number, the physician's name, source of the tissue (bladder, right ureter, left ureter, etc), time, and date.

Posttest

- The nurse takes vital signs and records the results. For patients who have undergone general anesthesia, the nurse continues to monitor the vital signs every 15 to 30 minutes until the patient is stable.
- The nurse assesses for pain or bladder spasms and administers prescribed medication as needed.

○ *Patient Teaching.* The nurse encourages extra oral fluids (4 to 6 glasses of water per day) to promote adequate hydration and the voiding of urine. Instruct the patient to void within 8 hours after the test. The nurse or the patient at home notifies the physician if the patient is unable to void within this time. Reassure the patient that it is normal to have a burning sensation on voiding and to see a small amount of blood or pink-tinged urine. These problems usually disappear after the third voiding.

○ *Patient Teaching.* At home, warm tub baths can help alleviate the patient's discomfort or pain of bladder spasms. Instruct the patient to avoid alcohol for 48 hours because of its irritant effect on the bladder mucosa. To prevent infection, the nurse instructs the patient to take the prescribed antibiotic.

◆ **Nursing Response to Complications**

The most common complications of cystoscopy are persistent bleeding, infection, and urinary retention. Because the patient usually goes home soon after the test, a review of abnormal problems should be provided, and the patient should be advised to notify the urologist when these problems occur.

Bleeding. After a cystoscopy, bleeding may be evident by persistent, painless hematuria, bright red urine, or the passage of blood clots. Notify the urologist or instruct the patient who has been discharged to call the urologist to report any of these findings.

Urinary obstruction. The urologist should be informed if the patient is unable to urinate within 8 hours of the procedure. The nurse palpates the bladder and reports the level where it is felt. The nurse also reports the patient's sensation of needing to void. The nurse anticipates the physician's need for a Foley catheter and catheterization tray.

Infection. The nurse assesses for infection and instructs the patient being discharged to report signs of infection, including fever, chills, flank or abdominal pain, or cloudy urine.

D-dimer and Fibrin/Fibrinogen Degradation Products

Also called: (FDP); Fibrin/Fibrinogen Breakdown Product (FBP)

SPECIMEN OR TYPE OF TEST: Whole Blood

PURPOSE OF THE TEST

The D-dimer test and the fibrin degradation products are tests that help determine whether a clot is present in the diagnosis of deep vein thrombosis, disseminated intravascular coagulation (DIC), or an acute myocardial infarction. They are also used in the diagnosis of hypercoagulable conditions that cause recurrent thrombosis.

BASICS THE NURSE NEEDS TO KNOW

In fibrinolysis, D-dimers are fragments of fibrin that appear in the blood when a thrombus (clot) dissolves or degrades. Fibrin degradation products are end products of the dissolving fibrin and fibrinogen.

These tests are used for screening to exclude the presence of a deep vein thrombus. When the results are in the normal range or negative, no thrombus is present. Elevated test results or the presence of D-dimer fragments is evidence that thrombus formation occurred and lysis of the thrombus is occurring. When the value is elevated, additional tests are needed to determine a specific diagnosis. The combination of elevated levels of fibrin/fibrinogen degradation products and D-dimer fragments is highly predictive of DIC. In DIC, the fibrin/fibrinogen degradation products value rises to greater than 40 µg/mL (SI: >40 mg/L).

Disseminated Intravascular Coagulation (DIC) Screen

D-dimer and fibrin/fibrinogen degradation products are part of the panel of tests to assess for DIC. The additional tests in this group include Prothrombin Time (see p. 525), Activated Partial Thromboplastin Time (see p. 42), Platelet Count (see p. 499), and Fibrinogen (see p. 315). DIC is a common and often severe coagulation disorder commonly precipitated by sepsis, severe tissue injury, or some complications of pregnancy. When the anticoagulation and fibrinolytic systems are overwhelmed by the underlying disorder, DIC can result. In DIC, the patient develops systemic microvascular thrombi and, as platelets and natural anticoagulant factors are depleted, the patient begins to bleed.

In laboratory testing, DIC causes the values of D-dimer and fibrin/fibrinogen degradation products to be elevated as a result of the lysis of the clot or clots. The loss of platelets and anticoagulants result in a prolonged prothrombin time and activated partial thromboplastin time. There is a decrease in the platelet count and fibrinogen value.

REFERENCE VALUES   D-dimers: <0.5 µg/mL *or* SI: <500 µg/L
Fibrin degradation products: <10 µg/mL *or* SI: <10 mg/L

HOW THE TEST IS DONE
Venipuncture is used to obtain a sample of venous blood.

SIGNIFICANCE OF TEST RESULTS
Elevated Values
Thrombotic disease
Deep vein thrombosis
Pulmonary embolism
Arterial thromboembolism
Thrombolytic-defibrination therapy
DIC
Sickle cell anemia crisis
Pregnancy
Malignancy
Surgery (postoperatively)

INTERFERING FACTORS
- None

NURSING CARE

Nursing actions are similar to those used in other venipuncture procedures (see Chapter 2), with the following additional measures.

Posttest
- When the laboratory result of the D-dimer or the FDP test is elevated, the nurse notifies the physician immediately. The nurse recognizes that the patient may have a thrombus or embolus. Nursing assessment should include identification of the location of impaired circulation. A deep vein thrombosis, particularly in the calf of the leg, may produce a positive Homans' sign. The patient's legs should be assessed, observing for swelling, redness, and pain in one leg. The patient may already have manifestations of a pulmonary embolus that resulted from the thrombus, with signs of shock, chest pain, and dyspnea.
- When the DIC panel shows the characteristic abnormal coagulation values associated with this illness, the nurse would immediately notify the physician. The nurse should assess the patient for signs of bleeding, including petechiae (multiple red hemorrhagic spots) or ecchymosis (bruising) of the skin, hematoma, or oozing of blood from a wound or venipuncture site. There may be hematuria, blood in the feces, or blood in nasogastric drainage.

The nurse assesses vital signs often because of the potential for shock. The patient may develop oliguria or anuria. Neurologic manifestations include severe headache, lethargy, or coma, and other alterations of neurologic status. The overt signs of bleeding are serious, but the more significant damage is to organs, which develop microthrombi, leading to ischemia and permanent tissue damage. The assessment findings vary with the severity of the condition but tend to worsen over a short time.

Dexamethasone Suppression Test

SPECIMEN OR TYPE OF TEST: Serum, urine

PURPOSE OF THE TEST

The dexamethasone suppression test assesses the hypothalamic-pituitary-adrenal axis. It usually is performed to identify Cushing's syndrome. With the dexamethasone test, Cushing's disease and ectopic production of adrenocorticotropic hormone (ACTH) and adrenal tumors can be differentiated.

BASICS THE NURSE NEEDS TO KNOW

Dexamethasone (Decadron) is a potent glucocorticoid. It will normally suppress ACTH secretion by the pituitary gland via the normal hormonal feedback mechanism. With the suppression of ACTH, the stimulation for cortisol secretion is suppressed in the adrenal cortex, resulting in a decrease in plasma cortisol and urinary corticosteroid levels.

High-dose dexamethasone testing can be helpful in distinguishing Cushing's disease (pituitary hypersecretion of ACTH) from adrenal tumors or ectopic secretion of ACTH. With high-dose dexamethasone, pituitary secretion of ACTH can be suppressed, with a resulting decrease in plasma cortisol levels. No change will occur with adrenal tumors or ectopic ACTH production.

REFERENCE VALUES   Serum cortisol: <5 μg/dL *or* SI: <138 nmol/L
Urine 17-hydroxycorticosteroid (17-OHCS): <4 ng/24 hr
Urine for free cortisol: <25 μg/24 hr

HOW THE TEST IS DONE

A variety of dexamethasone procedures are possible. Low-dose dexamethasone testing may be carried out overnight or over 2 days. Overnight testing requires the oral administration of dexamethasone at night (10 PM to 11 PM). The next morning, a plasma cortisol level is determined. With the 2-day method, dexamethasone is given orally every 6 hours for 2 days. A 24-hour urine specimen is obtained before and after administration (see discussion of 17-Hydroxycorticosteriods, p. 389), and a plasma cortisol test is performed 6 hours after the last dose of dexamethasone.

High-dose dexamethasone testing begins with obtaining a baseline plasma cortisol level, then giving dexamethasone orally at night, and obtaining another plasma cortisol level the next morning.

SIGNIFICANCE OF TEST RESULTS

Elevated Values
Ectopic corticotropin syndrome

Unchanged Values
Cushing's syndrome

Decreased Values
Cushing's disease

INTERFERING FACTORS
- Review discussions of 17-Hydroxycorticosteriods (p. 389), Free Cortisol (p. 319), and Cortisol, Total (p. 227).

NURSING CARE

Nursing actions are similar to those used in other venipuncture and urine collection procedures (see Chapter 2). Also, review discussions of 17-Hydroxycorticosteroids (p. 389), Free Cortisol (p. 319), and Cortisol, Total (p. 227).

Dipyridamole Scan

See Stress Testing, Cardiac on p. 558.

Dopamine

See Catecholamines, Plasma on p. 180.

Drugs of Abuse

Also called: (DAU); Preemployment Drug Screen
See also: Opiates, urinary on p. 463.

SPECIMEN OR TYPE OF TEST: Urine

PURPOSE OF THE TEST

This urine test is used to screen for the presence of drugs of abuse, often as a condition of preemployment or in cases of suspected overdose.

BASICS THE NURSE NEEDS TO KNOW

This test screens for the most commonly used drug substances or classes of drugs. The federally regulated workplace drug screen (under the Substance Abuse and Mental Health Services Administration -[SAMHSA]) includes five drugs: amphetamines, cannabinoids, cocaine metabolite, opiates, and PCP. The private sector workplace uses these same five drugs of abuse and additional others in a panel of tests. The additional tests can include barbiturates, benzodiazepines, methadone, methaqualone, ethyl alcohol, phencyclidine, and propoxyphene. The reference values may be lower for testing in the private sector workplace. When the drug test is positive or exceeds the cut-off value as measured by one method of laboratory analysis, a second test is done on the specimen, using a different and more sensitive method of analysis (Table 7). Both test results must be positive for the final report to be positive. If the screening is done for workplace purposes, the person should report any use of prescription opioids or amphetamines and the name of the prescribing physician. These medications will produce a positive test result, but the prescriptive use for medical purposes can be verified.

REFERENCE VALUES   Negative

HOW THE TEST IS DONE

A random specimen of urine is collected in a clean container with a lid.

SIGNIFICANCE OF TEST RESULTS

Positive Value
Use of a drug of abuse

INTERFERING FACTORS

- Dilution of the specimen
- Alteration of the specimen

TABLE 7 Drugs of Abuse Cutoff Values	
Screening Cutoff Value	**Second Testing Cutoff Value**
Amphetamines: 1000 ng/mL	Amphetamines: 500 ng/mL
	Methamphetamines: 500 ng/mL
Cannabinoids: 50 ng/mL	THC metabolite: 15 ng/mL
Cocaine metabolite: 300 ng/mL	Benzoylecgonine: 150 ng/mL
Opiates: 2000 ng/mL	Codeine 2000 ng/mL
	Morphine: 2000 ng/mL
	6-acetyl morphine (6 AM): 10 ng/mL
PCP: 25 ng/mL	25 ng/mL

(From Wu, AHB: *Tietz clinical guide to laboratory tests,* ed 4, Philadelphia, 2006, Saunders.)

NURSING CARE

Pretest

- When this test is needed for forensic purposes or for preemployment requirements, the nurse institutes the written protocol for collection and the paperwork for the custody and control form. Because individuals have been known to tamper with their specimen in hopes of passing the test, the nurse follows the protocol guidelines exactly to prevent tampering. Common methods of tampering with the specimen include a substitute donor or substitute urine sample, dilution of the specimen with water from the sink or toilet bowl and adding a chemical to the specimen. The laboratory will test for evidence of tampering.

During the Test

- The donor must provide photo identification or a positive identification from the employer representative. Outerwear, coat, purse, and briefcase remain outside of the collection area to prevent access to concealed tampering substances. The donor washes his or her hands before beginning the procedure. The donor should be observed voiding and collecting the urine, (a witnessed collection) as per the protocol. Alternatively, indirect observation may be acceptable by the observer who remains in the room, outside the door of the toilet stall, listening for unauthorized water use. Once the specimen is collected, the container is sealed with tape and the label is completed with a special patient number, time, and date.

Posttest

- If the voided specimen has an unusual color, odor, or appearance, the nurse records the description in the individual's record and on the form. The temperature strip shows a range of 32.5° to 37.7° C. The temperature of the specimen should be within that range. If it is outside that range, it is suspected of alteration or dilution (Strassinger & Di Lorenzo, 2008). The abnormal temperature result is recorded, a new specimen must be collected, and the supervisor is notified. On the Custody and Control form, signatures for the chain of custody are required to document whenever the custody of the specimen is transferred to the next person (donor, nurse or observer, transporter, laboratory personnel, the Medical Review Officer, and the employer or prospective employer).

Dual Energy X-Ray Absorptiometry

Also called: DXA; bone mineral density (BMD); Bone Densitometry;

SPECIMEN OR TYPE OF TEST: Radiography

PURPOSE OF THE TEST

Dual energy x-ray absorptiometry is a radiology procedure that measures bone mineral density. It is used as a screening test to predict risk of a fracture of the bone. It also establishes the diagnosis of osteoporosis and measures the initial severity of the condition, as well as the effectiveness of treatment.

BASICS THE NURSE NEEDS TO KNOW

Osteoporosis is a metabolic bone disease that causes the bones to become more porous or less dense. Because the bones become thin or brittle, they are at risk for fracture. Osteoporosis occurs most often in postmenopausal women older than age 65. It can also affect men over the age of 70.

Dual energy densitometry absorptiometry (DEXA) will detect a decrease in bone mineral density at a very early stage, before osteoporosis or fractures occur. If the procedure is done only once, the measurement of the patient's bone mineral density is compared with the values of the general population. If the patient has follow-up procedures performed over the years, the results are compared with previous findings and determine whether additional loss has occurred or improvement is demonstrated in response to therapy.

DEXA Test Values

The patient's bone mineral density measurement is usually compared with the average test value of young normal individuals (T score). It also can be compared with the average test value of individuals who are the same sex and age (Z score). The standard deviation (SD) is a statistical measurement that represents how much the patient's value is above (+) or below (−) the average score, which is 0.

Osteopenia means a low bone mass as measured by a test result that is between 1.0 and 2.5 SD below the average value (written as −1.0 SD to −2.5 SD). *Osteoporosis* is indicated by a test result that is −2.5 S.D below the average value, or lower.

Follow-up DEXA scans are done to monitor for changes in the bone mineral density measurements. T-scores or Z scores are not used. The patient's new bone mineral density measurements are compared with his or her previous BMD measurements. A mathematical calculation is used to compare the results and determine if there is any change. A decrease in the bone mineral density over time means there is increased risk of fractures (Dasher, Newton & Lenchik, 2010).

REFERENCE VALUES	T score of +1 to −1.0 SD
	Z score of +1 to −1.0 SD

HOW THE TEST IS DONE

X-ray beams are directed to pass through the body at specific sites and detectors on the opposite side receive the impulses and collect the raw data. The usual areas of imaging are the vertebrae of the lumbar spine, the neck of the femur, and the forearm (Figure 41). Computer calculations measure the bone density and calculate the test results as compared with standardized normal values.

SIGNIFICANCE OF TEST RESULTS

Osteopenia
Osteoporosis
Osteomalacia

INTERFERING FACTORS

- Incorrect positioning of the patient
- Metal prosthetic device
- Metallic items on the clothing or the body in the imaging area

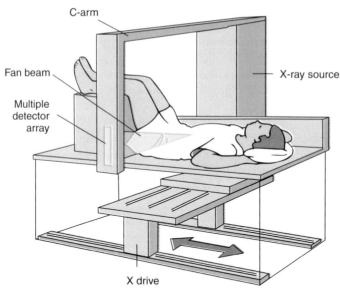

Figure 41. Dual x-ray absorptiometry. The DXA system is used to perform a scan of the lumbar spine (vertebrae L1-L4). During the imaging, the patient is centered on the scanner table with hips and knees flexed by using the positioning block. During the imaging, the C arm with its x-ray source and detectors move in the directions of the arrow. (From Frank ED, Long BW, Smith BJ: *Merrill's atlas of radiographic positioning and procedures,* ed 12, St Louis, 2012, Mosby.)

NURSING CARE

Health Promotion

The nurse can teach people over age 50 about the risks of osteoporosis and the benefits of the density scan. The goals of this screening test are early stage detection of decreased bone density and early intervention to prevent further bone loss and fractures of the bone. For all postmenopausal women, the risk of osteoporosis increases with age.

- As a screening test, The US Preventive Services Task Force (2011) recommends bone mineral density testing should be done routinely for all women age 65 and older. Screening is also recommended for younger women whose fracture risk is equal to or greater than a 65-year-old white woman who has no additional risk factors. The task force makes no recommendations for the screening of men.
- Some of the risk factors can be reduced or eliminated with changes in lifestyle (Box 5). These changes include not smoking, reducing alcohol intake to less than three drinks per day, increasing calcium intake to 1200 IU and vitamin D to 600 IU per day (for those older than 70, the vitamin D intake increases to 800 IU/ day), and increasing weight-bearing activity through daily activities such as walking, jogging, dancing, and other means of obtaining physical exercise.

Pretest

○ *Patient Teaching.* Instruct the patient to remove any jewelry or clothing that contains metal (buttons, belt, and clothing with a zipper) in the area to be imaged. It is not necessary to disrobe completely.

○ *Patient Teaching.* Explain that no noise, pain, or discomfort is associated with the procedure. Although the procedure uses radiation, the exposure and dose are minimal.

During the Test

- The patient is positioned on the imaging table and must not move during the imaging. For measurement of the bone density of the vertebrae, the patient is in the supine position, with the lower legs elevated on a boxlike cushion. This aligns the pelvis and spine in a flat position on the table. For measurement of the bone density of the femoral neck, the patient is supine, with the nondominant leg braced in a position of internal rotation. For measurement of the arm bones, the patient is seated in a chair and the arm is placed on the DEXA table.

Posttest

- The patient is informed of the test results by the health care provider. If the patient has osteopenia or osteoporosis, medication therapy helps increase bone mineral density. The treatment lowers the risk of a bone fracture in the patient who is vulnerable. The nurse assists the patient by teaching about the prescribed medication and the specific information about when and how to take the drug.

BOX 5	Common Risk Factors for Osteoporosis

- Age
- Female
- Postmenopausal
- Low body weight/small frame
- Race/ethnicity-white and Asian people
- Family history of osteoporosis
- Insufficient vitamin D intake
- Insufficient calcium intake
- History of fractures
- Tobacco
- Excess drinking of alcohol, daily

d-Xylose Absorption

Also called: Xylose Tolerance Test; Xylose Absorption Test

SPECIMEN OR TYPE OF TEST: Serum, Urine

PURPOSE OF THE TEST

This test is used in the diagnosis of malabsorption syndrome, and to evaluate the ability of the duodenum and jejunum to absorb carbohydrates.

BASICS THE NURSE NEEDS TO KNOW

One of the causes of intestinal malabsorption is a defect in the mucosal lining of the duodenum and jejunum that prevents or limits carbohydrate absorption. If unabsorbed, the carbohydrate passes through the intestinal tract and does not enter the blood. The concentration of sugar pulls fluid into the intestinal lumen by osmosis. This osmotic effect causes the patient to experience persistent diarrhea and abdominal cramping.

In this test, the patient ingests a prescribed amount of liquid d-xylose, a pentose sugar. If the intestinal tract is able to absorb the sugar, there will be a measured rise in blood glucose and a later rise in urinary glucose as the kidneys clear the glucose from the blood.

If there is a defect in the intestinal mucosa, the d-xylose will not be absorbed and the glucose levels in the blood sample and urine collection will have lower than normal values. Further diagnostic testing may be needed to determine the exact cause of the malabsorption.

REFERENCE VALUES

Whole Blood
Child (1 hour): >30 mg/dL *or* SI: >2.0 mmol/L
Adult (2 hours, 25-g dose): >25 mg/dL *or* SI: >1.7 mmol/L

Urine
Child: 16% to 44% of ingested dose/5 hr *or* SI: 0.16 to 0.44
   (fraction of ingested dose)
Adult (25-g dose): >4 g/5 hr *or* SI: >26.64 mmol/L/5 hr

HOW THE TEST IS DONE

To verify adequate renal function, blood specimens for blood urea nitrogen and creatinine determinations are drawn and a urinalysis is obtained in the early morning before the d-xylose test begins.

The recommended dose of d-xylose is 25 g. For adults, the full dose is preferred because it will detect less severe conditions. For children younger than age 12, the recommended dose is 5 g of d-xylose.

Venipuncture is used to collect two venous blood samples. One is done pretest for a baseline value and the other is drawn 1 or 2 hours after drinking the pentose sugar (1 hour later for children and 2 hours later for adults).

For adults and children older than age 12, the first urine is voided and discarded. Then all urine is collected for 5 hours in a dark bottle and kept refrigerated during the test.

SIGNIFICANCE OF TEST RESULTS

Decreased Values
Intestinal malabsorption (not related to pancreatic disease)
Whipple's disease
Bacterial overgrowth in the small intestine
Delayed gastric emptying
Vomiting
Ascites

INTERFERING FACTORS

- Failure to maintain pretest dietary restrictions
- Physical activity during the test
- Poor renal function
- Vomiting or diarrhea
- Rapid or delayed gastric emptying

▌ NURSING CARE

Nursing actions are similar to those used in other venipuncture and timed urine collection procedures (see Chapter 2), with the following additional measures.

Pretest

○ *Patient Teaching.* For 24 hours before the test, the patient should omit intake of all food that contains pentose sugar (fruits, jams, jellies, and fruit pastries). The pentose in these fruit products is similar to the d-xylose used in the test. If possible, the patient should discontinue all medications for 24 hours before the test because some of the medications alter intestinal motility. Adults should fast from food intake for 8 hours before the test and children should fast for 4 hours. Water intake is permitted and encouraged.

- The nurse ensures that the early morning laboratory test results are present in the patient's record. The physician is notified of abnormal renal function values that would alter the urine phase of the test.

During the Test

- At 8 AM, the patient drinks the prescribed dose of pentose mixed with 250 mL of water. This is followed by another 250 mL of water. At 9 AM, 250 mL of water is taken a third time, with water, as desired, thereafter. After ingestion of the d-xylose, the nurse observes the patient for vomiting or diarrhea. These problems would invalidate the test. If the test is to be rescheduled, a lower dose of d-xylose would be used.
- The patient voids at 8 AM and this specimen is discarded. For the next 5 hours, all urine is collected and refrigerated, using a brown or dark container.

○ *Patient Teaching.* The patient is instructed to remain lying down throughout the test, as physical activity will increase intestinal motility and alter the test results.

Posttest

- Blood specimens are labeled with correct patient identification including the time and date of each specimen. The urine sample is also labeled with correct patient identification and includes the time and date of the start and finish of the collection period. The specimens are sent to the lab immediately to prevent warming by the temperature of the room.

Echocardiogram

Also called: (ECHO); Heart Sonogram; Transthoracic Echocardiogram, Stress Echocardiogram

SPECIMEN OR TYPE OF TEST: Ultrasound

PURPOSE OF THE TEST

An echocardiogram is performed for a variety of diagnostic reasons, such as to evaluate abnormal heart sounds; to evaluate heart size, chamber size, and valvular function; and to detect tumors, pericardial effusion, septal defects, and wall motion abnormalities. It may be used to determine the cause of syncope by assessing the patient's ejection fraction and possible structural abnormalities.

BASICS THE NURSE NEEDS TO KNOW

An echocardiogram is a noninvasive test that uses ultrasound techniques to detect enlargement of the cardiac chambers or variations in chamber size during the cardiac cycle. Even with the advent of CT angiography, the echocardiogram is the gold standard to evaluate heart valves. When echocardiography has been integrated into stress testing, it is called *stress echocardiography* or *exercise echocardiography* (see Stress Testing, Cardiac p. 558). It is frequently used for risk stratification and to assess therapeutic outcomes for patients with coronary artery disease. Stress echocardiography is similar to stress testing, but with an echocardiogram being done at baseline and at each progressive level of exertion. It is especially helpful as a screening tool for women and for persons with a left bundle-branch block. If the patient is unable to use the treadmill or bicycle, stress can be induced with dobutamine or dipyridamole. Sometimes atropine is needed to reach the desired heart rate. *Dobutamine stress echocardiography* (DSE) is frequently used to assess "stunned" or "hibernating" myocardium.

A major limitation of the standard echocardiography is poor imaging because it is 2-dimensional. Improved visualization can be obtained with *real-time 3-D echocardiography* (RT3DE). While RT3DE improves image quality at the current time, its use is limited to guiding intracardiac procedures.

REFERENCE VALUES   No anatomic or functional abnormalities

HOW THE TEST IS DONE

An echocardiogram may be carried out at the bedside, in a special laboratory, in a clinic, or in a doctor's office. A transducer is placed over the third and fourth intercostal spaces to the left of the sternum. The transducer emits ultrasonic beams of high-frequency sound waves that are inaudible to the human ear. The transducer then picks up the echoes created by the deflection of the beams off the various heart structures. This creates a picture on the oscilloscope. The picture is created because the echo varies in intensity based on the differing densities of the structures.

SIGNIFICANCE OF TEST RESULTS

Abnormal Values

Abnormal heart valves

Aneurysm

Cardiomyopathy

Congenital heart disorders

Congestive heart failure

Idiopathic hypertrophic subaortic stenosis

Mural thrombi

Myocardial infarction

Pericardial effusion

Restrictive pericarditis

Tumor of the heart

E

INTERFERING FACTORS

- Chest wall abnormalities
- Excessive movement
- Obesity or very muscular patient
- Improper placement of transducer

NURSING CARE*

Pretest

○ *Patient Teaching.* The nurse informs the patient that the test is noninvasive. The patient is awake during the test and is usually in a recumbent position. The nurse informs the patient that an electromechanical transducer will be positioned on the chest. The patient will sense only the conduction jelly and the movement of the transducer. No pain or risk is involved.

During the Test

- The patient may be asked to breathe slowly or to hold his or her breath.
- Patient may be asked to change position.
- If anxiety is causing excessive wall motion, the nurse provides emotional support.

Posttest

- The nurse evaluates the patient's response to the procedure. The nurse cleanses the chest of conduction gel.
- See **Stress Testing, Cardiac** for care of the patient during a Stress Echocardiogram. In addition to posttest care, a post-exercise echocardiogram is done.

Ejection Fraction, Cardiac

See Catheterization, Cardiac on p. 221.

Electrocardiogram

Also called: (ECG); (EKG); 12-lead ECG or EKG; 15-lead ECG or EKG; 18-lead ECG or EKG

E

SPECIMEN OR TYPE OF TEST: Electrophysiology

PURPOSE OF THE TEST

The purpose of the 12-, 15-, and 18-lead ECG is to diagnose myocardial infarction, injury, and ischemia. An ECG is the most important, rapid, and cost-effective way to assess chest pain. It also assists in identifying hypertrophy, axis deviations, and electrolyte abnormalities, and distinguishes between ventricular and supraventricular tachycardia. Left versus right hypertrophy can be distinguished by comparing the morphologic characteristics of the QRS complex in leads V_1 and V_6, by determining axis deviation, and by interpreting the P-wave.

BASICS THE NURSE NEEDS TO KNOW

The electrocardiogram (ECG) is an invaluable tool in the assessment of the heart. It records the heart's electric activity. Several lead systems are available for the measurement of the electric activity of the heart: 12-, 15-, and 18-lead ECG. The electrochemical physiology characteristics are the same for each of these systems; that is, each uses electrodes on the body surface, amplifies changes in electric potentials, and provides a graphic recording. This is made possible by the body's fluid system, which acts as a conductor of electric forces. The 12-lead ECG is the system used most commonly; it presents a graphic recording of 12 electric planes of the heart. By manipulating the skin electrodes, 12 various views of the heart's electric activity are seen.

In a 12-lead ECG, leads I, II, and III are limb leads. In lead I, the negative electrode of the electrocardiograph is connected to the right arm, and the positive electrode is attached to the left arm. In lead II, the negative electrode is placed on the right arm, and the positive electrode is placed on the left leg. In lead III, the negative electrode is placed on the left arm, and the positive electrode is placed on the left leg. Leads I, II, and III form a triangle, which is called Einthoven's triangle (Figure 42).

The second set of three leads recorded by the electrocardiograph machine is called the augmented limb leads. In these leads, two limbs are attached to negative electrodes, and a third limb is attached to a positive electrode. If the positive electrode is placed on the right arm, the lead is called aVR (augmented voltage right arm). If the positive electrode is on the left arm, it is called aVL (augmented voltage left arm). When the positive electrode is on the left foot, it is called aVF (augmented voltage foot) (Figure 43).

The limb leads and augmented leads are called the standard leads. If one takes the three sides of Einthoven's triangle and moves them to the center, they form three intersecting lines of reference (Figure 44, *A*). If one superimposes the augmented limb leads, the lines of reference and the six limb leads form six intersecting lines (one every 30 degrees). Each limb and augmented lead records a different angle and, therefore, a different view of the same electric activity (Figure 44, B).

For the precordial, or chest, leads, the positive electrodes are applied to the person's chest and the negative electrode is applied to the limbs.

Usually, six chest leads are recorded. This is done by placing the positive electrodes at six different positions across the chest. The chest leads are identified as V_1 through V_6. The chest leads give various views of the horizontal plane of the left ventricle. The precordial leads can be visualized as spokes of a wheel, the center being the atrioventricular (AV) node (Figure 45).

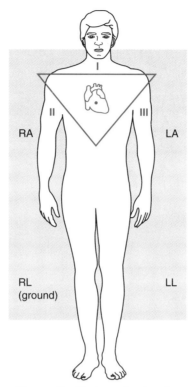

Figure 42. Einthoven's triangle.

15-Lead ECG

With growing recognition of right ventricular infarction, right-sided ECGs are increasing in frequency. Right ventricular infarctions have ST elevations of at least 1 mm in the right precordial leads V_{4r} and V_{5r}. Because the right coronary artery serves both the left ventricular inferior wall and the right ventricle, it is recommended that a right-sided or 15-lead ECG be done on any patient having an inferior wall myocardial infarction.

18-Lead ECG

Frequently, posterior wall infarctions were diagnosed by reciprocal changes seen on the 12-lead ECG. However, when a posterior wall infarction is suspected (an inferior wall myocardial infarction has occurred), three additional leads may be placed with the 15-lead ECG. These are the posterior leads V_7, V_8, and V_9.

REFERENCE VALUES   Normal sinus rhythm

HOW THE TEST IS DONE

For a 12-lead ECG, the technician, the physician, or the nurse places the patient in a supine position. Conduction jelly is placed on the electrodes (disposable electrodes already have jelly on the electrode), and the electrodes are applied. The electrocardiograph's electrode wires are

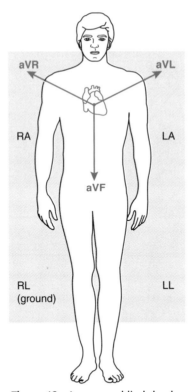

Figure 43. Augmented limb leads.

marked and color coded. It is essential that the chest leads be positioned correctly for accurate interpretation.

The chest leads are applied as follows (Figure 46):

V_1: Fourth intercostal space (ICS) at the right sternal border

V_2: Fourth ICS at the left sternal border

V_3: Midway between V_2 and V_4

V_4: Fifth ICS at the left midclavicular line

V_5: Fifth ICS at the anterior axillary line

V_6: Fifth ICS at the midaxillary line

Electrocardiographs vary. Older machines record one lead at a time. Newer machines simultaneously record the 12 leads and automatically mark them.

Leads for right ventricular assessment are placed at the right fifth intercostal space at the midclavicular line (V_{4r}), at the right intercostal space at the anterior axillary line (V_{5r}), and at the right fifth intercostal space at the midaxillary line (V_{6r}).

With the 18-lead ECG, a 15-lead ECG is taken, and then three chest electrodes are placed on the line level with the fifth ICS at the posterior axillary line (V_7). The next electrode is placed at the fifth ICS at the posterior midclavicular line (V_8), and the last electrode is placed at the fifth ICS, left of the spinal column (V_9).

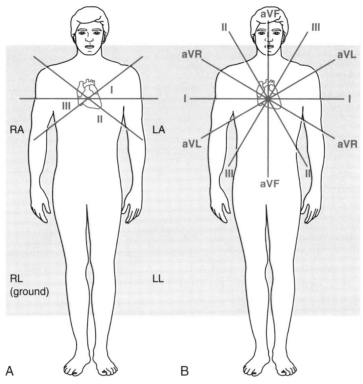

Figure 44. Intersecting limb leads and augmented leads.

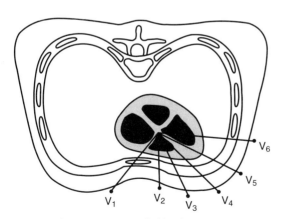

Figure 45. Precordial leads (V_1-V_6).

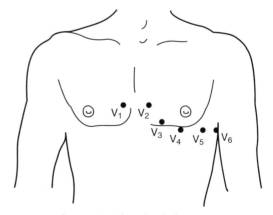

Figure 46. Chest lead placement.

E

SIGNIFICANCE OF TEST RESULTS

Axis deviations (right or left)
Conduction disturbances
Dysrhythmias
Hypertrophy of the ventricles
Electrolyte imbalances
Pericarditis
Pulmonary infarctions
Therapeutic drug effects or toxicity, or both
Myocardial ischemia
Myocardial infarction

Myocardial Infarction

As a myocardial infarction evolves, a sequence of electrocardiographic changes occurs. First, the ST segment changes. Elevation of an ST segment indicates myocardial injury. ST depression occurs as a reciprocal change in the ventricular wall opposite the infarction. The ST segment will return to normal within days or weeks after the infarction.

Within hours or days of the infarction, the T wave inverts. It reflects ischemic changes in the heart. The T wave will revert back to normal within weeks or months of the infarction.

Lastly, an abnormal Q wave appears in the leads directly over the transmural myocardial infarction. An abnormal Q wave is a Q wave in a lead in which a Q wave is not normally seen or one that is wider than 0.04 seconds or a third of the height of the QRS complex. A non-Q wave infarction occurs in the setting of a subendocardial infarction. A Q wave indicates myocardial necrosis and may remain for years after the infarction.

Table 8 summarizes which leads reflect which walls of the left ventricle. Note that because leads usually are not placed over the posterior wall of the heart, posterior infarctions are diagnosed by reciprocal changes. Right ventricular infarctions are assessed by performing a right-sided ECG.

INTERFERING FACTORS

- Patient movement, poor grounding, and poor skin contact can interfere with a clear recording of the ECG.
- Improper placement of the leads.

TABLE 8	Electrocardiographic Changes with Acute Myocardial Infarction	
	Lead Changes	**Reciprocal Changes**
Inferior wall	II, III, aVF	I, aVL
Lateral wall	I, aVL, V_5, V_6	V_1, V_2, V_3
Anterior wall	V_2, V_3, V_4	II, III, aVF
Anteroseptal	V_1, V_2, V_3, V_4	II, III, aVF
Posterior wall	V_7, V_8, V_9	V_1, V_2
Right ventricular	V_{4R}, V_{5R}	

NURSING CARE

Pretest

○ *Patient Teaching.* The nurse explains to the patient the purpose and procedure for the ECG. No risk is involved. No pretest restrictions are required.

- Because electrodes are applied to the four extremities and the chest, clothing should permit easy access. If the male patient's chest is excessively hairy, the sites may need to be shaved.

During the Test

- Establish a relaxed environment.
- Place the patient in a supine position.
- Apply electrodes with conduction jelly.
- The recording is made.
- If a 15- or 18-lead ECG is done, clearly identify the lead placement on the ECG recording.

Posttest

- Remove electrodes and wipe off conduction jelly.
- Help the patient to a comfortable position.

Electrocardiogram, Signal-Averaged

Also called: (SAECG)

SPECIMEN OR TYPE OF TEST: Electrophysiology

PURPOSE OF THE TEST

The cardiologist assesses the printout of the signal-averaged electrocardiogram (ECG) for late potentials, which place the patient at risk for sustained ventricular tachycardia (VT). A late potential is seen as a QRS complex that extends 20 to 60 msec into the ST segment.

BASICS THE NURSE NEEDS TO KNOW

Signal-averaged electrocardiography (SAECG) is a technique used to detect conduction defects that may precede VT. It is a noninvasive bedside test similar to a 12-lead ECG. With a signal-averaged ECG, the recording is obtained for 15 to 30 minutes, and the electric current from the heart is amplified 1000 times. The machine then integrates all these signals and removes extraneous electric signals.

REFERENCE VALUES   Normal cardiac rhythm and conduction times; normal Q–T interval

HOW THE TEST IS DONE

The procedure is similar to the 12-lead ECG, except that no limb electrodes are necessary and the six chest electrodes and ground lead are positioned differently on the chest.

SIGNIFICANCE OF TEST RESULTS

Late potentials

INTERFERING FACTORS

- Because the signal-averaged ECG averages the cardiac cycle of the patient, a relatively regular rhythm is needed during the test. Frequent premature atrial contractions or premature ventricular contractions will interfere with the results.
- Signal-averaged ECG is also unable to detect late potentials in patients with right or left bundle branch block.

NURSING CARE

The nursing actions are similar to those for an electrocardiogram (ECG) (p. 271). In addition, review the following.

Pretest

- The nurse checks with the physician regarding discontinuing or administering the patient's antiarrhythmic medication.

During the Test

- Keep the environment quiet.
- The nurse instructs others to stay out of the patient's room.

Electroencephalography

Also called: (EEG); Electroencephalogram

SPECIMEN OR TYPE OF TEST: Electrophysiology

PURPOSE OF THE TEST

The major applications of electroencephalography (EEG) are in the diagnosis of epilepsy and the determination of the type of epilepsy. It may be used to detect brain injury, evaluate sleep disorders, and to monitor function during brain surgery. It is also used to determine brain activity in the patient in deep coma and to help decide if a patient is brain dead.

BASICS THE NURSE NEEDS TO KNOW

EEG records the spontaneous brain activity that originates from brain cells on the surface of the brain. The fluctuations of electrical activity from the larger cortical areas of the brain pass through the cranial bones and the scalp. The voltage is detected by the electrodes and is converted to specific wave patterns that are seen on the computer screen.

In the process of *electric brain mapping*, the brain waves and patterns are demonstrated on the computer screen, allowing for the detection of abnormalities in a specific region of the brain.

The *video electroencephalography monitor* combines the recording of the EEG waveforms with videotaping to correlate the behavioral events with electroencephalographic seizure activity.

Normal EEG recordings are generally rhythmic and have waveforms of similar height and duration. The interpretation of the EEG considers the frequency of the predominant rhythm, the amplitude, any abnormal waves or wave groups, and the asymmetry between the right and left hemispheres.

REFERENCE VALUES Normal patterns of electric brain activity are seen.

HOW THE TEST IS DONE

Sixteen to twenty-five electrodes are applied to the scalp in a set pattern, using a paste that promotes conduction. The electrode wires are connected to an amplifier and recording machine. The images of the tracings are seen on the computer screen. The EEG procedure usually takes 30 to 90 minutes, but the sleep EEG is recorded all night.

SIGNIFICANCE OF TEST RESULTS

Abnormal Values
Seizure disorder
Intracranial hemorrhage
Mental retardation
Stroke or ischemic encephalopathy
Meningitis
Brain tumor
Drug or alcohol abuse
Infection (toxoplasmosis, rubella, cytomegalovirus, herpes simplex)

INTERFERING FACTORS

- Caffeine and alcohol
- Movements of the hands, body, or tongue
- Muscle contractions
- Drug intoxication (heroin, cocaine, marijuana, crack cocaine, lysergic acid diethylamide [LSD])
- Particular medications (narcotics, sedatives, tranquilizers, monoamine oxidase inhibitors, anticonvulsants, antihistamines)
- Low glucose level

NURSING CARE

Pretest
○ *Patient Teaching.* Instruct the patient to avoid caffeine and alcohol for 8 hours before the test because stimulants alter the electroencephalographic activity. A light meal and fluid intake are encouraged because a low blood glucose level also can alter the test results. Instruct the patient to shampoo his or her hair thoroughly before the test. Hair spray, mousse, or conditioner must not be used because they interfere with attachment of the electrodes and conductivity.
- The nurse or technician provides information about the test and offers support to the patient and family member, as applicable. The purpose is to reduce the patient's fear of the unknown because variables such as tense neck muscles and anxiety would alter the brain wave patterns.

Continued

	NURSING CARE—cont'd

- If a sleep-deprived EEG is performed to evaluate sleep disorder or seizures that occur during sleep, the patient may be instructed not to sleep on the night before the test. At the time of the test, a sedative may be given to promote sleep. If this form of EEG is used, the nurse informs the patient to have a responsible person available to drive him or her home after the test is completed.
- Because anticonvulsants, stimulants, and tranquilizers alter the electric activity of the brain, these medications may be withheld for 24 to 48 hours before the test begins, as determined by the physician. If the medications cannot be withheld because of the seriousness of the patient's seizure disorder, all medications taken in the 24- to 48-hour pretest period are documented on the requisition form.

During the Test

- Help the patient to relax in the reclining chair or on the bed. Inform the patient that the electrodes are attached to the scalp with a sticky paste. Reassure the patient that the electrodes and wires will not cause harm or a shock.
- Instruct the patient not to move the head or body and not to talk during the test. These muscle movements alter the electroencephalographic readings. For the neonate, place the head in a midline alignment. Children often are more relaxed and quiet if the parent remains in the room.
- Reassure the patient that the nurse is nearby with full visibility of the patient during the procedure. If a seizure occurs, the nurse is prepared to provide care during the episode.

Posttest

- Observe the patient for any further seizure activity.
- Remove the electrodes. The electrode paste is cleaned from the hair and scalp with acetone and cotton balls. Any residual paste can be removed at home by several hair washings with regular shampoo.
- Anticonvulsant medications that were withheld for the test are not automatically restarted at the same dosage. The previous orders are reviewed by the physician, and new orders are written.

Electrolyte Gap

See Anion Gap on p. 90.

Electrolytes, 24-Hour Urine

Includes: Sodium, Urine; Chloride, Urine; Potassium, Urine; Calcium, Urine; Magnesium, Urine

SPECIMEN OR TYPE OF TEST: Urine

PURPOSE OF THE TEST

Urine electrolytes are used to help monitor renal function, fluid and electrolyte balance, and acid-base balance. The urinary calcium level is used to evaluate bone disease, parathyroid disorders, nephrolithiasis, calcium metabolism, and idiopathic hypercalciuria.

BASICS THE NURSE NEEDS TO KNOW

Normally, the daily intake of food includes a renewing supply of electrolytes. The glomeruli filter the electrolytes from the blood, and the renal tubules resorb most of them for recirculation and redistribution as needed. Electrolyte excesses are not resorbed and are excreted in urine.

The normal urinary excretion of electrolytes is dependent on the amount of intake, the serum level of the electrolytes, and the state of hydration of the body. The equilibrium of water and electrolytes is controlled by renal and multiple endocrine functions. Any condition that causes a decrease in perfusion to the kidney will cause a decrease in electrolytes excreted in urine.

E

REFERENCE VALUES

Sodium
Male child (6-10 years): 41-115 mEq/24 hr *or* SI: 41-115 mmol/24 hr
Female child (6-10 years): 20-69 mEq/24 hr *or* SI: 20-69 mmol/24 hr
Male child (10-14 years): 63-117 mEq/24 hr *or* SI: 63-117 mmol/24 hr
Female child (10-14 years): 48-168 mEq/24 hr *or* SI: 48-168 mmol/24 hr
Adult: 40-220 mEq/24 hr *or* SI: 40-220 mmol/24 hr

Chloride
Infant: 2-10 mEq/24 hr *or* SI: 2-10 mmol/24 hr
Male child (6-10 years): 36-110 mEq/24 hr *or* SI: 36-110 mmol/24 hr
Female child (6-10 years): 18-74 mEq/24 hr *or* SI: 18-74 mmol/24 hr
Male child (10-14 years): 64-176 mEq/24 hr *or* SI: 64-176 mmol/24 hr
Female child (10-14 years): 36-173 mEq/24 hr *or* SI: 36-173 mmol/24 hr
Adult (<60 years): 40-220 mEq/24 hr *or* SI: 40-220 mmol/24 hr

Potassium
Infant: 4.1-5.3 mEq/24 hr *or* SI: 4.1-5.3 mmol/24 hr
Male child (6-10 years): 17-54 mEq/24 hr *or* SI: 17-54 mmol/24 hr
Female child (6-10 years): 8-37 mEq/24 hr *or* SI: 8-37 mmol/24 hr
Male child (10-14 years): 22-57 mEq/24 hr *or* SI: 22-57 mmol/24 hr
Female child (10-14 years): 18-58 mEq/24 hr *or* SI: 18-58 mmol/24 hr
Adult: 25-125 mEq/24 hr *or* SI: 25-125 mmol/24 hr

Calcium
Infant and child: 6 mg/kg/day or less *or* SI: 0.15 mmol/kg/day or less
Adult (normal calcium intake): 100-300 mg/day *or* SI: 2.5-7.5 mmol/day
Adult (low calcium intake): 50-100 mg/day *or* SI: 1.25-3.75 mmol/day
Adult (calcium-free diet): 5-40 mg/day *or* SI: 0.13-1 mmol/day

Magnesium
Adults: 6.0-10.0 mEq/L *or* SI: 3-5 mmol/day

HOW THE TEST IS DONE

A 24-hour urine specimen is collected in a large, clean urine collection container. Urine is kept refrigerated or on ice during the collection period. Alternative methods include a 12-hour urine collection or a single random urine sample for electrolyte testing. If a 24-hour urine test for protein or creatinine clearance is also ordered, these tests can be performed simultaneously with the urine electrolyte test, using the same specimen.

SIGNIFICANCE OF TEST RESULTS

Elevated Values

Sodium and Chloride
Increased sodium chloride intake
Adrenal insufficiency
Addison's disease
Nephritis (salt-wasting)
Renal tubular acidosis
Diuretic therapy
Acute or chronic renal failure

Potassium
Increased potassium intake
Cushing's syndrome
Aldosteronism
Renal tubular disease
Metabolic acidosis
Adrenocorticotropic hormone or cortisone treatment

Calcium
Hyperparathyroidism
Vitamin D toxicity
Malignancy of bone, breast, bladder
Renal tubular acidosis
Skeletal immobility
Multiple myeloma
Nephrolithiasis
Multiple myeloma
Paget's disease
Sarcoidosis

Magnesium
Addison's disease
Chronic alcoholism
Cisplatin therapy
Diuretic therapy

Decreased Values

Sodium and Chloride
Decreased sodium chloride intake
Cushing's syndrome

Nephrotic syndrome
Prerenal azotemia
Severe vomiting, diarrhea
Intestinal fistula
Severe burns
Excessive sweating
Metabolic acidosis
Potassium
Addison's disease
Acute glomerulonephritis
Pyelonephritis
Nephrosclerosis
Metabolic alkalosis
Prolonged vomiting and diarrhea
Calcium
Hypoparathyroidism
Celiac disease
Inadequate nutrition
Cancer, bone
Nephrosis
Steatorrhea
Acute nephritis
Vitamin D-resistant rickets

INTERFERING FACTORS

- Failure to collect all the urine during the 24-hour collection period
- Failure to refrigerate the specimen
- For magnesium testing: contact with a metal bedpan or urinal

NURSING CARE

Pretest
- Obtain a urine collection container from the laboratory for the collection of all urine in the 24-hour (or 12-hour, if ordered) test period.

○ *Patient Teaching.* If the test is used to evaluate nephrolithiasis, the nurse instructs the patient to eat the usual diet for 3 days before the test. If the patient is already receiving a calcium-restricted diet as part of the calcium stone prevention treatment, instruct the patient to maintain the dietary restriction before and during the test period.

○ *Patient Teaching.* If thiazide diuretics are used to prevent formation of calcium stones, the nurse instructs the patient to continue the medication before and during the test. Thiazides are effective in lowering the urine calcium levels, and the benefits of the medication can be evaluated.

During the Test
○ *Patient Teaching.* Instruct the patient to void at 8 AM and discard the specimen. The test begins immediately thereafter, and all urine is collected for the next 24 hours, including the

Continued

| NURSING CARE—cont'd

8 AM specimen of the next morning. The nurse needs to remind the patient periodically that all urine must be collected.

- Keep the urine in the refrigerator or on ice throughout the collection period.
- Instruct the patient to use the special laboratory container to collect the urine. If a bedpan or urinal is used for voiding, it must be made of plastic, not metal.
- Ensure that the patient's name, identification number, the date and time of the start and finish of the test are written on the label and the requisition form.

Posttest

- Arrange for prompt transport of the chilled specimen to the laboratory.

Electromyography and Nerve Conduction Studies

Also called: (EMG); (NCS); Electrodiagnostic Studies

SPECIMEN OR TYPE OF TEST: Electrophysiology

PURPOSE OF THE TEST

These tests help distinguish among the causes of weakness and paralysis. The tests are used to identify the particular nerve or muscle group that is involved, to localize the site of the abnormality, to evaluate the severity, and to distinguish a sensorimotor nerve disorder from a pure motor disorder.

BASICS THE NURSE NEEDS TO KNOW

When a patient complains of muscle weakness, muscle spasms, paralysis, or loss of sensation, the cause may be disease of the muscle or nervous system or a problem with neuromuscular transmission at the junction between the nerves and the muscle fibers. Electromyography and nerve conduction studies are two diagnostic tests that help identify the physiologic location and severity of the problem.

Electromyography

This procedure records the electric potential of various muscles in a resting state, during stimulation, and during voluntary contraction of the muscles. The normal tracings of muscle potential demonstrate characteristic patterns and the tracings are examined for amplitude, duration, form, and abundance. Characteristic abnormal patterns demonstrate that the problem is neurologic in origin, such as denervation, or muscular in origin, such as muscle inflammation.

Nerve Conduction Studies

These studies measure motor conduction velocity and sensory conduction. Motor conduction velocity is the timed measurement of conduction as a stimulus moves along a nerve between two points. Sensory conduction measures the voltage or strength of the nerve stimulus in sensory nerve endings.

REFERENCE VALUES	The muscle shows minimal activity at rest Nerve conduction time is within normal limits

HOW THE TEST IS DONE

Electromyography

Needle electrodes are inserted into specific muscles and connected to stimulator and recorder devices. As the electric stimulus is initiated, the results appear on an oscilloscope, video screen, or are photographed. Linear tracings of the electromyography are recorded.

Nerve Conduction Studies

The stimulator is placed on the skin, directly over the particular nerve to be evaluated (Figure 47). Recording electrodes are placed over the distal aspect of the same nerve, at a measured distance from the stimulator. The different placements of the recorders provide for measurement of sensory and motor nerve conduction time.

SIGNIFICANCE OF TEST RESULTS

Abnormal Findings

Amyotrophic lateral sclerosis
Muscular dystrophy
Herniated lumbar disk
Myasthenia gravis
Guillain-Barré syndrome
Poliomyelitis
Carpal tunnel syndrome
Inflammatory myositis

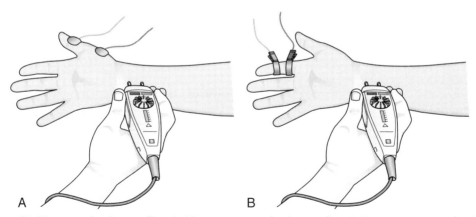

Figure 47. Nerve conduction studies. **A,** Motor nerve conduction studies. **B,** Sensory nerve conduction studies. In this illustration, the median nerve is evaluated to determine quality of nerve transmission along motor and sensory pathways that enervate the fingers. In carpal tunnel syndrome, the median nerve is compressed in the wrist and causes impaired sensory and motor functions in the hand and fingers. (Redrawn from Gooch CL & Weimer LH., (2007) The electrodiagnosis of neuropathy: Basic principles and common pitfalls. *Neurologic Clinics, 25*, (1), 1-28.)

Brachial plexus injury
Myopathy (endocrine, metabolic, toxic, congenital)
Lumbosacral plexus injury
Nerve trauma
Diabetic neuropathy
Hypothyroidism

INTERFERING FACTORS

* Acute anxiety

NURSING CARE

Pretest

   Electromyography. Current prothrombin time and INR blood values are usually required of patients who are receiving anticoagulant therapy. As long as the results are in the therapeutic range, the test can be performed. The nurse ensures that the laboratory results are in the patient's record. The patient is also asked if he or she has a pacemaker. The pacemaker is acceptable, but awareness of it will allow for correct interpretation of the data.

   Nerve Conduction Studies. For nerve conduction studies, no pretest blood work is needed.

* After the physician has explained one or both procedures, the patient must sign a written consent that is placed in .his or her record.

O *Patient Teaching.* For both electromyography and nerve conduction studies, instruct the patient to shower before the test. This will remove the body oil from the surface of the skin. No skin cream or lotion should be used afterward.

O *Patient Teaching.* For electromyography, inform the patient that the insertion of the needles and the small shocks are painful. Reassurance and empathy are helpful in promoting the patient's tolerance and acceptance. If possible, encourage the parent of a child patient to comfort the child during the procedure.

   For nerve conduction studies, inform the patient that the examiner will use electrode paste to apply the sensors to the skin over the distal motor and then sensory aspects of a particular nerve. The stimulator is placed on the skin over the proximal part of the nerve. A series of small shocks will be delivered with increasing intensity, to obtain accurate data about how well the motor and sensory portions of the nerve function when stimulated.

During the Test

* For grounding, a metal plate is placed under the patient's body in the area being tested. The physician cleanses the skin with antiseptic before inserting or placing the electrodes.

   Electromyography. As the needle electrode is inserted, reassurance is given that the pain will be brief and minimal. Continuous reassurance throughout the procedure is very helpful to the patient and reduces the level of anxiety. Once inserted, the needle is gradually advanced across the diameter of the muscle. At appropriate intervals during EMG, the patient is asked to perform various voluntary muscle contractions. Then the needle is withdrawn from that muscle site and is repositioned in another direction in the muscle. The sequence is then repeated, for a total of 2 to 4 times. The test may be of one muscle or of several muscles, depending on the suspected clinical diagnosis.

* The recordings of the results are in the form of linear tracings of muscle activity during (1) insertion of the needle electrode; (2) at rest, identifying spontaneous muscle activity; and (3) during voluntary activity (Daube & Rubin, 2009).

Nerve conduction studies. Although there are no needle insertions in this test, the shocks are small, but somewhat painful. The examiner provides empathy to help the patient tolerate the brief procedure.

Posttest

- In electromyography, the needle electrodes are removed gently and slowly. To control for bleeding, pressure is applied to the puncture site for 1-2 minutes. If pain persists at the puncture site, the patient is instructed to apply warm compresses.
- In nerve conduction studies, the sensors are peeled off and electrode paste is removed from the skin.

Electrophysiologic Studies, Cardiac

Also called: (EPS)

SPECIMEN OR TYPE OF TEST: Radiography

PURPOSE OF THE TEST

Electrophysiologic studies are performed to diagnose dysrhythmias, to identify causes of ectopy and reentry phenomenon, and to determine a person's risk for lethal ventricular dysrhythmias. They are used to determine appropriate therapy for patients who have not obtained the desired effect from usual therapies and in whom noninvasive evaluation techniques have not provided the information necessary to determine which therapy or combination of therapies will be effective.

BASICS THE NURSE NEEDS TO KNOW

Electrophysiologic studies are invasive procedures performed in special laboratories or in cardiac catheterization laboratories. These studies require the insertion of catheters via femoral, brachial, or jugular vein access to the right and sometimes the left side of the heart. Several procedures are included: atrial stimulation, ventricular stimulation, His bundle studies, and ventricular mapping.

REFERENCE VALUES	Normal cardiac rhythm; normal conduction and interval times, no reentry pathways noted

HOW THE TEST IS DONE

Several procedures are included in the category of electrophysiologic studies. The patient may have one or all the studies performed based on the clinical state. During the test, three or four multipolar intracardiac catheters are inserted percutaneously. One is positioned high in the atrium, one in the low-septal right atrium, one in the coronary sinus, and one in the right ventricle.

Conduction intervals are measured to locate conduction delays by *programmed electrical stimulation* (PES). Atrial pacing is carried out to assess sinoatrial node response, atrioventricular node response, and His bundle and Purkinje conduction. If indicated, *atrial extrastimulus testing*

(AEST) is performed. With this test, a premature atrial stimulus is initiated to assess atrial and atrioventricular node response. Atrial flutter or atrial fibrillation may be initiated. The focus or reentry pathway may then be identified. In some patients, *His bundle electrographic studies* are performed to evaluate His bundle conduction.

Ventricular extrastimulus testing (VEST) is performed to assess ventricular dysrhythmias. Ventricular tachycardia (VT) may be induced. If a right ventricular stimulus does not induce VT, a left-sided stimulation may be carried out. This requires the insertion of a multipolar pacing catheter through an artery. When VT is induced, its response to overdrive pacing or drugs, or both, can be evaluated. If the patient has recurrent VT, *ventricular endocardial mapping* may be performed to localize the origin of the dysrhythmia. If ventricular mapping is performed, VT is induced, and the ectopic focus is delineated by multiple intracardiac tracings.

If the electrophysiologic studies involve evaluation of drug responses, the test must be repeated, because only one drug or combination of drugs can be assessed at a time. If this is necessary, catheters are left in place between testings.

SIGNIFICANCE OF TEST RESULTS

Electrophysiologic studies may identify dysrhythmias, conduction abnormalities, and appropriate treatment for these disturbances.

INTERFERING FACTORS

- Inability to produce arrhythmia
- Altered autonomic tone from supine position

NURSING CARE

Pretest
- Verify that an informed consent has been obtained.
- The nurse assists with the precatheterization evaluation: blood tests, including prothrombin time test and a partial thromboplastin time test; an electrocardiogram (ECG); and a chest radiograph if the procedure will be performed on an outpatient basis. An echocardiogram may be ordered to assess possible risk.
- The nurse assesses the patient's fears and anxieties. Correct any misperceptions and reassure the patient that the nurses and physician will be continuously present during the procedure.
- ○ *Patient Teaching.* The nurse instructs the patient about the purpose and procedure for the study. Inform the patient to report any chest pain, dizziness, or shortness of breath. The patient is instructed to take nothing by mouth after midnight, except if the EPS study is planned for the late afternoon. In that case, a clear liquid breakfast may be taken.
- The nurse checks with the physician if cardiac drugs are to be withheld. Usually antiarrhythmic medications are withheld for at least 24 hours.
- The nurse prepares the site of catheter access according to laboratory protocols. The femoral vein is commonly used for the percutaneous insertion of the electrode catheters. Usually both sides of the groin are prepared.
- Instruct the patient to void before going to the catheterization laboratory.
- To reduce the anxiety, the nurse premedicates the patient as prescribed.
- Encourage the patient to wear his or her glasses to the catheterization laboratory.

E

During the Test
- The patient is awake. The nurse provides emotional support and reinforces explanations given about the procedure.
- Continuous cardiac monitoring is maintained.
- A local anesthetic is given by the physician, after the insertion site (usually the right side of the groin) is prepared and draped. The physician inserts the electrode catheters using fluoroscopy visualization.
- The patient may be asked to cough during the procedure.
- When tachyarrhythmias are produced, the nurse assesses the patient's responses and reports any indication of hemodynamic instability. Overdrive pacing may be used to treat ventricular tachycardia.

Posttest
- The nurse monitors the patient's vital signs and cardiac rhythm according to hospital protocol.
- Observe the insertion site for signs of bleeding and hematoma. If bleeding is present, the nurse exerts pressure just proximal to the puncture site with a gloved hand for a minimum of 15 minutes.
- The nurse evaluates the patient's psychological response to the procedure and its findings.
- Assess for complications: pain, adverse drug reaction, cardiac perforation, cardiac tamponade, dysrhythmias, and heart blockers.
- Observe for late complications: thromboembolism and infection including pericarditis.

○ *Patient Teaching.* If the study is done as an outpatient procedure, instruct the patient to (1) not drive for 24 hours; (2) avoid heavy lifting, sports, and strenuous housework for 3 days; and (3) avoid baths until the wound is healed. Instruct the patient that after 24 hours, he or she may shower and change the dressing.

◆ **Nursing Response to Complications**
The nurse needs to assess for and report any observations indicating complications, which may occur during and after the EPS study. Complications include dysrhythmias, vasovagal reaction, and pericardial effusion.

Dysrhythmias. The purpose of the EPS studies includes the production of dysrhythmias; however, other nondiagnostically produced dysrhythmias may occur especially during the insertion and removal of the electrode catheters. The nurse continuously monitors the cardiac rhythm during the procedure. Notify the physician and anticipate treatment based on established protocols.

Vasovagal Response. A vasovagal response may occur because of the insertion or withdrawal of the electrode catheters. The patient may experience diaphoresis, pallor, nausea, vomiting, bradycardia, and hypotension. The nurse takes frequent vital signs and informs the physician of patient status.

Pericardial Effusion. Because of the insertion of catheters, a small ventricular puncture may occur, causing a pericardial effusion. Small leaks usually seal themselves. Very rarely, the ventricular leak may lead to cardiac tamponade. Cardiac tamponade is an emergency. As blood accumulates in the pericardial sac, the heart is restricted. The nurse will observe signs of a decrease in cardiac output and muffled heart sounds. Notify the physician immediately. The blood in the pericardial sac must be aspirated to restore an adequate cardiac output.

Endoscopic Retrograde Cholangiopancreatography and Pancreatic Endoscopy

Also called: (ERCP)
Includes: Endoscopic ultrasound, Biliary and pancreatic cytology studies

SPECIMEN OR TYPE OF TEST: Endoscopy

PURPOSE OF THE TEST

Endoscopic retrograde cholangiopancreatography (ERCP) is used to investigate the cause of obstructive jaundice, persistent abdominal pain, or both, associated with biliary or pancreatic disorder. Biliary and pancreatic cytology identifies the cell type from the secretions or tissue biopsy specimens.

BASICS THE NURSE NEEDS TO KNOW

Bile from the liver and gallbladder and secretions from the pancreas drain through the common bile duct into the small intestine. If there is obstruction in the biliary ducts, cystic duct, or common duct or at the ampulla of Vater, the bile flow into the intestine is impeded and the patient develops obstructive jaundice. If there is blockage of the flow of pancreatic secretions, inflammation of the pancreas occurs. Because these organs and ducts are very close to each other, endoscopic visualization and radiography of the biliary and pancreatic ducts are needed to determine the cause of the problem and its precise location.

Endoscopic Ultrasound

The endoscope has an ultrasound probe that is attached to the tip of the instrument to provide imaging of tissue that is 3 to 4 inches beneath the surface of the lumen. The ultrasound imaging is particularly useful in detection and sizing of a stone in the common bile duct. It also provides imaging detail about the depth and size of a polyp, stricture, ulcer, or tumor. In the staging of a malignant tumor, the endoscopic ultrasound is very useful for determining the depth of the cancerous growth and its possible spread to surrounding tissues and lymph gland (Rumack, Wilson & Charboneau, 2005).

ERCP is a highly accurate method to diagnose pathology of the common bile duct, sphincter of Oddi, and the pancreatic duct. After the diagnostic phase is completed, endoscopic interventions are often performed. These can include removal by crushing or retrieving a common bile duct stone, sphincterotomy, dilation of a stricture in the bile duct, or placement of stents to reestablish drainage of bile or pancreatic secretions.

REFERENCE VALUES   ERCP: The anatomy of the common duct and pancreatic duct are normal, with no evidence of obstruction from stone, stricture, or tumor
Biliary cytology: Normal; no malignant cells are present in the biliary biopsy tissue or secretions
Pancreatic cytology: Normal; no malignant pancreatic cells are present in the biopsy tissue or secretions

HOW THE TEST IS DONE
ERCP

After the patient receives conscious sedation, the endoscopist passes the fiberoptic endoscope through the mouth, esophagus, and stomach and into the duodenum. An intravenous dose of glucagon may be given to relax the intestine and sphincter of Oddi. At the ampulla of Vater, a small cannula (a special tube on the end of the endoscope) is inserted into the ampulla and then, in turn, into the common duct and the pancreatic duct (Figure 48). Fluoroscopy (a type of x-ray) is used to guide the placement of the instrument. Once the cannula is in the common duct, radiopaque contrast is instilled and multiple radiographs are taken. To help with the gravity flow of the contrast medium, the patient is assisted in changing positions, and the table is tilted so that all branches of the biliary tree are filled and visible. Once the biliary duct examination is completed, the physician relocates the cannula into the pancreatic duct and the radiograph procedure is repeated.

Biliary and Pancreatic Cytology

When cytology (a study of the cells and their pathology) examination of the biliary or pancreatic tissue and secretions is indicated, the specimens are collected after the cannula is in the appropriate duct. To stimulate the flow of pancreatic secretions, the patient is given an intravenous bolus of secretin. The endoscope is used to aspirate a sample of the secretions; a collection of the cells can be done by brushing technique or biopsy.

SIGNIFICANCE OF TEST RESULTS
Abnormal Biliary Findings
Common bile duct stone
Stenosis of the papilla
Fibrosis or stricture

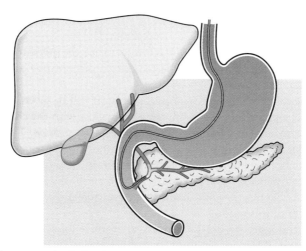

Figure 48. Endoscopic retrograde cholangiopancreatography. The endoscope is passed through the upper gastrointestinal tract. At the level of the duodenum, the papilla is located and the cannula is inserted through it. The cannula tip is then advanced to obtain images in the common bile duct (endoscopic retrograde cholangiography). On completion of that phase of the examination, cannula is moved and inserted into the pancreatic duct for imaging (endoscopic retrograde pancreatography).

Biliary duct tumor (benign or malignant)
Primary biliary cirrhosis
Sclerosing cholangitis
Leakage of cystic duct, post-laparoscopic cholecystectomy
Lymphoma
Liver metastases or cirrhosis

Abnormal Pancreatic Findings
Acute pancreatitis
Chronic pancreatitis
Pancreatic pseudocyst
Cancer
Fistula
Abscess

INTERFERING FACTORS

- The patient who cannot cooperate or relax during the examination
- Severe, acute pancreatitis
- Acute biliary obstruction
- Acute myocardial infarction
- Pancreatic pseudocyst
- Esophageal or gastric outlet obstruction
- Hepatitis B infection

NURSING CARE

Pretest
- Once the physician has explained the procedure, the patient must sign a written consent. The nurse enters the consent into the patient's record.
- ○ *Patient Teaching.* Provide preprocedure teaching so that the patient can relax during the 1-hour examination. The nurse instructs the patient to discontinue all food and fluids for 6 hours before the test.
- Because ERCP is uncomfortable, intravenous medication will be given to promote relaxation and relief of pain. The patient will be aware enough to assist with the changing from prone to lateral position and to remain immobile during the viewing process. The nurse assesses vital signs and documents the baseline values. Question the patient regarding any history of a reaction to the contrast medium used during a previous radiograph study. Inform the physician of any positive history and record the assessment findings related to allergy.
- Before the procedure begins, the endoscopy nurse tests all equipment for correct mechanical function and proper illumination.
- One hour before the start of the procedure, an intravenous infusion is started in the patient's arm or hand. When infection in the gallbladder is suspected, systemic antibiotics are started and continued into the postprocedure period.
- Intravenous diazepam (Valium), meperidine (Demerol), or fentanyl (Sublimaze) are given to the patient to provide relaxation and pain relief. Alternatively, a bolus (concentrated) dose

of midazolam (Versed) may be ordered. Midazolam exerts a powerful, rapid enhancement of the narcotic and provides sedation and anesthesia. Atropine is given to reduce the motility of the intestinal tract.

- The side effects of diazepam and midazolam are central nervous system and respiratory depression. To prevent respiratory depression and/or cardiac arrest, the intravenous analgesics are given very slowly over a 1- to 2-minute period. Naloxone (Narcan) is kept on hand to reverse the respiratory depressive effect of meperidine or fentanyl, but it is ineffective against diazepam. Once the administration of medication begins, the nurse monitors the vital signs and respiratory status frequently. In many endoscopy units, automated blood pressure, pulse oximetry, and cardiac monitors are used. Because the risk of apnea exists, resuscitation equipment must be readily available.
- Before inserting the endoscope, the physician anesthetizes the patient's mouth and throat with topical anesthetic spray. The patient's tongue will then feel thick and it will be difficult to swallow. An oral brace is inserted into the mouth to keep it open and a suction catheter is inserted to remove the saliva.
- The patient wears a lead shield over the thyroid gland. The nurse and physician wear lead body shields and thyroid shields because of their repeated exposure to radiation during the procedure.

During the Test

- The nurse continues to monitor the patient's cardiac and respiratory status frequently. Oxygen administered by nasal cannula helps prevent hypoxemia (a low oxygen level in the blood). As the endoscope is manipulated by the physician, the patient may experience a vasovagal reflex, as indicated by sudden bradycardia (a slow heartbeat, less than 60 beats per minute). Atropine sulfate medication is kept on hand to overcome the effects of the bradycardia.
- The nurse assists the patient with turning, positioning, and relaxation.
- For cytology analysis, two vials of the biliary or pancreatic secretions are collected, as indicated. The first tube is discarded because the secretions contain contrast medium. The nurse labels and identifies the second specimen of fluid, including the time and date of retrieval. The laboratory request form contains the identifying information of the patient's name, identifying patient number, name of the physician, the date and time of the collection, and the identification of the specimen and procedure used. The specimen is packed on ice and sent to the laboratory quickly. This cooling process and prompt delivery minimizes the deterioration of any cells in the fluid. Tissue biopsy samples are placed in a sterile jar with a fixative solution and are labeled in the same manner as the fluid secretions.

Posttest

- Until the patient is stable, the nurse monitors the cardiovascular and respiratory status every 15 minutes.
- The patient ingests nothing by mouth until the gag reflex and swallowing ability return, at which point clear liquids are started; a light meal can follow shortly thereafter. In the first hour or so, colicky abdominal pain can occur because of the air that was inserted in the intestinal tract during the procedure. It will disappear as food intake returns.

○ *Patient Teaching.* For discharge teaching, the nurse instructs the patient to notify the physician of any severe or prolonged symptoms of abdominal pain, fever, nausea, or vomiting.

◆ **Nursing Response to Complications**

Because of the tissue manipulation during the procedure and the already compromised state of the patient's health, complications can occur. The overall complication rate for ERCP is

Continued

NURSING CARE—cont'd

5.0%, with a greater proportion resulting from therapeutic ERCP and a lesser proportion from a diagnostic ERCP (Colton & Curran, 2009). The complications can begin within 1 hour or up to 2 days later. Abnormal assessment findings, should they appear, are indications of a serious problem that requires medical intervention. The nurse notifies the physician of abnormal findings and records the data in the patient's record.

Sepsis. Sepsis (the presence of microorganisms and their toxins in the blood and other tissues) is a serious complication of this procedure. The nurse's assessment findings would include moderate abdominal pain, fever, chills, and jaundice. When infection is suspected, the nurse should check the recent laboratory results for leukocytosis (an elevated white blood cell count) and abnormal liver values.

Pancreatitis. Pancreatitis (inflammation of the pancreas) is also a possible complication of ERCP. Nursing assessment findings include acute epigastric pain, abdominal distention, a "board-like" abdomen, nausea, and vomiting. The serum amylase value is often elevated after the ERCP procedure and is not significant by itself. However, the presence of clinical symptoms in addition to an elevated serum amylase is significant and indicates a serious pancreatic inflammation.

End-Tidal Carbon Dioxide

See Capnogram on p. 165.

Epinephrine

See Catecholamines, Plasma on p. 180.

Epstein-Barr Virus, Serology

Also called: Epstein-Barr titer

SPECIMEN OR TYPE OF TEST: Serum

PURPOSE OF THE TEST

These serologic tests are used to diagnose acute or chronic Epstein-Barr viral infection in patients with infectious mononucleosis in whom heterophil antibody titers are negative.

BASICS THE NURSE NEEDS TO KNOW

There are now eight identified types of herpes virus that cause infectious illness. As presented in Table 9, the Epstein-Barr virus is a herpesvirus that is responsible for most cases of infectious mononucleosis. The virus is transmitted through close contact with infected saliva. Infectious mononucleosis causes fever, swollen lymph glands, malaise, headache, fatigue, and sore throat.

TABLE 9 Herpes Viruses, Infection, and Diagnostic Testing

Virus Type	Infection	Diagnostic Tests
Herpes simplex 1	"Cold sores," infection of the mouth, lips, pharynx, conjunctiva, or skin; encephalitis (adult); disseminated infection (neonate)	Antigen detection; cell culture; nucleic acid amplification (PCR) from vesicle fluid or cells from tissue scraping
Herpes simplex 2	Genital herpes, disseminated infection (neonate)	Antigen detection; cell culture from vesicle fluid or cells from tissue scraping; nucleic acid amplification –polymerase chain reaction (PCR)
Epstein-Barr virus	Infectious mononucleosis, Burkitt's lymphoma, nasopharyngeal cancer, oral hairy cell leukoplakia (in HIV-infected patients)	Serology testing (EBV) antigen and antibody detection; nucleic acid amplification (PCR)
Cytomegalovirus	Infectious mononucleosis, retinitis (in HIV-infected patients); interstitial pneumonia, hepatitis or encephalitis (in organ transplant patients)	Serology testing (CMV antigen and antibody detection); nucleic acid amplification (PCR) from blood or tissue specimen; cell culture
Varicella-Zoster virus	Chickenpox (varicella), shingles (herpes zoster)	Cell culture from vesicle fluids or cells; antigen detection; nucleic acid amplification (PCR)
Herpesviruses 6 and 7	Roseola, interstitial pneumonia (in organ transplant patients)	Nucleic acid amplification (PCR) in blood specimen; cell culture
Herpesvirus 8	A factor in the development of Kaposi's sarcoma	Antigen detection; nucleic acid amplification (PCR) of cellular material from tissue, blood marrow, bone, semen, and saliva

In the blood, Epstein-Barr virus infects the B lymphocytes and stimulates DNA synthesis to form three antigens. These antigens are viral capsid antigen (VCA), Epstein-Barr nuclear antigen (EBNA), and early antigen (EA). In the immunologic response to combat the infection, the body makes antibodies to the specific antigens.

Antibody Formation
The antibody VCA immunoglobulin M (VCA-IgM) appears in the blood before and during the acute phase of illness. It remains in the blood for 1 to 2 months and then disappears. The antibody VCA immunoglobin G (VCA-IgG) also elevates and peaks in the blood at an early stage of illness. In the convalescent stage, it declines but then persists for life at a lower, positive value. This antibody is the most often used test and is reported as the standard Epstein-Barr virus titer. It is the marker for current or prior infection.

The EA antibodies appear a few weeks after the onset of symptoms and then gradually disappear from the blood. The IgG type, however, may persist for several years after an acute infection.

The EBNA antibody (anti-EBNA) appears in the blood several weeks to months after the onset of symptoms of infection. The antibody titer remains elevated for life.

In summary, elevated (positive) titers) for VCA-IgG, VCA-IgM, and EA-IgG are diagnostic for acute infectious mononucleosis. Positive titers of VCA-IgG and antibody to EBNA are diagnostic for past Epstein-Barr infection.

Several of the Epstein-Barr antibody titers also are elevated in certain malignant disorders. These cancers are Burkitt's lymphoma and nasopharyngeal cancer. Tissue biopsy will be needed to confirm the malignancy.

REFERENCE VALUES   Antibodies to viral capsid antigen (VCA-IgM): Negative, <1:10;
(VCA-IgG): Negative, <1:10
Antibody to Epstein-Barr nuclear antigen (anti-EBNA): Negative, <1:5
Antibodies to early antigen (anti-EA): Negative, <1:10

HOW THE TEST IS DONE
Venipuncture is used to collect a specimen of venous blood.

SIGNIFICANCE OF TEST RESULTS
Elevated Values
Infectious mononucleosis
Oral hairy leukoplakia (in HIV-infected patients)
Burkitt's lymphoma
Nasopharyngeal cancer

INTERFERING FACTORS
• None

NURSING CARE

Nursing measures include care of the venipuncture site as presented in Chapter 2, with the following additional measures.
Pretest
• Schedule this test to be performed at the onset of illness and again after 2 to 3 weeks. This scheduling provides data during the acute and convalescent phases of illness.
Posttest
• On the requisition request, include the date of the onset of illness.

Erythrocyte Sedimentation Rate

Also called: (ESR); Sed Rate

SPECIMEN OR TYPE OF TEST: Blood

PURPOSE OF THE TEST

The erythrocyte sedimentation test is useful in monitoring disease activity in inflammatory and infectious conditions. It is helpful in the diagnosis and monitoring of temporal arteritis and polymyalgia rheumatica.

BASICS THE NURSE NEEDS TO KNOW

The erythrocyte sedimentation rate (ESR) test is a nonspecific measurement of inflammation and infection in the body. When venous blood is placed in a vertical tube, the erythrocytes act like sediment; over time, they fall to the bottom of the tube. In normal conditions, as the erythrocytes settle, they exhibit a characteristic rouleau formation, meaning that they form a stack. The test results measure the distance that the erythrocytes fall in a column of anticoagulated blood in 1 hour. Because the test is not sensitive or specific, the results may be elevated in various conditions. Thus it cannot be used for diagnosis or in screening of asymptomatic individuals. It may be helpful in monitoring the response to treatment of an inflammatory or infectious disorder.

Elevated Values

In inflammatory or infectious conditions, the rouleau formation is greater, the sedimentation rate is faster, and the ESR is elevated. The abnormal, elevated value for females is greater than 30 mm/hour and for males is greater than 20 mm/hour. A rise in the ESR is usually reflective of the severity of the inflammatory or infectious condition. The ESR result will also rise with conditions that increase the level of fibrinogen or proteins in the blood and in anemia that is increasing in severity.

Decreased Values

Microcytes (abnormally small red blood cells) have a slower sedimentation rate than normal. Additionally, erythrocytes with irregularities or abnormal shape exhibit less rouleau formation. When a low plasma fibrinogen level exists, erythrocyte sedimentation is less and the ESR value is proportionately lower.

REFERENCE VALUES | Adult (Westergren Method)
Male: 0-15 mm/hr
Female: 0-20 mm/hr

HOW THE TEST IS DONE

Venipuncture is used to obtain a sample of venous blood.

SIGNIFICANCE OF TEST RESULTS

Elevated Values
Polymyalgia rheumatica
Temporal arteritis
Rheumatoid arthritis
Multiple myeloma

Rheumatic fever
Waldenström's macroglobulinemia
Anemia

Decreased Values
Sickle cell anemia
Polycythemia
Spherocytosis
Hypofibrinogenemia

INTERFERING FACTORS
• None

NURSING CARE

Nursing actions are similar to those used in other venipuncture procedures (see Chapter 2), with the following additional measures.

Pretest
• Because many medications, including salicylate and heparin, can alter lab values, list all medications taken by the patient on the requisition request. In some cases, the medication may be withheld until after the test.

Posttest
• Ensure that the specimen is sent promptly to the lab. The specimen must be analyzed within 4 hours of collection.

Erythropoietin

Also called: (EPO)

SPECIMEN OR TYPE OF TEST: Serum

PURPOSE OF THE TEST
Measurement of erythropoietin is performed to investigate some anemias and the anemia of end-stage renal disease. It also may be used to differentiate between primary and secondary polycythemia vera or to detect the recurrence of an erythropoietin-producing tumor.

BASICS THE NURSE NEEDS TO KNOW
Erythropoietin is a hormone manufactured primarily by the kidneys. Its action is to regulate erythropoiesis, meaning that it stimulates or promotes the proliferation, differentiation, and maturation of erythrocyte precursor cells of the bone marrow. In normal kidneys, the stimuli to produce erythropoietin are hypoxia and decreased renal oxygenation.

Elevated Values
In chronic iron deficiency anemia and other types of anemia and after a moderate blood loss, the erythropoietin level is elevated as the kidneys respond to the need for more red blood cells and oxygen. The erythropoietin level rises dramatically in pregnancy and with erythropoietin-producing tumors.

Decreased Values

In cases of end-stage renal disease or after bilateral nephrectomy, erythropoietin is greatly reduced, and as a result, erythropoiesis by the bone marrow is limited. Anemia results from the impaired function of the bone marrow.

REFERENCE VALUES   Children and adolescents: 1.0-21.0 mU/ml *or* SI: 1.0-21.0 IU/L
Adults: 5-30 mU/mL *or* SI: 5-30 IU/L

E

HOW THE TEST IS DONE

Venipuncture is used to collect a sample of venous blood.

SIGNIFICANCE OF TEST RESULTS

Elevated Values

Anemias
Secondary polycythemia
Pulmonary fibrosis
Chronic obstructive pulmonary disease
Erythropoietin-producing tumor
Cerebellar hemangioblastoma
Renal tumor
Pheochromocytoma
Polycystic kidney disease
Early renal transplant rejection

Decreased Values

End-stage renal failure
Primary polycythemia (polycythemia vera)

INTERFERING FACTORS

• Pregnancy

NURSING CARE

Nursing actions are similar to those used in other venipuncture procedures (see Chapter 2). No specific patient instruction or intervention is needed.

Esophagogastroduodenoscopy

Also called: (EGD)
Includes: Endoscopic Ultrasound

SPECIMEN OR TYPE OF TEST: Endoscopy

PURPOSE OF THE TEST

The purposes of this upper gastrointestinal endoscopy procedure include: (1) identification and biopsy of abnormal tissue, (2) determination of the exact site and cause of upper gastrointestinal bleeding, (3) evaluation of the healing of gastric ulcers, (4) evaluation of the stomach and duodenum after gastric surgery, and (5) investigation of the cause of *dysphagia* (difficulty swallowing), *dyspepsia* (epigastric discomfort after meals), gastric outlet obstruction, or epigastric pain.

BASICS THE NURSE NEEDS TO KNOW

In esophagogastroduodenoscopy (EGD), the fiberoptic endoscope provides direct visualization of the lumen and mucosal lining of the esophagus, stomach, and duodenum in all surface areas. Tissue abnormalities are observed for their location, size, shape, appearance, and position (Figure 49). Tissue or secretion samples are obtained by biopsy, scrapings, or aspiration, and are sent for lab analysis.

Endoscopic Ultrasound

An ultrasound probe is attached to the tip of the endoscope. It provides imaging of the esophageal, gastric, and duodenal tissue that lies beneath the mucosa of the intestinal lumen. Because the instrument can provide images of the tissue to a depth of 3 to 4 inches, it is used to help with the staging of esophageal and gastric cancer, including the full thickness of the intestinal wall and the organs and lymph nodes of the nearby area. It provides imaging guidance when taking biopsy specimens. Endoscopic ultrasound is particularly helpful in providing images of esophageal varices that lie deep into the submucosa, and in imaging the depth of an ulcer crater (Scholton, 2010; Rumach, Wilson & Charboneau, 2005).

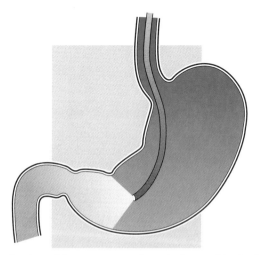

Figure 49. Endoscopic visualization of the upper gastrointestinal tract. The flexible tube, the fiberoptic filaments within the tube, and the light are used to evaluate the mucosal surface of the esophagus, stomach, and duodenum for inflammation, erosion, ulceration, bleeding, stricture, and abnormal tissue.

REFERENCE VALUES   No abnormal structures or tissues are observed in the esophagus, stomach, or duodenum.

HOW THE TEST IS DONE

The endoscope is a long, flexible fiberoptic tube with light and a lens for magnification at the distal end and a viewing eyepiece at the proximal end. Within the channels of the endoscope, there are various instruments to obtain biopsy samples, cell brushings, aspiration of fluid samples for analysis, ultrasound imaging, suction, and cautery. The endoscope is usually passed through the mouth (oral EGD) and esophagus to the stomach and duodenum. These adult patients receive conscious sedation and a local anesthetic throat spray to help them tolerate the procedure and cooperate during the examination. Infants and small children usually require general anesthesia.

A newly developed ultrathin endoscope may be used for a transnasal approach. This endoscope can be used for patients with a cardiac history who require an EGD examination. With the transnasal approach, there is less stimulation of the sympathetic nervous system, less elevation of the patient's blood pressure and pulse, and less risk that the procedure will induce a cardiac arrhythmia or other cardiovascular complication. The use of the ultrathin endoscope requires topical anesthesia of the nasal cavity and pharynx, but no sedative or conscious sedation is needed (Mori, Ohashi, Tatebe, et al, 2008).

As either type of endoscope is advanced into position, the tip is flexed and rotated in all directions. This allows for the examination of the entire mucosal surface of the upper gastrointestinal tract. Ultrasound images of abnormal tissue are obtained. Biopsy and fluid samples are taken, as needed. The viewing continues as the endoscope is gradually withdrawn (Figure 50).

SIGNIFICANCE OF TEST RESULTS

Gastric or duodenal ulcer
Tumor, benign or malignant
Stenosis, esophageal or pyloric

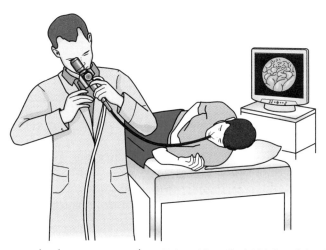

Figure 50. **Esophagogastroduodenoscopy procedure.** (Adapted from Sivak MV: *Gastrologic endoscopy,* Philadelphia, 1987, Saunders.)

Hiatal hernia
Inflammation (esophagitis, gastritis)
Mallory-Weiss tear of esophagus
Varices, esophageal or gastric

INTERFERING FACTORS

- Failure to maintain nothing-by-mouth status
- Unstable or life-threatening cardiac or pulmonary status
- Known or suspected perforation of the stomach or intestine
- Shock
- Recent heart attack

NURSING CARE

Pretest

- Schedule this test at least 2 days after an upper gastrointestinal series so that residual barium will not interfere with the visual examination.
- A signed consent is needed and the document is entered in the patient's record.

○ *Patient Teaching.* The nurse instructs the patient to maintain a nothing-by-mouth status for 6 to 8 hours before the test. If the patient uses aspirin or NSAIDs for minor pain relief, or is on anticoagulant therapy, these medications may be discontinued before the examination. They could increase the risks of bleeding during certain EGD procedures, but most of the EGD procedures are considered low risk for bleeding complications (Greenwald, 2007).

- If conscious sedation will be used, advise the patient to have a responsible adult provide transportation home after discharge. During pretest teaching, review the written posttest instructions with the patient. This timing is best because the conscious sedation will disrupt comprehension and memory for a short period after the test is over.
- The nurse obtains the pretest coagulation profile test results, which include prothrombin time, partial thromboplastin time, bleeding time, and platelet count. The lab results are placed in the patient's record and the nurse informs the physician of any abnormal results. The patient must have normal coagulation ability to avoid a bleeding complication during the procedure. On the morning of the test, the nurse takes vital signs, including temperature, pulse respirations, and blood pressure. The results are entered in the patient's record.
- Assist the patient to remove and store eyeglasses, dentures, jewelry, and clothing. Provide a surgical gown for the patient to wear.

During the Test

- Before the procedure begins, the endoscopy nurse tests all equipment for correct mechanical function and proper illumination.
- Atropine is given to reduce the motility of the intestinal tract. Intravenous diazepam (Valium) and meperidine (Demerol) are given to the patient to provide relaxation and pain relief. Alternatively, a bolus dose of midazolam (Versed) may be ordered. Midazolam exerts a powerful, rapid enhancement of the narcotic and provides sedation and anesthesia. Fentanyl (Sublimaze) may be used instead of meperidine.
- The side effects of diazepam and midazolam are central nervous system and respiratory depression. To prevent respiratory depression or cardiac arrest, the intravenous analgesics

are given very slowly over a 1- to 2-minute period. Naloxone (Narcan) is kept on hand to reverse the respiratory depressive effect of meperidine or fentanyl, but it is ineffective against diazepam. Once the administration of medication begins, the nurse monitors the vital signs and respiratory status frequently. In many endoscopy units, automated blood pressure, pulse oximetry, and cardiac monitors are used. Because the risk of apnea exists, resuscitation equipment must be readily available.

- The nurse assists the patient into a left lateral recumbent position. Oxygen may be delivered by nasal cannula to help prevent hypoxia from the respiratory depression associated with conscious sedation.
- Before inserting the endoscope, the physician anesthetizes the patient's mouth and throat with topical anesthetic spray. The patient's tongue will then feel thick and it will be difficult to swallow. An oral brace is inserted into the mouth to keep it open and a suction catheter is inserted to remove the saliva.
- The nurse assists with the collection of tissue specimens. Tissue samples are placed in sterile collection jars with preservative. They are labeled with the patient's name, date, and the source of the tissue specimen (e.g., gastric biopsy tissue). The requisition form also includes the patient's identification data, source of the tissue, procedure, physician's name, and date.

Posttest

- Until the patient is stable, the nurse monitors the cardiovascular and respiratory status and the level of alertness of the patient every 15 minutes, for about 1 hour.
- The patient ingests nothing by mouth until the gag reflex and swallowing ability return. Oral fluids can then be started.

○ *Patient Teaching.* For discharge teaching, the nurse reviews the protocol with the patient, as follows: Use throat lozenges or saline gargle to relieve any discomfort in the throat, no driving for 4 to 6 hours, and full resumption of food and fluids, as desired.

◆ **Nursing Response to Complications**

The incidence of complication during or after an EGD procedure is quite rare. During the procedure, the patient may experience respiratory depression or cardiac arrhythmia. The hypoxia and low respiratory rate usually occurs because of the conscious sedation medications, and the arrhythmia may occur as a result of the hypoxia. Perforation may also occur, usually in the esophagus, as the endoscope is passed through a narrow space. Bleeding can occur from the perforation or from a biopsy site. Although these complications occur during the test, the patient may not experience symptoms until later. With signs of complication, the nurse performs a careful assessment and notifies the physician of abnormal results.

Respiratory Depression. When assessing for respiratory depression, abnormal findings include a respiratory rate of less than 12 breaths/min and tachycardia (a pulse rate >120 beats/min). The patient breathes shallowly, and the color of the skin turns pale or cyanotic.

Cardiac Arrhythmia. When assessing for a cardiac arrhythmia, the abnormal findings include an irregular pulse (premature atrial or ventricular contractions or atrial fibrillation).

Perforation and Bleeding. In the event of perforation or bleeding, abnormal assessment findings include hematemesis (usually bright red color blood in the vomitus), persistent pain on swallowing and breathing, pain in the mediastinum or epigastric area, and fever. The nurse should pay particular attention to the patient's description of the pain and dysphagia, including the location and the severity of the complaint.

Esophagography

Also called: Barium swallow

SPECIMEN OR TYPE OF TEST: Radiography

PURPOSE OF THE TEST

The esophagogram is used to identify abnormalities in the structure and function of the oropharynx and esophagus during swallowing.

BASICS THE NURSE NEEDS TO KNOW

The esophagogram may be performed as a separate barium study or as part of the upper gastrointestinal series. *Dysphagia* (difficulty swallowing) is the most common problem investigated by this procedure. The cause can be an obstruction in the esophagus or a neuromuscular deficit that interferes with swallowing and slows the transit time for the passage of food to the stomach. The normal transit time from the oropharynx to the stomach is 6 to 15 seconds. The esophagogram provides data about the mucosa, filling defects, swallowing dynamics, and peristalsis of the esophagus.

A speech pathologist may participate or perform a modified esophagogram with the radiologist. The purpose is to identify the stronger areas of pharyngeal and esophageal muscle function that can improve swallowing ability. The data are used in rehabilitation therapy and swallow therapy for the patient who has neuromuscular deficits that impair swallowing ability.

Imaging

The procedure uses a digital fluoroscope to provide rapid spot images (4 to 6 images per second). Videotaping of the oropharynx and esophagus during swallowing is also done. The oral contrast media are preparations of thin and thick barium solutions in single contrast studies. Double contrast studies use the ingestion of an effervescent pill that dissolves in the esophagus, releasing carbon dioxide gas bubbles; this is immediately followed by the oral ingestion of thick barium solution. As the gas is released, it distends the walls of the esophagus and together with the barium provides greater clarity to the images.

REFERENCE VALUES   No mucosal, structural, or functional abnormalities are visualized.

HOW THE TEST IS DONE

The patient takes repeated swallows of barium liquid with or without air contrast to provide for imaging of the passage of contrast medium during swallowing and peristaltic movement (Figure 51). During the study, the patient is instructed to change body positions, including standing erect, moving and turning the head, and lying supine and prone. Instructions about when to hold a breath are also given. At the end of the study, the patient performs the Valsalva maneuver to help identify gastroesophageal reflux. Imaging is done throughout the examination.

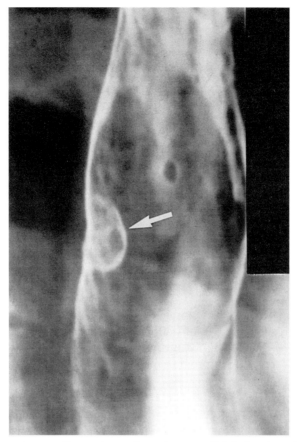

Figure 51. **Esophagogram image of an early esophageal cancer.** This lesion *(arrow)* appears as a relatively small mass in the lumen of the midesophagus. (Courtesy of Seth N. Glick, MD, Philadelphia, PA.)

SIGNIFICANCE OF TEST RESULTS

Swallowed foreign body
Neuromuscular weakness or incoordination
Esophageal stricture
Esophageal spasm
Hiatal hernia
Polyps, tumor, cancer
Esophageal varices
Ulcers or peptic esophagitis
Gastroesophageal reflux disease (GERD)

INTERFERING FACTORS

• Jewelry and metallic objects in the imaging field

NURSING CARE

Pretest
- The patient signs a written consent for the test and the consent is entered into the patient's record.

○ *Patient Teaching.* No food or dietary restrictions are needed in the pretest period (Frank, Long & Smith, 2007). At the radiology setting, the patient will remove all clothes, jewelry, and metallic objects above the waist. A surgical gown is worn.

Posttest
- A laxative is given to help eliminate the barium from the intestinal tract. Inform the patient that the feces will appear gray or whitish for 24 to 72 hours until all barium is expelled.

Estriol, Free, Unconjugated

Also called: E_3; uE_3

SPECIMEN OR TYPE OF TEST: Blood

PURPOSE OF THE TEST

In the later stages of pregnancy, the results of the serial estriol test may be used to evaluate fetal well-being and placental function, especially in the high-risk pregnancy. It also is used as part of the multiple marker screening test to detect Down syndrome.

BASICS THE NURSE NEEDS TO KNOW

During pregnancy, estriol is the predominant estrogen present in the serum. Because this hormone is synthesized by the placenta, the serum value is considered a measure of the integrity and well-being of the fetal-placental-maternal unit. The serum level rises progressively during a normal pregnancy. Therefore, the number of weeks of gestation is a necessary consideration in the interpretation of the test result. When the test results are declining or at a lower-than-normal level, the fetus is considered to be in danger. Immediate further investigation of the status of fetal health is indicated.

Multiple Marker Screening for Down Syndrome

Pregnant women can be tested for fetal Down syndrome in the first or early in the second trimester. Unconjugated estriol is part of the second-trimester quadruple testing (Quad tests). These blood tests are done between the 15th to 22nd week of the pregnancy and consist of alpha fetoprotein, human chorionic gonadotrophin, unconjugated estriol, and inhibin A.

When Down syndrome affects the fetus, the quadruple marker screening test demonstrates characteristic changes in the second trimester of pregnancy. The alpha fetoprotein result is 25% lower than normal and the unconjugated estriol result is 30% lower than normal. Both human chorionic gonadotrophin and inhibin A rise to twice the normal value. Pregnancy ultrasound must be done first to obtain an accurate gestational age.

The quadruple marker screening test detects 81% of fetal Down syndrome pregnancies, with a 7% false positive rate of error (Peterson. 2006). A false positive result means that the test results are positive for Down syndrome or other fetal abnormality but in reality, the fetus is normal. For positive results of this screening test, follow-up testing by ultrasound and possible amniocentesis is recommended.

REFERENCE VALUES

> Non Pregnant female and male: <2.0 ng/mol *or* <6.9 nmol/L
> Pregnancy
> 22 weeks of gestation: 2.6-8.0 mcg/mL *or* SI: 9-27.8 nmol/L
> 26 weeks of gestation: 2.5-13.5 mcg/L *or* SI: 8.7-46.8 nmol/L
> 30 weeks of gestation: 3.5-19.0 mcg/L *or* SI: 12.1-65.9 nmol/L
> 34 weeks of gestation: 5.3-18.3 mcg/L *or* SI: 18.4-63.5 nmol/L
> 38 weeks of gestation: 8.6-38.0 mcg/L *or* SI: 29.8-131.9 nmol/L
> 40 weeks of gestation: 9.6-28.9 mcg/L *or* SI: 33.3-17-100.3 nmol/L

E

HOW THE TEST IS DONE

Venipuncture is used to obtain a sample of maternal venous blood.

SIGNIFICANCE OF TEST RESULTS

Decreased Values

Diabetes mellitus
Fetal growth retardation
Fetal encephalopathy
Intrauterine death
Down syndrome
Fetal chromosomal disorder

INTERFERING FACTORS

- Recent radioisotope scan

NURSING CARE

Nursing actions are similar to those used in other venipuncture procedures (see Chapter 2), with the following additional measures.

Pretest

- Schedule this test before or 7 days after any radioisotope scan. When serial tests are done, the blood should be drawn at the same time of day for each visit.
- On the lab requisition form, include the patient's information of maternal age, gestation age as calculated by ultrasound, diabetic status, and maternal weight.

Estrogen Receptor (ER)

See Biopsy, Breast on p. 118.

Exercise Challenge Test

See Pulmonary Function Studies on p. 528.

Fasting Blood Sugar

See Glucose, Fasting on p. 340.

Fasting Plasma Glucose

See Glucose, Fasting on p. 340.

Fecal DNA Assay

SPECIMEN OR TYPE OF TEST: Feces

PURPOSE OF THE TEST

The fecal DNA assay is used as a screening test to detect genetic mutations in epithelial cells of the colon. The mutations are associated with precancerous adenomatous polyps and adenocarcinoma of the colon (colorectal cancer).

BASICS THE NURSE NEEDS TO KNOW

Cancer of the colon is believed to develop over a period of many years, as a benign polyp mutates and becomes a malignant tumor. During this time period, several genetic mutations develop, affecting both oncogene and tumor suppressor genes. As rapidly growing epithelial cells shed continuously into the fecal matter, the cells contain the DNA mutations. The cells are degraded, but the altered DNA markers remain intact in the feces (Sanford & McPherson, 2009).

Precancerous polyps only bleed intermittently, making it difficult to detect their presence by fecal occult blood testing. The fecal DNA assay test has a much higher sensitivity than the fecal occult blood test because of the continuous presence of DNA mutations in the feces. However, of all who have a positive fecal DNA test result, only 2% were shown to have colorectal cancer when the follow-up colonoscopy was performed (Sanford & McPherson, 2009).

Currently, the high cost of the test and less insurance coverage for this method of testing make it difficult to use this test for mass screening for all people. In addition, only reference laboratories are equipped to analyze the specimens. There are no current recommendations as to how often a person should be screened by this method of testing (Mahon, 2009).

REFERENCE VALUES   Negative

HOW THE TEST IS DONE

A special test collection kit must be used. The patient defecates into a large special container that fits over the toilet seat. The container with the feces is placed inside a larger container with a lid. The container is mailed to the reference laboratory, using the required cooler with its freezer packet inside.

SIGNIFICANCE OF THE TEST RESULTS

Positive Values

Precancerous polyp

Colorectal cancer

INTERFERING FACTORS

- Warming of the fecal matter

| NURSING CARE

Pretest

- The collected fecal matter must not contain urine, toilet paper, or toilet water.

Posttest

- The freezer pack must be included in the cooler with the specimen. Warming of the specimen will invalidate the results.
- If the test result is positive, the patient is advised to consult with his or her physician. A follow-up colonoscopy is recommended.

Fecal Elastase-1

Also called: Pancreatic Elastase-1

SPECIMEN OR TYPE OF TEST: Feces

PURPOSE OF THE TEST

The fecal elastase-1 test is used to detect pancreatic insufficiency and support the diagnosis of cystic fibrosis in infancy. It also is used to detect moderate to severe chronic pancreatitis in adults.

BASICS THE NURSE NEEDS TO KNOW

Elastase is an enzyme normally found in pancreatic secretions. The enzyme enters the small intestine via the pancreatic duct and functions to emulsify dietary fats so they can be absorbed. Most of the enzyme enters the colon and is evacuated in feces. When the pancreatic secretion is reduced, there is a lower amount of elastase in the feces. A fecal elastase-1 value of 100 to 200 µg/g indicates a moderate pancreatic insufficiency from any cause and a value of less than 100 µg/g indicates severe pancreatic insufficiency.

Fecal elastase-1 is the best marker of pancreatic insufficiency in patients with cystic fibrosis. Pancreatic insufficiency can be the first presenting symptom of cystic fibrosis. Infants with cystic fibrosis may demonstrate a severe decrease in the stool elastase-1 value at 4 weeks of age. The addition of pancreatic enzyme supplement in food will not affect the fecal elastase test results.

REFERENCE VALUES   Fecal elastase-1: >200 µg/ g

HOW THE TEST IS DONE
A random sample of stool is collected.

SIGNIFICANCE OF THE TEST RESULTS

Elevated Values
Acute and relapsing chronic pancreatitis

Decreased Values
Cystic fibrosis
Pancreatic insufficiency
Malabsorption
Inflammatory bowel disease

INTERFERING FACTORS
• Contamination of the specimen

NURSING CARE

Nursing actions are similar to those used in the stool collection procedure (see Chapter 2). A random sample of formed stool is collected. No other nursing measures are needed.

Fecal Occult Blood Tests

Also called: FOBT

SPECIMEN OR TYPE OF TEST: Feces

PURPOSE OF THE TEST
This test detects small amounts of blood in the feces. It is used as a screening test for the early diagnosis of precancerous polyps and adenocarcinoma of the colon.

BASICS THE NURSE NEEDS TO KNOW
Occult blood refers to blood that is present in feces, but is not visible. In some cases, the blood is not seen because the amount is small and mixed in the feces. Also, precancerous polyps bleed intermittently and blood is not always present in a single specimen. There are two basic test methods to screen for detection of fecal occult blood. These are: the older Guaiac method (Hemoccult Sensa™) and the newer fecal immunochemical test method (FIT). Both methods provide for collection of the fecal samples at home. The specimens can then be mailed or taken to the physician's office or laboratory for analysis. Each of these FOBT methods has been approved as a screening test for colorectal cancer and when this method of screening is used, the test should be done annually (Mahon, 2009). If the FOBT result is positive, a colonoscopy is recommended.

Guaiac Method

This method detects the heme molecule and hemoglobin in the fecal sample. The heme molecules in the feces react to the guaiaconic acid on the test card or strip of paper. Once the reagent of ethanol and hydrogen peroxide is used, a peroxidase reaction occurs. The appearance of a blue color is a positive test result. The source of the bleeding could be from anywhere in the gastrointestinal tract and this method cannot determine the location. The patient will collect three fecal samples on three separate days to improve detection of intermittent bleeding in at least one of the samples.

This method has many false-positive results. A false positive means that the test showed a positive value, but the patient did not have occult blood in the feces. Eating red meat will cause a positive result because the red meat and blood contain animal hemoglobin and heme molecules. Some fruits and vegetables contain a vegetative source of peroxidase and will cause a false-positive result. Some medications and alcohol can cause slight bleeding in the intestinal mucosa and bleeding from that source cannot be distinguished from bleeding from a polyp or tumor (Box 6). Vitamin C, as a supplement or in citrus fruits, can cause a false-negative test result. A false negative means that the test result is negative, but the patient actually has blood in the fecal sample.

Immunochemical Method

This method is based on antihuman hemoglobin antibodies that react with the undegraded globulin molecules of hemoglobin in the feces. In the test, immunochemicals are placed in contact with the fecal smears. If hemoglobin is present in the feces, there will be an antibody response and a pink color test line will appear on the testing strip. This test method only detects hemoglobin that originated from a bleeding site in the colon. It cannot detect hemoglobin that came from bleeding sites in the upper gastrointestinal tract or small intestine. It does not react to peroxidase from fruits and vegetables or from hemoglobin that comes from eating red meat. The FIT test has many fewer false-positive results than tests using the guaiac method (Sanford & McPherson, 2009).

BOX 6	Food, Medication, and Other Restrictions for the Guaiac Method—Fecal Occult Blood Test
Food	**Medications**
Horseradish	Aspirin
Turnips	Nonsteroidal antiinflammatory drugs
Red meat	Vitamin C
Artichokes	Steroids
Broccoli	Reserpine
Cauliflower	Chemotherapy drugs
Black grapes	
Melon	**Other**
Bananas	Alcohol
Plums	
Pears	

F

REFERENCE VALUES   Negative for occult blood

HOW THE TEST IS DONE

Guaiac method: Specimens of three separate stools are collected on three separate days. Using an applicator stick, a small sample of feces from each day is smeared on individual collection cards or papers. The three samples are then taken or mailed to the physician or laboratory for chemical analysis.

Immunochemical method: One stool specimen is obtained. Applicator sticks are used to take two small samples of feces from two separate places in the stool. The feces are spread thinly on separate collection cards and then are taken or mailed to the physician or laboratory for analysis.

SIGNIFICANCE OF TEST RESULTS

Positive Values
Guaiac Method
Esophageal varices
Hiatal hernia
Mallory Weiss tears in the esophagus
Gastritis
Peptic ulcer
Intussusception
Dysentery
Crohn's disease
Parasitic disease
Benign polyps of the colon
Diverticular disease
Arteriovenous formation in the colon
Adenocarcinoma of the colon
Polyps in the colon
Kaposi's sarcoma
Immunochemical Method
Arteriovenous formation in the colon
Adenocarcinoma of the colon
Precancerous polyps in the colon

INTERFERING FACTORS

Guaiac Method
- Recent dietary intake of animal protein, vegetable peroxidase, or vitamin C
- Recent intake of alcohol and some medications that cause intestinal irritation

Guaiac Method and Immunochemical Method
- Presence of toilet bowl cleaner that contains chlorine
- Presence of urine, soap, or toilet paper

| NURSING CARE

Health Promotion

The nurse can educate and encourage healthy people older than age 50 to have an annual fecal occult blood test. Many people do not have a routine health screening performed for various reasons. Health education can correct the perceptions of the public such as: "I have no symptoms and feel well, so I do not need the test." With cancer of the colon and precancerous polyps, detection can occur before symptoms are experienced.

Pretest

○ *Patient Teaching. Guaiac method only*: Instruct the patient to avoid the foods presented in Box 6 for 3 days before the test. Vitamin C must be omitted for 5 days before the test. If possible, the medications that cause intestinal irritation should be stopped for 7 days before the test. To avoid intestinal irritation, alcohol should also be omitted.

○ *Patient Teaching. Immunochemical method only:* There are no dietary or medication restrictions.

○ *Patient Teaching.* The nurse instructs the patient about how to collect a stool specimen. The reader is referred to Chapter 2 for additional information about collection procedure.

- For both methods of testing, specific laboratory instructions by the manufacturers also are included with the test kits.

Posttest

- Once the specimens are collected, the cards can remain at room temperature until they are mailed or delivered to the testing location.
- If the fecal occult blood test is positive, further diagnostic testing is essential. A colonoscopy will be needed to determine the cause of the bleeding in the colon. The nurse provides caring support to the patient and strongly encourages that the patient complete the additional diagnostic testing that is prescribed.

Ferritin

See Iron Studies on p. 400.

Fetal Fibronectin

Also called: fFN

SPECIMEN OR TYPE OF TEST: Cervicovaginal Secretions

PURPOSE OF THE TEST

This test is used to determine the risk of a preterm (early) delivery in symptomatic and asymptomatic pregnant women.

BASICS THE NURSE NEEDS TO KNOW

Fibronectin is a glycoprotein that is present in various tissues, including the placenta and amniotic fluid. It has adhesive properties and in pregnancy helps the placenta bond to the uterine wall. In normal physiology, fetal fibronectin is present in cervicovaginal secretions of the pregnant woman before 21 weeks of gestation. It then disappears from the fluid and reappears at 37 weeks' gestation. In the late phase of pregnancy, the adhesive bond loosens and additional fibronectin leaks into the secretions, predicting the onset of labor.

Pregnant women are screened for fetal fibronectin between the 24th and 30th week of pregnancy. In this time frame, there should be only minimal levels of fibronectin in the cervicovaginal secretions. When an asymptomatic woman has a negative fetal fibronectin result, it is unlikely that preterm labor will occur in the next 7 days. If she has meaningful symptoms of suspected preterm labor and has a negative fFN value, she is at low risk to deliver in the next 7 days. The fetal fibronectin measurement has a very high 99% negative predictive value that is both specific and accurate (Pelaez, Fox & Chasen, 2008).

For the woman who has symptoms of labor and also has an elevated (positive) fetal fibronectin value, there is a high risk that she will have preterm delivery before 34 weeks or within the next 7 days. The positive fFN value is not as effective in predicting risk because only 26% of those with preterm labor symptoms and a positive fFN value will deliver prematurely within 7 days after the test (Wax, Partin & Pinette, 2010). The majority of the patients who have a positive value will repair the disruption of the placental-uterine bond that caused the leakage of fibronectin and they will continue with the pregnancy successfully (Wu, 2006).

The positive fFN result is considered very useful because with the early warning of the risk of preterm labor and possible delivery of a premature infant, medical intervention can help delay labor and allow the fetus more time to mature. When fetal lungs have time to mature fully, the complication of respiratory distress syndrome (RDS) in the neonate is avoided.

REFERENCE VALUES   Negative; <50 ng/mL

HOW THE TEST IS DONE

A dry speculum is inserted in the vagina. No water or lubricant is used because these substances and any tissue manipulation before or during pelvic examination would alter the laboratory results. A special swab is rotated across the cervix and posterior fornix to collect cervicovaginal secretions.

SIGNIFICANCE OF TEST RESULTS

Positive Value
Preterm labor

INTERFERING FACTORS

- Sexual intercourse within the past 24 hours
- Manipulation of the cervix during the pelvic examination
- Placenta previa
- Placental abruption
- Vaginal bleeding

NURSING CARE

Pretest

- When this test is performed, it should be done before a digital examination or cervical ultrasound procedure. Ask the patient if she had sexual intercourse within the past 24 hours, because this activity would also manipulate the cervix and cause a false-positive result.

During the Test

- After the secretions are collected, the swab is placed in the special collection tube with a buffer solution. The shaft of the swab must be broken at the scored line even with the top of the tube. The cap is pushed into the tube with the top of the shaft aligned with the hole in the center of the cap. The specimen is correctly labeled with the patient's identification, date, type of specimen, and the physician's name. The specimen may be analyzed in the central laboratory or by a rapid, desktop analyzer at the point of care.

Posttest

- If the fetal fibronectin test result is negative, the patient is not expected to have a preterm delivery in the next 7 days.
- If the test result is positive, and premature labor is predicted, the patient will be observed and will undergo additional assessment, including the monitoring for fetal contractions. The nurse monitors vital signs, including the maternal temperature and the fetal heart rate, and the results are recorded. Tocolytic medication may be prescribed to suppress the onset of labor, and antenatal corticosteroids may be prescribed to help the fetal lungs mature.

○ *Patient Teaching.* When the patient is to be discharged home, the nurse implements a plan for discharge instruction. This includes instructing the patient to continue with prenatal visits to her health care provider. Guidelines regarding the patient's activity are individualized and reviewed with the patient. The patient also is taught to recognize the signs of preterm labor and what to do if it occurs.

Fibrinogen

Also called: Factor I

SPECIMEN OR TYPE OF TEST: Blood

PURPOSE OF THE TEST

The measurement of fibrinogen is used to help diagnose bleeding disorders, including afibrinogenemia, disseminated intravascular coagulation (DIC), and fibrinolysis.

BASICS THE NURSE NEEDS TO KNOW

Fibrinogen is a coagulation protein that is a vital contributor to the meshwork that binds platelets to form a clot. When vascular or tissue injury occurs, fibrinogen levels increase in the early phase of coagulation. Within 24 hours of the injury, the fibrinogen level rises dramatically. At the site of vascular disruption, adhesive proteins and fibrinogen bind the platelets together and plug the break in the vascular wall. As the clotting process progresses, fibrinogen converts to fibrin. The fibrin threads provide stability for the clot.

Elevated Values

An increased amount of fibrinogen normally occurs during acute injury and in pregnancy. In abnormal conditions, the fibrinogen value rises, and an unwanted thrombus or embolus can occur.

Decreased Values

Afibrinogenemia means that there is no detectable fibrinogen in the blood. This condition is an inherited, autosomal dominant disorder caused by various genetic mutations. It will affect the neonate and is evidenced by umbilical cord bleeding or severe bleeding at another site. *Hypofibrinogenemia* means that there is a decreased level of fibrinogen in the blood and a test value of less than 100 mg/dL will decrease clotting ability. Excess bleeding occurs because of a slower process of clot formation. The condition may be inherited as an autosomal dominant disorder caused by various genetic mutations, or it may be acquired. *Dysfibrogenemia* means that the fibrogen is present but does not function properly when trying to form a clot. The dysfunction is an autosomal dominant inherited condition caused by various genetic mutations. It may also be an acquired condition because of advanced liver disease. Dysfibrogenemia causes bleeding in the adult or it may be asymptomatic.

The fibrinogen test measures the quantity of fibrinogen in the blood (afibrinogenemia and hypofibrinogenemia), but does not measure the quality of fibrinogen activity (dysfibrogenemia). The fibrinogen test may be ordered as part of a disseminated intravascular coagulation (DIC) panel of coagulation tests. In DIC, the fibrinogen level is severely decreased (see also DIC Screen, pp. 259-260).

REFERENCE VALUES	Adult: 150-400 mg/dL *or* Clauss method: 1.5-4 g/L
▽ Critical Values	60 ng/L *or* less[*]

[*]Varies with the guidelines that are developed by individual institutions.

HOW THE TEST IS DONE

Venipuncture or capillary puncture is used to obtain the sample of blood.

SIGNIFICANCE OF TEST RESULTS

Elevated Values

Sepsis, infection
Inflammation
Malignancy
Traumatic injury
Pregnancy
Oral contraceptive use
Afibrinogenemia
Hypofibrinogenemia
DIC
Liver disease

INTERFERING FACTORS

- Heparinization
- Pregnancy (third trimester)
- Recent surgery

F

NURSING CARE

Nursing actions are similar to those used in other venipuncture or capillary puncture procedures (see Chapter 2), with the following additional measures.

Pretest

- For the patient who receives intermittent doses of heparin, schedule this test at least 1 hour after the medication is administered. In some methods of analysis, a recent heparin dose alters the test result.

During the Test

- When drawing the blood, the intravenous catheter line with a heparin lock should not be used, because the heparin flush procedure and residual heparin would invalidate the result of this test.

Posttest

- For the patient with a suspected bleeding disorder, assess the venipuncture or capillary site for signs of bleeding or ecchymosis. To promote clotting, the nurse uses sterile gauze to apply pressure to the site, or raises the patient's arm above the head while maintaining pressure on the site.

▼ **Nursing Response to Critical Values**

The nurse must notify the physician of a decrease to the critical value range because the patient is at risk for bleeding or hemorrhage. The nurse assesses the patient for signs of abnormal bleeding, including petechiae (small red hemorrhagic spots in the skin), ecchymosis (bruising), hematuria, blood in the feces, or bleeding in the oral cavity. Ongoing reassessments at intervals are indicated. Baseline vital signs should be taken and monitored at intervals thereafter.

Fibrin Breakdown Products

See D-dimer and Fibrin Breakdown Products on p. 259.

Fine-Needle Biopsy of the Lung

See Biopsy, Lung, Percutaneous, Needle on p. 127.

Folic Acid

Also called: Folate

SPECIMEN OR TYPE OF TEST: Serum

PURPOSE OF THE TEST

This test is used to detect folic acid deficiency and monitor replacement therapy. It is also used to investigate the cause of megaloblastic anemia.

BASICS THE NURSE NEEDS TO KNOW

Folic acid is one of the B vitamins important in the synthesis of protein and in the maintenance of a normal level of mature red blood cells in the blood. It is a necessary ingredient for DNA synthesis in the bone marrow and in other rapidly dividing cells, such as the lining of the intestinal tract and the neurologic system of the developing fetus. The natural intake of folic acid is from dietary sources. Food that is rich in folic acid includes liver, green leafy vegetables, legumes, and citrus fruits or juices. The body's demand for folic acid is greatest in adolescence, the first trimester of pregnancy, and during lactation. To assist in overcoming the dietary deficiencies, the U.S. government regulations require that bread and grain products be fortified with folate.

Decreased Values

The deficiency of folic acid affects DNA synthesis in the bone marrow. Fewer new red blood cells are produced and they are defective. If the problem is uncorrected, the patient develops anemia. In the mouth, the patient develops painful glossitis, or a loss of surface epithelium of the tongue. The loss of epithelium in the intestinal tract can cause gastritis, nausea, and constipation.

In the pregnant female, the deficiency is correlated with neural tube defect in the fetus, including anencephaly, spinal bifida, encephalocele, myelomeningocele, and others. Neural tube defect in the fetus occurs in the first trimester of pregnancy. .

Folate deficiency is usually due to a problem with dietary intake. The population groups who are most vulnerable to the deficiency include people who are poor, the elderly, and pregnant women. Folate deficiency is prevalent in cases of alcoholic liver disease. Other causes of folate deficiency are due to intestinal disorders that interfere with absorption of this vitamin. Some medications cause folate deficiency by acting as folate antagonists or impairing the absorption of this vitamin. The medications include anticonvulsants, methotrexate and other chemotherapy drugs, and oral contraceptives.

REFERENCE VALUES*   5-16 ng/mL *or* SI: 11-36 nmol/L

*The reference value depends on the laboratory method of analysis.

HOW THE TEST IS DONE

Venipuncture is performed to obtain a sample of blood.

SIGNIFICANCE OF TEST RESULTS

Decreased Values

Megaloblastic anemia
Malnutrition
Pregnancy

Adult celiac disease
Regional enteritis
Malabsorption
Alcoholism

INTERFERING FACTORS

- Hemolysis
- Exposure to sunlight

▎ NURSING CARE

Nursing actions are similar to those used in other venipuncture procedures (see Chapter 2), with the following additional measures.

Pretest

- The nurse should ensure that this test is done before blood transfusion is given or folate replacement is started. These factors would elevate the patient's serum value.
- If the patient takes medications, they should be listed on the lab requisition form.
- ○ *Patient Teaching.* The nurse instructs the patient to fast from food for 8 hours.

Posttest

- When folate deficiency is detected, additional data are needed to determine the cause of the deficiency and the existence of megaloblastic anemia before specific interventions are selected. Other blood tests to evaluate the problem include the complete blood count (CBC), hemoglobin, hematocrit, and mean corpuscular volume (MCV).
- The nurse assesses for signs of anemia that include pallor and fatigue or lethargy and shortness of breath. Glossitis, a reddened, sore tongue, is visible in examination of the oral cavity. The nurse can also do a nutritional assessment, especially for those patients who are pregnant, have cancer, receive chemotherapy treatment, or who are maintained on phenytoin (Dilantin), as well as those who are in the vulnerable age and economic groups.

Health Promotion

Women who are trying to become pregnant or who just became pregnant are encouraged to take extra folic acid. The ideal time is 1 month before conception to the end of the first trimester. This is will help prevent neural tube defect in the developing fetus. The daily requirement of folic acid is 400 μg for nonpregnant women and 600 μg during pregnancy. The increased amount can be obtained by taking one multivitamin tablet daily. The patient should be taught to eat folate-rich food, but dietary intervention is insufficient to replace depleted folate stores and correct the anemia that has already occurred.

Free Cortisol

SPECIMEN OR TYPE OF TEST: Urine

PURPOSE OF THE TEST

Free cortisol is evaluated to determine excessive production of glucocorticoids by the adrenal cortex. It is also used to evaluate the hypothalamus-pituitary-adrenal (HPA) axis.

BASICS THE NURSE NEEDS TO KNOW

When secreted by the adrenal cortex, cortisol binds with corticosteroid-binding globulin (CBG) and, to a much lesser degree, albumin. Only a small amount of cortisol (10%) circulates unbound or in the free state, which is the biologically active form. Free cortisol is normally excreted in the urine in small amounts.

If excessive secretion of cortisol occurs, the CBG-binding sites are filled, causing an increase in free cortisol; therefore, the urinary excretion increases. Because of this, an increased secretion of urinary free cortisol is helpful in diagnosing Cushing's syndrome. It is not helpful in diagnosing adrenal insufficiency, because it is not sensitive at low levels, and low levels are relatively common in healthy individuals.

CBG is produced by the liver. Liver failure will affect CBG and, therefore, free cortisol levels. CBG is influenced by other factors. CBG levels increase in hyperthyroidism, diabetes, and high-estrogen states such as pregnancy. Genetic disorders may cause an increase or decrease in CBG. Hypothyroidism, protein deficiency, and renal failure may cause a decrease in CBG and influence free cortisol levels.

Salivary cortisol level tests may be conducted, since salivary levels correlate with free cortisol values. Timing of salivary level tests may vary. Often a *midnight salivary cortisol* (MSC) test is done.

REFERENCE VALUES   20-90 μ g/24 hr *or* SI: 55-248 nmol/24 hr

HOW THE TEST IS DONE

A 24-hour urine specimen is collected and analyzed by radioimmunoassay (RIA) or by competitive protein-binding assay.

SIGNIFICANCE OF TEST RESULTS

Elevated Values

Cushing's syndrome
Adrenal or pituitary tumor
Ectopic adrenocorticotropic hormone (ACTH) production
Stress, including critical illness

Decreased Values

Addison's disease
Hypothyroidism

INTERFERING FACTORS

- Stress
- Decrease in creatinine clearance
- Physical activity
- Failure to collect all the urine during the 24-hour period
- Failure to store urine on ice or in a refrigerator
- Medications such as amphetamines, morphine sulfate, phenothiazines, reserpine, and steroids

F

NURSING CARE

Nursing actions are similar to those used in other timed urine collections (see Chapter 2), with the following additional measures.

Pretest

○ *Patient Teaching.* The nurse instructs the patient to avoid strenuous physical activity. The patient is taught how to collect the specimen.

During the Test

- At the start of the test, the nurse instructs the patient to void at 8 AM and discard this urine. The collection period starts at this time, and all urine is collected for 24 hours, including the 8 AM specimen of the following morning.
- Keep the urine refrigerated or on ice throughout the collection period.

Posttest

- On the requisition slip and specimen label, write the patient's name and the time and date of the start and finish of the test period. Arrange for prompt transport of the cooled specimen to the lab.

Free Thyroxine

Also called: FT_4; Free T_4; Unbound T_4

SPECIMEN OR TYPE OF TEST: Serum

PURPOSE OF THE TEST

Free thyroxine is used to diagnose hyperthyroidism and hypothyroidism. It is especially helpful when abnormal thyroxine-binding globulin levels exist.

BASICS THE NURSE NEEDS TO KNOW

The majority of thyroxine (see section on Thyroxine, Total, p. 578) is carried by thyroid-binding globulin, albumin, and prealbumin. It is free thyroxine (FT_4), which is not bound, that is biologically active and converts to triiodothyronine (T_3) in the peripheral circulation. The ability to measure free thyroxine has replaced a classic test called *protein-bound iodine*.

Frequently, because of the expense of an FT_4 test, free thyroxine may be evaluated by the *free thyroxine index* (FT_4I), which is an estimated value. The FT_4I is calculated by multiplying the total T_4 by the thyroid hormone-binding ratio (THBR). The normal value for an adult is 4.2 to 13.0 (no units of value).

REFERENCE VALUES Newborns: 2.6-6.3 ng/dL *or* SI: 33.5-81.3 pmol/L
Adults: 0.9-2.7 ng/dL *or* SI: 11.5-35 pmol/L

HOW THE TEST IS DONE

Venipuncture is performed.

SIGNIFICANCE OF TEST RESULTS

Elevated Values
Acute psychiatric disorders
Hyperthyroidism

Decreased Values
Anorexia nervosa
Hypothyroidism

INTERFERING FACTORS
- Medications such as carbamazepine, exogenous thyroid therapy, heparin, phenytoin, salicylates, and radioisotopes

NURSING CARE

Nursing actions are similar to those used in other venipuncture procedures (see Chapter 2), with the following additional measures.

Pretest
- The nurse checks with the lab. Depending on the lab methodology used, radionuclide scans may need to be scheduled after the blood is drawn for this test.
- The nurse checks with the physician if a serum albumin level is desired at the same time.

Free Triiodothyronine

Also called: FT_3; Free T_3

SPECIMEN OR TYPE OF TEST: Serum

PURPOSE OF THE TEST
Free triiodothyronine is used to diagnose hyperthyroidism and hypothyroidism.

BASICS THE NURSE NEEDS TO KNOW
Triiodothyronine is a hormone secreted by the thyroid gland. Most of the hormone is bound to thyroid-binding globulin. Some triiodothyronine is in the free state; that is, unbound. The unbound or free triiodothyronine is the biologically active form of the hormone.

REFERENCE VALUES   260-480 pg/dL *or* SI: 4.0-7.4 pmol/L

HOW THE TEST IS DONE
Venipuncture is performed.

SIGNIFICANCE OF TEST RESULTS

Elevated Values
Hyperthyroidism

Decreased Values
Hypothyroidism
Late pregnancy

INTERFERING FACTORS

- Exogenous thyroid therapy
- Radioisotopes within 7 days
- Glucocorticoids

G

NURSING CARE

Nursing actions resemble those of other venipuncture procedures, as presented in Chapter 2, with the following additional measures.

Pretest

- The nurse checks with the lab. Depending on the lab methodology used, radionuclide scans may need to be scheduled after the blood is drawn for this test.
- The nurse checks with the physician if a serum albumin level is desired at the same time.

Gamma-Glutamyltransferase

Also called: GGT

SPECIMEN OR TYPE OF TEST: Serum

PURPOSE OF THE TEST

The gamma-glutamyltransferase test is used to detect hepatobiliary disease.

BASICS THE NURSE NEEDS TO KNOW

Gamma-glutamyltransferase (GGT) is an enzyme that is amply present in liver tissue. When there is damage to those hepatocytes that manufacture bile, the enzyme will release through the cell membranes and be absorbed into the blood. In addition, with cholestasis (stasis or obstruction of the flow of bile) within the liver or biliary system, the GGT level in the blood will rise early in the course of illness and remain elevated for as long as the dysfunction persists. In cases of biliary duct obstruction, the GGT value may rise from 5 to 50 times the upper limit of the normal value. In cases of hepatitis, the rise is more moderate and may be 5 times the upper limit of normal.

In the range of reference values, there are differences related to gender, age, and ethnicity. The values for adult males are 25% higher than adult females. People of African ancestry have normal values that are double the values of those who are white, for all age groups.

REFERENCE VALUES

Premature newborn: 56-233 U/L *or* SI: 56-233 U/L at 37° C
Newborn-3 weeks: 10-103 U/L *or* SI: 10-103 U/L at 37° C
3 weeks-3 months: 4-111U/L *or* SI: 4-111 U/L at 37° C
1-5 years: 2-23 U/L *or* SI: 2-23 U/L at 37° C
6-15 years: 2-23 U/L *or* SI: 2-23 U/L at 37° C
16 years-Adult: 2-35 U/L *or* SI: 2-35 U/L at 37° C
Adult: 5-40 U/L *or* SI: 5-40 U/L at 37° C

HOW THE TEST IS DONE

A venipuncture is performed to collect a sample of venous blood.

SIGNIFICANCE OF TEST RESULTS

Cancer of the liver (primary, metastatic)
Intrahepatic cholestasis
Hepatitis, infectious, alcoholic
Cirrhosis
Cholestasis
Biliary tract obstruction
Biliary cirrhosis
Pancreatitis
Cancer of the pancreas

INTERFERING FACTORS

- Alcohol ingested before the test
- Use of medications such as estrogen, phenytoin, and acetaminophen

NURSING CARE

Nursing actions are similar to those used in other venipuncture procedures (see Chapter 2), with the following additional measures.

Pretest

○ *Patient Teaching.* Instruct the patient to abstain from alcohol intake before the test. The patient should also fast from food for 8 hours before the test. The food and alcoholic intake would elevate the test result.

- If the patient takes medications that interfere with the accuracy of the test, the nurse should document the medications on the laboratory requisition form. Patients who must take these medications should not suspend the dosage schedule.

Gastrin

SPECIMEN OR TYPE OF TEST: Serum

PURPOSE OF THE TEST

Serum gastrin is a test used to help diagnose Zollinger-Ellison syndrome and gastrinoma.

BASICS THE NURSE NEEDS TO KNOW

Gastrin is a hormone manufactured by specific cells in the gastric mucosa. Gastrin functions to stimulate the production of gastric acid and intrinsic factor and stimulates gastric motility and pancreatic secretions. When the pH of gastric secretions rises to a less acidic value, gastrin secretion is stimulated. Conversely, when the pH of gastric acid falls to a more acidic value, the gastrin value declines. This interaction protects the stomach from overacidification from excess gastrin production. Older adults may have an age-related decrease in gastric acid production that causes a slightly more elevated level of gastrin.

Elevated Values

A gastrinoma is a pancreatic or duodenal endocrine tumor. It produces large amounts of gastrin and the serum value can rise to greater than 1000 pg/mL (SI: 1000 ng/L). This can cause increased gastric acid production and multiple peptic ulcers. When all three of these factors are present, the diagnosis of Zollinger-Ellison syndrome is made. In disorders with low or absent gastric acid production, such as pernicious anemia, postsurgical vagotomy, and atrophic gastritis, the physiologic response is to increase the production of gastrin.

G

REFERENCE VALUES   Newborn, 0-4 days: 120-183 pg/mL *or* 57-87 pmol/L
Child: <10-125 pg/mL *or* SI: <5-59 pmol/L
Adult (16-60 years): 25-90 pg/mL *or* SI: 12-43 pmol/L
Adults >60 years: <100 pg/mL *or* <48 pmol/L

HOW THE TEST IS DONE

Venipuncture is performed to obtain a sample of venous blood.

SIGNIFICANCE OF TEST RESULTS

Zollinger-Ellison syndrome
Chronic atrophic gastritis
Pernicious anemia
Gastric ulcer
Pyloric obstruction
Gastric cancer

INTERFERING FACTORS

- Recent radioisotope scan
- Failure to maintain a nothing-by-mouth status
- Recent gastroscopy

▌ NURSING CARE

Nursing actions are similar to those used in other venipuncture procedures (see Chapter 2), with the following additional measures.

Continued

NURSING CARE—cont'd

Pretest
- Schedule this test before gastroscopy and any nuclear scan. The gastroscopy can irritate the gastric mucosa and the radioisotopes would interfere with the lab method of analysis of the blood.
- ⊙ *Patient Teaching.* Instruct the patient to fast from food for at least 12 hours before the test. This is because any recent intake of protein causes an elevation of the serum gastrin level.

Posttest
- Ensure that the specimen is sent to the lab without delay. Gastrin is unstable at room temperature and delay would invalidate the test result.

Gated Blood Pool Studies

Also called: Gated Blood Pool Ventriculography, Technetium 99 Ventriculography; (MUGA); Multiple Gated Acquisition Angiography

SPECIMEN OR TYPE OF TEST: Radionuclide Imaging

PURPOSE OF THE TEST

A gated blood pool study is performed to assess ventricular function by evaluating wall motion and determining ejection fraction of the heart. It may be used for prognosis following an acute myocardial infarction because a resting left ventricular ejection fraction (LVEF) of 30% or less during the first 24 hours after a coronary occlusion correlates with a high mortality rate.

BASICS THE NURSE NEEDS TO KNOW

A gated blood pool study is a noninvasive method of assessing myocardial function, particularly wall motion of the left ventricle. It also permits evaluation of left ventricular ejection fraction without invasive catheterization. Gated blood pool studies are being replaced by echocardiography (see pp. 270) and gated-SPECT myocardial perfusion imaging. GSPECT (gated single proton emission computed tomography) provides the evaluation of LV function and myocardial perfusion in one study. See pp. 488 for discussion of myocardial perfusion studies.

REFERENCE VALUES	Normal wall motion Ejection fraction: 55%-75% Response to exercise: Increase in ejection fraction greater than 5%

HOW THE TEST IS DONE

The procedure for the gated blood pool study is similar to that for myocardial imaging. The red blood cells are tagged with technetium 99m pyrophosphate, a gamma-emitting radionuclide. Because the bound technetium cannot diffuse through cell membranes, it remains in the blood. Its emissions are more concentrated in body cavities with large blood volumes, including the heart chambers.

During the procedure, the patient is monitored with a cardiac monitor, and the ECG is synchronized with the imaging equipment. Multiple images can be obtained. Results usually report the "first pass," which analyzes the radiotracing during the initial flow through the heart. In addition, a "gated" analysis is performed, which reports cardiac chamber responses of 200 to 300 cardiac cycles. Because left ventricular size can be measured at the end of diastole and systole, the ventricular ejection fraction can be measured. After a gated analysis, the patient may be reassessed with exercise stress testing.

SIGNIFICANCE OF TEST RESULTS

Hypokinesis (slightly diminished wall motion)
Akinesis (absence of wall motion)
Dyskinesia (paradoxical wall motion or bulging)
Decreased ejection fraction

INTERFERING FACTORS

- Uncooperative patient
- Inconsistent cardiac rate or rhythm
- Failure to follow dietary restrictions

NURSING CARE

Pretest

○ *Patient Teaching.* The nurse instructs the patient about the purpose and the procedure of the test. Explain to the patient that only a slight amount of radioactive substance is necessary, which will be excreted within hours. Patient needs to know to follow instructions regarding position changes. If an exercise stress test is included, explain the procedure. The nurse also instructs the patient to wear comfortable, loose clothes and to avoid any heavy meals for 3 to 4 hours before the test.

- Check with the physician, but cardiac medications are usually continued.
- If the gated blood pool study is being conducted with a stress test, assess for contraindications. These include chest pain, hypertension, thrombophlebitis, second or third degree heart block, serious dysrhythmia, severe heart failure, and neurologic, musculoskeletal, or vascular problems that would impede mobility.

○ *Patient Teaching.* Ask the patient to inform the staff if he or she experiences any chest pain, shortness of breath, or nausea during the testing procedure.

During the Test

- Patient is maintained on a cardiac monitor. A blood pressure cuff is applied for periodic assessment.
- The patient is placed in the supine position and instructed to remain still. The gamma-ray camera is positioned close to the patient's chest.
- A peripheral intravenous line is established. One or two doses of a tracer material are injected by the physician.

Posttest

- Evaluate the patient's physical and emotional response to the testing.
- The patient may resume normal diet and medications.
- Tracer elements will be excreted within hours. To handle patient's urine, the nurse will use Standard Precautions, wearing gloves and washing his or her hands afterward.
- See section on Perfusion studies, Cardiac (p. 488) for Nursing Responses to Complications.

Genetic Sonogram

Includes: Nuchal translucency (NT)

SPECIMEN OR TYPE OF TEST: Ultrasound

PURPOSE OF THE TEST

The genetic sonogram is used to help identify the presence or absence of fetal abnormalities that are characteristic of Down syndrome.

BASICS THE NURSE NEEDS TO KNOW

Amniocentesis and chorionic villus sampling are two invasive diagnostic procedures that identify the presence or absence of Down syndrome through chromosome analysis. The chromosome analysis is highly accurate but these two procedures present a small, but possible risk to fetal well-being. The current approach to diagnostic testing for Down syndrome is to use alternative nonrisk test methods to exclude Down syndrome and to reserve the invasive procedures for those who have abnormal test results. With advances in ultrasound technology, the genetic sonogram is a noninvasive ultrasound procedure to help assess for Down syndrome in the first or second trimester of pregnancy. There is no single test that will identify Down syndrome in the fetus with 100% accuracy. Therefore, multiple tests are used in combination to improve the accuracy of the results (H.S. Cuckle, personal communication, October 27, 2010).

Genetic Sonogram

This ultrasound examination consists of a series of fetal images of specific tissues that help demonstrate or exclude Down syndrome. The complete genetic sonogram includes various ultrasound images of the fetus, searching to identify characteristic Down syndrome abnormalities including nuchal translucency and thickening, short femur and humerus, an absent or underdeveloped nasal bone, and sandal gap deformity of the toes. Nuchal translucency is the best and most accurate marker that is predictive of Down syndrome. The other physical characteristics, called short markers, vary in sensitivity (the ability to detect the abnormality) and accuracy in interpreting the results.

Nuchal translucency imaging is best when done in between the 11th and 14th week of gestation, as one of the recommended combined first trimester screening tests. The combined first trimester screening tests consist of nuchal translucency ultrasound imaging, human chorionic gonadotrophin (p. 193), and pregnancy-associated plasma protein A (p. 514).

For interpretation, the test results are considered as a combined result rather than as single entities. When nuchal translucency, the most sensitive of the triple markers is included, the combined first trimester screening tests have a 90% detection rate of Down syndrome and a 5% false-positive rate (Sonek & Nicolaides, 2010). The second trimester quadruple marker screening tests also assesses for indicators of Down syndrome and neural tube defects. The included tests are serum alpha-fetoprotein (p. 62), human chorionic gonadotrophin (p. 193), unconjugated estriol (p. 306), and inhibin A. The more complete genetic sonogram, including nuchal translucency, may be done late in the first trimester, or in the early part of the second trimester, in the follow-up of abnormal results of the combined first trimester screen or second trimester quadruple marker screening tests.

Nuchal Translucency

Nuchal translucency or nuchal fold thickness is the most effective and accepted soft marker as an indicator of chromosomal disorder of the fetus, and Down syndrome in particular. It has higher sensitivity and a lower rate of a false-positive finding than the other soft markers. There is a 4.7% false-positive rate with the nuchal translucency measurement. A false-positive result means that the tests indicate abnormality, but in reality, the fetus is normal.

The nuchal tissue is located in the back of the fetal neck. Nuchal fold translucency is measurable by ultrasound in the 11th to 14th week of gestation; the tissue appears translucent because of fluid or edema. On the sonogram image, the thickness of the translucent tissue of the nuchal fold is measured from the outer surface of the occipital bone to the exterior of the fetal scalp (Figure 52). When the measurement is greater than the reference value, it is an indicator of risk for Down syndrome, cardiac anomalies, and other fetal defects (Sonek and Nicolaides, 2010).

Likelihood Ratio

The results are presented as a mathematical score called the Likelihood Ratio (LR). When the likelihood ratio is a large number, the data is considered very convincing. If the likelihood ratio is less than 1 or near zero, the data is considered not very convincing and the abnormal condition is not very likely (McGee, 2007). In the evaluation of the genetic sonogram, the calculation of the likelihood ratio includes the modifiers of maternal age, gestational age of the fetus, test sensitivity, and false-positive percentage. The presence of multiple abnormal images and additional structural defects in the fetus will increase the likelihood ratio score. Abnormal results are greater than 1. Scores of 2 to 5, 5 to 10, or greater than 10 in the likelihood ratio are considered as a small, moderate, or high probability of Down syndrome, respectively.

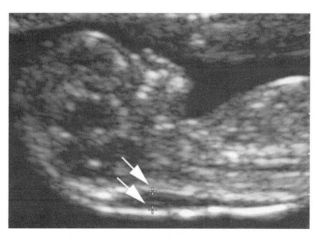

Figure 52. Nuchal translucency. Abnormally large nuchal translucency measurement *(arrows)* of 4.1 mm. This fetus had trisomy 21. (From Rumack C, Wilson SR, Charboneau JW: *Diagnostic ultrasound,* ed 3, St Louis, 2005, Mosby.)

REFERENCE VALUES | Likelihood ratio score: <1
Nuchal translucency average measurement (10-12 weeks): 2.5 mm
or less (Rumack et al, 2005)*

*The measurement in millimeters changes with gestational age, so the measurement may be reported in terms of MoM (multiples of the normal median) (Bahado-Singh & Argoti, 2010).

HOW THE TEST IS DONE

Transabdominal ultrasound is used to obtain the various images of the fetus. If the imaging results are not effective, a second ultrasound testing will be done, using the transabdominal or possibly transvaginal approach.

SIGNIFICANCE OF THE TEST RESULTS

Abnormal Results

Down syndrome
Other chromosomal disorders

INTERFERING FACTORS

• None

NURSING CARE

Pretest
• The American College of Obstetricians and Gynecologists (2007) now recommends that pregnant women of all ages be offered screening tests in the first trimester. This means that it is highly likely that more women will undergo this screening early in their pregnancy, recognizing that the purpose of the screening is to identify risk of having a baby with Down syndrome. The woman should have a clear understanding that the first trimester screening is highly accurate but does not provide a final diagnosis. There can be inaccuracy and false-positive findings. One nursing research study (Hawthorne & Ahern, 2009) identifies that some patients contemplating nuchal translucency testing experience anxiety about the possibility that their baby may not be normal. Other patients recognize they are at high risk (such as older than 35 years) and view the nuchal translucency imaging as a way to rule out a major concern.
• The blood tests that are part of first trimester screening should be scheduled just before or on the same day as the sonogram. Some ultrasound centers perform the blood tests as well, and the combined results are discussed with the patient on the same day, following the completion of the testing.
• The patient's signed consent is required for the ultrasound procedure. The nurse enters the document into the patient's record.

Posttest
• A positive finding is presented in terms of risk of having a Down syndrome baby. Genetic counseling is important to help the prospective parents understand the results, the level of risk, and to begin to make decisions (Pergament, 2010). The first decision is to obtain

G

additional information by having either a chorionic villus sampling or amniocentesis with a chromosomal analysis of the fetus.

- Based on all the test results, the prospective parents ultimately will have to make informed decisions about the future of the pregnancy, aided by their genetic counselor. For the prospective parents, the discussions and decisions are difficult. Many opt for an abortion (Chasen, 2010). Other women continue the pregnancy, but additional genetic malformations, spontaneous fetal death or death of the neonate in the early postdelivery period can occur. Alternatively, the child may have Down syndrome and live with special needs or disabilities. In some cases when the screening tests are abnormal but with a low likelihood ratio score and normal chromosomal results, the child is born as a normal neonate without Down syndrome (Rumack et al, 2005).

Genetic Testing for Cystic Fibrosis

Also called: Cystic Fibrosis; DNA Detection

SPECIMEN OR TYPE OF TEST: Blood, Buccal Mucosal Cells, Amniotic Fluid, Chorionic Villus Cells

PURPOSE OF THE TEST

This test screens for the genetic mutation of cystic fibrosis that reveals carrier or disease status.

BASICS THE NURSE NEEDS TO KNOW

Cystic fibrosis is an inherited autosomal-recessive genetic disorder. In the heterozygous (carrier) form, the individual has one mutated gene for cystic fibrosis, but does not have the disease or symptoms of the disease. In the homozygous form, the individual inherits two mutated cystic fibrosis genes, one from each carrier parent. This individual inherits cystic fibrosis disease. When both reproductive partners have the heterozygous form of the genetic mutation, each pregnancy has a one in four chance (25% risk) of conceiving a child with cystic fibrosis disease (Figure 53). Cystic fibrosis most commonly affects Caucasian people and the subgroup of

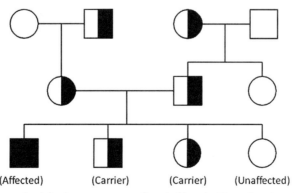

(Affected)   (Carrier)   (Carrier)   (Unaffected)

Figure 53. Autosomal recessive inheritance pattern of cystic fibrosis. (From Goetzinger KR, Cahill AG: An update on cystic fibrosis screening, *Clin Lab Med* 30 (3):534, 2010.)

Ashkenazi Jewish people. Cystic fibrosis also affects people who are African American, Asian, or Hispanic, but occurs less frequently.

The genetic mutation occurs on chromosome 7 and alters the gene called CF transmembrane conductance regulator (CFTR). If the paired CTFR genes are absent or have a mutation, the child with cystic fibrosis will have multiple alterations for fluid and electrolyte transport to cells including dehydrated secretions, thick mucus in the lungs, poor secretion of pancreatic enzymes, altered intestinal function, and increased sodium chloride in sweat (Goetzinger & Cahill, 2010). There are over 1000 identified CFTR mutations in cystic fibrosis. The standard screening panel consists of testing for 23 of the most common mutations.

The genetic testing for cystic fibrosis is not 100% sensitive. One hundred percent sensitivity would mean that the cystic fibrosis mutation will be detected in every tested person who has the mutation. In the current state of genetic testing for cystic fibrosis, there are some false-negative results. False negative means that some people who have a negative test result actually are positive for the CFTR mutation and the mutations have not been identified. The sensitivity in genetic testing for cystic fibrosis varies among different racial and ethnic groups. The sensitivity or true positive detection rates are: Caucasians 80% to 88%, African American 65% to 69%, Ashkenazi Jewish 94% to 97%, Hispanic 57% to 72%, and Asian 30% to 49% (Goetzinger & Cahill, 2010).

Carrier Screening for Cystic Fibrosis

To identify the carriers of this genetic mutation, genetic screening is offered to the female before conception or at the time of the first prenatal visit to her doctor. Because in the United States it is increasingly difficult to identify a single race or ethnic background, the current recommendation is to offer CF testing to all women, regardless of ethnic or racial status (Goetzinger & Cahill, 2010).

If the woman tests positive for this mutation, she is given the information and genetic counseling. Then, her reproductive partner is offered testing. Alternatively, both partners may be tested simultaneously. If the partner also tests positive, both are given genetic counseling. They receive a thorough explanation of cystic fibrosis and their risk of transmitting the disease or the genetic carrier status to their offspring. They are also counseled that DNA testing does not always identify the genetic mutations when they actually exist.

Fetal Screening for Cystic Fibrosis

If the fetus is to be tested genetically for the disease, chorionic villus sampling is done at 10 to 13 weeks' gestation or amniocentesis is done at 15 to 20 weeks' gestation. If the fetus tests positive for the homozygous genetic mutation of cystic fibrosis disease, the couple is given the information and counseling by the genetics counselor and their physician. They have a choice to terminate the pregnancy or carry the baby to term and prepare for the delivery of a child who will have many health care needs.

REFERENCE VALUES   **No detected genetic mutation for cystic fibrosis**

HOW THE TEST IS DONE

Blood: Venipuncture is used to collect a sample of venous blood.

Cell sample: Within the mouth, a sample of buccal cells from the inner surface of the cheek is collected, using a swab, scoop, or mouth rinse. The specimen is placed in a sterile container.

SIGNIFICANCE OF TEST RESULTS

Heterozygous mutation for the cystic fibrosis gene (carrier)
Homozygous mutation for the cystic fibrosis gene (disease)

INTERFERING FACTORS

• None

NURSING CARE

Nursing actions are similar to those used in other venipuncture procedures (see Chapter 2), with the following additional measures.

Pretest
• After the physician has explained this genetic screening test and its significance to the patient, a signed patient's consent is needed to perform the genetic testing.
• If the patient expresses apprehension or anxiety about the possible results of the genetic testing, the nurse can provide empathy and support. It is important to know one's health status or risk so that potential decisions are based on fact and information. The risk to have a child with cystic fibrosis disease is much greater when there is a family history of cystic fibrosis or when both reproductive partners are carriers.

During the Test
• The laboratory requisition form should state additional information including the patient's ethnicity and pertinent family history regarding cystic fibrosis.

Posttest
Health Promotion
Screening for the genetic mutation of the cystic fibrosis gene is now offered to all pregnant women, regardless of ethnicity. The nurse encourages all women of childbearing age to have the test done early in the prenatal period. Some women and their partners may choose to have the test done when they are planning a pregnancy but have not yet conceived.

Glomerular Filtration Rate

Also called: GFR

SPECIMEN OR TYPE OF TEST: Urine, Blood

PURPOSE OF THE TEST

GFR is used to evaluate renal function and to stage chronic renal disease.

BASICS THE NURSE NEEDS TO KNOW

GFC cannot be measured directly, but is estimated by evaluating marker clearance through the kidneys. Creatinine or insulin may be used as markers.

REFERENCE VALUES* 130 mL/min/1.73m^2
Staging of chronic renal failure, according to the National Kidney
    Foundation:
Stage 1: >90 mL/min
Stage 2: 60-89 mL/min
Stage 3: 30-59 mL/min
Stage 4: 15-29 mL/min
Stage 5: <15 mL/min

*Varies with formula used.

HOW THE TEST IS DONE

GFR is not a direct measurement, but is estimated using formulas. Two formulas frequently used are the Cockcroft-Gault and the MDRD study equation. Both formulas require the patient's age in years, sex, and weight. The MDRD equation adjusts for the patient who is African American.

SIGNIFICANCE OF TEST RESULTS

Decreased Values
Chronic renal failure

INTERFERING FACTORS

See Creatinine Clearance on pp. 231.

NURSING CARE

See Creatinine Clearance on pp. 233.

Glucagon

SPECIMEN OR TYPE OF TEST: Plasma

PURPOSE OF THE TEST

Glucagon levels are assessed in suspected pancreatic tumors, chronic pancreatitis, and familial hyperglucagonemia.

BASICS THE NURSE NEEDS TO KNOW

Glucagon is produced and secreted by the alpha cells of the islets of Langerhans of the pancreas. Glucagon stimulates the breakdown of stored glycogen and maintains gluconeogenesis. Glucagon is secreted in response to hypoglycemia, helping to meet glucose needs of tissues between intakes of food.

REFERENCE VALUES*	Infant: 0-1750 pg/mL *or* SI: 0-1750 ng/L
	Child: 0-148 pg/mL *or* SI: 0-148 ng/L
	Adult: 20-100 pg/mL *or* SI: 20-100 ng/L

*Varies with laboratory

HOW THE TEST IS DONE

Venipuncture is performed and the specimen is placed on ice and sent to the lab immediately.

SIGNIFICANCE OF TEST RESULTS

Elevated Values

Acute pancreatitis
Cirrhosis of the liver
Diabetic ketoacidosis
Glucagonoma
Hypoglycemia
Parasympathetic stimulation
Pheochromocytoma
Renal failure, chronic
Stress, high levels
Sympathetic stimulation

Decreased Values

Chronic pancreatitis
Cystic fibrosis
High fatty acid levels
Hyperglycemia
Insulinoma
Pancreatic tumors

INTERFERING FACTORS

- Stress
- Prolonged fasting
- Radioactive scan within 2 days
- Medications, such as catecholamines, insulin, and glucocorticoids

NURSING CARE

The nurse takes actions similar to those used in other venipuncture procedures as described in Chapter 2, with the following additional measures.

Pretest

○ *Patient Teaching.* The nurse instructs the patient to fast for 10 to 12 hours before the blood is drawn.

Continued

> ▌ **NURSING CARE—cont'd**
>
> ○ *Patient Teaching.* Explain to the patient the need to rest for 30 minutes before the test.
> - The nurse takes a medication history and determines if any interfering drugs should be withheld until after the blood is drawn.
> - Schedule any radioactive scans after the glucagon determination is obtained.
>
> **Posttest**
> - Place the specimen on ice and send it to the lab immediately. (Not all laboratories require the specimen to be placed on ice.)
> - The patient can resume a normal diet and medication regimen.

Glucose, Capillary

Also called: Self-Blood Glucose Monitoring; (SBGM); Capillary Bedside Glucose Monitoring; (CBGM); Capillary Sugar Monitoring

SPECIMEN OR TYPE OF TEST: Blood

PURPOSE OF THE TEST

Capillary glucose monitoring is carried out to assess and manage patients with diabetes mellitus. It may be used in hospitals to monitor other hyperglycemic patients, such as those on hyperalimentation or high-dose glucocorticoid therapy. Capillary glucose evaluation is *not* used to diagnose diabetes mellitus, but it may indicate a need to assess plasma glucose levels. It is usually used as part of aggressive treatment for diabetes. Most health care providers recommend that patients with type 1 diabetes mellitus check their capillary glucose levels three to four times a day; some may need more frequent checks. It is not clear how often patients with type 2 diabetes should check their capillary glucose levels; however, SBGM can help identify hypoglycemia in patients on sulfonylurea and other hypoglycemic agents. Controlling the blood glucose level in diabetes very strictly has been shown to lower the complications of the disease.

BASICS THE NURSE NEEDS TO KNOW

Capillary glucose monitoring has revolutionized the management of patients with type 1 diabetes mellitus. Capillary glucose monitoring determines the glucose level of whole blood (which is lower than serum or plasma levels). It evaluates current status, permitting more accurate management and therapy. It has replaced urine glucose testing as the preferred technique to determine insulin replacement requirements in hospitals and in the home.

In the past to perform capillary glucose monitoring, a drop of capillary blood was dropped onto a reagent strip, and the glucose level was determined by the color changes on the strip. The color change was then compared with a color chart. Because the visual method is subjective and some diabetics have visual impairment, glucose meters (glucometers) are currently used.

For type 1 and type 2 diabetics, regular capillary glucose testing will produce greater control, with more effective long-term treatment. Capillary glucose testing can help the diabetic maintain control during periods of stress, for example, illness, pregnancy, and surgery. Usually, the patient with type 1 diabetes will monitor the capillary glucose level before each meal and at bedtime. The patient with type 2 diabetes should follow their health provider's recommendation on assessing their SGBM because these recommendations vary.

Nurses need to teach their patients how to monitor capillary glucose, including how to use and care for the glucose meter and reagent strips and how to check the reliability of the meter. This information needs to be reinforced periodically.

REFERENCE VALUES   60-110 mg/dL *or* SI: 3.3-6.1 mmol/L

G

HOW THE TEST IS DONE

There are many different glucose monitors on the market today. Most measure whole blood obtained by a finger stick. Glucometers must be approved by the U.S. Food and Drug Administration. Most health insurers will cover the cost of the glucometer, test strips, and lancets. However, the copay must be covered by the patient. Be aware if the person does not have any insurance and make appropriate referrals. Cost of glucometers and the equipment differ. Encourage the patient to be consumer-wise and shop around for the best prices.

In selecting a glucometer, besides cost, other factors are important such as size and weight of the meter, the size of the digital read out, size of the blood sample needed, ability to trend/track results, and pain/discomfort. The size of the sample needed for the glucometer may affect patient comfort. The higher the gauge of the lancet, the finer the point. The finer the point, the smaller the blood sample. For those with poor vision, an audio or "talking" meter may be necessary.

When teaching a patient how to self-monitor their glucose, emphasize the importance of following the manufacturer's directions. It is best to instruct the patient on using the equipment they will use at home.

New technology for glucose monitoring is being developed that does not require a blood sample. These new monitors, called continuous glucose monitoring (CGM), include disposable subcutaneous probes placed under the skin. These sensors transmit to a receiver every 1 to 5 minutes a reading of the person's interstitial glucose level. The receiver can be attached to a belt or carried in a pocket. CGMs have alarms, a sound or vibration, to warn the patient of hyperglycemia or hypoglycemia. The new technology may decrease the number of finger sticks required, but does not replace them. The CGM need to be checked at least twice daily with whole blood glucometers. The CGM systems are expensive, since the sensors must be changed frequently (every 3 to 7 days).

SIGNIFICANCE OF TEST RESULTS

Elevated Values
Acromegaly
Chronic pancreatitis
Cushing's syndrome
Diabetes mellitus
Hyperthyroidism
Hyperosmolar coma
Pheochromocytoma
Stress

Decreased Values

Addison's disease

Advanced liver disease

Alcohol intake when fasting

Excessive exogenous insulin

Islet cell adenoma

Leucine sensitivity

Malnutrition

INTERFERING FACTORS

- Failure to follow the manufacturer's guidelines

NURSING CARE

Many different glucose meters are on the market. It is essential to follow the manufacturers' guidelines for their use. In addition, a number of lancing devices are available.

Pretest

- Glucose meters should be checked daily in hospitals and once a week or when opening a new vial of strips at home, using a quality control solution containing a known amount of dissolved glucose in water. The meter should also be tested if it is dropped or if the meter reading does not correlate with clinical assessments.
- When a fasting blood glucose determination is obtained, a capillary glucose level also can be obtained and the two measures compared. A variance of less than 15% is acceptable. Since plasma glucose levels are higher than whole blood levels, the nurse and patient need to know whether the glucose monitor used by the patient provides whole or plasma glucose measures.
- If the battery in the meter has worn out, recalibrate the meter with the plastic calibration strip provided in the reagent vial according to the manufacturer's guidelines.
- Check the code numbers on the glucose meter and on the reagent strip to ensure that they are the same. Check the expiration date on the reagent strip container and discard outdated strips.
- The nurse wears gloves for this procedure because blood contact is possible.

During the Test

- Instruct the patient to wash his or her hands in warm water and soap. The warm water will help dilate the vessels.
- Hospital protocol may require the patient's finger to be wiped with an alcohol swab (this is usually not done in the home). If alcohol is used, it must be allowed to dry out or it will affect the results and increase the painfulness of the procedure.
- Have the reagent strip on hand, and puncture the skin. The puncture site should be on the side of the fingertip. The middle of the fingertip is more sensitive to pain, and the side has more capillaries. Instruct the patient to rotate sites.
- Let the drop of blood fall on the reagent strip so that the entire pad at the tip is covered with blood. Do not smear the blood or try to add another drop.

- Time the wiping of the strip, if required, and the insertion of the strip into the meter according to the manufacturer's guidelines. Timing is essential for accurate measurement. Some manufacturers require that a cotton ball be used to wipe the reagent strip.
- Insert the strip into the meter (Figure 54). Read and document the results.
- Instruct the patient on how to dispose of the lancet in a heavy plastic container, for example, an empty detergent bottle.

Posttest

- Administer insulin as ordered. If the patient is hypoglycemic, give glucose, as prescribed.

◯ *Patient Teaching.* Instruct the patient to keep an accurate record of the glucose level and insulin replacement. This record should be brought to the physician, diabetic nurse specialist, or clinic on the next visit.

- New, more sophisticated meters will keep a record of glucose values, which can be accessed by the health care provider.

◯ *Patient Teaching.* The procedure for teaching the capillary glucose testing to the patient in the home is the same as that for capillary bedside monitoring. The above nursing implementation integrates the teaching required. Emphasis must be placed on the patient having an opportunity to practice self-blood glucose monitoring.

◯ *Patient Teaching.* Tell the patient to follow the manufacturer's instructions exactly. Unfortunately, the hospital glucometer may not be the same as the one the patient will use at home. The community health nurse needs to assess the patient's ability to apply hospital learning to the home environment. Reinforce learning. Periodically, the community health nurse needs to observe the patient's technique to ensure accurate test results.

G

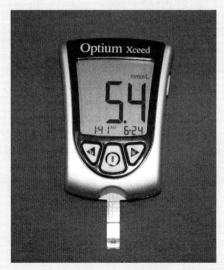

Figure 54. Glucometer. (From Gregory P, Ward A, eds: *Saunders' paramedic textbook*, ed 3, Oxford, 2011, Mosby.)

Glucose, Fasting

Also called: Fasting Blood Sugar (FBS); Fasting Plasma Sugar (FPS)

SPECIMEN OR TYPE OF TEST: Whole Blood, Serum, Plasma

PURPOSE OF THE TEST

Fasting glucose is evaluated to diagnose and manage patients with diabetes mellitus. The fasting glucose level also is obtained as supportive data in many diagnoses because metabolic factors will influence glucose use and storage. Certain therapies may be evaluated by checking the fasting blood glucose level (e.g., hyperalimentation and exogenous glucocorticoid therapy).

BASICS THE NURSE NEEDS TO KNOW

To meet cellular needs, the body has developed complex mechanisms to take in, use, and store nutrients. A serum glucose level determination reflects the ability of the body to perform its metabolic tasks. Glucose levels are not static; they vary after eating, so a fasting blood glucose (FBS) level determination is desirable. Many factors influence blood glucose, but testing is most frequently used to diagnose and manage diabetes mellitus.

With age, the norms for blood and plasma glucose levels are adjusted by 1 mg/dL per year of life after age 60.

A single elevated fasting plasma glucose test is not considered diagnostic when symptoms are not present, but the test should be repeated. If the second fasting blood glucose level test result is elevated (>126 mg/dL or SI: 6.99 mmol/L), it supports the diagnosis of diabetes mellitus. A blood glucose level between 100 and 125 mg/dL suggests impaired fasting glucose (IFG).

REFERENCE VALUES	Neonate: 30-60 mg/dL *or* SI: 1.7-3.3 mmol/L
	Infant: 40-90 mg/dL *or* SI: 2.2-5.0 mmol/L
	Children <2 years: 60-100 mg/dL *or* SI: 3.3-5.6 mmol/L
	Children 2 years to adult: Whole blood: 60-110 mg/dL *or* SI: 3.3-6.1 mmol/L
	Plasma or serum: 70-110 mg/dL *or* SI: 3.9-6.1 mmol/L
	Adult: 65-100 mg/dL *or* SI: 3.5-5.6 mmol/L
	Elderly individuals: 80-150 mg/dL *or* SI: 4.4-8.3 mmol/L
▽ **Critical Values**	<50 mg/dL or >500 mg/dL *or* in neonates, <30 mg *or* >300 mg/dL

HOW THE TEST IS DONE

After a 12-hour fast, venipuncture is performed. Usually a plasma sampling is performed because it reflects glucose levels in interstitial tissue and is not affected by the hematocrit.

SIGNIFICANCE OF TEST RESULTS

Elevated Values
Acromegaly
Chronic pancreatitis
Cushing's syndrome

Diabetes mellitus
Hyperthyroidism
Hyperosmolar coma
Pheochromocytoma
Stress

Decreased Values
Addison's disease
Advanced liver disease
Alcohol intake when fasting
Excessive exogenous insulin
Islet cell adenoma
Leucine sensitivity
Malnutrition

INTERFERING FACTORS

- Noncompliance with fasting
- Vigorous exercise
- Stress
- Medications, such as acetaminophen, arginine, benzodiazepines, β-blockers, epinephrine, ethacrynic acid, furosemide, glucocorticoids, glucose, hypoglycemic agents, insulin, lithium, MAO inhibitors, oral contraceptives, phenothiazines, phenytoin, and thiazide diuretics

NURSING CARE

Nursing actions are similar to those used in other venipuncture procedures (see Chapter 2), with the following additional measures.

Pretest

○ *Patient Teaching.* The nurse instructs the patient to fast for 12 hours before the blood is drawn. Instruct the patient who is taking insulin or hypoglycemic agents to stop the medication until after the blood is drawn.

- The nurse observes the patient for clinical manifestations of hypoglycemia.

Posttest

- The nurse ensures that the patient receives food and medications that were withheld.
- Send blood to the lab because it needs to be centrifuged within 30 minutes for serum and plasma levels.

Health Promotion

The American Diabetes Association recommends that the fasting plasma glucose (FPG) be used to evaluate patients. It also recommends that women at risk for gestational diabetes mellitus (obesity, history of GDM, or a family history of diabetes) should have an FPG at her first prenatal visit.

▽ **Nursing Response to Critical Values**

A low fasting plasma sugar (FPS) result indicates hypoglycemia. Notify the physician. If the patient is alert and not in danger of aspiration, give glucose by mouth. If the patient is unconscious, or if aspiration is likely, prepare to give 50% glucose intravenously as ordered.

Continued

NURSING CARE—cont'd

High FPS indicates hyperglycemia, usually related to diabetes ketoacidosis or a hyperosmolar coma. Notify the physician. Change any glucose-containing infusion the patient is receiving to a nonglucose solution. Prepare to give short-acting insulin as ordered. Assess ketone levels.

◆ **Nursing Response to Complications**

Because a fasting glucose determination requires that the patient maintain a nothing-by-mouth status, hypoglycemia may occur.

Hypoglycemia. Indications of hypoglycemia are: pallor, diaphoresis, tachycardia, palpitations, hunger, paresthesia, vagueness, confusion, slurred speech, somnolence, convulsions, and coma. If signs of hypoglycemia occur, the nurse should check the patient's capillary glucose level and obtain a specimen for a plasma glucose level. If the patient is awake and able to swallow, glucose is given orally. Notify the physician.

Glucose Loading Test

See Growth Hormone Suppression Test on p. 355.

Glucose, Postprandial

Also called: 2-Hour Postprandial Blood Sugar

SPECIMEN OR TYPE OF TEST: Plasma

PURPOSE OF THE TEST

The 2-hour postprandial glucose test is performed to support the diagnosis of diabetes mellitus and to evaluate the management of a patient with diabetes mellitus.

BASICS THE NURSE NEEDS TO KNOW

In healthy individuals, the ingestion of food raises the blood glucose level, which is a potent stimulant for insulin release. The insulin level peaks in less than an hour. Normally, within 1½ to 2 hours, the glucose level will return to baseline. It may take slightly longer in older individuals for the value to return to a baseline level. The 2-hour postprandial glucose test evaluates whether the individual has an adequate insulin response to intake. A diabetic is considered in good control if the 2-hour postprandial glucose level is less than 130 mg/dL. In an undiagnosed case, a 2-hour postprandial glucose level greater than 140 mg/dL indicates that an oral glucose tolerance test (OGTT) should be performed.

REFERENCE VALUES	Fasting plasma glucose: <140 mg/dL *or* SI: <7.8 mmol/L Values may be slightly elevated in elderly patients
▽ **Critical Values**	>200 mg/dL *or* 11 mmol/L

HOW THE TEST IS DONE

Two hours after a meal is ingested, venipuncture is performed.

SIGNIFICANCE OF TEST RESULTS

A 2-hour postprandial glucose determination greater than 140 mg/dL is consistent with the diagnosis of diabetes mellitus. Diagnosis is not made with a 2-hour postprandial glucose test; an elevation indicates a need for a fasting plasma sugar or glycosylated hemoglobin assay.

INTERFERING FACTORS

- Noncompliance with dietary requirements
- Cushing's disease or Cushing syndrome
- Infection
- Malabsorption syndrome
- Malnutrition
- Severe stress
- Medications, such as arginine, β-adrenergic blockers, epinephrine, glucocorticoids, glucose administered intravenously, hypoglycemic agents, insulin, lithium, phenothiazines, and phenytoin.

NURSING CARE

Nursing actions are similar to those used in other venipuncture procedures (see Chapter 2), with the following additional measures.

Pretest

◯ *Patient Teaching.* Instruct the patient to eat normally before the test, but not to eat or drink for 2 hours after the meal is ingested.

◯ *Patient Teaching.* Instruct patient to rest between meals and when a specimen is drawn.

During the Test

- The patient ingests a meal containing at least 75 to 100 g of carbohydrate.
- Venipuncture is performed to obtain a blood glucose level 2 hours after the meal.

Posttest

- The patient resumes a normal diet.

Glucose-6-Phosphate Dehydrogenase Screen

Also called: G-6-PD Screen

SPECIMEN OR TYPE OF TEST: Whole Blood

PURPOSE OF THE TEST

This test is used to detect a G-6-PD enzyme defect in erythrocytes and determine this cause of hemolytic anemia.

BASICS THE NURSE NEEDS TO KNOW

Genetic defects in erythrocyte metabolism are responsible for many forms of hemolytic anemia. The deficiency of the glucose-6-phosphate dehydrogenase (G-6-PD) enzyme in the erythrocyte is the most common cause of sudden hemolysis and is commonly associated with chronic hemolytic anemia. With deficient or diminished enzyme activity, the erythrocytes have a shorter life span. The deficiency of this enzyme is hereditary and linked to the X chromosome. In the United States, this type of hemolytic anemia is seen most frequently in African Americans and is usually a mild to moderate condition. A more severe form of the disorder affects individuals from southeast Asia, the Mideast, central Africa, and countries of the Mediterranean. With today's increasing worldwide migration of people, this genetic disorder can occur almost anywhere in the world.

In individuals with G-6-PD deficiency, a sudden, acute episode of severe hemolytic anemia usually is triggered by particular conditions. The ingestion of fava beans is the most common trigger that affects children and adults. Particular medications can trigger an episode of acute hemolysis, including sulfonamides, antimalarial drugs, aspirin, and large doses of vitamin C. The illnesses that can trigger hemolytic episodes are usually acute bacterial or viral infections or diabetic acidosis. Neonates with this genetic disorder are very vulnerable during a severe episode of hemolysis because of the high bilirubin level and the danger of kernicterus. Some individuals have a mild or moderate condition, but it will recur, particularly if the triggering factor is not eliminated. Finally, some people have this genetic disorder, but never experience hemolytic anemia.

REFERENCE VALUES	Newborn: 7.8-14.4 U/g Hb *or* 0.50-0.93 MU/mol Hb Adult: 5.5-9.3 U/g Hb *or* 0.35-0.60 MU/mol Hb

HOW THE TEST IS DONE

Venipuncture or capillary puncture is used to collect a specimen of venous blood.

SIGNIFICANCE OF TEST RESULTS

Decreased Values

G-6-PD anemia, mild to moderate
G-6-PD anemia, severe

INTERFERING FACTORS

• Sudden, severe hemolysis episode in the patient

NURSING CARE

Nursing actions are similar to those used in other venipuncture procedures (see Chapter 2), with the following additional measures.

Posttest

• If the patient is diagnosed with G-6-PD deficiency, he or she needs to understand which triggering factors can cause an episode of anemia, and eliminate the causative food or medication. The patient should also be instructed to avoid aspirin or nonprescription medications that contain aspirin.

- In cases of severe hemolysis, the nurse should assess for severe pallor and possible abdominal pain. Later, jaundice will occur and the indirect bilirubin level rises. Severe episodes last about 7 to 12 days, and then the condition recedes. For mild or severe episodes, the nurse encourages the patient to rest because fatigue accompanies anemia. In addition, extra fluid intake will help promote renal function and urinary output. A nutritious diet will help in the recovery process as the patient begins to manufacture new erythrocytes.
- In hemolytic anemia of the newborn that is caused by this hemoglobin deficiency, the hyperbilirubinemia will usually respond to phototherapy treatment. Exchange transfusions may be needed.

G

Glucose Tolerance Test

Also called: GTT; Oral Glucose Tolerance Test (OGGT); Intravenous Glucose Tolerance Test (IVGGT)

SPECIMEN OR TYPE OF TEST: Plasma

PURPOSE OF THE TEST

The glucose tolerance test is performed to confirm the diagnosis of diabetes mellitus and gestational diabetes.

BASICS THE NURSE NEEDS TO KNOW

Fasting plasma glucose level determinations, if repeated, are usually adequate to diagnose diabetes mellitus if the plasma glucose level is greater than 126 mg/dL. However, if the fasting blood glucose levels are questionable, and clinical indications make diabetes mellitus likely, an oral glucose tolerance test (OGTT) or an intravenous glucose tolerance test (IVGTT) may be performed. Other indications include delivery of an infant weighing more than 9 lb (4.1 kg), frequent vaginal yeast infections, and impotence in males.

The *IVGTT* is similar to the OGTT. An IVGTT is not usually used to diagnose diabetes mellitus. Its use is limited to research or when the patient has a problem with gastrointestinal absorption. It is not preferable to the OGTT because it bypasses normal glucose absorption and, therefore, normal changes in gastrointestinal hormones. Patient preparation for the IVGTT is the same as that for the OGTT, except that the glucose load (0.5 g/kg of ideal body weight) is given intravenously over 2 to 3 minutes. The fasting blood glucose levels after the IVGTT are similar to those after an OGTT, except that the 30-minute ingestion fasting blood glucose level tends to be higher.

The OGTT confirms the diagnosis of diabetes mellitus if the 2-hour blood glucose level is greater than 200 mg/dL and at least one other blood glucose determination is greater than 200 mg/dL. Blood glucose levels between the diagnostic criteria and normal values are called *impaired glucose tolerance* (IGT).

REFERENCE VALUES   Baseline fasting blood glucose level: 70-105 mg/dL *or*
SI: 3.9-5.8 mmol/L
30-minute blood glucose level: 110-170 mg/dL *or* SI: 6.1-9.4 mmol/L
60-minute blood glucose level: 120-170 mg/dL *or* SI: 6.7-9.4 mmol/L
90-minute blood glucose level: 100-140 mg/dL *or* SI: 5.6-7.8 mmol/L
120-minute blood glucose level: 70-120 mg/dL *or* SI: 3.9-6.7 mmol/L

HOW THE TEST IS DONE

After the ingestion of a glucose load, venous blood samplings for plasma glucose are obtained at the time of ingestion and then at 30, 60, 90, and 120 minutes after the glucose load is given.

SIGNIFICANCE OF TEST RESULTS

Diabetes mellitus
Impaired glucose tolerance

INTERFERING FACTORS

- Noncompliance with dietary and fasting requirements
- Alcohol ingestion
- Being bedridden
- Cushing's syndrome or Cushing's disease
- Infection
- Malabsorption syndrome
- Malnutrition
- Pregnancy
- Severe stress
- Smoking
- Medications such as amphetamines, arginine, β-adrenergic blockers, diuretics, epinephrine, glucocorticoids, glucose administered intravenously, insulin, lithium, oral contraceptives, oral hypoglycemic agents, phenothiazines, phenytoin, and salicylates

NURSING CARE

Nursing actions are similar to those used in other venipuncture procedures (see Chapter 2), with the following additional measures:

Pretest

- The nurse takes a medication history to determine if any interfering drugs are being taken. Check with the physician to determine if medications should be withheld. Oral hypoglycemic agents are withheld for 2 weeks before an OGTT is performed. The nurse also questions the patient regarding any recent acute illnesses. The OGTT should be delayed for at least 2 weeks after an acute illness.

○ *Patient Teaching.* Instruct the patient to take in at least 150 to 250 g of carbohydrates per day for 3 days before the test to optimize insulin secretion.

○ *Patient Teaching.* Instruct the patient not to drink or eat for 8 hours before the test begins. The patient is also instructed to avoid stimulants and not to smoke or perform any unusual activity for 8 hours before the test.

During the Test

- A fasting blood glucose determination is performed (usually in the early morning between 7 AM and 9 AM).
- Within 5 minutes of obtaining the baseline fasting blood glucose level, the patient drinks 75 g of glucose in 300 mL of water. Children are given 1.5 g of glucose per kilogram of ideal body weight. The glucose solution should be ingested within 5 minutes.
- Venipunctures are performed to obtain blood glucose readings at 30, 60, 90, and 120 minutes after the glucose solution is ingested. If a hypoglycemic reaction is suspected, a 3-hour blood specimen is obtained.
- The nurse observes the patient for a hyperglycemic or hypoglycemic reaction.
- The patient may drink water during the collection period.

Posttest

- The patient resumes taking medications that were withheld.
- A normal diet and activity level are resumed.

Health Promotion

The American Diabetes Association recommends that pregnant women at the 24th to 28th week of gestation have an OGTT done using 50 g of glucose. If any abnormality results, a repeat OGTT is done with 100 g of glucose. Many recommend that any pregnant woman at risk for gestational diabetes have the OGTT done in the 16th to 18th week of pregnancy and repeat the test at the 24th to 28th week.

Glucose, Urinary

Also called: Self-Monitoring of Urine Glucose; (SMUG); Urinary Sugar

SPECIMEN OR TYPE OF TEST: Urine

PURPOSE OF THE TEST

When capillary glucose monitoring is not possible, urinary glucose is measured to determine insulin and dietary requirements of patients with diabetes mellitus. Urinary glucose levels only provide a rough estimate of current blood glucose levels.

BASICS THE NURSE NEEDS TO KNOW

As serum glucose levels rise, the renal threshold for glucose will be reached and glucose will "spill out" into the urine. The presence of glycosuria (glucose in the urine) once played a major role in regulating the diet and insulin therapy of patients with diabetes mellitus. The urine was checked four times a day (before each meal and at bedtime) and insulin coverage given depending on how much glucose was spilled.

Today, patients with type 1 diabetes mellitus and some patients with type 2 diabetes mellitus are regulated by self-capillary blood glucose monitoring. Capillary glucose monitoring is superior to urinary glucose testing because it reflects the patient's current glucose status, whereas urine reflects the blood glucose level at the time the urine was formed.

If the patient is planning to use self-monitoring of urinary glucose (SMUG) to manage his or her diabetes, the renal glucose threshold must be determined; otherwise, the patient may be overtreated or undertreated.

REFERENCE VALUES   Negative

HOW THE TEST IS DONE

The test is done by dipping a dipstick into fresh urine.

SIGNIFICANCE OF TEST RESULTS

Glucosuria may be a result of the following:
Diabetes mellitus
Chronic renal failure
Cushing's syndrome
Thyroid disorders
Fanconi's syndrome
Hyperalimentation
Pregnancy

INTERFERING FACTORS

- Failure to use fresh urine
- Urine heavily contaminated with bacteria
- Dipstick exposed to air, light, heat, or moisture
- Medications, such as acetylsalicylic acid, chloral hydrate, glucocorticoids, isoniazid, levodopa, lithium, methyldopa, penicillin G, probenecid, salicylates, streptomycin, tetramycin, and thiazide diuretics

NURSING CARE

Because this test is used for self-monitoring, patient education is an essential part of the nursing role.

Pretest

○ *Patient Teaching.* Instruct the patient to collect the specimen in a clean container.

During the Test

○ *Patient Teaching.* Instruct patient to follow the manufacturer's guidelines. Frequently used dipsticks are: Clinistix, Diastix, and Multistix.

- The dipstick is dipped in urine. The waiting time is indicated by the manufacturer.
- Compare the color change with the chart provided and record the results.

Posttest

- Clean the equipment with soap and water and rinse thoroughly.
- Store the dipstick in a dry, cool place in its original container.

- Document the results on a flow sheet.
- Adjust insulin dosage as ordered based on the results.
- Provide the patient with the opportunity to practice SMUG.
- The community health nurse assesses the patient's ability to apply hospital learning to the home and reinforces the learning. Periodically, the community health nurse needs to observe the patient's technique to ensure that test results are accurate. Periodic evaluation of the patient's visual acuity is necessary because the patient must use a color chart to determine the glucose level. Instruct the patient to document results and any insulin taken based on the results and to bring the record to the physician, nurse practitioner, or diabetes clinic at each visit.

G

Glycosylated Hemoglobin Assay

Also called: Glycohemoglobin (GHb); Glycated Hemoglobin; Hemoglobin A_{1c}; Hb A

SPECIMEN OR TYPE OF TEST: Blood

PURPOSE OF THE TEST

The American Diabetes Association (ADA) in 2010 recommended the use of A_{1c} as a means of diagnosing diabetes mellitus. The ADA determined an A_{1c} of 5.7 to 6.4 percent as prediabetes and an A_{1c} of 6.5 or above as diagnostic of diabetes mellitus.

A glycosylated hemoglobin determination is also performed to measure a patient's diabetic control over a period of weeks or months. The maximum period for evaluation of control is the life span of the red blood cells (120 days).

BASICS THE NURSE NEEDS TO KNOW

Glycosylated hemoglobin refers to hemoglobin that has hooked up with glucose. The major glycosylated hemoglobin is hemoglobin A_{1c}, which is approximately 4% of the total hemoglobin. The other glycosylated hemoglobins are phosphoxylated glucose (A_{1a}) and phosphoxylated fructose (A_{1b}).

The reaction between glucose and hemoglobin is based on the blood glucose concentration. The higher the glucose concentration, the higher the percentage of glycosylated hemoglobin. Because the reaction is not reversible, once the glucose adheres to the hemoglobin it remains glycosylated. Since the life span of a red blood cell is normally 120 days, measuring the glycosylated hemoglobin can assist in diabetic control assessment. It is not affected by recent changes in diet or medication, as fasting blood glucose levels are, so the physician can determine diabetic control over a period of weeks or months. The guidelines of the American Diabetes Association recommend that the A_{1c} test be done routinely in the management of patients with type 1 diabetes and that the patient's goal should be less than 7%.

The reliability of the test is based on normal hemoglobin levels. If a person has an abnormal hemoglobin value, the accuracy of the HbA_{1c} is suspect. An example of this is the sickle cell trait. Also, any condition that shortens or lengthens the life of the red blood cells will make the results questionable.

REFERENCE VALUES*
Normal, healthy person: <5.5% of total hemoglobin *or*
SI: 0.05-0.08 (fraction of total hemoglobin)
Diabetic under control: <7% of total hemoglobin
Hemoglobin A_{1a}: 1.8% of total hemoglobin
Hemoglobin A_{1b}: 0.8% of total hemoglobin
Hemoglobin A_{1c}: 3%-6% of total hemoglobin

▼ Critical Values   6.5% *or* above for undiagnosed person

*Note: A_{1c} levels are usually 0.13% higher in young African Americans and 0.21% higher in African Americans over 40 years old.

HOW THE TEST IS DONE
Venipuncture is performed.

SIGNIFICANCE OF TEST RESULTS
Elevated Values
Poorly controlled diabetes mellitus
Hyperglycemia

INTERFERING FACTORS
- Acetylsalicylic acid (chronic ingestion)
- Anemia
- Chronic renal failure
- Clotting of specimen
- Fetal-maternal transfusion
- Hemodialysis
- Hemorrhage
- Hemolytic disease
- Phlebotomies
- Thalassemias
- Vitamin C and E

NURSING CARE

Nursing actions are similar to those used in other venipuncture procedures (see Chapter 2), with the following additional measures.
Health Promotion
Patients who have diabetes need to be aware of the need to keep close glycemic control of their condition to prevent complications. The nurse encourages the patient to follow up on prescribed glycosylated testing. The nurse teaches the patient about lowering the A_{1c} to 7% or less to reduce the risk of microvascular and neuropathologic complications.

Gonorrhea Tests

Also called: *Neisseria gonorrhoeae* tests
Includes: Genital culture; DNA testing for *Neisseria gonorrhoeae*

PURPOSE OF THE TEST

The testing is done to diagnose *N. gonorrhoeae* as the causative organism of gonorrhea, a sexually transmitted disease.

SPECIMEN OR TYPE OF TEST: Purulent Discharge; Microbiology

BASICS THE NURSE NEEDS TO KNOW

Gonorrhea, a bacterial infection, is the second most frequent sexually transmitted disease in the United States. The infection is transmitted from infected individuals to the sexual partner. Those who have multiple sexual partners and unprotected sexual intercourse are more likely to acquire and transmit the infection.

With infection, the male has symptoms of a purulent urethral discharge and dysuria. Infected females have a purulent endocervical discharge and dysuria, but as many as 50% of the infected women may be asymptomatic (Mahon, Lehman & Manuselis, 2011). Both males and females may acquire a gonococcus infection of the pharynx or the anal/rectal canal during sexual intercourse that involves these locations. Gonococcal ophthalmia neonatorum can be acquired by the baby during vaginal delivery by the infected mother. The incidence of this cause of infection is rare in the United States because of legal mandates that ophthalmic antimicrobial medication be administered to all newborns to prevent infection.

For identification of this bacterium, blood testing is not useful. The culture specimen is the gold standard method to visualize and identify the organism. It is highly accurate with excellent specificity and sensitivity results. Testing for susceptibility is also done in the laboratory to identify which antibiotics would be effective for eradication of the bacteria. The gonococcus has developed resistance to many antibiotics already, so that selection of a specific medication is guided by the laboratory findings. Other methods of laboratory testing include direct microscopic visualization of a smear of the secretions on a prepared slide. Nucleic acid assay testing can be done on urine, cervical, or urethral secretions to detect the antigen of the gonococcus or the DNA of the bacteria.

REFERENCE VALUES | Culture: negative; no growth
DNA analysis: negative for gonococcus
Antigen *or* antibody for gonococcus: negative

HOW THE TEST IS DONE

The genital culture of the secretions is obtained with a cervical swab for females or a urethral swab for males. A throat culture or an anal/rectal culture specimen is obtained by culture swab for male or female, as needed.

A first void urine specimen or a swab of the cervical or urethral secretions can be tested by nucleic acid detection for *N. gonorrhoeae*. Rapid testing, point of care can detect the antibody to *N. gonorrhoeae*. Recently approved antigen testing can be done in the laboratory.

For further information and discussion, see Culture, genital on p. 239.

Growth Hormone

Also called: (GH); somatotropin; (STH); hGH

SPECIMEN OR TYPE OF TEST: Serum

PURPOSE OF THE TEST

Growth hormone levels are evaluated to diagnose growth disorders and possible pituitary tumors. Abnormal linear growth may be a result of several factors: genetics, chronic disease, malnutrition, and so forth. Growth hormone levels will assist in determining the cause of the growth disorder and thereby influence therapy and prognosis.

BASICS THE NURSE NEEDS TO KNOW

Growth hormone is synthesized and secreted by the anterior pituitary gland under the direction of the hypothalamus. The hypothalamus controls growth hormone secretion via somatostatin (growth hormone release-inhibiting hormone) and growth hormone releasing hormone. The primary function of growth hormone is the promotion of linear growth, which it does by stimulating the production of somatomedin, which is produced by a variety of organs.

During linear growth and afterward, growth hormone influences protein, carbohydrate, and fat metabolism. It increases protein synthesis, decreases protein catabolism, and activates lipolysis. Excessive growth hormone will decrease carbohydrate use and glucose uptake by the cells.

REFERENCE VALUES

Cord blood: 8-41 ng/mL *or* SI: 8-41 µg/L
Newborns: 5-53 ng/mL *or* SI: 5-53 µg/L
Infants: 2-10 ng/mL *or* SI: 2-10 µg/mL
Child: Undetectable-16 ng/mL *or* SI: 0-16 µg/L
Adult female: Undetectable-10 ng/mL *or* SI: 0-10 µg/L
Adult male: Undetectable-5 ng/mL *or* SI: 0-5 µg/L

HOW THE TEST IS DONE

A venous blood sample is drawn.

SIGNIFICANCE OF TEST RESULTS

Elevated Values
Pituitary tumor
Hypothalamic tumor
Ectopic GH secretion

Acromegaly
Gigantism
Malnutrition
Cirrhosis
Severe stress
Anorexia nervosa

Decreased Values
Dwarfism
Metastatic or anoxic pituitary destruction

INTERFERING FACTORS

- Failure to fast for 8 to 12 hours before the test
- Administration of radioactive scan within 7 days
- Stress
- Medications, such as amphetamines, arginine, β-blockers, chlorpromazine, corticosteroids, dopamine, glucagon, insulin, levodopa, and oral contraceptives

NURSING CARE

Nursing actions are similar to those used in other venipuncture procedures (see Chapter 2), with the following additional measures.

Pretest
- Obtain a drug history to determine if any interfering medication is being taken.
- The nurse inquires if the patient has undergone any recent radioactive scans.
- ○ *Patient Teaching.* The nurse instructs the patient to limit activity and not eat or drink for 8 to 12 hours before the specimen is collected. Bedrest is maintained for 30 minutes before the specimen is drawn.

During the Test
- The nurse takes actions similar to those for other venipuncture procedures.

Posttest
- The patient can resume diet and the medications that were withheld.
- Send the specimen to the lab on ice.
- The nurse informs the patient that normal activity may be resumed.

Growth Hormone Stimulation Test

Also called: Arginine Test; Insulin Tolerance Test (ITT)

SPECIMEN OR TYPE OF TEST: Serum

PURPOSE OF THE TEST

The growth hormone stimulation test is usually performed to evaluate children and infants with retarded growth. It is also used to support the diagnosis of a pituitary tumor. A variety of stimulants can be used to stimulate the secretion of the growth hormone, including arginine, glucagon, propranolol, insulin, levodopa, exercise, and corticotropin-releasing hormone (CRH). Arginine and insulin are the most frequently used stimulants. When insulin is used as the stimulant, the test is called an insulin tolerance test (ITT).

The *insulin tolerance test* is used to distinguish primary versus secondary adrenocorticoid insufficiency by measuring adrenocorticotropic hormone (ACTH) levels, as well as growth hormone levels. ITT is considered the gold standard for evaluating the hypothalamic-pituitary-adrenal (HPA) axis.

BASICS THE NURSE NEEDS TO KNOW
Review the preceding section on growth hormone.

REFERENCE VALUES

With arginine: >7 ng/mL *or* SI: >7 µg/L
With insulin (with serum glucose of <40 mg/dL): >20 ng/mL *or* SI: >20 µg/L
With propranolol and glucagon: >10 ng/mL *or* SI: >10 µg/L

HOW THE TEST IS DONE
Depending on the substance used, slight variations exist in the method. With arginine, a baseline sample of venous blood is obtained. A venous infusion of arginine is then administered. After the arginine infusion is completed (in approximately 30 minutes), 30 minutes are allowed to pass. Three venous samples are then obtained at 30-minute intervals.

If an ITT is done, a baseline venous sample is taken, after which 0.05 to 0.15 U/kg of insulin is given intravenously over 2 to 3 minutes. Venous samples are taken at 15, 30, 45, 60, 90, and 120 minutes after the administration of insulin. Blood glucose levels must fall to below 40 mg/dL within 1 hour after the insulin is given for an accurate evaluation.

SIGNIFICANCE OF TEST RESULTS
Elevated Values
No growth hormone deficiency

Decreased Values
Pituitary dwarfism
Pituitary tumors

INTERFERING FACTORS
- Failure to comply with fasting or activity restrictions
- Alcohol
- Medications such as amphetamines, β-blockers, calcium gluconate, estrogen, spironolactone, and steroids

NURSING CARE

Nursing actions are similar to those used in other venipuncture procedures (see Chapter 2), with the following additional measures.

Pretest

- Assess patients at risk if a growth hormone stimulation test with insulin is planned. This includes patients with cardiovascular disease, epilepsy, a history of a cerebrovascular accident, or adrenal insufficiency.
- The nurse obtains a medication history to determine if any interfering drug is being taken. The nurse also checks with the physician about withholding any interfering medication.

○ *Patient Teaching.* The nurse instructs the patient to limit physical activity and not to eat or drink for 12 hours before the test.

○ *Patient Teaching.* Instruct the patient not to drink alcohol for 24 hours before the blood is drawn.

- The nurse reassures the patient and instructs him or her to lie down quietly for 90 minutes before the blood is drawn.

During the Test

- An intravenous catheter (saline lock) is inserted to eliminate the need for multiple venous punctures.
- A baseline venous sample is taken.
- If arginine is used, an infusion is given over 30 minutes in the arm opposite the saline lock used for blood sampling. Thirty minutes after the arginine infusion is completed, three additional blood specimens are obtained at 30-minute intervals.
- If insulin is used, regular insulin is given over 2 to 3 minutes. Blood specimens are drawn at 15, 30, 45, 60, 90, and 120 minutes.
- The nurse observes the patient carefully. Stop the test if serious signs of hypoglycemia occur (e.g., vertigo, chest pain).

Posttest

- The patient can resume the medication schedule, diet, and physical activities.
- Ensure that the patient who received insulin as a stimulant has adequate food intake.

Growth Hormone Suppression Test

Also called: Glucose Loading Test

SPECIMEN OR TYPE OF TEST: Serum

PURPOSE OF THE TEST

This test usually is performed to assess an increase in growth hormone levels and to confirm the diagnoses of gigantism in children and acromegaly in adults.

BASICS THE NURSE NEEDS TO KNOW

The growth hormone suppression test is performed after high levels of growth hormone are found. Normally, the ingestion of glucose causes a decrease in the secretion of growth hormone. In patients with hypersecretion of growth hormone, however, a significant decrease does not occur.

REFERENCE VALUES   Growth hormone levels decrease to undetectable to <3 ng/mL *or* SI: <3 mcg/L in 30-120 minutes

HOW THE TEST IS DONE

A baseline venous blood sample is drawn. The patient ingests a glucose solution. After 1 to 2 hours, another blood sample is drawn.

SIGNIFICANCE OF TEST RESULTS

If high growth hormone levels are maintained:
Acromegaly
Gigantism

INTERFERING FACTORS

- Noncompliance with activity restrictions and fasting
- Radioactive scans within the previous week
- Medications, such as amphetamines, arginine, β-blockers, chlorpromazine, dopamine, glucagon, histamine, insulin, levodopa, nicotinic acid, and steroids

NURSING CARE

Nursing actions are similar to those used in other venipuncture procedures (see Chapter 2), with the following additional measures.

Pretest
- The nurse obtains a medication history to ensure that any interfering drug has not been taken.
- Question the patient or check the patient's chart for any recent radioactive scans.
- *Patient Teaching.* The nurse instructs the patient about the need to avoid physical activity for 10 to 12 hours before the test and to lie quietly for 30 minutes before the blood is drawn.
- *Patient Teaching.* Instruct the patient not to eat or drink for 12 hours before the sample is taken.

During the Test
- Explain the purpose of the two venipunctures.
- After the first specimen is obtained in the early morning, the nurse instructs the patient to drink the glucose solution slowly to minimize nausea.
- Ensure that the second specimen is obtained 1 to 2 hours after the ingestion of glucose.

Posttest
- The patient resumes normal diet and activity.

Guthrie Screening Test

See Phenylalanine, Blood on p. 493.

Haptoglobin

Also called: Hp

SPECIMEN OR TYPE OF TEST: Serum

PURPOSE OF THE TEST

Haptoglobin measurement is useful in the workup for hemolytic conditions. It also is used for monitoring of acute reactions that involve hemolysis of erythrocytes.

BASICS THE NURSE NEEDS TO KNOW

When erythrocytes undergo hemolysis by normal or abnormal processes, circulating haptoglobin binds to the free hemoglobin. These newly formed complexes cannot be filtered through the renal glomeruli so hemoglobin cannot be excreted in the urine. As the complexes are broken down, iron is conserved and stored for use in the manufacture of new erythrocytes.

Elevated Values

Increases in serum haptoglobin may occur in conditions of inflammation, infection, or tissue destruction.

Decreased Values

A decreased value is more useful as a laboratory test. Decreased values occur with conditions of abnormal hemolysis of red blood cells. The decrease may be gradual, chronic, or sudden and severe in occurrence. In acute hemolysis, a severe decline in haptoglobin will occur. As the red blood cells are destroyed, available haptoglobin is rapidly consumed by the reticuloendothelial system.

REFERENCE VALUES   Negative
Newborn: 5-48 mg/dL *or* SI: 50-580 mg/L
Adult: 26-185 mg/dL *or* SI: 260-1850 mg/L
Adult >60 years:
Male: 35-164 mg/dL *or* SI: 350-1640 mg/L
Female: 40-175 mg/dL *or* SI: 400-1750 mg/L

HOW THE TEST IS DONE

Venipuncture is used to collect a specimen of venous blood.

SIGNIFICANCE OF TEST RESULTS

Elevated Values

Acute rheumatoid arthritis
Nephrotic syndrome
Trauma
Infection
Advanced malignancy

Decreased Values
Hemolytic transfusion reaction
Sickle cell anemia
Thalassemia
G-6-PD deficiency
Hereditary spherocytosis
Hematoma formation
Folate deficiency
Malaria
Liver disease

INTERFERING FACTORS

• Hemolysis of the specimen

| NURSING CARE |

Nursing actions are similar to those used in other venipuncture procedures (see Chapter 2), with the following additional measures.

Pretest

• This test may be used to monitor for a blood transfusion reaction. If prescribed, ensure that the haptoglobin specimen is drawn before starting the transfusion. A repeat test may be ordered at the conclusion of the transfusion.

Posttest

• The nurse compares the current results with the patient's baseline value to monitor for the level and direction of change. The physician is notified of a sudden or severe decrease in this laboratory value. The cause of an abnormal laboratory value will determine the interventions that are needed.

• The nurse should assess any fresh sample of urine for change in color. If the haptoglobin level is decreased, free hemoglobin will be filtered out of the blood into the urine. Hemoglobin changes the color of the urine to dark red or brown.

Helicobacter pylori Tests

SPECIMEN OR TYPE OF TEST: Blood, Breath, Feces, Gastric Biopsy

PURPOSE OF THE TEST

This test establishes the presence of *Helicobacter pylori* infection that can cause chronic, active gastritis and peptic ulcers.

BASICS THE NURSE NEEDS TO KNOW

H. pylori is a gram-negative bacillus that resides under the mucosal layer, attached to the gastric epithelial tissue. It causes gastritis, is the main cause of ulcers in the stomach, and may be one cause of gastric cancer. The infection is usually acquired in childhood, particularly in people who are poor or who reside in developing countries where poor sanitary conditions and a lack of running water prevail. If the infection has not been eradicated in childhood, it remains as a lifelong infection, with or without symptoms. There are several different tests to confirm the *H. pylori* infection and to document its eradication. The tests are classified as noninvasive and invasive.

Noninvasive Testing

Serology Antibody Test

This frequently used blood test identifies the elevated level of immunoglobulin G (IgG) antibody to the *H. pylori* antigen in the symptomatic patient. The positive test result indicates current or past infection. After treatment, it cannot document that infection has been eliminated.

Urea Breath Test

If *H. pylori* is present, the organism produces a unique enzyme, urease. Radiolabeled carbon urea is administered to the patient orally. The urease converts the carbon urea to ammonia and radiolabeled carbon dioxide (CO_2) gas. The radiolabeled CO_2 enters the blood and is then exhaled by the lungs. The test measures the radiolabeled CO_2 in the exhaled air, demonstrating that the patient has an infection with *H. pylori*. When the urea breath test is conducted 7 days or more after completing the prescribed course of antibiotics, a negative result is proof that the infection has been eradicated. The test is highly accurate and widely used.

H. pylori Antigen Test

The antigen of *H. pylori* can be detected in the fecal matter of the infected patient. It can also be used to evaluate the patient's response to treatment. After treatment, a negative test result confirms that the infection has been eradicated.

Invasive Testing

Esophagogastroduodenoscopy with Tissue Biopsy

During the endoscopy procedure, the gastric and duodenal mucosa are examined, and a biopsy is taken of suspicious lesions and areas of inflammation or ulceration. In the laboratory, biopsy tissue slides are prepared and stained for microscopic examination. When present, the characteristic *H. pylori* bacteria are seen and identified. Additional laboratory tests on the biopsy samples are done, including those identified below. This testing approach is very accurate.

Rapid Urease Test. *H. pylori* produces a unique enzyme called urease. The urease can be detected by chemical analysis of the tissue sample. The presence of urease presumes the presence of *H. pylori*.

PCR-DNA. From the tissue specimen, polymerase chain reaction (PCR) technique amplifies the DNA sequence of *H. pylori* bacillus. The microbe is identified by its DNA blueprint.

Tissue Culture. After the tissue specimen is cultured, the culture plates are read at intervals of 1, 3, and 5 days to identify the presence of colonies of *H. pylori* bacilli.

REFERENCE VALUES

Serology, IgG antibody: Negative
Urea breath test: Negative
Stool antigen: Negative
Tissue biopsy: Negative
Rapid urease test: Negative for *H. pylori*
PCR-DNA: Negative
Tissue culture: No *H. pylori* growth

HOW THE TEST IS DONE

Antibody Serology

Venipuncture is performed to obtain a sample of venous blood.

Urea Breath Test

The patient ingests a capsule of radiolabeled carbon urea (C^{13} or C^{14}). Exhalation breath samples are collected in a special collection container every 5 minutes for 30 minutes. The measurement of the radiolabeled CO_2 is done by scintillation scanner.

***H. pylori* Antigen**

A stool sample is collected.

Tissue Biopsy

During an esophagogastroduodenoscopy (EGD) procedure, biopsy specimens are obtained.

SIGNIFICANCE OF TEST RESULTS

Positive Values

H. pylori infection
Chronic gastritis
Peptic ulcer disease
Gastric cancer

INTERFERING FACTORS

- Recent antimicrobial therapy
- Current bismuth preparation
- Current proton pump inhibitor medication

NURSING CARE

Pretest
- *Serology antibody.* Nursing actions are similar to those used in other venipuncture procedures (see Chapter 2), with the following additional measures.
- *Breath test.* Inform the client that a small amount of low-dose radiation will be in the capsule, but it will be exhaled within hours and the brief exposure will not harm the patient.
- ○ *Patient Teaching.* Instruct the patient that 7 days before the breath test, he or she should stop taking antibiotics, bismuth-containing medication (Pepto-Bismol), and proton pump inhibitor medication, such as omeprazole (Prilosec), lansoprazole (Prevacid), esomeprazole (Nexium), or rabeprazole (Aciphex).
- *H. pylori antigen* test. Instruct the patient to collect a random stool sample to be brought to the laboratory. Further discussion of the stool collection procedure is presented in Chapter 2.
- *Tissue biopsy.* The reader is referred to the nursing discussion for the procedure of esophago-gastroduodenoscopy (see p. 299)

Posttest

After treatment with antibiotics, follow-up testing for *H. pylori* antigen in the feces may be done to verify that the infection has been eradicated. This testing should occur no sooner than 4 weeks post treatment.

Hematocrit

Also called: (Hct); Microhematocrit

SPECIMEN OR TYPE OF TEST: Blood

PURPOSE OF THE TEST

The hematocrit is useful in the evaluation of blood loss, anemia, hemolytic anemia, polycythemia, and dehydration.

BASICS THE NURSE NEEDS TO KNOW

The hematocrit is a measurement of the proportion of whole blood volume occupied by erythrocytes. The value is expressed as a percentage or fraction of cells to whole blood. For example, a hematocrit value of 40% means that there are 40 mL of erythrocytes in 1 dL of blood.

Elevated Values

The hematocrit rises if the number or size of the erythrocytes increases or when the plasma fluid volume is reduced. When the fluid volume is decreased, the red blood cells become concentrated in the smaller fluid volume. The blood is thicker or has increased viscosity.

Decreased Values

The hematocrit falls to less than the reference value when an excessive loss of erythrocytes occurs, as in hemolytic anemia or after excessive bleeding. It also can occur because fewer red blood cells are made or the erythrocytes are microcytic (smaller). The hematocrit also can decrease because of excessive intravenous fluids or fluid retention that creates greater plasma volume. The fluids exert a dilution effect, meaning that normal numbers of red blood cells are in a larger amount of fluid. In bleeding or hemorrhage, the hematocrit drops several hours after the bleeding episode. The severity of the drop in value correlates directly with the amount of red blood cells that are lost.

REFERENCE VALUES	Male: 41.0%-51.0% *or* SI: 0.41-0.51 (volume fraction) Female: 36.0% -45.0% *or* SI: 0.36-0.45 (volume fraction)
▽ Critical Values	>65% (SI: >0.65 [volume fraction]) *or* <21% (SI: <0.21) [volume fraction])

HOW THE TEST IS DONE

Venipuncture or skin puncture is done to collect a sample of blood.

SIGNIFICANCE OF TEST RESULTS

Elevated Values

Polycythemia vera
Secondary polycythemia
Addison's disease
Acute thermal injury

Extreme physical exertion
Dehydration

Decreased Values
Recent hemorrhage
Anemia
Fluid overload
Fluid retention
Cirrhosis
Hemolytic anemia

INTERFERING FACTORS

• None

NURSING CARE

Pretest
Nursing actions are similar to those used in other venipuncture or fingerstick procedures (see Chapter 2), with the following additional measures.
• The nurse informs the patient that blood will be drawn at intervals to monitor his or her condition.

During the Test
• Ensure that the blood sample is not taken from a vein in the hand or arm with an intravenous line. Hemodilution with intravenous fluids will lower the hematocrit value falsely.

Posttest

Elevated Hematocrit
When the patient's condition is due to dehydration and the hematocrit is elevated, fluid and electrolyte replacement is usually administered intravenously, as prescribed. The nurse ensures that the correct solution and the correct amount of solution are given in the prescribed period. If the patient's medical condition allows, the nurse encourages the patient to take extra fluids orally. As the patient is rehydrated, the hematocrit value will fall toward the normal value.

Decreased Hematocrit
When the patient is hemorrhaging or has just had a severe bleeding episode, the hematocrit value decreases. After transfusion replacement of packed cells or whole blood, the nurse monitors the hematocrit results for a rising value. The hematocrit value, however, is not reliable immediately after an acute blood loss or blood transfusion. The changes will occur a few hours later.
• Because the loss of blood or fluids often results in hemodynamic instability, the nurse measures and records vital signs at regular and frequent intervals. Abnormal findings would include *hypotension* (a low blood pressure), *tachycardia* (a rapid pulse), and *dyspnea* (labored breathing).
• When the patient has excess fluid volume, often with edema, the underlying cause must be diagnosed and treated medically. In cases such as cirrhosis, congestive heart failure, and renal failure, the hematocrit falls because the normal number of red blood cells is diluted in excess plasma. The nurse carries out the medical treatment protocol that often includes

medications, fluid restrictions, and salt restrictions. As excess fluid is excreted, the hematocrit rises toward a more normal reference value.

▼ Nursing Response to Critical Values

When the hematocrit rises to a critical value or higher, the patient is at great risk of developing a myocardial infarction or a stroke because of increased viscosity. Those who are most vulnerable are patients with preexisting cardiovascular disease. When the hematocrit decreases to a critical value or lower, the patient may go into shock, particularly when there is associated blood loss or hemorrhage. The nurse notifies the physician immediately of a hematocrit result that is in the critical value range.

The nurse also starts frequent and regular monitoring of vital signs and assessment of the patient's overall condition. The patient may complain of intense chest pain or exhibit signs of neurologic abnormality, including loss of consciousness, *aphasia* (impairment or loss of speech), *hemiparesis* (weakness in one side of the body), and *hemiplegia* (paralysis on one side of the body).

H

Hemoglobin

Also called: Hgb, Hb

SPECIMEN OR TYPE OF TEST: Whole Blood

PURPOSE OF THE TEST

The hemoglobin is used to measure the severity of anemia or polycythemia, and it monitors the response to treatment of anemia. It is also used to calculate the mean corpuscular hemoglobin (MCH) and mean corpuscular hemoglobin concentration (MCHC) values.

BASICS THE NURSE NEEDS TO KNOW

Hemoglobin is the oxygen-carrying compound contained in each erythrocyte. The large amount of hemoglobin and the broad surface area of each erythrocyte enable the red blood cells to have a large oxygen-carrying capacity and to function with great efficiency.

Elevated Values

An elevated hemoglobin value may be a result of either excess production of erythrocytes by the bone marrow or dehydration. In excess production of erythrocytes, the hemoglobin rises because it is present in additional cells. In dehydration, the red blood cell counts and hemoglobin are relatively high because of the normal number and quality of cells that are concentrated in a smaller amount of fluid.

Decreased Values

An individual generally is considered anemic when the hemoglobin value for the male is less than 13 g/dL (SI: <130 g/L) and for the female, less than 11 g/dL (SI: <110 g/L). The low hemoglobin value can be caused by a low red blood cell count, by a lack of hemoglobin in each erythrocyte, or by fluid retention. The low red cell count may be a lack of production by the bone marrow, a loss of red blood cells in bleeding, or a loss of red blood cells from *hemolysis* (rapid destruction of the erythrocytes). The lack of hemoglobin in the erythrocytes is often due to a lack of iron, an essential mineral used to make heme, the iron-containing molecule of hemoglobin. In fluid retention, red blood cell counts and hemoglobin values are normal, but the cells are diluted in a greater amount of fluid.

REFERENCE VALUES	Newborn (1 day): 17.3-21.5 g/dL *or* SI: 173-215 g/L
	Infant (5-7 months): 10.8-12.2 g/dL *or* SI: 108-122 g/L
	Child (5 years): 11.7-13.7 g/dL *or* SI: 117-137 g/L
	Male: 14.0-18.0 g/dL *or* SI: 140-180 g/L
	Female: 12..0-15.0 g/dL *or* SI: 120-150 g/L

▼ **Critical Values**   7.0 g/dL *or* SI: 70.0 g/L

H

HOW THE TEST IS DONE
Venipuncture or capillary puncture is used to obtain a sample of blood

SIGNIFICANCE OF TEST RESULTS
Elevated Values
Polycythemia vera
Secondary polycythemia
Acute thermal injury
Dehydration
Hemoconcentration

Decreased Values
Recent bleeding/hemorrhage
Fluid retention
Hemolysis of red blood cells
Pregnancy
Anemia

INTERFERING FACTORS
- White blood cell count greater than 100×10^3 µL (SI: $>100 \times 10^9$/L)

NURSING CARE

Nursing actions are similar to those used in other venipuncture or capillary puncture procedures (see Chapter 2), with the following additional measures.
Pretest
- The nurse informs the patient of the need for additional lab testing to monitor his or her condition. When the patient had a severe bleeding episode, the hemoglobin measurement is taken at regular intervals. The decreased results indicate the severity of the blood loss. Likewise, after transfusion replacement of packed cells or whole blood, this test is used to monitor for a rise in the value. Ensure that the tests are performed at the indicated times.

During the Test

- Ensure that the blood sample is not taken from the arm that has an intravenous line in place. The intravenous infusion would dilute the blood and alter the test value.

Posttest

- When the hemoglobin level is decreased, the nurse can assess abnormal physical responses that include dizziness, pallor, and fatigue associated with physical activity. When the decline in hemoglobin occurs slowly over time, the patient may not experience symptoms of anemia, particularly when resting. With physical activity, however, the patient may report breathlessness or palpitations.
- There are numerous causes for an abnormal hemoglobin value. Laboratory testing will be needed to determine the specific cause and appropriate medical therapy. Additional specific nursing interventions will be implemented when the medical diagnosis is made.

▽ **Nursing Response to Critical Values**

The nurse notifies the physician of a severe decrease in the reference value. The decrease in hemoglobin means that less oxygen can be transported. The lungs and heart must work harder to get as much oxygen to cells as possible. As a result, both the pulse and respiratory rate will increase.

H

Hemoglobin Electrophoresis

SPECIMEN OR TYPE OF TEST: Blood

PURPOSE OF THE TEST

Hemoglobin electrophoresis is used to detect *hemoglobinopathy* (a genetic disorder of hemoglobin) and identify the type of anemia that results from the abnormal hemoglobin. It is also one of the tests used to identify sickle cell hemoglobin and differentiate between sickle cell trait and disease.

BASICS THE NURSE NEEDS TO KNOW

In the body, the manufacture of the various types of globin that bind with iron to make hemoglobin is genetically determined. The specific gene clusters to make alpha-type globins are located on chromosome 16 and the cluster of genes to make beta-type globins are located on chromosome 11. Mutations or absence of some of these genes will result in altered production or function of hemoglobin in the red blood cells of the affected individual. The genetic mutation of one or more genes can be transmitted to the offspring of the individual in an autosomal recessive inheritance pattern.

In the normal adult, the three types of hemoglobin found in erythrocytes are HbA, HbA_2, and HbF. Using the electrophoresis method, the test separates the normal from the abnormal hemoglobin types and measures the percentage amounts of each type.

There are more than 700 *variants* (abnormal or altered types) of hemoglobin, identified by letters other than HbA, HbA_2, and HbF. Hemoglobinopathy is the general term used to describe altered hemoglobin and some forms of hemolytic anemia. The specific hemoglobinopathy affects either the structure of the hemoglobin molecules or causes a decreased synthesis of hemoglobin, as in the various thalassemias. Of all the abnormal variants, HbS, or sickle cell hemoglobin, is the most predominant. Another common variant is HbC. Some conditions are asymptomatic or mild because the genetic defect of hemoglobin is a heterozygous (mixed) type, or trait condition. In the *heterozogous* (trait) condition, the mutant gene is inherited from one, but not both parents. In the *homozygous* (pure) state that produces the disease, the individual inherits the mutant gene from both parents.

Hemoglobin A$_2$

Although this is normal hemoglobin, it is only a small proportion of the total hemoglobin in healthy individuals. Hemoglobin electrophoresis evaluates the amount of HbA$_2$ in the investigation of β-thalassemia trait and differentiates β-thalassemia diseases from iron deficiency anemia. The β-thalassemia diseases are a group of disorders that produce a range of conditions varying from no clinical change to severe hypochromic, microcytic anemia. The amount of HbA$_2$ is increased in the β-thalassemia trait. Abnormal elevations of HbA$_2$ may include up to 7% of the total hemoglobin content.

Hemoglobin F

HbF is the hemoglobin present in fetal life. During infancy and early childhood, it is gradually replaced by HbA and HbA$_2$. By age 3, only 2% or less of HbF remains and the rest of the hemoglobin is HbA and HbA$_2$. Adults can have abnormal quantities of HbF in a condition called hereditary persistence of fetal hemoglobin. The homozygous state produces mildly microcytic, hypochromic erythrocytes without anemia. The hemoglobin electrophoresis test reveals 100% HbF. The heterozygous state does not cause anemia, but hemoglobin electrophoresis reveals 30% to 40% HbF.

Hemoglobin S

In the homozygous state, HbS produces the disease of sickle cell anemia, a type of severe hemolytic anemia that causes many health problems throughout life. In the heterozygous form, or sickle cell trait, hemoglobin electrophoresis demonstrates 30% to 35% HbS. Sickle cell trait produces no disease or hematologic abnormality unless the person experiences hypoxia, acidosis, or *thrombosis* (a blood clot).

Hemoglobin C

In the homozygous state of HbC disease, a mild hemolytic anemia often exists, but it is usually asymptomatic. On electrophoresis, no HbA is present. Most of the hemoglobin is HbC, with smaller quantities of other forms of hemoglobin. In the heterozygous state, 30% to 40% of the hemoglobin is type HbC.

REFERENCE VALUES   HbA: 95%-98%
HbA$_2$: 1.5%-3.7%
HbF: 0%-2%
HbC: Absent
HbS: Absent

HOW THE TEST IS DONE

Venipuncture or capillary puncture is used to collect a sample of blood.

SIGNIFICANCE OF TEST RESULTS

Elevated Values

β-thalassemia minor or major
Hereditary persistence of fetal hemoglobin
Sickle cell disease
Sickle cell trait
HbC disease
HbC trait
Megaloblastic anemia

Decreased Values

Deficiency of HbA$_2$
Sideroblastic anemia
Untreated iron deficiency anemia
Hereditary persistence of fetal hemoglobin

INTERFERING FACTORS

- Blood transfusion in the preceding 4 months
- Hemolysis of the erythrocytes

H

NURSING CARE

Nursing actions are similar to those used in other venipuncture or finger stick procedures (see Chapter 2), with the following additional measures.

Pretest

- Ask the patient about any transfusion of blood received within the preceding 4 months. A recent transfusion would make the findings of the test inconsistent.

Posttest

Health Promotion

In all states of the U.S. and its territories, screening for sickle cell disease is mandated for all newborns, regardless of ethnicity (US Preventive Services Task Force, 2007).

- The genetic counselor and the physician discuss the abnormal results with the parents of the infant, providing counseling and education
- The nurse also provides support to the parents who have an infant who tested positive for sickle cell trait or disease. Parents may not understand the difference between trait and disease. The parents often have feelings of concern, guilt, fear, and worry about the well-being of the infant. In discharge planning, encourage the parents to keep the follow-up appointments with the pediatrician for additional testing and specific follow-up care for the infant.
- When one child of the family tests positive for the trait or disease, the nurse encourages testing of all members of the family. If the individual knows his or her genetic status regarding this mutation, he or she can make informed decisions regarding health and reproduction.

Hemosiderin, Urinary

SPECIMEN OR TYPE OF TEST: Urine

PURPOSE OF THE TEST

Urinary hemosiderin is used to identify hemolytic anemia that is associated with hemolysis of red blood cells.

BASICS THE NURSE NEEDS TO KNOW

Hemosiderin granules are indicators of hemoglobin in the urine resulting from significant acute or chronic intravascular hemolysis. With the lysis of many erythrocytes, free hemoglobin is converted to ferritin and hemosiderin by the kidneys. The kidneys then remove the hemosiderin and those granules are present in the cells or casts in urinary sediment. The hemosiderin appears in the urine on the second or third day after the hemolytic episode. Urinary hemosiderin may also be caused by the excretion of excess iron, as from hematochromatosis.

The presence of hemosiderin in urine may not be detected by a urine reagent strip. In the laboratory analysis, however, the urinary sediment is stained with Prussian blue stain. If hemosiderin is present, the iron in urinary hemosiderin appears as blue-stained granules. The results are seen by microscopic examination of the slides that contain urinary cells and casts.

REFERENCE VALUES   Negative

HOW THE TEST IS DONE

A random sample of 30 to 60 mL of urine is collected in a clean container with a lid.

SIGNIFICANCE OF TEST RESULTS

Positive Values

Blood transfusion reaction
Chronic hemolytic anemia
Mechanical trauma to erythrocytes
Exposure to oxidant drugs or chemicals
G-6-PD deficiency
Thalassemia major
Severe megaloblastic anemia
Sickle cell anemia
Hematochromatosis
Severe infectious organisms (malaria, *Clostridium perfringens*)

INTERFERING FACTORS

• None

H

> **NURSING CARE**
>
> The procedure for collection of a random urine specimen is found in Chapter 2.

Hepatitis A Antibodies

Also called: HAV, ab; Anti-HAV
Includes: Hepatitis A antibody IgG, Hepatitis A antibody IgM

SPECIMEN OR TYPE OF TEST: Serum

PURPOSE OF THE TEST

The hepatitis A antibodies identify the hepatitis A virus as the cause of asymptomatic or acute infection of the liver. The specific antibody type distinguishes between current and past infection.

BASICS THE NURSE NEEDS TO KNOW

The hepatitis A virus is usually transmitted by the fecal-oral route, primarily after ingestion of virus-contaminated water or food. Increasingly, it can be transmitted via the parenteral route. The spread of the infection often originates with infected food handlers and children. In addition, there is risk of transmission via sexual intercourse with an infected person, in day care facilities, with IV drug abuse, and in recent international travel to countries where hepatitis A is endemic. Although the virus is found in the feces of an infected individual for about 3 weeks before there are symptoms of illness, the diagnosis is delayed until there are clinical symptoms, abnormal liver function tests, and identification of the hepatitis A antibodies in the blood.

Two types of hepatitis A antibodies can be measured: the immunoglobin M (IgM) type and the immunoglobin G (IgG) type. The IgM type, also called anti-HAV IgM, appears early in the course of illness. This antibody is present in the blood within 1 week after the patient develops symptoms and may persist for as long as 1 to 2 years. The IgM type is the test used to diagnose the acute infection. The IgG type, also called anti-HAV IgG, begins to rise after 4 weeks of infection and persists for life (Figure 55).

REFERENCE VALUES Hepatitis A antibody
IgM type: Negative
IgG type: Negative

HOW THE TEST IS DONE

A venipuncture is performed to collect a specimen of venous blood.

SIGNIFICANCE OF TEST RESULTS

Elevated Values
Hepatitis A antibody:
IgM: Current hepatitis A infection, acute or convalescent stage
IgG type: Past exposure to hepatitis A infection.

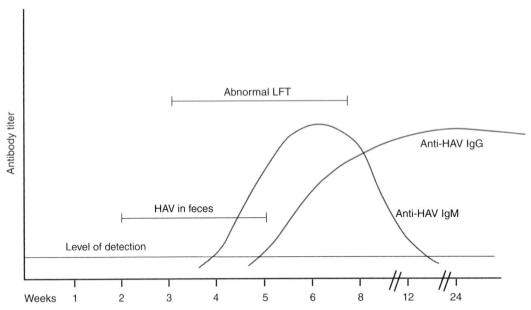

Figure 55. Serologic evaluation of hepatitis A virus infection showing the rise and fall of antibodies. *LFT*, Liver function test. (From Mahon CR, Lehman DC, Manuselis G: *Textbook of diagnostic microbiology*, ed 4, Philadelphia, 2011, Saunders.)

INTERFERING FACTORS
• Recent administration of radioisotopes

NURSING CARE

Nursing measures are similar to those used in other venipuncture procedures (see Chapter 2), with the following additional measures.

Pretest
• Apply standard precautions. Hepatitis A infection is contagious and the virus is present in the feces before the patient feels any symptoms.

○ *Patient Teaching.* Since immediate family members are exposed to the infected patient, the nurse instructs them to wash their hands often, particularly before meals and after toileting. The patient should not handle or prepare food while ill with the infection.

Hepatitis B Tests

Includes: Hepatitis B Surface Antigen (Also called: HBsAg)
Hepatitis B Surface Antibody (Also called: HBsAb; Anti-HBs)
Hepatitis B Core Antibody (Also called: Anti-HBc-IgM)
Hepatitis Be Antibody (Also called: Anti-HBe, total; HBe Ab)
Hepatitis B Virus DNA Assay (Also called: HBV DNA)

SPECIMEN OR TYPE OF TEST: Serum

PURPOSE OF THE TESTS

The various hepatitis B tests identify specific hepatitis B antigens and antibodies in the blood and help determine the stage of illness, including acute infection, convalescence, chronic infection, carrier of the disease, or past infection. Additionally, the hepatitis B surface antibody test is used to verify immunity after vaccination.

BASICS THE NURSE NEEDS TO KNOW

Hepatitis B is a viral illness that is transmitted from person to person primarily by contact with infected blood, but also by the exchange of body fluids, including semen, vaginal secretions, and saliva. The most common incidences of transmission occur during heterosexual and male homosexual intercourse, intravenous drug use, and by the infected mother to her baby at the time of delivery. Nurses and other health care workers who are not immunized against hepatitis B infection are vulnerable because of the potential for contact with infected blood, body fluids, and instruments such as needles that are contaminated with infected blood.

Once the infection is in the blood, the virus migrates to the liver and enters hepatocytes (liver cells), damaging and destroying them. The human body can recognize the various viral antigens and produces specific antibodies to destroy those antigens. Most of the hepatitis B laboratory tests detect the presence of the antigens and corresponding antibodies that emerge and persist or disappear at different times throughout the course of an illness (Figure 56). In addition, the hepatitis B virus-DNA testing identifies the virus by its genetic makeup. During the course of illness and recovery, the various test results are used at different time intervals for diagnosis, monitoring of the patient's response to treatment, and prognosis.

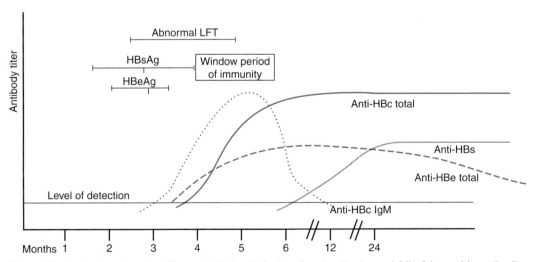

Figure 56. Serologic evaluation of hepatitis B virus infection showing the rise and fall of detectable antibodies in acute infection with resolution. (From Mahon CR, Lehman DC, Manuselis G: *Textbook of diagnostic microbiology,* ed 4, Philadelphia, 2011, Saunders.)

Hepatitis B Surface Antigen

A positive laboratory value for this antigen indicates the acute stage of illness when the patient is most infectious. It is the first marker of hepatitis B to appear in the blood, some 2 to 4 weeks before the liver function tests are elevated and 5 weeks before the patient begins to have symptoms. The antigen level will rise and peak during the acute phase of illness. It should then begin to decline and eventually disappear during convalescence, over a 12-week period of time. If however, the hepatitis B surface antigen remains elevated for 4 to 6 months or more and does not decline, it means that the patient now has a chronic hepatitis B infection or is a carrier and is potentially infectious.

Hepatitis B Surface Antibody

This antibody appears several weeks to months after the hepatitis B surface antigen has disappeared from the blood. The antibody remains in the blood during convalescence and may or may not disappear after recovery. Vaccination to prevent hepatitis B infection is widely available in the United States. Once the immunization process is completed, testing can be done to confirm the immune status. The positive result (>10 U/L) of the hepatitis B surface antibody test confirms immunity from future infection.

Hepatitis B Core Antibody-IgM

This is the earliest antibody to emerge in hepatitis B infection and confirms the diagnosis. The IgM antibody type is the marker of acute infection with a high level of infectivity. It is detectable in the blood for about 5 months. As the IgM type declines, the IgG type should appear in the blood as a marker of convalescence and resolution of the infection. The laboratory testing can measure only the IgM antibody or it can measure the total hepatitis B core antibody, consisting of both the IgM and IgG types. The value of total hepatitis B core antibody remains elevated for years after the illness. The lengthy time is an indicator of a resolved infection or of chronic hepatitis B virus infection. Retesting will be needed several months to years later to differentiate between complete resolution and chronic infection.

Hepatitis Be Antigen and Antibody

The hepatitis Be antigen appears early in the infectious process, but is not used for testing during the acute phase of illness. The hepatitis Be antibodies emerge a few months after exposure to the hepatitis B virus and remain elevated for several years. Both the HBe antigen and antibody tests are used together to evaluate patients who are chronically infected with the hepatitis B virus.

Hepatitis B Virus DNA

This test method identifies the presence in the blood of the DNA of the hepatitis virus and measures the viral load (the number of copies of the virus in the blood per measured volume or tissue sample). The measurement of the viral load is the determinant of the degree of infectivity; the quantity of viral load fluctuates over time.

The test is used to detect active hepatitis B virus infection in patients whose hepatitis B surface antigen detection is falsely negative. A false negative means that the original antigen test result was negative, but the patient is actually positive for the infection. DNA testing is a very sensitive and accurate detector of infection. DNA testing can also serve to evaluate the response to hepatitis B treatment with medications. In preliver and postliver transplantation, the DNA testing of liver biopsy tissue samples is used to detect low-level hepatitis virus infection.

REFERENCE VALUES   Negative

HOW THE TEST IS DONE

Venipuncture is used to obtain a sample of blood.
Liver biopsy may be done to obtain a sample of liver tissue.

SIGNIFICANCE OF THE TEST RESULTS

Positive Values

Hepatitis B surface antigen: acute or chronic infection with high or low infectivity
Hepatitis Be antigen: chronic infection with high or low infectivity
Hepatitis B core antibody, total: convalescent stage or past infection
Hepatitis B core antibody-IgM: acute infection, high or low infectivity
Hepatitis B surface antibody: convalescence or past infection; immunization
Hepatitis Be antibody: acute or chronic infection with low infectivity
Hepatitis B-DNA: acute, convalescent or chronic infection

INTERFERING FACTORS

• None

NURSING CARE

Nursing actions are similar to those used in other venipuncture procedures (see Chapter 2), with the following additional measures.

During the Test

• Venipuncture is always performed with gloves, and used needles must be discarded carefully, according to agency protocol. In delivery of nursing care to the patient who has or is suspected of having hepatitis, extra attention to technique should help prevent needlestick injury or contact with blood from splashes.

Posttest

• In giving care and in handling blood and body fluids, always use standard precautions. Hepatitis B infection is contagious and the virus is present in the blood and body fluids for weeks to months before the patient has symptoms of hepatitis. Although most patients recover completely from a hepatitis B infection, the virus remains in the blood and body fluids for months during the acute phase or for years later if they are carriers of chronic infection.

Health Promotion

The nurse provides health instruction to parents of newborn babies and young children by recommending vaccination for hepatitis B, along with all other recommended childhood vaccinations. Hepatitis B vaccination consists of a series of three injections given at timed intervals. The recommendation is that the first dose be given to the neonate at birth and before discharge from the hospital. The second dose is given 1 to 2 months later. The third dose is given at 6 months of age. Because of increased emphasis on vaccination of infants, children, and adults, there has been a dramatic decline in the incidence of hepatitis B virus infection in the United States during the past 30 years.

H

Hepatitis C Tests

Includes: Hepatitis C Antibody (Anti-HCV; HCV Antibody)
Hepatitis C-RNA Assay (HCV-RNA)
Hepatitis C Core Antigen (HCV-Ag)

SPECIMEN OR TYPE OF TEST: Serum

PURPOSE OF THE TEST

Hepatitis C antibody is used to diagnose chronic hepatitis C infection. It is also used to screen the blood of potential donors, with rejection of the blood of potential donors who have positive results.

Hepatitis C-RNA confirms the diagnosis of hepatitis C virus infection in acute or chronic stages of illness and monitors the response to treatment.

Hepatitis C core antigen can be used to detect acute and current infection in an early stage of the disease.

BASICS THE NURSE NEEDS TO KNOW

The HCV infection is transmitted in infected blood and body fluids. The most common occurrence is in intravenous drug users who shared contaminated needles. In this high-risk population, the HCV infection is highly likely to become a chronic infection. Chronic HCV infection is the cause of a significant number of cases of cirrhosis of the liver, and primary cancer of the liver. The virus can also infect health care workers and patients who receive hemodialysis treatments because of the transmission of the virus in the blood. Needlestick injuries or perinatal transmissions account for a small percentage of the hepatitic C infections. In the United States before there was effective screening of blood donors for hepatitis C antibodies, contaminated blood transfusions were a major route of transmission of the hepatitis C virus.

The *hepatitis C antibody test* is the first test performed to detect the presence of the hepatitis C virus infection. Depending on the method of analysis used, the antibodies will be detected in the blood from 9 to 12 weeks after the patient is infected. The HCV antibody test is very highly accurate in identifying the patient with a chronic stage of the illness. It cannot however, identify hepatitis C in the acute stage of illness. If hepatitis C is suspected, but the antibody test is negative, a follow-up hepatitis C-RNA assay test is then used to detect the presence of the hepatitis C virus at the earlier stage of acute infection.

After effective treatment to eliminate the hepatitis C infection, this antibody test will remain positive for 15 to 20 years until it gradually returns to a negative value. The presence of a positive hepatitis C virus antibody test does not imply immunity to future infection.

The *hepatitis C-RNA* test is the most specific and accurate test that identifies the virus by detecting the genetic material of the virus in the patient's blood. The test can detect the virus within 2 weeks of acquiring the infection. It also measures the viral load, meaning a count of how many viral particles are in the blood. There are six different types (genotypes) of the hepatitis C virus; the hepatitic C-RNA identifies which genotype the patient has. Four out of the six genotypes will require a lower dose of medication and a shorter duration of treatment to eradicate the hepatitis C virus. The hepatitis C-RNA monitoring is done to evaluate the effectiveness of the 12 weeks of antiviral medications. When the treatment is effective, the hepatitis C-DNA test should begin to show a reduction in the viral count and then become negative within 6 months.

Hepatitic C core antigen can be detected in the blood within 2 weeks of acquiring the infection. It has an early response in acute illness that is very similar in timing to the detection of the hepatitis C virus-RNA. With effective treatment of the infection, the antigen will disappear from the blood. It is not as sensitive as the hepatitis C virus-DNA test at detecting the low measurement of residual virions that may still be present.

REFERENCE VALUES   Hepatitis C antibody: Negative
Hepatitis C virus-RNA: Negative
Hepatitic C core antigen: <2 pg/mL

HOW THE TEST IS DONE
Venipuncture is performed to collect a sample of blood.

SIGNIFICANCE OF TEST RESULTS
Positive Values
Hepatitis C infection, acute or chronic

INTERFERING FACTORS
• Recent vaccination for influenza will cause the antibody test to show a false-positive value.

NURSING CARE

Nursing measures are similar to those used in other venipuncture procedures (see Chapter 2), with the following additional measures.
Posttest
• Apply standard precautions until the specific diagnosis is made and continue these precautions when the hepatitis C core antigen or RNA tests are positive. Hepatitis C infection is contagious, when the virus is in the blood and body fluids.

Hepatitis Delta Tests

Includes: Hepatitis D Antigen (HDAg), Hepatitis D Antibody (anti-HD)

SPECIMEN OR TYPE OF TEST: Serum

PURPOSE OF THE TEST
Hepatitis D antigen may be used to diagnose a hepatitis delta virus coinfection with the hepatitis B infection during the acute stage of illness.

Hepatitis D antibody may be used to diagnose the hepatitis D virus as a superinfection in the patient who is a hepatitis B carrier.

BASICS THE NURSE NEEDS TO KNOW

Testing for hepatitis D antigen is no longer recommended as routine. The antigen test can be used as an optional test for the patient who has an acute stage of hepatitis B infection and who demonstrates a positive hepatitis B surface antigen test. The antibody IgM or IgG testing may be done for all carriers of chronic hepatitis or when the chronic carrier of hepatitis B infection has an exacerbation of hepatitis. If needed, testing for the presence and amount of hepatitis D-RNA may also be done.

The hepatitis D virus is transmitted in the blood and blood fluids. In endemic areas, it is also transmitted by contact with the mucosa of the infected person. The most frequent groups who are at risk of acquiring the infection are intravenous drug users and men who have sex with men. The hepatitis D virus has defective RNA and because of the defect, the virus can only cause liver cell infection and damage when it coexists with hepatitis B antigen. With coinfection or superinfection with hepatitis B, the patient will have a more severe hepatitis infection that often leads to cirrhosis of the liver.

H

REFERENCE VALUES   Negative

HOW THE TEST IS DONE

Venipuncture is used to obtain a sample of blood.

SIGNIFICANCE OF THE TEST RESULTS

Elevated Values

Hepatitis D virus coinfection or superinfection with hepatitis B

INTERFERING FACTORS

• None

█ NURSING CARE

Nursing actions are similar to those used in other venipuncture procedures (see Chapter 2). Nursing care is the same as for patients with hepatitis B infection.

Hepatitis E Virus

Includes: Hepatitis E antibody IgM (HEV-IgM), Hepatitis E antibody IgG (HEV-IgG)

SPECIMEN OR TYPE OF TEST: Serum

PURPOSE OF THE TEST

The hepatitis E antibody IgM test identifies hepatitis E infection in the acute illness stage. The hepatitis E antibody IgG identifies hepatitis E infection in the convalescent stage of illness.

BASICS THE NURSE NEEDS TO KNOW

Hepatitis E infection is infrequent in the United States, but is more prevalent or endemic in countries of Africa, Southeast and Central Asia, the Middle East, Central America, and Mexico. Individuals who have a recent history of travel to countries where there is no water purification or sanitary disposal of human waste may develop the infection after they return home. The infection is transmitted by the fecal-oral route. It occurs when the person drinks unpurified water that has fecal contamination with the hepatitis E virus or eats contaminated, uncooked food such as raw shellfish, salad greens, and fresh fruit that has no peel or skin.

The incubation period is 2 to 9 weeks before the acute illness appears. Once the person is infected, the virus infects the liver and causes abnormal liver function test results. The virus is found in the blood, bile secretions, and feces (Bashir, Hussain, Hassain & Elahi, 2009). Most patients with this infection recover with only supportive care. Pregnant women, however, are particularly vulnerable to severe infection. They are more prone to develop liver failure and the death rate in pregnant women with hepatitis E infection is many times higher than it is in nonpregnant adults.

H

REFERENCE VALUES   **Negative**

HOW THE TEST IS DONE

Venipuncture is used to obtain a sample of blood

SIGNIFICANCE OF THE TEST RESULTS

Elevated Values

Hepatitis E virus infection, acute, convalescent

INTERFERING FACTORS

• None

NURSING CARE

Nursing actions are similar to those used in other venipuncture procedures (see Chapter 2), Nursing care measures are the same as those for hepatitis A infection.

Hepatic-Biliary Scan

Also called: Liver-Biliary Scan; Cholescintigraphy; HIDA scan

PURPOSE OF THE TEST

This nuclear scan is used to diagnose acute cholecystitis. It is also used to examine the biliary tract for patency or locate the site of an obstruction. It can locate the site of bile leakage, postoperatively. In the jaundiced neonate, it can differentiate between biliary atresia and neonatal hepatitis.

SPECIMEN OR TYPE OF TEST: Radiology; Nuclear Scan

BASICS THE NURSE NEEDS TO KNOW

When a hepatic-biliary scan is done with normal results, a radiopharmaceutical (a ^{99m}Tc-IDA agent) is injected intravenously. This tracer passes from the circulatory system into the liver where it attaches to hepatocytes throughout the organ. Then the radionuclide releases from the hepatocytes and attaches to a shared transport medium with bile. Thus the tracer will travel along the same route with bile, from liver to duodenum. Visualization of the uptake, filling, and excretion of the radiotracer in the liver, gallbladder, and biliary tract is done at timed intervals. The gamma camera detects the concentration of radioactivity and converts the information into physiologic images (Figure 57). When there is normal function, it takes 35 minutes to 1 hour to complete the transit of the radiopharmaceutical from time of injection to entry into the duodenum. In abnormal conditions, the images will demonstrate

H

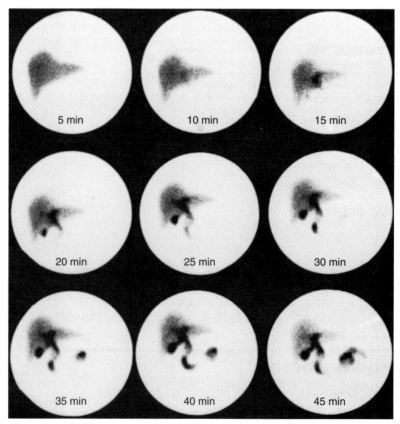

Figure 57. Normal hepatobiliary scan, using a ^{99m}Tc-IDA radionuclide. Imaging of the liver occurs at 5 minutes after the radionuclide is injected into the vein. Imaging of the gallbladder and common bile duct occurs by 20 minutes. Small bowel activity is seen by 35 minutes, as the radionuclide passes into the duodenum. (From Mettler FA, Guiberteau MJ: *Essentials of nuclear medicine imaging*, ed 5, Philadelphia, 2006, Saunders.)

delayed transit or blockage of the radiopharmaceutical at a particular anatomic location in the liver-biliary tract. With delayed filling or no visualization of the gallbladder, the scan can take up to 4 hours to complete.

In acute cholecystitis, most patients have edema and inflammation in the cystic duct and gallbladder. The images show no visualization of the gallbladder because the flow of the radiopharmaceutical cannot reach its destination. In chronic cholecystitis, the gallbladder does fill with the radiopharmaceutical, but it is very delayed in doing so. With blockage in the common duct, the radiopharmaceutical will appear in the proximal section of the common duct but there will be no visualization distal to the obstruction or of the excretion of the radionuclide in the duodenum. The blockage may be caused by a tumor, common duct stone, or inflammation, but the nuclear scan cannot identify the cause.

REFERENCE VALUES	Normal anatomic structure and physiologic function in the liver-biliary system

HOW THE TEST IS DONE

A radionuclide is injected intravenously and a gamma camera detects the radioactivity as the tracer passes through the patient's liver, biliary tract, gallbladder, and duodenum. The camera will process the information and convert it into visual images of the organs and biliary tract. The imaging is done at timed intervals and may take from 1 to 4 hours to complete the study. (See also: Nuclear Scans, p. 455)

After 1 hour of scanning, if there is no visualization of the gallbladder, the patient will be given an intravenous morphine infusion to assist the flow of bile and radionuclide into the gallbladder. The morphine causes a contraction of the sphincter of Oddi and with the resultant backup of bile in the common duct, the pressure in that duct rises. Then the flow of bile and the radiotracer are more likely to be diverted into the gallbladder where the pressure is lower. By using morphine, the imaging process can be shortened to 2 hours time, instead of waiting 4 hours for the gallbladder visualization to occur or not.

SIGNIFICANCE OF THE TEST RESULTS

Abnormal Values

Acute cholecystitis
Chronic cholecystitis
Biliary tract obstruction
Leakage in a biliary duct, postoperatively
Biliary atresia, neonate

INTERFERING FACTORS

- Recent x-ray with barium
- Impaired liver function (bilirubin level >20 mg/dL)
- Recent narcotic administration
- Failure to maintain NPO status

NURSING CARE

Nursing actions are similar to those used in other venipuncture procedures (see Chapter 2), with the following additional measures.

Pretest
- After the physician informs the patient about the scan, the patient signs an informed consent. The consent is entered into the patient's record.
- The patient must be NPO for 2 to 4 hours before the scan. Four hours of fasting is preferred.
- The patient will be instructed to remove all clothes and put on a hospital gown. All jewelry and metallic items must be removed from the torso.

During the Test
- Other than the intravenous catheter insertion, there is no discomfort with this test.
- The patient is positioned supine on the scanner table, with the gamma camera overhead.
- An intravenous line is placed in a vein in the antecubital fossa of the arm. The intravenous radionuclide will be injected and imaging begins within 5 minutes.

Posttest
- For the disposal of any urine or feces, the nurse wears gloves and then performs a thorough handwashing. The patient's radionuclide is excreted in urine and feces for several days, although the radioactivity level is minimal after a few hours. The body waste can be disposed of in the toilet.

○ *Patient Teaching.* The nurse instructs the patient to wash his or her hands after voiding or a bowel movement. Parents and others should wash their hands after changing the diapers of an infant who has had a liver-biliary scan. The patient is reassured that the amount of radioactivity is negligible, but that it can remain on the hands unless they are washed.

HER-2/*neu* Receptor

See Biopsy, breast on pp. 118-119.

High-Density Lipoproteins

See Lipid Profile on p. 417.

Histamine Challenge Test

See Pulmonary Function Studies on p. 528.

Histoplasmosis, Antigen and Antibody Tests

SPECIMEN OR TYPE OF TEST: Serum, Urine, Cerebrospinal Fluid

PURPOSE OF THE TEST

These tests are used to help diagnose severe histoplasmosis infection and monitor the patient's response to treatment.

BASICS THE NURSE NEEDS TO KNOW

Histoplasmosis is a fungal disease caused by the *Histoplasma capsulatum* organism. The histoplasmosis infection results from the inhalation of spore-laden dust containing the infected excreta of birds, bats, chickens, or turkeys. Many people may be asymptomatic and the infection is self-limited. Others, however, experience acute illness as the spores cause pulmonary infection. Additionally, the infection can also become chronic in the lungs and chest or disseminated in any organ of the body. Patients who are immunocompromised are vulnerable to develop the disseminated form of the disease.

    In acute infection, the antigen and antibodies appear in the blood. However, the antibodies do not appear for 2 to 6 weeks after the infection starts. The antibodies may be from current or past infection. In disseminated infection, the antigen and antibodies appear in the blood, urine, and cerebrospinal fluid. The disease is difficult to identify, so more than one test may be needed for diagnosis.

H

REFERENCE VALUES

Antigen test, blood <1.0 ; negative
Antibody test: serum: <1:4, negative
Culture, blood, urine, or cerebrospinal fluid: negative
DNA probe: negative for *Histoplasma capsulatum*

HOW THE TEST IS DONE

Serum (antigen and antibody tests): A venipuncture is performed to collect a sample of blood.
Urine (antigen test): A random sample of urine is placed in a plastic urine container.
Urine culture: (See Culture Urine on p. 252)
CSF (antigen test or culture): During a lumbar puncture, a sample of CSF is collected in a sterile
    CSF tube (See Lumbar Puncture and Cerebrospinal Fluid Analysis on p. 421)

SIGNIFICANCE OF TEST RESULTS

Positive/Elevated Value
Histoplasmosis

INTERFERING FACTORS

- Positive value for rheumatoid factor
- Other fungal infections
- Histoplasmin skin test

▌NURSING CARE

Nursing measures are similar to those used in other venipuncture procedures (see Chapter 2), with the following additional measures.

Pretest
- When histoplasmosis is suspected, ask the patient if he or she has had any recent exposure to the feces of birds. Cleaning out the chicken coop is a common source of infection. By geographic region, this infection is endemic in the Ohio and Mississippi River valleys (Figure 58). Also ask the patient if he or she has had a histoplasmosis skin test performed recently. A recent skin test can cause a positive antibody result.

Posttest
- The nurse monitors the patient's vital signs, including temperature. When the client is symptomatic, he or she develops a fever and flulike manifestations of infection. The illness can infect the lungs and pericardium, causing chest pain and pleuritic pain.
- ○ *Patient Teaching.* Remind the patient to have a histoplasmosis antibody blood test in 2 to 6 weeks to evaluate the convalescent phase of the infection.
- ○ *Patient Teaching.* When the patient has mild to moderate infection, reinforce that the antifungal medication regime is to be followed for 12 weeks. For disseminated infection, the medication is taken for 24 months and for immunocompromised patients, treatment is for life.
- ○ *Patient Teaching.* Repeated antigen and antibody testing will be needed every 3 months to monitor the response to the medication treatment and to detect a relapse or recurring infection.

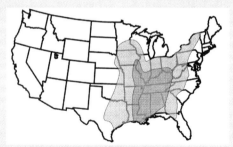

Figure 58. Geographic distribution of cases of histoplasmosis in the United States. The region that is most endemic is shaded darkest and the area that is less endemic is shaded more lightly. (From McPherson RA, Pincus MR: *Henry's clinical diagnosis and management by laboratory methods,* ed 21, Philadelphia, 2007, Saunders.)

Holter Monitoring

Also called: Ambulatory Monitoring

SPECIMEN OR TYPE OF TEST: Electrophysiology

⊙ PURPOSE OF THE TEST

The primary purpose of Holter monitoring is dysrhythmia detection. This procedure is helpful in identifying conduction defects and responses to therapeutic measures. It may be used to evaluate patients with low left ventricular ejection fractions to assess for nonsustained ventricular tachycardia and those who would benefit from an implanted cardiac defibrillator.

BASICS THE NURSE NEEDS TO KNOW

Holter monitoring permits the recording of cardiac electric activity over time (usually 24 hours) with an electronic recording device. It allows the patient to perform normal daily activities so that cardiac responses to these activities can be determined.

REFERENCE VALUES   Normal rate and rhythm; no ectopy, reentry phenomenon, or changes in segments of the ECG with exercise or medication, or both

HOW THE TEST IS DONE

With Holter monitoring, electrodes are applied to the patient's chest (placement varies with desired leads) and attached to an electronic recording device. Most recorders permit simultaneous recording of two channels (frequently leads II and V_5 are chosen; Figure 59). Recorders are equipped with an event marker, which alerts the scanning technician that the patient experienced some symptom. A diary is kept by the patient, who records daily activities and the times at which they were performed, when and what medications were taken, and the presence and time at which symptoms occurred. The recordings are analyzed at 60 to 120 times real time by a microcomputer program. Any abnormalities are then recorded on the usual electrocardiograph paper.

If symptoms are rare, the recording may be done for several days.

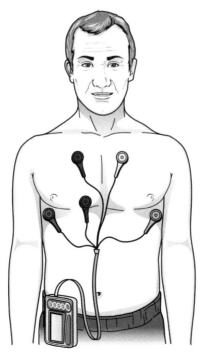

Figure 59. Holter monitor.

SIGNIFICANCE OF TEST RESULTS
Abnormal Values
Conduction disturbances
Dysrhythmias

INTERFERING FACTORS
- Failure of patient to keep records of events and medications taken
- Poor connection or failure of the recorder to capture the cardiac rhythm

NURSING CARE

Pretest
- The nurse checks the Holter monitor's indicator light to determine if the battery is functioning.
○ *Patient Teaching.* The nurse informs the patient regarding the purpose of the Holter monitoring and the vital role he or she plays in obtaining the needed information.
○ *Patient Teaching.* The patient is instructed by the nurse to keep a diary of activities and is taught how to trigger the event marker. Demonstrate and have the patient redemonstrate how to trigger the recorder.
○ *Patient Teaching.* Instruct the patient to keep the recorder dry. Patient should avoid bathing and showering.
During the Test
- Apply electrodes to the chest. Shave the site if the chest is hairy.
- Remind the patient to trigger the marker whenever pain or other symptoms occur.
- Give the patient a writing pad to record activities during the test time.
Posttest
- Remove electrodes and cleanse the site.
- Return recorder device for rhythm evaluation.
- The nurse checks the skin for signs of irritation.

Homocysteine

Also called: Total Homocysteine

SPECIMEN OR TYPE OF TEST: Plasma, Serum

PURPOSE OF THE TEST
Homocysteine levels may be done to identify people at risk for myocardial infarction or stroke.

BASICS THE NURSE NEEDS TO KNOW
Homocysteine is an intermediate amino acid, which increases with vascular disease. It has been associated with increased risk for coronary artery disease, myocardial infarction, peripheral vascular disease, and stroke. It appears to promote the progression of atherosclerosis.

REFERENCE VALUES

Plasma
Child <8 µmol/L
Adult: 5-15 µmol/L

Serum
5%-10% higher than plasma levels

HOW THE TEST IS DONE

A fasting venous sample is obtained by venipuncture.
Send specimen to the lab immediately.

SIGNIFICANCE OF TEST RESULTS

Increased Values
Atherosclerosis
Cardiovascular disease
Deficiency in B_6, B_{12}, folic acid, and riboflavin
Hypothyroidism
Inborn errors of cobalamin and folate metabolism
Medications: metformin, niacin, L-dopa, diuretics
Renal insufficiency

Decreased Values
Hyperthyroidism
Medications: estrogens, simvastatin

INTERFERING FACTORS

* Ingestion of regular and decaffeinated coffee
* Delay in sending specimen to the laboratory immediately
* Smoking
* Medications: corticosteroids, cyclosporine, phenytoin

NURSING CARE

Nursing measures are similar to those used in other venipuncture procedures (see Chapter 2), with the following additional measures.
Pretest
⭕ *Patient Teaching.* Instruct patient to fast for 8 to 10 hours before the blood is drawn.
⭕ *Patient Teaching.* Instruct patient to avoid drinking coffee.

Homovanillic Acid

See Catecholamines, Urinary on p. 182.

Human Immunodeficiency Virus Tests

Also called: HIV; Acquired Immune Deficiency Syndrome (AIDS)

SPECIMEN OR TYPE OF TEST: Blood

PURPOSE OF THE TEST

The HIV tests are used to diagnose the infection and to monitor the response to treatment. They also are used to screen blood donated for transfusion purposes.

BASICS THE NURSE NEEDS TO KNOW

The two types of HIV are HIV-1 and HIV-2. HIV-1 is the more prevalent type in the United States. HIV infection is transmitted by contaminated blood; by contaminated needles, as in intravenous drug use; by unprotected sexual intercourse with an infected person; and from an infected pregnant woman to her fetus.

Antibody Tests

The ELISA (enzyme-linked immunosorbent assay) method is commonly used to detect anti-HIV antibodies in the patient's serum. Once the virus enters the patient's body, the virions attach to C4+ cells and they begin to replicate at a fast rate. Each copy of the virus contains p24 antigens. Within 21 or 22 days, antibodies to HIV can be identified in the serum in response to the presence of the antigens. Positive results of ELISA testing are followed up with a confirmatory second test, usually the Western Blot method or immunofluorescent assay (IFA) method of analysis. With the second test, the positive result confirms the diagnosis of HIV infection. A negative result in the second test excludes HIV infection as a diagnosis. The antibody tests can be used to screen donor blood or blood products.

Rapid Tests

Rapid testing is an approved method for the detection of the HIV antigen. The point-of- care testing can be done in community settings, including physicians' offices, health care clinics, HIV counseling centers, drug treatment centers, and prisons. The screening test is performed and results are available within 30 minutes. The rapid analysis of the blood helps identify the large group of individuals who are infected with HIV and do not know it. The positive rapid test result is confirmed by follow-up testing by Western Blot method. When both tests are positive, the diagnosis of HIV infection is confirmed.

Other rapid tests include the OraQuick™ test, which uses oral fluid for the specimen sample. The test identifies the presence of the HIV antigen and the results are available in 20 minutes or less. A different home collection kit guides the person to perform a finger stick to collect drops of capillary blood. The blood is applied to filter paper, and when dried, the specimen is mailed to the laboratory. The person calls in to the laboratory in 3 to 7 days to obtain the results. For both of these types of tests performed at home, the person receives educational telephone counseling and guidance before the testing and after the test result is known.

Antigen Test

The p24 core antigen is present in every HIV virion. In laboratory analysis, the antigen will be detected in the patient's blood 14 days after exposure and before the antibodies have formed. Thus the antigen test can be used for diagnosis in the early stage of HIV infection.

HIV-RNA

This test detects the RNA genetic material of the HIV virus that is in infected T-lymphocytes and other types of human cells. It is used to test neonates born to mothers who have HIV infection. It is also used for donor screening before the donor's blood is taken for transfusion purposes. This method identifies the HIV infection at an earlier time than all other tests. The presence of HIV-RNA can be detected 12 days after the virus has infected the patient.

The *viral load* is a term that refers to the quantity of HIV-RNA in the blood. Viral load is a powerful predictor of the progression of the disease. Of the various RNA detection tests that are available, the viral load count can detect from 400 to 750,000 copies of the virus per milliliter. The viral load count also is used to measure the response to therapy. The viral load is measured before the medication regime begins to establish a baseline value. The HIV-RNA measurement of viral load is repeated 2 to 8 weeks after the start of medications and every 3 to 6 months thereafter. The goal of medication therapy is to reduce the viral load to an undetectable level within 12 to 24 weeks. Treatment failure occurs when that goal is not reached, or the viral load begins to increase after it was previously undetectable. The medications need to be changed and the changes are guided by resistance testing.

H

CD4$^+$

CD4$^+$ lymphocytes (T lymphocytes) are the immune system cells that are killed by the HIV virus. The CD4$^+$ measurement of 200 cells/mm^3 (200$\times$ 10^9/L) or lower determines that the chronic HIV infection has progressed to acquired immune deficiency syndrome (AIDS). The person is severely immunosuppressed and is at risk to develop opportunistic infections or cancer. Generally, treatment for AIDS begins when the CD4$^+$ cell count is at 350 cells/mm^3 (350 $\times$ 10^9/L) or lower. However, the decision to start antiretroviral therapy varies when including consideration of other clinical factors. The CD4$^+$ count is repeated in 2 to 8 weeks after treatment begins and serial monitoring will be done every 3 to 6 months thereafter to measure the immune system's response to the medications. When the medications are effective, the cell count should rise modestly and stabilize (Romanelli & Matheny, 2009).

HIV Drug Resistance Assay

Two test approaches are used to detect drug-resistant HIV infection. One method identifies the specific genetic mutation of the HIV virus that causes resistance to particular antiretroviral medications. The other method estimates the concentration of specific antiretroviral drugs needed to stop the viral replication and lower the viral load count. The resistance testing is done at the time of detection of the virus, again at the time when antiretroviral medications will be prescribed, and later when treatment failure begins to occur.

REFERENCE VALUES   HIV antibody: Negative
p24 Antigen test: Negative
HIV-RNA: No HIV-RNA detected
Viral load: No HIV-RNA copies detected
CD4$^+$ (T4) lymphocytes: 800-1100 cells/mm^3

HOW THE TEST IS DONE

All tests except the rapid antibody tests use venipuncture to collect a sample of whole blood.

Rapid antibody tests: Venipuncture or finger stick puncture is used to collect a sample of whole blood.

In the OraQuick™ test, a swab is used to collect cells and oral fluid from gingival surfaces. The swab is placed into a vial that contains developing solution. After 20 minutes or less, a positive result is indicated by red-purple lines that appear in the window of the device.

SIGNIFICANCE OF TEST RESULTS

Positive Values

HIV infection
AIDS

Decreased Values

CD4$^+$: AIDS

INTERFERING FACTORS

With the OraQuick™ method, noncompliance with oral and mouth care instructions

NURSING CARE

Nursing measures are similar to those used in other venipuncture procedures (see Chapter 2), with the following additional measures:

Pretest

- A special consent for HIV testing is not recommended. The routine general consent for medical care includes HIV testing. When screening for HIV is done routinely, the patient should be informed, including the explanation of the infection and the test results. The screening is voluntary and patient has the right to "opt out" or decline to have the screening test. If he or she declines, an opt-out declination form is signed and placed in the patient's record.
- If the nurse draws the blood, standard precautions are used. This means the nurse wears gloves when in contact with blood or body fluids. Needles are disposed of in the puncture-proof container. Proper hand-washing is performed after the gloves are removed.

○ *Patient Teaching.* If the OraQuick™ HIV-1 oral specimen collection device is to be used, the nurse instructs the patient to discontinue food and fluid intake for 2 hours before the test. The patient should also avoid brushing the teeth, using mouthwash, rinsing the mouth with water, and chewing gum during the 2-hour period. These activities could alter the cellular surface of the tissues and interfere with the accuracy of the test result.

Posttest

- Once the patient has a confirmed diagnosis of HIV infection, he or she will need a medical appointment to begin treatment.
- Inform the patient that he or she cannot donate blood. If appropriate, instruct that intravenous needles must not be shared.

○ *Patient Teaching.* The nurse explains that safe sex practices or abstaining from sexual intercourse will help prevent transmission of the infection to others.

○ *Patient Teaching.* The patient should be taught and encouraged to continue with regular periodic examinations and follow-up laboratory testing. In addition, the obstetrician of the pregnant female patient should be informed of the positive test results.

○ *Patient Teaching.* The nurse teaches the patient to seek health care assistance for symptoms of AIDS, including recurrent respiratory or skin infections, fatigue, diarrhea, weight loss, fever, lymphadenopathy, or a combination of these conditions. The nurse also can assist the patient with education, supportive counseling, and by encouraging referral for prompt medical assistance.

Health Promotion

The CDC recommends that all people ages 13 to 64 receive an HIV screening test routinely. Patients with tuberculosis should be screened for HIV infection before starting treatment with medication and routinely thereafter. All patients who are seeking treatment for a sexually transmitted disease (STD) should be screened for HIV infection. Repeat testing is indicated if the patient returns with another STD infection or when he or she has a new sexual partner. All pregnant women should have a prenatal screening test for HIV and repeat testing in the third trimester. If the woman is in labor and the HIV status is unknown, a rapid HIV test can be done.

Human Papilloma Virus Testing

See Papanicolaou Smear on pp. 470.

Hydrocortisone, Serum

See Cortisol, Total on p. 227.

17-Hydroxycorticosteroids

Also called: 17-OHCS

SPECIMEN OR TYPE OF TEST: Urine

PURPOSE OF THE TEST

17-OHCS levels are obtained to assess adrenal function.

BASICS THE NURSE NEEDS TO KNOW

17-Hydroxycorticosteroids (17-OHCS) are urinary steroids (cortisol and cortisone metabolites) used to assess adrenal function. An increase in 17-OHCS in the urine reflects an increase in plasma cortisol. With the direct measurement of plasma cortisol and free cortisol, the frequency of 17-OHCS determinations has significantly decreased.

When assessing 17-OHCS values, it is necessary to consider the patient's body type. Obese or muscular individuals will have higher 17-OHCS levels than those with normal body types because of an increase in cortisol metabolism. To adjust to body type, some clinicians correlate the 17-OHCS to the creatinine clearance.

REFERENCE VALUES*   Children <8 years: <1.5 mg/24 hr *or* SI: <4.14 µmol/24 hr
Children (8-12 years): <4.5 mg/24 hr *or* SI: <12.4 µmol/24 hr
Adult female: 2.5-10 mg/24 hr *or* SI: 6.9-27.6 µmol/24 hr
Adult male: 4.5-12 mg/24 hr *or* SI: 12.4-33.1 µmol/24 hr

*Varies with laboratories

HOW THE TEST IS DONE

A 24-hour urine specimen is obtained.

SIGNIFICANCE OF TEST RESULTS

Elevated Values

Adrenal cancer
Cushing's syndrome
Extreme stress
Hyperthyroidism
Pituitary tumor
Obesity
Severe hypertension
Acromegaly

Decreased Values

Addison's disease
Hypothyroidism
Starvation
Liver failure
Renal failure
Pregnancy
Congenital adrenal hyperplasia
Hypotension

INTERFERING FACTORS

- Failure to collect all the urine during the 24-hour collection period
- Failure to keep specimen on ice or refrigerated
- Medications such as chloral hydrate, chlorpromazine, colchicine, erythromycin, estrogens, oral contraceptives, paraldehyde, quinidine, quinine, reserpine, and spironolactone

NURSING CARE

Nursing measures are similar to those used in other timed urine collections (see Chapter 2), with the following additional measures.

Pretest
- Take the patient's medication history to assess for interfering medications.

○ *Patient Teaching.* The nurse explains the collection procedure to the patient, especially the need to collect all the urine for 24 hours.

○ *Patient Teaching.* Instruct the patient to avoid excessive physical activity during the testing period.

During the Test

- At the start of the test, the nurse instructs the patient to void at 8 AM and discard this urine. The collection period begins at this time, and all the urine is collected for 24 hours, including the 8 AM specimen of the following morning. The nurse needs to remind the patient during the collection period to save all the urine.
- Keep the urine and collection container refrigerated or on ice during the collection period.

Posttest

- On the requisition form and specimen label, write the patient's name and the time and date of the start and finish of the test period.
- Arrange for prompt transport of the cooled specimen to the laboratory.

Hysterosalpingography

Also called: (HSG); Hysterosalpingogram

SPECIMEN OR TYPE OF TEST: Radiography

PURPOSE OF THE TEST

Hysterosalpingography is used to assess the patency of the fallopian tubes as part of infertility studies of the female. It also can identify abnormal development of the uterus and the presence of a uterine fistula.

BASICS THE NURSE NEEDS TO KNOW

As part of the infertility workup in the female, the hysterosalpingogram is performed to identify anatomic abnormality of the uterus or occlusion of the fallopian tubes. The lumen of each of these structures is visualized by either fluoroscopy or x-ray. The tubes can be blocked because of external compression from an abdominal or pelvic abnormality, or internal blockage from scarring. The uterus may have an anatomic abnormality, such as that caused by incomplete development of the uterus, or a congenital abnormality resulting from intrauterine exposure to diethylstilbestrol.

In normal anatomy, the radiopaque dye is instilled into the uterine cavity. Then, the effects of gravity and positional changes promote the flow of dye through the uterus and fallopian tubes and on into the abdominal cavity. If the contrast material does not enter the abdominal cavity, one or both tubes are blocked (Figure 60). The test requires 30 to 45 minutes to complete.

REFERENCE VALUES   Normal flow of dye through the uterus and fallopian tubes

H

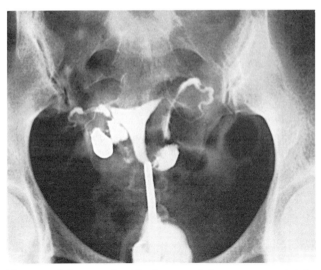

Figure 60. Abnormal hysterosalpingography. The hysterosalpingogram reveals bilateral, dilation, and fluid-filled areas in the fallopian tubes. The obstruction of both tubes is the end-stage of an earlier infection called salpingitis, or pelvic inflammatory disease. The uterus is normal. (From Frank ED, Long BW, Smith BJ: *Merrill's atlas of radiographic positioning and procedures*, ed 12, St Louis, 2012, Mosby.)

HOW THE TEST IS DONE

Radiopaque, water-based contrast medium is instilled into the uterus and fluoroscopic or x-ray films provide visualization of the interior surfaces of the uterus and fallopian tubes.

SIGNIFICANCE OF TEST RESULTS

Abnormal Values

Partial or complete obstruction of the fallopian tubes
Fibroid tumor of the uterus
Adhesions
Uterine fistula
Foreign body (e.g., intrauterine device)
Uterine malformation

INTERFERING FACTORS

- Menstruation
- Pregnancy
- Active uterine bleeding
- Pelvic inflammatory disease
- Allergy to the contrast medium

NURSING CARE

Pretest

- The nurse schedules this test during the early part of the menstrual cycle, before ovulation occurs. This prevents interference with ovulation, irradiation of the oocytes, or the possibility of an early phase of pregnancy. The patient will have a pretest laboratory screening for gonorrhea and chlamydia infection. These infections would postpone this radiology study. Ensure that the patient has no current vaginal bleeding. When bleeding or infection exist, the contrast material could be absorbed into the vasculature, or its flow could introduce microorganisms into the fallopian tubes.
- The nurse identifies any patient with a history a sensitivity reaction to the contrast medium. If a positive history exists, the sensitivity is documented in the patient's record and reported to the physician. Plans are made to premedicate the patient with prescribed steroids or an antihistamine, or both.
- Once the patient is informed of the procedure, obtain written consent and place it in the patient's record.

○ *Patient Teaching.* In the pretest preparation, instruct the patient to take the prescribed laxative on the night before the test. Antibiotics are often prescribed to prevent infection in the fallopian tubes. The patient takes the first dose on the day before the examination and continues taking the medication for 5 to 7 days following the examination. On the morning of the procedure, the patient performs cleansing enemas until the returns are clear. The patient should fast from eating a meal before the scheduled examination.

- The nurse assists the patient in removing all clothes and putting on a hospital gown. Vital signs are taken and the results are recorded in the patient's record.

○ *Patient Teaching.* The patient is instructed to void to empty the bladder. This prevents displacement of the uterus and fallopian tubes by an enlarged bladder.

During the Test

- The nurse places the patient in the lithotomy position.
- The nurse provides reassurance as the physician inserts the vaginal speculum, cleanses the cervix with povidone-iodine, and inserts the cannula. As the contrast material is instilled, the patient may experience temporary sensations of nausea, dizziness, bradycardia, or uterine cramping.
- Between radiographic images, the nurse helps the patient change position so that the contrast medium flows through the fallopian tubes.

Posttest

- The nurse monitors and records the patient's vital signs. On discharge, the patient is instructed to gradually return to pretest activity levels.

◆ **Nursing Response to Complications**

A sensitivity reaction to the contrast medium can occur. The reaction is usually mild.

Mild Sensitivity Reaction. The nurse assesses for hives and urticaria. The patient would develop redness and some swelling in the skin. The patient complains of itching. The blood pressure can demonstrate hypotension. In cases of mild allergic reaction, the nurse reports the findings to the physician and prepares to administer diphenhydramine hydrochloride (Benadryl), as prescribed.

Immunoglobin E Antibody

Also called: IgE antibody test, (IgE)

SPECIMEN OR TYPE OF TEST: Serum

PURPOSE OF THE TEST

This test measures the amount of IgE antibody in the blood and the identification of the specific antigen(s) that caused the IgE level to rise. The test identifies sensitivity to one or more specific antigens and confirms or excludes allergy as the cause of the patient's symptoms.

BASICS THE NURSE NEEDS TO KNOW

There are many sources of allergy in the home and environment that have the potential to cause an allergic response in sensitized individuals. Common allergens are foods, pollens, mold spores, dust mites, animal dander and proteins, insect bites, parasites, and particular medications (see box 4 on p. 59).

Immunoglobin E is the allergy antibody. The IgE antibodies in nonallergic individuals exist at very low levels in the blood. If, however, the individual is allergic to a particular substance and is exposed to it, the IgE antibody level usually rises in the blood, demonstrating sensitivity to the allergen.

The allergen-specific IgE antibody test method uses *in vitro* testing to identify offending allergens for the individual patient. This means that a blood sample is drawn and in the laboratory specific allergens are mixed with the serum sample to measure the IgE response. The IgE testing is the newer and more accurate method of testing.

The radioallergosorbent test (RAST) method is no longer used, but the term RAST has continued in use as a general name for IgE antibody testing. To avoid confusion, the RAST colloquialism for IgE testing should be discontinued (Cox, Williams, Sicherer, 2008).

If additional testing is needed to identify specific allergens that cause a positive response in sensitized patients, the skin prick, intradermal injection, or patch test methods testing may be done. (See Allergy testing, p. 58 and Patch Test, Skin, p. 480).

REFERENCE VALUES

IgE Antibody (fluorescent enzyme immunoassay method):
<0.35-100 kU/L
Note: there are three different manufacturers of the testing materials and the normal values and test results are based on which product was used.

HOW THE TEST IS DONE

Venipuncture is used to collect a specimen of blood.

SIGNIFICANCE OF TEST RESULTS

Elevated Values
Sensitivity to specific allergens

INTERFERING FACTORS

• None

NURSING CARE

Pretest

- A complete clinical history and physical examination must be done to help identify possible allergens, recent exposure or contact with these allergens, and the type of physical symptoms that resulted. The patient's age, occupation, hobbies, and employment are also noted.

○ *Patient Teaching*

- Instruct the patient to continue taking the antihistamine or corticosteroid medications as prescribed. Current use will not interfere with this blood test.
- Reassure the patient that the test is safe and will not worsen the current symptoms.

Posttest

- If the patient has tested positive to specific IgE antibodies and the clinical history and physical examination also indicates exposure to the allergen, additional skin testing methods may be employed to confirm the medical diagnosis. Once the allergy is confirmed and the specific allergen is identified, the goals of treatment for the patient will be to avoid future contact or exposure to the allergen; use prescribed medications to lessen the symptoms of the allergic response.

Impedance Cardiography

See Catheterization, Cardiac on p. 221.

Influenza Tests

Includes: Influenza A, Influenza B, H1N1

PURPOSE OF THE TEST

The testing identifies influenza A and B viruses and differentiates them from other causes of acute respiratory infections. The results help with the diagnosis and provide guidance for medical treatment.

SPECIMEN OR TYPE OF TEST: Nasal secretions

BASICS THE NURSE NEEDS TO KNOW

The influenza viruses A and B cause worldwide acute respiratory infection in seasonal patterns. In North America the flu season occurs from November to April. H1N1 is one subtype of the influenza A virus. The influenza A virus mutates every year and result in outbreaks of the flu annually. The influenza B virus mutates less frequently and outbreaks occur every few years. The method of transmission from person to person is by respiratory droplet and probable hand contact with contaminated objects such as doorknobs.

These viruses initially infect various animals, birds, or mammals, such as pigs or chickens. As the virus gradually adapts and mutates, it becomes transmissible to humans. Because humans have no resistance to the mutant strain, outbreaks occur quickly and spread in epidemic and pandemic patterns of illness.

The influenza virus has an envelope that surrounds the core genetic material. The envelope contains various H and N type antigens. As the RNA of the influenza A virus mutates, it changes the structure of the H and N antigens and a new strain of the virus occurs. The outbreak of the flu of 2009-2011 is a type A H1N1 influenza infection (Mahon, Lehman & Manuselis, 2011).

Patients with the flu have high fever, a nonproductive cough, and muscle aches. The complication of pneumonia can develop and death can occur. Pregnant women are very vulnerable to severe illness and complication with this current strain of A/H1N1 influenza. Morbidly obese people may also have a high risk of complications.

Laboratory testing detects the type A and B types of influenza, but at this time there is no test for the subgroup of H1N1. The rapid tests are most accurate during the busiest part of the flu season and are least accurate at the beginning and end of the flu season. Not every patient is tested.

There are various methods to identify the virus and most can distinguish between type A and type B. Some of the tests are not practical in the clinical setting because of the lengthy delay before the results are known. For example, viral culture takes 5 to 10 days to obtain the results and reverse transcriptase-PCR method takes 1 to 2 days to complete the testing. In this discussion, only the tests that are most useful are included. The antibody test results are available in 2 to 4 hours and the results of rapid tests are available in 15 minutes or less (Lewandewski, 2009c).

REFERENCE VALUES
Direct fluorescent antibody (DFA): negative
Enzyme immunosorbent antibody (EIA): negative
Rapid tests: negative

HOW THE TEST IS DONE

The best method is to collect samples of nasal secretions or nasal washings by swab or aspiration. Throat swabbing or bronchial washings may also be obtained.

SIGNIFICANCE OF THE TEST RESULTS

Positive Values

Influenza A or B

INTERFERING FACTORS

• Use of a generic swab that is not part of the test kit.

▌NURSING CARE

Pretest

All nurses and employees who give patient care should be vaccinated before the start of every flu season. When flu is suspected, the nurse wears a mask and asks the patient to wear one also. The nurse monitors the vital signs including blood pressure, pulse, respirations, and temperature. The patient's history and the results of the physical examination provide important information for the diagnosis. The results are recorded in the patient's record.

Posttest

○ *Patient Teaching.* If the patient has the flu, the nurse teaches the patient, family, and caregiver to wash their hands frequently. Respiratory etiquette is reinforced. In the home, washing of dirty dishes and utensils should be done promptly. The patient's bed linens need to be changed often and the dirty linens washed.

Health Promotion

The nurse teaches that everyone older than 6 months should have the flu vaccine, annually.

Insulin

Also called: Immunoreactive Insulin

SPECIMEN OR TYPE OF TEST: Serum, plasma

PURPOSE OF THE TEST

Insulin levels are determined to assess for insulin-producing tumors, to confirm suspected insulin-resistant states, and as part of the evaluation of glucocorticoid insufficiency. It is not recommended for routine testing of patients with diabetes mellitus.

BASICS THE NURSE NEEDS TO KNOW

Insulin is a protein hormone produced and secreted by the pancreas. It has a short half-life (3 to 5 minutes) and is broken down by the liver and kidneys. Insulin is secreted in response to food intake. It increases in concentration within 10 minutes of eating, peaks in 30 to 45 minutes, and returns to baseline levels within 90 to 120 minutes. Normally, insulin levels increase as blood glucose levels increase.

Without insulin, carbohydrate, protein, and fat metabolism are affected, resulting in hyperglycemia and metabolic acidosis.

REFERENCE VALUES | Fasting
Newborn: 3-20 µU/mL *or* SI: 21-139 pmol/L
Adult: 5-25 µU/mL *or* SI: 35-174 pmol/L

1 Hour After Eating
50-130 µU/mL *or* SI: 347.3-902.8 pmol/L

2 Hours After Eating
<30 µU/mL *or* SI: <208.4 pmol/L

HOW THE TEST IS DONE

Insulin levels may be assessed by random venous sampling or during a glucose tolerance test. A specimen is obtained by venipuncture.

SIGNIFICANCE OF TEST RESULTS

Elevated Values

Acromegaly
Cushing's syndrome
Hyperinsulinism
Insulinoma
Insulin overdose
Liver disease
Pancreatic lesions
Vagal stimulation

Decreased Values

Type 1 diabetes mellitus
Hypopituitarism

INTERFERING FACTORS

- Noncompliance with test protocol
- Insulin antibodies
- Medications such as ACTH, catecholamines, colchicine, diazoxide, oral contraceptives, phenytoin, steroids, sulfonylureas, thyroid hormones, vinblastine, and radioisotopes
- Obesity

NURSING CARE

Nursing care varies according to whether a fasting sample is used or the insulin level is being obtained as part of the glucose tolerance test (GTT). See pp. 345 for discussion of GTT.

Pretest

- The nurse takes a medication history to determine if any interfering drugs are being taken. Check to determine if these drugs are to be withheld. If the patient is receiving insulin therapy, the insulin is withheld until the test is performed.
- Assess the patient's stress level, which may increase endogenous glucocorticoid secretion.

○ *Patient Teaching.* If a fasting insulin sample is to be drawn, the nurse instructs the patient not to eat or drink for 7 hours before the blood is drawn.

During the Test

- Observe the patient for hyperglycemia if insulin is withheld and for hypoglycemia because of the fasting state.
- If performed with a GTT, a blood sample for insulin is obtained each time a glucose level specimen is drawn.

Posttest

- Send the specimen to the laboratory immediately because it must be centrifuged within 30 minutes and frozen until the assay can be performed.
- The patient resumes normal medication schedule and diet therapies.

Insulin Tolerance Test

See Growth Hormone Stimulation Test on p. 353.

Insulin-Induced Hypoglycemia Test

See Metyrapone Stimulation Test on p. 447.

International Normalized Ratio (INR)

See Prothrombin Time on p. 526

Intravenous Glucose Tolerance Test

See Glucose Tolerance Test on p. 345.

Intravenous Pyelogram

See Computed Tomography, Kidneys, Ureters, and Bladder on p. 218

Intrinsic Factor Antibody

Also called: IF Antibody

SPECIMEN OR TYPE OF TEST: Serum

PURPOSE OF THE TEST

This test is performed to differentiate pernicious anemia from other causes of megaloblastic anemia. It also helps determine the cause of a decreased cobalamin (vitamin B_{12}) level.

BASICS THE NURSE NEEDS TO KNOW

Intrinsic factor is a glycoprotein manufactured by the parietal cells of the gastric mucosa. The function of intrinsic factor is to bond with ingested vitamin B_{12} and then facilitate absorption of the vitamin in the ilium. Vitamin B_{12} is needed by the bone marrow in the manufacture of new red blood cells. Without available intrinsic factor, the patient develops pernicious anemia, a megaloblastic anemia.

Interference with the function of intrinsic factor is caused by intrinsic factor antibodies. These antibodies are autoimmune complexes that are present in many cases of pernicious anemia. Two types of intrinsic factor antibody exist. Type 1, the "blocking" antibody, interferes with the bonding of intrinsic factor to vitamin B_{12}. Type 2, the "binding" antibody, interferes with the attachment of the intrinsic factor vitamin B_{12} complex to the ileal receptor sites.

HOW THE TEST IS DONE
Venipuncture is used to obtain a sample of blood.

SIGNIFICANCE OF TEST RESULTS
Positive Values
Pernicious anemia
Hyperthyroidism (Graves' disease)
Diabetes mellitus (insulin dependent)

INTERFERING FACTORS
- Recent radioisotope scan
- Recent vitamin B_{12} injection

NURSING CARE

Nursing measures are similar to those used in other venipuncture procedures (see Chapter 2), with the following additional measures.
Pretest
- Schedule this test before any radioisotope scan. The radioisotopes of the nuclear scan would interfere with the radioimmunoassay method of analysis used in this test.
- Instruct the patient to withhold any injection of vitamin B_{12} for 48 hours before the test. Recent injection of this vitamin could cause a false-positive result.

Iron Studies

Includes: Serum Iron (Fe); Transferrin (Tf); Siderophilin; Total Iron-Binding Capacity (TIBC); Transferrin Saturation; Iron Saturation

SPECIMEN OR TYPE OF TEST: Serum

PURPOSE OF THE TEST
These tests provide an estimate of total iron storage and information regarding the nutritional status of the individual. They help distinguish between iron deficiency anemia and the anemia of chronic disease. They also confirm the presence of iron overload and hematochromatosis.

BASICS THE NURSE NEEDS TO KNOW
Iron is an inorganic ion that is essential to many vital body processes, including erythropoiesis (the manufacture of red blood cells) and as a component of hemoglobin, which is needed for the transport of oxygen to tissues. In normal physiology, the total iron content remains

relatively constant throughout life. The source of iron intake is from food or mineral supplement. The body has an efficient method to conserve the iron from senescent erythrocytes and reuse it in erythropoiesis and hemoglobin synthesis (Figure 61).

Iron overload occurs in some types of anemia, in liver disease, in excessive iron replacement therapy, and after multiple transfusions. Iron deficiency occurs when the supply of iron is insufficient to meet the body's demand and the iron reserves are also depleted. The source of the problem can be insufficient intake, impaired absorption, blood loss, or increased demand because of pregnancy or lactation (Table 10).

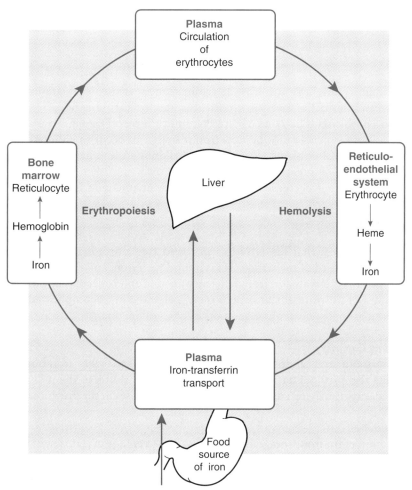

Figure 61. The use and conservation of iron. Some iron is readily available in the plasma and bone marrow for the synthesis of hemoglobin and erythropoiesis. After the hemolysis of old or damaged erythrocytes, the body is very efficient in the conservation and storage of iron in the liver and bone marrow. Whenever the immediate supply of iron is low, the liver releases the stored iron for erythropoiesis.

TABLE 10	Sources of Iron Deficiency, with Conditions That Cause Iron Deficiency Anemia		
Insufficient Intake	**Impaired Absorption**	**Blood Loss**	**Increased Demand**
Fad diets	Gastric surgery	Gastrointestinal bleeding	Pregnancy
Pica	Celiac disease	Excessive menstruation	Lactation
Poverty	Achlorhydria		

Laboratory Testing

No single test fully measures iron deficiency, iron overload, and iron storage. A battery of several tests, including the complete blood count (See Complete Blood Count on p. 208), is used to provide a complete assessment. The laboratory assessment of iron stores includes serum iron, transferrin, total iron-binding capacity, transferrin saturation, and ferritin.

Serum Iron

As a single laboratory test, a serum iron determination is used to evaluate iron toxicity. The elevated value can rise to the level of a critical value, indicating serious iron toxicity. Iron overload is also a problem for patients who receive multiple blood transfusions and discontinue their medication for iron chelation therapy. Iron toxicity can occur in children who ingest the iron pills in an accidental poisoning. Fatalities in children occur when the iron serum level is greater than 1800 µg/dL *or* greater than 322.2 µmol/L.

The serum iron value is decreased in iron deficiency anemia and in the anemia associated with chronic disease.

Transferrin

This is the major protein that binds serum iron and transports it in the blood. In normal physiology, about one third of the transferrin is bound with iron, and the remainder is available in reserve. Transferrin is elevated in iron deficiency anemia and is decreased with iron overload. It is a useful index of nutritional status because it is elevated in uncomplicated iron deficiency but is in the normal to low-normal range in other types of anemia.

Total Iron-Binding Capacity

This is the maximum iron-binding capacity of transferrin and other iron-binding globulins. The serum value also provides data regarding the nutritional status of the individual. The total iron-binding capacity rises in iron deficiency anemia and decreases in the presence of iron overload.

Transferrin Saturation

This is a calculation of the iron storage, expressed as the percentage of transferrin that is saturated with iron. The value is decreased in iron deficiency, but a value of less than 15% indicates iron deficiency erythropoiesis.

Ferritin

This is a reliable indicator of total iron storage. The level is decreased in iron deficiency anemia and elevated in iron overload. When a ferritin determination is combined with other iron studies, the results differentiate among the different types of microcytic, hypochromic anemias. Iron deficiency anemia is indicated by a serum ferritin value of less than 10 ng/mL (SI: <10 µg/L).

REFERENCE VALUES

Serum Iron
Newborn: 100-250 µg/dL *or* SI: 17.9-44.8 µmol/L
Infant: 40-100 µg/dL *or* SI: 7.2-17.9 µmol/L
Child: 50-120 µg/dL *or* SI: 9-21.5 µmol/L
Adult female: 50-120 µg/dL *or* SI: 9-21.5 µmol/L
Adult male: 60-150 µg/dL *or* SI: 10.7-26.9 µmol/L

Transferrin
Newborn: 130-275 mg/dL *or* SI: 1.3-2.75 g/L
Child (3 months-16 years): 203-360 mg/dL *or* SI: 2.03-3.6 g/L
Female: 250-380 mg/dL *or* SI: 2.50-3.80 g/L
Adult (16-60 years): Male: 215-365 mg/dL *or* SI: 2.15-3.65 g/L
Adult (>60 years): 190-375 mg/dL *or* SI: 1.9-3.75 g/L

Total Iron-Binding Capacity
250-400 µg/dL *or* SI: 44.8-71.6 µmol/L

Transferrin Saturation
20%-50% *or* SI: 0.20-0.50 fraction saturation

Ferritin
Newborn: 25-200 ng/mL *or* SI: 25-200 µg/L
Infant (2-5 months): 50-200 ng/mL *or* SI: 50-200 µg/L
Child (6 months-15 years): 7-140 ng/mL *or* SI: 7-140 µg/L
Adult female: 10-120 ng/mL *or* SI: 10-120 µg/L
Adult male: 20-250 ng/mL *or* SI: 20-250 µg/L

▽ **Critical Values**   Serum iron: 62.7 µmol/L

HOW THE TEST IS DONE
Venipuncture is used to collect a sample of venous blood.

SIGNIFICANCE OF TEST RESULTS
Elevated Values
Serum Iron
Anemias (pernicious, aplastic, hemolytic)
Hematochromatosis
Thalassemia
Multiple transfusions
Iron poisoning, child
Lead poisoning
Vitamin B_6 (folate) deficiency
Acute leukemia

Transferrin
Iron deficiency anemia
Elevated estrogen levels (oral contraceptives)
Pregnancy
Total Iron-Binding Capacity
Hypochromic anemias
Chronic blood loss
Iron deficiency anemia
Dietary deficiency, infants, children
Acute hepatitis
Ferritin
Thalassemia
Iron overload, toxicity
Hemochromatosis
Liver disease, infectious hepatitis, alcoholism
Leukemia
Transferrin Saturation
Hemochromatosis
Vitamin B_6 deficiency
Excessive iron intake
Aplastic anemia

Decreased Values
Serum Iron
Iron deficiency anemia
Laennec's cirrhosis
Hypothyroidism
Acute or chronic infection
Malignancy
Starvation
Transferrin
Inflammation or necrosis
Malignancy
Malnutrition
Multiple myeloma
Hepatocellular diseases
Nephrotic syndrome
Transferrin Saturation
Iron deficiency anemia
Anemia of chronic infection
Malignancy, stomach, small intestine
Total Iron-Binding Capacity
Anemias, hemolytic, pernicious
Chronic infection
Hemochromatosis
Ferritin
Iron deficiency anemia

INTERFERING FACTORS

- Recent administration of radioisotopes (ferritin)
- Hemolysis (serum iron, iron saturation)
- Lipemia (transferrin)
- Recent blood transfusion (serum iron)
- Oral iron medication therapy

NURSING CARE

Nursing measures are similar to those used in other venipuncture procedures (see Chapter 2), with the following additional measures.

Pretest

- To obtain the most accurate results, these lab tests should be scheduled before or a few days after a blood transfusion. The blood tests should be done before any nuclear scans because the radioactive isotopes of the scan interfere with the radioimmunoassay method for testing of ferritin. They also should be performed in the morning. Serum iron has a diurnal rhythm, with the highest value in the early morning. The serum iron values fluctuate widely between day and night and also different days.
- If the patient takes an iron supplement, the nurse includes this information on the requisition form.

○ *Patient Teaching.* The nurse instructs the patient to fast from food and fluids for 8 hours before the test for transferrin levels. Lipemia interferes with the transferrin values.

Posttest

Elevated Value of Iron. The patient who has chronic renal failure and is treated by hemodialysis therapy is vulnerable to development of a chronically elevated serum iron level. The patient who receives multiple transfusions as treatment for a chronic form of anemia will also develop elevated iron and ferritin values and receive an overload of iron. The nurse monitors the laboratory results for elevations of these values and notifies the physician of the abnormal results. After the serum ferritin value reaches more than 1000 µg/L, oral iron chelation treatment is indicated (Ault & Jones, 2009).

Once the physician establishes the diagnosis and the cause of the iron and ferritin values, the oral medication Exjade (deferasirox) is prescribed as the chelating agent. The medication is taken once a day, every day and maintains a lower level of serum iron on a sustained basis.

Decreased Value of Iron. In iron deficiency anemia, the nurse assesses for changes in the patient, including pallor, fatigue, and elevated pulse and respirations. A nutritional assessment provides information about the patient's food intake, particularly related to sources of iron.

○ *Patient Teaching.* The nurse can teach the patient to increase the intake of dietary sources of iron, including red meat, liver, egg yolk, whole grain bread, fortified cereals, and dried fruits such as raisins. If an oral iron supplement is prescribed, the patient is taught to take the iron tablet or liquid after meals or with a snack. This helps avoid gastric irritation. Replacement iron therapy will cause some constipation and black color of the feces.

Continued

NURSING CARE—cont'd

▽ **Nursing Response to Critical Values**

The iron value of 350 µg/dL or above is considered to be a critical value indicating a severe iron toxicity. The nurse notifies the physician immediately and assesses the patient for vomiting and severe abdominal pain. The patient will develop metabolic acidosis and an increased anion gap.

With an extreme critical value of 1000 µg/dL (SI: 179 µmol/L), the problem of acute iron toxicity has become far more severe. Unless the problem is reversed, the patient is likely to develop shock and cardiovascular collapse, leading to death. In this extreme situation, the nurse prepares to administer the chelating agent deferoxamine mesylate (Desferal) by the intravenous route, as prescribed by the physician. The medication is mixed in an intravenous solution and administered by a slow and controlled infusion rate. If the medication is administered too rapidly, it will cause hypotension and shock, worsening the problem.

Ketone Bodies, Blood

Also called: Ketones

SPECIMEN OR TYPE OF TEST: Serum, Plasma, Whole Blood

PURPOSE OF THE TEST

Serum ketone levels are measured to evaluate ketoacidosis in patients with diabetes mellitus and for patients with ketoacidosis due to alcoholism, starvation, or high-protein diets. For patients with ketoacidosis associated with diabetes mellitus, ketone levels may be used to determine insulin requirements.

BASICS THE NURSE NEEDS TO KNOW

Serum ketone levels may be measured to distinguish between diabetic ketoacidosis and hyperosmolar coma. With diabetic ketoacidosis, incomplete fatty acid metabolism leads to increasing ketones in the blood. Patients with hyperosmolar coma and extremely high levels of serum glucose produce minimal to no measurable ketones. The mechanism of maintaining nearly normal ketone levels in hyperosmolar coma is not known. It is theorized that these patients have sufficient insulin to break down fatty acids or are glucagon resistant. Without adequate insulin, three major ketone bodies accumulate in the blood: acetone, acetoacetate acid, and β-hydroxybutyric acid.

REFERENCE VALUES   Negative: <2 mg/dL *or* SI: <0.34 mmol/L as acetone *or*
SI: <0.2 mmol/L as acetoacetate

HOW THE TEST IS DONE

Venipuncture is performed.

SIGNIFICANCE OF TEST RESULTS

Elevated Values

Alcoholic ketoacidosis
Decreased caloric intake (dieting)
Eclampsia
Isopropanol poisoning
Propranolol poisoning
Starvation
Uncontrolled diabetes mellitus
Gierke's disease

INTERFERING FACTORS

- Hemolysis of specimen

NURSING CARE

The nurse's duties are similar to those performed in other venipuncture procedures, as presented in Chapter 2.

K

Ketones, Urinary

Also called: Acetoacetate; Acetones

SPECIMEN OR TYPE OF TEST: Urine

PURPOSE OF THE TEST

Urine is tested for ketone bodies to evaluate the patient with diabetes mellitus and to diagnose carbohydrate deprivation. The concentration of urine ketones can be used to adjust insulin requirements in diabetic patients, assist in the diagnosis of diabetic ketoacidosis, and to monitor patients on low-carbohydrate diets.

BASICS THE NURSE NEEDS TO KNOW

Without adequate insulin, three major ketone bodies accumulate in the blood and are excreted in the urine. These ketone bodies are acetone, acetoacetic acid, and β-hydroxybutyric acid. Ketones form as fats and fatty acids are broken down.

A variety of commercial products are available to test for ketones in the urine. Popular products include Ketostix and Keto-Diastix. These products measure acetone and acetoacetate acid levels, but not β-hydroxybutyric acid, which may be the dominant ketone in patients with poorly controlled diabetes mellitus.

Urinary ketone testing is usually performed in conjunction with capillary or urinary glucose testing. It may be carried out randomly to evaluate a suspected diagnosis of uncontrolled diabetes mellitus or periodically during the day to regulate insulin coverage. Ketones should be checked in diabetic patients during acute illness, severe stress, and pregnancy.

REFERENCE VALUES   Negative

HOW THE TEST IS DONE

With the Ketostix or Keto-Diastix, the reagent strip is dipped in the urine. The color change of the strip is compared with the chart provided by the manufacturer to determine the presence and concentration of ketones. Review the manufacturer's guidelines for the use of their product.

SIGNIFICANCE OF TEST RESULTS

Elevated Values
Alcoholic ketoacidosis
Fever
High-fat diet
Hypermetabolic states
Starvation
Uncontrolled diabetes mellitus

INTERFERING FACTORS

- Using products that have been exposed to light or are outdated
- Bacteria in the urine
- Highly acidic urine
- Diets low in carbohydrates and fat
- Medications: ascorbic acid, levodopa
- Inability to see color changes

NURSING CARE

Health Promotion
The nurse instructs the patient with diabetes mellitus to check his or her urinary ketones whenever the glucose level is more than 300 mg/dL (SI: 16.7 mmol/L) or he or she is experiencing an acute illness. Instruct the patient to be aware of possible indications of ketoacidosis, such as nausea, vomiting, or abdominal pain, and to check urinary ketones if these symptoms occur.

- If a diabetic patient is pregnant, the nurse instructs her to inform the manager of her diabetes. During pregnancy, urinary ketones will be assessed periodically.

During the Test
- Instruct the patient to void into a clean, dry container.
- Check voided urine within 60 minutes.
- The method of checking for ketones varies with the product. Follow the manufacturer's guidelines.

Posttest
- Document the results, usually on a flow chart.
- Adjust insulin dosage as ordered based on the results.

Lactate Dehydrogenase (LDH)

See Cardiac Markers on p. 175.

Lactate Dehydrogenase, Isoenzymes

See Cardiac Markers on p. 175.

Lactic Acid

Also called: Lactate; l-Lactate; Blood Lactate

SPECIMEN OR TYPE OF TEST: Venous

PURPOSE OF THE TEST

Lactate levels are most frequently used to support the diagnosis of cellular hypoxia. Lactate levels can also predict survival in severe shock states.

BASICS THE NURSE NEEDS TO KNOW

Elevated lactic levels cause a form of metabolic acidosis called lactic acidosis. Lactate levels in the blood result from the balance of production and clearance. There are two types of lactic acidosis. Type A lactic acidosis is due to a lack of cellular oxygenation. If the cells do not receive adequate oxygen, anaerobic metabolism will occur. Lactic acid is the by-product of anaerobic metabolism. Rising lactate levels indicate a need to examine O_2 transport and consumption. Type B lactic acidosis is due to the overproduction and/or decreased ability of the liver to remove lactate.

REFERENCE VALUES	8.1-15.3 mg/dl *or* SI: 0.9-1.7 mmol/L
▽ Critical Values	>4 mmol/L

HOW THE TEST IS DONE

A venipuncture is performed. Arterial blood may also be used, but there is no significant difference between arterial and venous lactate measures.

For shock states, a random sample may be obtained.

SIGNIFICANCE OF TEST RESULTS

Elevated Values
Type A
Shock states
Severe hypoxia
Severe anemia

Prolonged seizures/shivering
Mesenteric ischemia
Type B
Alcoholism
Diabetes mellitus
Liver failure
Malignancy
Renal failure
Many medications: metformin, salicylates carbonic anhydrase inhibitors

Decreased Values
Hypothermia

INTERFERING FACTORS

- Noncompliance with dietary and activity restrictions
- The drugs acetaminophen (large dose), ethanol (large dose), epinephrine, fructose, morphine, and sorbitol

NURSING CARE

Nursing measures are similar to those used in other venipuncture procedures (see Chapter 2), with the following additional measures.

Pretest

⊙ *Patient Teaching.* The nurse instructs the patient not to eat or drink for 12 hours before the test and to ingest no alcohol for 24 hours before the blood is drawn.

⊙ *Patient Teaching.* Instruct the patient to lie quietly for 2 hours before the blood is drawn.

- For shock states, a random sample may be obtained.

During the Test

- No tourniquet should be applied, and the patient should not clench the fist.

Posttest

- Send the specimen to the laboratory immediately.
- Advise the patient to resume a normal diet and activity level.

▽ **Nursing Response to Critical Values**

High lactate levels (>4 mmol/L) indicate higher mortality rates. Report elevated values to the physician.

Lactose Tolerance Test

SPECIMEN OR TYPE OF TEST: Blood, Urine

PURPOSE OF THE TEST

This test identifies lactose intolerance-lactate deficiency. It is used in the workup for abdominal distention, chronic diarrhea, and abdominal cramps associated with the ingestion of milk. It is also used to investigate the cause of malabsorption.

BASICS THE NURSE NEEDS TO KNOW

Lactose is a sugar present in milk and milk products. For the intestinal absorption of lactose, the person must have lactase enzymes to break down the lactose into simpler sugars. These sugars are then absorbed through the villi of the small intestine and enter the blood circulation. This process results in a normal rise of the plasma glucose level to greater than 30 mg/dL (SI: >1.7 mmol/L) over the normal fasting value of glucose.

When the lactase enzyme is deficient, the client is lactose intolerant. Varying amounts of lactose cannot be absorbed and the sugar remains in the lumen of the intestine. Sugar attracts water into the lumen by osmosis, causing diarrhea. Bacterial fermentation of the sugar causes gas formation, bloating, abdominal cramps, and distention. The lactose intolerance may range from mild to severe, and often worsens with aging.

Abnormal Findings

Glucose Measurements

With lactase deficiency, only some of the simple sugar is absorbed and reaches the blood. There is a small increase in the plasma glucose, but it does not reach the reference value of this test. In the lactose tolerance test, the abnormal findings are described as a flat glucose curve or a decreased plasma glucose value. The test is often repeated 2 days later and the higher test result is the one that is used for diagnosis.

Abnormal test results may not indicate lactose intolerance, but can be the result of other causes of intestinal malabsorption or inflammatory disease.

L

REFERENCE VALUES	Plasma glucose: (an increase over the fasting serum glucose value) >30 mg/dL *or* SI: >1.7 mmol/L

HOW THE TEST IS DONE

The fasting patient takes an oral dose of lactose mixed with 400 mL of water. Venipuncture is used to take serial blood samples at timed intervals for 90 minutes.

SIGNIFICANCE OF TEST RESULTS

Lactose intolerance
Crohn's disease
Ulcerative colitis
Small bowel resection
Sprue
Viral or bacterial bowel infection
Giardiasis

INTERFERING FACTORS

- Failure to maintain dietary restrictions
- Delayed emptying of the stomach
- Vomiting
- Diabetes mellitus

NURSING CARE

Nursing measures are similar to those used in other venipuncture procedures (see Chapter 2), with the following additional measures.

Pretest

⦿ *Patient Teaching.* Instruct the patient to discontinue food intake for 8 hours before the test. In addition, there can be no eating during the test since food would alter the baseline glucose value. There can be no smoking or gum chewing before or during the test because these activities would alter the gastric motility and gastric emptying; both would alter the test results.

During the Test

• Assess the patient for any signs of watery diarrhea, abdominal cramps, or nausea because the dosage of lactose can exacerbate symptoms.

Posttest

• The patient can resume eating in 2 hours, after all the blood test samples are obtained.

• For the patient who is medically diagnosed with lactose intolerance, there is a need for nutritional instruction to modify the diet. The goals are to alleviate the abdominal symptoms and, at the same time, maintain calcium intake.

⦿ *Patient Teaching.* If the patient is diagnosed with lactose intolerance, the nurse or dietitian can teach the patient to restrict the intake of milk (lactose). Milk and food that contain milk or milk products cause varying degrees of abdominal discomfort among people. A lactase enzyme supplement may be helpful, but does not substitute for lactose restriction in the diet. The patient should also be taught that many nondairy foods contain lactose, including bread, baked goods, and biscuit and pancake mixes, among others. The nurse also teaches the patient to read the ingredient labels to avoid hidden sources of lactose.

• Most adults can tolerate 8 to 12 oz (1 glass) of milk daily and should be encouraged to continue ingesting the amount that can be tolerated. This will provide some calcium and other needed vitamins and minerals (A, D, riboflavin, and phosphorus). Soy and rice milk are tolerated well. Calcium supplementation in tablet form can be given so that the patient receives 1200 to 1500 mg of calcium per day.

Laparoscopy, Pelvic

Also called: Peritoneoscopy

SPECIMEN OR TYPE OF TEST: Endoscopy

PURPOSE OF THE TEST

Laparoscopy is used to investigate the cause of pelvic pain, to detect infected fallopian tubes, endometriosis or an ectopic pregnancy, to identify a pelvic mass, or to determine if cancer is present.

BASICS THE NURSE NEEDS TO KNOW

The laparoscope is a fiberoptic endoscope used to visualize the size and shape of the ovaries, uterus, and fallopian tubes. The peritoneal cavity and peritoneum are observed for signs of infection, abscess, or adhesions. Biopsy of abnormal tissue may be performed.

REFERENCE VALUES   No abnormalities of the ovaries, fallopian tubes, uterus, or peritoneal cavity are noted.

HOW THE TEST IS DONE

When general or regional anesthetic is used, the surgeon inflates the peritoneal cavity with 2 to 3 L of carbon dioxide. When local anesthetic and conscious sedation are used, the abdomen is insufflated with nitrous oxide gas. The gas distends the abdominal wall and provides space for the instruments. The laparoscope is inserted through a small incision just below the umbilicus, and the organs are visualized. If a biopsy, culture, or other surgical procedure is performed, a second incision is made in the lower abdomen for insertion of additional instruments.

SIGNIFICANCE OF TEST RESULTS

Abnormal Values

Ovarian cyst
Endometriosis
Ectopic pregnancy
Uterine fibroid tumors
Pelvic abscess
Pelvic inflammatory disease
Adhesions
Abnormality of the fallopian tubes
Malignancy

INTERFERING FACTORS

- Failure to maintain a nothing-by-mouth status
- Obesity
- Adhesions
- Anticoagulation therapy

NURSING CARE

Pretest
- After the patient has been informed about the procedure by the physician, the nurse obtains written consent from the patient and places the form in the patient's record. Ensure that all preoperative laboratory work is completed and that the results are posted in the record.

○ *Patient Teaching.* The nurse instructs the patient to discontinue all food and fluids for 8 hours before the procedure is performed.

- At the time of the surgery, the patient removes all clothes and puts on a hospital gown. The nurse identifies the patient by two forms of identification. Vital signs are taken and recorded, including temperature, blood pressure, pulse, and respirations. The nurse also verifies that the patient has not had anything to eat or drink in the past 8 hours.

Continued

| **NURSING CARE—cont'd** |

During the Test
- The nurse places the patient in the lithotomy position, with the legs supported in stirrups.
- An indwelling catheter is inserted into the bladder and connected to the urinary collection system. This keeps the bladder deflated and protects it from trauma or injury.
- The nurse provides reassurance to the patient until the anesthetic is administered.
- If a biopsy specimen is obtained, place the tissue in a glass container with preservative. The label is applied directly to the container with the patient's name, identification number, the physician's name, date, procedure, and type of the tissue. The requisition form has the same identifying information..

Posttest
- The nurse assesses the patient by monitoring the vital signs every 30 minutes for 4 hours or until they are stable. The small dressing(s) should remain dry and intact. Once the urinary catheter is removed, the nurse monitors the patient for resumption of voiding and urinary output.
- Once the patient is alert, the nurse encourages ambulation and the oral intake of fluids. Carbonated beverages are avoided for 24 to 36 hours. With the excess carbon dioxide in the abdomen, the intake of carbonated beverage can cause vomiting.
- The nurse provides pain medication as needed. Some pain in the abdomen and shoulder is to be expected for 24 to 36 hours. The cause is the carbon dioxide gas, which will gradually be absorbed and exhaled from the lungs.

○ *Patient Teaching.* The nurse instructs the patient to restrict physical activity for a few days until the incisions are healed. The patient is taught to notify the physician of increasing abdominal pain, fever, or abnormal drainage.

Lead, Blood

Also called: Pb

SPECIMEN OR TYPE OF TEST: Blood

PURPOSE OF THE TEST

This test is used to detect and measure the level of lead in the blood. It is also used as a screening test for people who are at risk for elevated lead levels.

BASICS THE NURSE NEEDS TO KNOW

Lead is a heavy metal in the environment that can enter the human body orally, through respiration of dust that contains lead, and by absorption through the skin. *Plumbism*, or lead toxicity, can occur as an acute condition because of recent exposure, or as a chronic accumulation of lead, over time. An elevated lead level in the body is highly toxic, causing damage to the bone marrow, the neurologic system, and kidneys. The blood test is able to measure recent exposure to lead but cannot evaluate the amount of lead already deposited in tissues from past exposure.

In children, the primary source of elevated lead levels is exposure to lead-based paint. The risk is highest for children of low socioeconomic status and with a history of inadequate nutrition including a lack of iron, calcium, and zinc. When a child is screened for a blood lead level, a value of greater than 45 to 69 µg/dL (SI: >2.17-3.33 µmol/L) indicates substantial exposure. At this level, current CDC guidelines for children recommend that an environmental investigation and control of hazard be done within 48 hours and that chelation therapy for the child be started immediately to help remove the lead from the body.

The majority of adults who have high blood lead levels were exposed through their work. Occupational exposure includes manufacturing of storage batteries, mining of lead and zinc ores, smelting, painting, wall paper hanging, and renovation, restoration or demolition of old houses (CDC, 2009). Based on Occupational Safety and Health Administration (OSHA) requirements, the adult with an occupational exposure and a blood lead level of greater than 50 mcg/dL (SI: >2.20 µmol/L) should be removed from the work setting to undergo medical evaluation and possible chelation therapy.

REFERENCE VALUES	Infant and Child: <10 µg/dL *or* SI: <0.48 µmol/L Adult: <25 µg/dL *or* SI: <1.21 µmol/L
▽ Critical Values	Children and Adult: >69 µg/dL *or* SI: >3.33 µmol/L Toxic Concentration 100 µg/dL or higher *or* SI: 4.83 µmol/L or higher

HOW THE TEST IS DONE
Venipuncture is used to collect a sample of blood.

SIGNIFICANCE OF TEST RESULTS
Exposure to lead
Lead toxicity, acute

INTERFERING FACTORS
• None

NURSING CARE

Nursing measures are similar to those used in other venipuncture or capillary puncture procedures (see Chapter 2), with the following additional measures.
Pretest
Health Promotion
For routine screening, the Centers for Disease Control and Prevention (CDC) currently recommends that all children ages 1 to 6 have an annual screening for lead levels. The nurse can teach parents the importance of the test and the need to detect lead content in the child's body at an early stage.

Continued

| NURSING CARE—cont'd

Posttest

- When the lead level is elevated, the nurse should assess the patient for signs of toxicity. At low to moderate levels of lead in the blood, the child will develop loss of some mental acuity, developmental lags, hearing loss, and growth delay. At moderate elevations, the child develops anemia, abdominal colic, and neuropathy. A nutritional assessment may also be indicated. In the adult, moderate elevations cause an elevation of the systolic blood pressure, a loss of hearing, infertility, and neuropathy.

O *Patient Teaching.* The nurse can teach the patient or family members about the sources of lead that may be in the patient's environment and the importance of removing the contaminants. The nurse can also advise the family to seek the assistance of the local health department regarding detection of the sources of lead exposure and advice on how to correct the problem.

▽ **Nursing Response to Critical Values**

At a blood lead level of 69 µg/dL (SI: >3.33 µmol/L) or higher, the patient is at serious risk for developing severe anemia and neurologic damage. The patient must be admitted to the hospital and undergo immediate chelation therapy for acute lead poisoning. The nurse notifies the physician of this elevated result.

Leukocyte Count

See White Blood Cell Count on p. 637

Lipase

SPECIMEN OR TYPE OF TEST: Blood

PURPOSE OF THE TEST

Lipase is a test to diagnose acute pancreatitis and can identify other sources of pancreatic disease.

BASICS THE NURSE NEEDS TO KNOW

Lipase is a pancreatic enzyme needed to help digest fatty acids. In pancreatic inflammation, this pancreatic enzyme cannot flow into the intestine because of inflammation or blockage in the pancreas, pancreatic duct, common bile duct, or intestine. Once there is obstruction of the flow, the lipase is secreted into the blood and the serum level rises. In pancreatic disorders, both serum lipase and serum amylase values are elevated on the first day of acute pancreatitis, but the lipase remains elevated in the blood for a few days longer than amylase.

REFERENCE VALUES   Adult: <200 units/L *or* SI: <3.4 µkat/L

HOW THE TEST IS DONE

Venipuncture is performed to collect a specimen of blood.

SIGNIFICANCE OF TEST RESULTS

Elevated Values

Acute pancreatitis
Chronic pancreatitis
Pancreatic cyst or pseudocyst
Pancreatic duct obstruction
Peritonitis
Strangulated or perforated bowel
Blunt force trauma to the abdomen
Colic from gallstone

INTERFERING FACTORS

- Heparin
- Narcotics
- Failure to maintain a nothing-by-mouth status

NURSING CARE

Nursing measures are similar to those used in other venipuncture procedures (see Chapter 2), with the following additional measures.

Pretest

○ *Patient Teaching.* Instruct the patient to discontinue food for 8 hours before the test.

Posttest

- If the patient has an elevated lipase value, assess for abdominal symptoms. Abdominal pain can range from mild to severe intensity. Nausea, vomiting, and jaundice may occur. Additional nursing assessments depend on the cause and severity of the problem.

Lipid Profile

Also called: Lipid Panel; Lipoprotein-Cholesterol Fractionation; Serum Lipids

SPECIMEN OR TYPE OF TEST: Serum

PURPOSE OF THE TEST

Lipid levels are used to identify individuals at risk for coronary artery disease (CAD) and as an evaluation tool to determine the effectiveness of "heart healthy" changes in lifestyle.

L

BASICS THE NURSE NEEDS TO KNOW

Most lipids are bound to protein in the blood and are called lipoproteins. Lipoproteins are usually measured to identify persons at risk for CAD. In the lab, lipoproteins are separated by electrophoresis. Fractionation of the lipoproteins is then performed according to their density. The following groups have been identified:

Very low-density lipoproteins (VLDL), which are made up of 70% triglycerides

Low-density lipoproteins (LDL), which are made up of 45% cholesterol (low-density cholesterol)

High-density lipoproteins (HDL) (high-density cholesterol)

A high correlation exists between elevated VLDL and LDL levels and CAD. Research has shown that HDL may help prevent CAD because it seems to inhibit the uptake of LDL.

REFERENCE VALUES*

Cholesterol, Total
<200 mg/dL *or* SI: <5.18 mmol/L

LDL
Child: <110 mg/dL *or* SI: <2.85 mmol/L
Adult: <100 mg/dL *or* SI: <2.59 mmol/L
Patient at high risk for cardiovascular disease: ≥190mg/dl *or* ≥4.92mmol/L

HDL
Male: >40 mg/dL *or* SI: >1.04 mmol/L
Female: >55 mg/dL *or* SI: 1.42 mmol/L
Approximately 10 mg/dl *or* 0.20 mmol/L higher in African Americans

LDL:HDL ratio
<3

Triglycerides
<150 mg/dl *or* <1.70 mmol/L

*Vary with reference group.

HOW THE TEST IS DONE

A venipuncture is necessary for a lipid profile. If a low-density cholesterol level determination is performed as a screening test, a drop or two of blood is obtained from a finger stick using a sterile lancet, and the blood is collected in a capillary pipette.

SIGNIFICANCE OF TEST RESULTS

Cholesterol

Elevated Values
Alcoholism
Arteriosclerosis
Diabetes mellitus
Hepatitis (early stage)
High-fat diet

Hypothyroidism
Nephrotic syndrome
Obstructed bile duct
Pancreatitis
Genetic factors

Decreased Values
Hyperalimentation
Hyperthyroidism
Liver disease
Malabsorption
Malnutrition

HDL
Elevated Values
Alcoholism
Diabetes mellitus
Exercise
Myxedema
Nephrotic syndrome
Pancreatitis

Decreased Values
Arteriosclerosis
Hyperalimentation
Hypothyroidism
Malabsorption
Malnutrition

LDL
Elevated Values
Alcoholism
Diabetes mellitus
Nephrotic syndrome
Pancreatitis

Decreased Values
Arteriosclerosis
Hyperalimentation
Malabsorption
Malnutrition

Triglycerides
Elevated Values
Alcoholism
Arteriosclerosis
Diabetes mellitus

L

Myxedema
Nephrotic syndrome
Pancreatitis

Decreased Values
Hyperalimentation
Malabsorption
Malnutrition

INTERFERING FACTORS

- Diet affects the results of a lipid profile and fractionation outcome. Has the patient been dieting to lose weight? If the patient has had a recent physical trauma or myocardial infarction, results will also be affected.
- Smoking may affect results.
- Medications such as estrogen, steroids, birth control pills, and hypolipid agents cause an inaccurate lipid picture.
- Alcohol intake
- High triglycerides will affect low-density cholesterol levels.
- For cholesterol screening, eating a diet high in saturated fats will affect the results.

NURSING CARE

Health Promotion
The nurse encourages people between the ages of 45 and 65 to have their cholesterol level checked every 5 years. This is to identify those at risk for atherosclerosis and CAD. A strong family history of CAD may indicate an earlier need for evaluation.

- Nursing measures are similar to those used in other venipuncture or capillary procedures (see Chapter 2), with the following additional measures.

Pretest

○ *Patient Teaching.* The nurse instructs the patient to fast for 10 to 12 hours before the blood sample is taken. If only a low-density cholesterol screening is planned, instruct the patient to refrain from eating a high-fat diet for 12 hours before the blood is drawn.

○ *Patient Teaching.* Avoid physical activity immediately before the blood is drawn.

- Inquire if the patient has been on his or her normal diet for the last 2 to 3 weeks.

Posttest

- Review results with the patient. The nurse needs to assess patients with elevated low-density cholesterol or high triglycerides for other modifiable risk factors for CAD, such as smoking, obesity, sedentary lifestyle, and hypertension.
- To reach lipid goals, diet and exercise education may be necessary. If significantly elevated, medication with diet and exercise is usually ordered.
- Home cholesterol screening is available. The reported accuracy for the home cholesterol test kits is 98%, which is consistent with tests done in physicians' offices. The accuracy of the home cholesterol test depends on the ability of the user to follow the manufacturer's guidelines. A major problem with home testing is the ability of the patient to understand and interpret the results.

- Before home cholesterol testing is taught, assess the person's medical history. The test is not recommended for anyone with a bleeding disorder or who is receiving anticoagulation therapy. Instruct the person to avoid vitamin A, acetaminophen, and mesalamine for at least 4 hours before the test. Warn the patient to check the packing of the kit for breaks and not to use the test if the foil package is not intact or if sterility of the lancet is questionable.
- ○ *Patient Teaching.* Home cholesterol testing requires capillary blood. Instruct the person to wash the hands before testing in warm soap and water. Warn the person not to use alcohol or hydrogen peroxide to clean the skin. Instruct the patient to obtain the blood sample from the side of a fingertip, which has fewer pain sensors and a better blood supply than the center. Instruct the patient to follow the manufacturer's guidelines. Multiple steps are required, with different timings at different steps. Inform the person that cholesterol levels will be affected by diet. One test result is not adequate. Repeating the test is recommended. Instruct the person to notify his or her physician or nurse practitioner if results are greater than 200 mg/dL.

Lipoproteins

See Lipid Profile on p. 417.

Liver-Biliary Scan

See Hepatic-Biliary Scan on pp. 377-380

Low-Density Lipoproteins

See Lipid Profile on p. 417

Lumbar Puncture and Cerebrospinal Fluid Analysis

Also called: (LP); Spinal Tap, CSF Analysis
Includes: ß-Amyloid protein 42, tau protein

SPECIMEN OR TYPE OF TEST: Cerebrospinal fluid

PURPOSE OF THE TEST

Lumbar Puncture

This procedure is performed to measure the pressure of the cerebrospinal fluid, to detect obstruction in the circulation of this fluid, and to obtain a sample of the cerebrospinal fluid for cellular, chemical, and microbiologic analysis.

Cerebrospinal Fluid Analysis

These laboratory tests are performed to confirm the diagnosis of infection in the central nervous system or to identify a tumor or hemorrhage in the brain, spinal cord, or surrounding lining of the neurologic tissues. It may be performed to confirm a chronic central nervous system infection, such as neurosyphilis or meningitis, or an inflammatory or autoimmune disorder affecting the central nervous system, such as multiple sclerosis. In the future, biochemical markers in the cerebrospinal fluid may be used to identify early-stage Alzheimer's disease.

BASICS THE NURSE NEEDS TO KNOW

Lumbar Puncture

This procedure is used to obtain the sample of cerebrospinal fluid for analysis. It involves the insertion of a sterile spinal needle between the lumbar vertebrae into the subarachnoid space. The level of the tap is usually in the fourth or fifth lumbar interspace. This avoids any damage to the spinal cord that ended at L-1 or L-2

Cerebrospinal Pressure

Once the needle is in the subarachnoid space, the pressure of the fluid is measured by a manometer, connected to the spinal needle. An opening pressure of <180 mm H_2O is normal. Then the fluid in the manometer will rise to its final pressure reading. An opening pressure reading greater than 200 mm H_2O is abnormal. If the pressure is normal, a specimen of up to 20 mL can be removed. Because children have less total fluid in proportion to age and body size, the specimen sample must be considerably smaller. If the child's opening pressure is higher or lower than normal, the amount of the specimen is limited to 1 to 2 mL.

Analysis of the Cerebrospinal Fluid

Appearance

The normal cerebrospinal fluid is clear and colorless, with a viscosity similar to that of water. Cloudy fluid is caused by an increased number of cells in the fluid. Gross blood may be present and is caused by a traumatic tap, a subarachnoid hemorrhage, or an intracerebral hemorrhage.

Microscopic Examination

The normal total cell count is low in adults and children of all ages. When a high elevation of leukocytes exists, the cause is often bacterial meningitis. A cloudy specimen is associated with a white blood cell count of more than 200 cells/µL. A very high count may be greater than 50,000 cells/µL.

The cerebrospinal fluid may be cultured to identify the infectious agent. Immunologic examination also may be performed to detect the specific microbial antigen present in bacterial or fungal meningitis. Immunologic testing may include the testing performed to confirm neurosyphilis. DNA-PCR technique can identify the genome of the mycobacterium of tuberculosis or the particular virus causing viral meningitis. DNA identification of the bacterial or fungal organism is not yet possible.

Malignant cells indicate a primary or metastatic tumor. Cytologic examination may be performed to identify the cells of the primary or metastatic tumor. The cells are shed from a malignant tumor that has extended into the ventricles or subarachnoid space. Metastases are commonly from melanoma, leukemia, lymphoma, or cancer of the breast, lung, or gastrointestinal tract.

Differential Cell Count   Normally, lymphocytes and monocytes are the predominant cells in cerebrospinal fluid. In bacterial meningitis, the neutrophil count is greatly elevated. In other causes of meningitis (fungal, tubercular, viral), an increased lymphocyte and monocyte count occurs. Multiple sclerosis is associated with an increase in lymphocytes and plasma cells. Malignant cells may also be present.

Chemical Analysis

Glucose   The glucose concentration is proportionate to the level of blood glucose. Within a period of 2 hours before the spinal tap, the glucose level in the cerebrospinal fluid is normally 60% to 70% of the blood level. To interpret the glucose level of the cerebrospinal fluid correctly, a blood specimen for glucose must be drawn 30 to 60 minutes before the spinal tap is performed. Higher-than-normal values of glucose in the cerebrospinal fluid reflect hyperglycemia. Lower-than-normal values (<40 mg/dL) of glucose in the cerebrospinal fluid occur with many forms of meningitis, neoplasm, inflammatory disorder, and other conditions.

Protein   Some protein is normally present in the cerebrospinal fluid, but an excessive increase or decrease is indicative of a problem. The increased level may be the result of increased permeability of the blood-brain barrier, allowing protein to pass into the cerebrospinal fluid. It may also be the result of poor resorption of the protein or of an increase in immunoglobulin synthesis. Decreased protein values occur when an increase in water resorption occurs, such as with increased intracranial pressure or with leakage of the cerebrospinal fluid as the result of head trauma. Because a measurement of cerebrospinal fluid protein does not indicate the cause of abnormality, there are numerous additional protein tests that can be performed to help with specificity.

Oligoclonal Bands   If present, oligoclonal bands are detected by protein electrophoresis performed on the cerebrospinal fluid. The presence of these bands is abnormal and supports the diagnosis of inflammatory or autoimmune disorder that affects the central nervous system. A positive test result is very common in patients with multiple sclerosis.

β-Amyloid Protein 42 and Tau Protein   These two proteins of the cerebrospinal fluid are potential biochemical markers to identify early-stage Alzheimer's disease. If Alzheimer's disease is present, the ß-amyloid protein 42 is decreased or is significantly lower than the normal value. At the same time, the tau protein level rises significantly. When both tests are used in combination, the abnormal results appear to be sensitive indicators of Alzheimer's disease before clinical symptoms are overt. Medical research continues to explore the role of these two proteins as clinical markers of Alzheimer's disease (Kelley & Minegar, 2009; Ringman, Younkin, Practico et al, 2008.)

REFERENCE VALUES

Cerebrospinal Fluid Analysis
Pressure: <180 mm H_2O (lateral recumbent position)
Appearance: Clear, colorless

Leukocyte Count
Neonate-1 year: 5.0-21 cells/µL *or* SI: 5-21 $\times$ 10^9/L
Adult: 0-5 cells/µL *or* SI: 0-5 $\times$ 10^3 cells /mL

Continued

Differential Count
Neonate
Lymphocytes: 5%-35% *or* SI: 0.05-0.35 number fraction
Monocytes: 50%-90% *or* SI: 0.50-0.90 number fraction
Neutrophils: 0%-8% *or* SI: 0.00-0.08 number fraction
Adult
Lymphocytes: 60%-80% *or* SI: 0.60-0.80 number fraction
Monocytes: 10%-40% *or* SI: 0.10-0.40 number fraction
Neutrophils: 0%-15% *or* SI: 0.00-0.15 number fraction

Glucose
60% of the patient's plasma glucose concentration
Adult 40-70 mg/dL *or* SI: 2.2-3.9 mmol/L
Child 60-80 mg/dL *or* 3.3-4.4 mmol/L

Total Protein
Adult: 8-32 mg/dL *or* SI: 80-320 mg/L
Newborn-1 year: 40-120 mg/dL *or* 400-1200 mg/L

Oligoclonal Bands
Negative

ß-Amyloid 42 protein
394.6 pg/mL

Tau protein, total
148 pg/mL

▼ **Critical Values**

Cerebrospinal fluid pressure: >300 mm H_2O
Bacterial, fungal mycobacterial, yeast or viral culture: positive
DNA-PCR of virus or mycobacterium: positive

HOW THE TEST IS DONE

Lumbar Puncture

Under sterile conditions and using local anesthetic, the physician inserts a spinal needle between the lower lumbar vertebrae and into the subarachnoid space (Figure 62). After pressure measurements are determined by manometer readings, spinal fluid is collected in three or more sterile tubes.

SIGNIFICANCE OF TEST RESULTS

Elevated Values
Intracranial Pressure
Brain tumor
Intracranial hemorrhage
Hydrocephalus

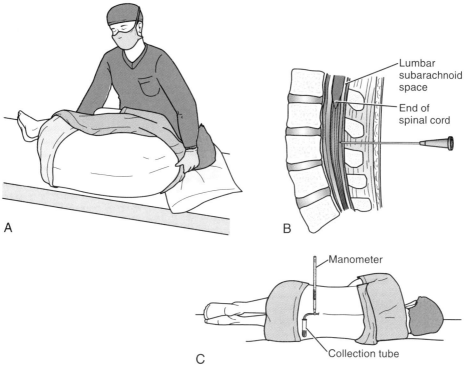

Figure 62. **A,** Patient position for lumbar puncture. **B,** The spinal needle is inserted into the subarachnoid space. From the flow of fluid out of the needle hub, samples of cerebrospinal fluid are collected in sterile tubes. **C,** The manometer measures the opening pressure and monitors the pressure during the lumbar puncture procedure.

Cerebral edema
Meningitis
Leukocytes
Bacterial meningitis
Neutrophils
Bacterial meningitis
Encephalomyelitis
Cerebral abscess
Cerebral hemorrhage
Cerebral infarction
Metastatic tumor
Lymphocytes
Meningitis
Multiple sclerosis
Parasitic infection
Glucose
Hyperglycemia

Total Protein
Meningitis
Stroke
Extradural abscess
Endocrine disorder
Trauma
Tumor
Herniated disk
Multiple sclerosis
Neurosyphilis
Oligoclonal Bands
Multiple sclerosis
Systemic lupus erythematosus
Neurosyphilis
Jakob-Creutzfeldt disease
T-Tau
Alzheimer's disease
Frontotemporal dementia

Decreased Values
Glucose
Acute or chronic meningitis
Meningoencephalitis
Systemic hypoglycemia
Subarachnoid hemorrhage
Neurosyphilis
Sarcoidosis (meningeal)
Total Protein
Trauma
Dural tear
Increased intracranial pressure
ß-Amyloid 42
Alzheimer's disease
Frontotemporal dementia
Vascular dementia
Jakob-Creutzfeldt disease
Amyotrophic lateral sclerosis

INTERFERING FACTORS

- Infection of skin or epidural abscess at the site of the proposed spinal tap
- Increased intracranial pressure
- Spinal block (incomplete or complete)
- Bleeding disorder

NURSING CARE

Pretest

- After the physician explains the test to the patient, obtain written consent from the patient and enter it into the patient's record.
- The patient's recent coagulation profile test result should be in the record and reviewed. A platelet count of less than 20,000/ μL, or a prolonged prothrombin time or thromboplastin time will result in prolonged bleeding into the tissues or cerebrospinal fluid. If the patient is maintained on anticoagulation therapy, the clotting profile is brought back to the reference range before the lumbar puncture procedure is done. Warfarin (Coumadin) is discontinued 5 to 7 days before the procedure and low molecular weight heparin is discontinued 12 to 24 hours before the lumbar puncture.
- The nurse verifies that a fasting plasma glucose test was done a few hours before the spinal tap.
- If needed, assist the patient in removing all clothing and putting on a hospital gown. Baseline vital signs are taken and recorded in the patient's record.
- Place the patient in a lateral recumbent position with his or her back at the edge of the bed or examining table. The patient's neck and knees are flexed toward the chest. The flexion of the spine widens the intervertebral spaces.

During the Test

- The nurse assists with the preparation of the equipment and sterile field, the antiseptic cleansing of the skin, and the preparation of the local anesthetic. Usually, 1 to 2 mL of lidocaine is administered subcutaneously by the physician.
- Instruct the patient to remain absolutely still during the insertion of each needle. The nurse holds the patient in position to help prevent movement. Provide reassurance to the patient as the needles are inserted. The administration of the anesthetic causes a stinging sensation. Brief pain also occurs as the spinal needle penetrates the dura and enters the subarachnoid space.
- Assist the patient in placing the legs in extension for the pressure reading. The nurse also assists with the collection of the cerebrospinal fluid. The tubes are marked "1," "2," "3," and so on, in the order in which they are collected. The first tube is used for chemical and immunologic analysis because blood or tissue fluid will not alter these test results. The second tube is used for microbial analysis, and the third tube for microscopic examination of cells. If only a small amount of fluid is drawn, it is placed in a single tube, and the physician prioritizes the tests.
- Every specimen tube must have a label that contains the patient's name, identification number, procedure and type of specimen, date, and physician's name. The requisition form has the same information as the labels. Arrange for immediate delivery of the specimen to the laboratory. With delay, lysis of the white blood cells results in a false decrease in the cell count and microbial organisms will be destroyed.

Posttest

- For the patient's record, the nurse verifies the time of the procedure, the position of the patient, the opening and final pressure readings, the color of the fluid, and the overall condition of the patient during the procedure.
- For nursing assessment, record all findings regarding vital signs every 30 minutes until they are stable. At the same time, assess the patient's level of consciousness and responsiveness.

Continued

▌ NURSING CARE—cont'd

Assess the puncture site for swelling, redness, bleeding, hematoma formation, or leakage of cerebrospinal fluid. At regular intervals, assess the patient's motor ability in the lower legs. If paresis (weakness) in the legs occurs, notify the physician immediately. The cause may be due to spinal blockage or severe compression of the cord. The paresis can progress to paralysis.

- Spinal headache (postlumbar puncture syndrome) sometimes occurs 24 to 48 hours after the procedure, although the incidence is much lower when a thinner or "atraumatic" needle is used for the lumbar puncture. A spinal headache usually causes pain in the back of the head, neck, and upper back, along with dizziness, orthostatic hypotension, as well as nausea, vomiting, and increased sweating. The symptoms are worsened when the patient stands erect and disappear when the patient is lying flat.

- Bedrest and increased fluid intake do not prevent spinal headache. Postprocedure, the patient may resume ambulation when ready. Recent research shows that there is no difference in the incidence of spinal headaches if the patient remains on bedrest or ambulates early (Williams, Lye & Umapathy, 2008). Extra fluid intake is encouraged in the belief that the fluids help replace the volume of fluid removed from the subarachnoidal space.

▽ **Nursing Response to Critical Values**

Increased Intracranial Pressure. An opening intracranial pressure reading of 300 mm H_2O or higher is considered a critical value. With a pressure reading at this very elevated level, the patient is in danger of a cerebellar herniation of the brain, with possible fatal consequences. Under these circumstances, the physician only removes a very small fluid sample.

The nurse assesses the patient for signs of increased intracranial pressure in the posttest period also. Abnormal findings include deteriorating levels of consciousness, including stupor or coma. Additionally, the patient may develop bradycardia, elevated blood pressure, slow or irregular respirations, and papillary changes. These findings are ominous and are reported to the physician immediately.

Infection. A positive culture or Gram stain with microscopic analysis of the cerebrospinal fluid that identifies meningitis is a very critical value. Isolation precautions will be instituted and antimicrobial treatment is started, as prescribed. The nurse assesses for high fever and the patient's complaints of pain in muscles (myalgia), headache, back pain, and photophobia (sensitivity to light). The nurse also assesses the patient's level of consciousness and any signs of meningeal irritation including a positive Kernig's or Brudzinski's sign. Seizures may occur. Abnormal assessment findings are reported to the physician immediately.

Lung Scans

Also called: Ventilation Scan; Perfusion Scan; Ventilation-Perfusion Scan (V/P scan); V/Q Scan; Ventilation-Perfusion Scintigraphy

SPECIMEN OR TYPE OF TEST: Radiography

PURPOSE OF THE TEST

Ventilation studies may be performed to evaluate patients with decreased pulmonary function. V/Q scans are usually carried out to diagnose pulmonary emboli.

BASICS THE NURSE NEEDS TO KNOW

For adequate oxygenation, the lungs must receive adequate alveolar ventilation and blood flow to the ventilated alveoli. Thus, two types of lung scans exist: a *ventilation scan* and a *perfusion scan*. Ventilation scans are performed to evaluate the distribution of gas within the lungs. The patient inhales a radioactive gas, and a scanner records the distribution of the gas as it enters and leaves the lungs. Perfusion scans evaluate arterial pulmonary blood flow. A radioactive dye is given intravenously, and a scintillation camera records the distribution of the dye as it passes through the right side of the heart to the pulmonary arterial bed.

Ventilation and perfusion scans (V/Q scans) may be performed together so that they can be compared to identify mismatching of ventilation and perfusion. V/Q scans are most often ordered to confirm the diagnosis of pulmonary emboli. The diagnosis of pulmonary emboli is difficult to confirm. Clinically, pulmonary emboli may be suspected because of chest pain, dyspnea, and hemoptysis, but pulmonary emboli are associated with other pulmonary and cardiac disorders, which makes the diagnosis difficult to confirm. Although pulmonary angiography is a diagnostic tool for pulmonary emboli, it is invasive. A V/Q scan is less invasive and therefore has fewer complications. It permits an evaluation of V/Q mismatching. Figure 63 demonstrates how alveolar-capillary blood flow must interface for adequate oxygenation.

When the radioactively tagged albumin is given intravenously, it circulates through the pulmonary vasculature. If a pulmonary artery is occluded, the part of the lung served by that vessel does not "take up" the radioisotope, and the scan is positive. The scan can verify a pulmonary occlusion. It cannot verify that the tissue is necrotic (pulmonary infarction). With the ventilation scan, decreased areas of ventilation are lighter, indicating poorly ventilated lung tissue. Additional information about Nuclear Scans is presented on p. 455.

L

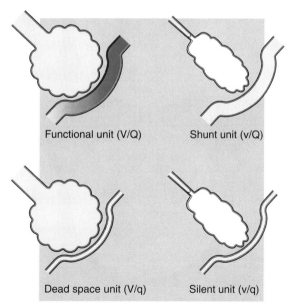

Functional unit (V/Q)   Shunt unit (v/Q)

Dead space unit (V/q)   Silent unit (v/q)

Figure 63. Alveolar-capillary interface. *V,* ventilated unit; *Q,* perfused unit; *v,* unventilated unit; *q,* unperfused unit.

While ventilation/perfusion scans were the tool of choice for diagnosing pulmonary embolism, multidetector computed tomography (MDCT) is replacing the scan. However, ventilation/perfusion scans are especially useful for patients with renal failure or those who have a history of allergy to contrast medium.

REFERENCE VALUES   Normal ventilation and perfusion
Ventilation-perfusion ratio of 0.85 or greater

HOW THE TEST IS DONE

Usually the ventilation scan is done first. With a ventilation scan, xenon-133 is most frequently used. If possible, the patient is positioned upright. Multiple scans are taken during (1) wash-in, as the radioactive gas builds up in the lung; (2) equilibrium, as the gas reaches its plateau within the lung; and (3) washout, as the radioactive gas is exhaled (Figure 64).

For a perfusion scan, albumin is tagged with a radioisotope, usually technetium-99, and given intravenously. As the tagged albumin passes through the right side of the heart into the pulmonary artery, a radiation detector scan of the lungs shows the diffusion of the radioactive albumin throughout the pulmonary vessels (Figure 65).

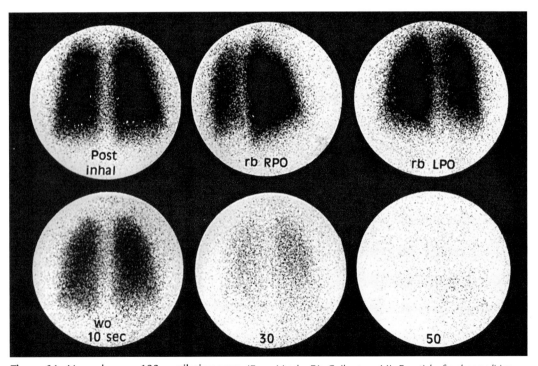

Figure 64. Normal xenon-133 ventilation scan. (From Mettler FA, Guiberteau MJ: *Essentials of nuclear medicine imaging*, ed 5, Philadelphia, 2006, Saunders.)

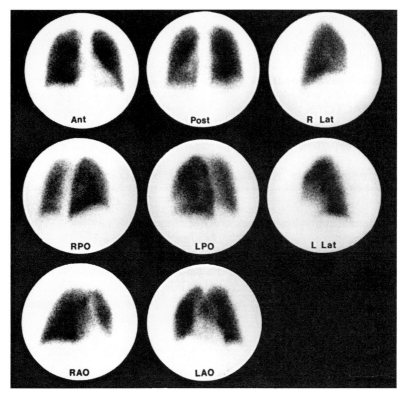

Figure 65. Normal perfusion lung scan in the standard eight projections. (From Mettler FA, Guiberteau MJ: *Essentials of nuclear medicine imaging,* ed 5, Philadelphia, 2006, Saunders.)

SIGNIFICANCE OF TEST RESULTS

Abnormal Values

Pulmonary Vascular Occlusion Resulting from the Following:

Thrombus

Cysts

Abscesses

Carcinomas

Necrotizing pneumonia

Inadequate Ventilation Resulting from the Following:

Atelectasis

Chronic obstructive pulmonary disease

Adult respiratory distress syndrome

Retained secretions

Pleural effusion

Pneumonia

Pneumothorax

Ventilation/Perfusion mismatch

Pulmonary embolism

Congenital pulmonary vascular abnormalities
Veno-occlusive diseases
Vasculitis
Lung cancer
Tuberculosis mediastinal adenopathy

INTERFERING FACTORS

- Uncooperative patient
- Severe pulmonary hypertension

NURSING CARE

Pretest
- Determine if patient is pregnant, because of the risks associated with radiation exposure.
- Schedule other radionuclide tests for 24 to 48 hours after the perfusion scan.
- *Patient Teaching.* Inform the patient about the procedure and ensure his or her cooperation.
- *Patient Teaching.* The nurse explains to the patient that the ventilation scan must be performed in the nuclear medicine department. Some hospitals have portable perfusion scanners.
- *Patient Teaching.* Advise the patient that with the ventilation scan, the inhaled gas should be held in the lungs for 20 seconds when the patient is instructed to do so.

During the Test
- Maintain the patient in an upright position for the ventilation scan. This position is maintained for at least 15 minutes.
- If the patient is unable to maintain the upright position, a supine position may be used with the gamma camera underneath the patient.
- After the radioactive gas is inhaled, encourage the patient to hold the breath for 20 seconds.
- After the ventilation scan is completed, the perfusion scan is done.
- Radiolabeled albumin is given to the patient intravenously.
- Six different views of the chest are obtained: anterior, posterior, right and left lateral, and right and left oblique.

Posttest
- The nurse evaluates the patient's response to the test. Most patients need to rest.

Lyme Disease Tests

Also called: Tests for *Borrelia burgdorferi*

SPECIMEN OR TYPE OF TEST: Serum; Cerebrospinal Fluid; Synovial Fluid, Skin

PURPOSE OF THE TEST

These tests are used to help diagnose the infection of Lyme disease.

BASICS THE NURSE NEEDS TO KNOW

Lyme disease is an infection caused by the spirochete *B. burgdorferi*. The infection is transmitted to the person by a bite from an infected tick. The infection progresses in two stages. In the early stage, most patients develop a characteristic bulls-eye rash and flulike symptoms.

In the late stage, the spirochete infects different tissues of the body including the heart, joints, and brain. The infection is difficult to diagnose because the symptoms vary among individuals.

Antibodies

In response to the infection, the immune system develops specific antibodies that can be detected by serologic testing of the blood. Unfortunately, antibodies to the spirochete do not appear in the blood until weeks after the tick bite, so antibody test results may not be positive until the late stage of the disease. The IgM antibodies do not start to develop until 10 days after the tick bite and the antibodies appear in the blood 3 to 6 weeks later. The IgG antibodies do not appear in the blood until 4 to 6 months later. If the patient has meningitis from Lyme disease, the cerebrospinal fluid may demonstrate the antibodies to *B. burgdorferi*.

DNA Identification

Using polymerase chain reaction (PCR) amplification technology, fragments of the DNA of the *B. burgdorferi* spirochete can be detected and identified from the patient's serum, cerebrospinal fluid, synovial fluid, or skin biopsy. This method is very specific and accurate in the identification of the spirochete at an early stage of infection.

REFERENCE VALUES   Negative for *B. burgdorferi*

L

HOW THE TEST IS DONE

Venipuncture is used to obtain a specimen of blood. Arthrocentesis is used to obtain a specimen of synovial fluid. Lumbar puncture is used to obtain a specimen of cerebrospinal fluid.

SIGNIFICANCE OF TEST RESULTS

Positive Value

B. burgdorferi infection

INTERFERING FACTORS

- Treatment with antibiotics before the testing is done.

NURSING CARE

Nursing measures are similar to those used in other venipuncture procedures (see Chapter 2), with the following additional measures.

Pretest

- Testing should be done before antibiotic therapy is initiated.
- In obtaining a nursing history, the patient may or may not remember a tick bite. After becoming infected, the skin rash appears within a month. The patient may have a travel or work history that included walking through high grass in a field or at the edge of a forest where ticks are found.

Continued

Posttest
Health Promotion
All people who undertake outdoor activity in tall grass or near the edge of a forest or park should take personal protective measures to prevent tick bites. These include the use of insect repellant with DEET, and wearing long pants and boots that protect the ankles and overlap the pant legs. Long-sleeved shirts and gloves protect the arms and hands when the individual is working in infested areas. The individual should inspect his or her skin for ticks daily. The dog in the household is also inspected daily for ticks embedded in the skin or lying in the fur.

Magnesium, Serum

Also called: Mg

SPECIMEN OR TYPE OF TEST: Blood

PURPOSE OF THE TEST

The measurement of serum magnesium helps to evaluate electrolyte disorders, hypocalcemia, hypokalemia, and acid-base imbalance. It also is used to monitor patients who have a cardiac disorder because low magnesium levels are dangerous to these individuals. The test is performed to monitor the pregnant patient with severe toxemia during the intravenous administration of magnesium sulfate.

BASICS THE NURSE NEEDS TO KNOW

Magnesium is one of the major intracellular cations of the body. Almost all magnesium is stored in soft tissue, muscle, and bone, with only 1% of the total magnesium present in the serum and extracellular fluid. Magnesium is obtained from food. The serum level is maintained in homeostatic balance by the functions of gastrointestinal absorption and excretion and renal resorption and excretion. Excess magnesium is removed from the body in feces and urine.

Elevated Values
Hypermagnesemia is an elevation of the serum value of magnesium in the blood. Most cases of hypermagnesemia are caused by advanced renal failure, with a decreased glomerular filtration rate and a resultant rise in the serum value of magnesium. The elevation also can occur from a high dosage of intravenous magnesium.

Decreased Values
Hypomagnesemia is a low level of magnesium in the blood. The deficiency of magnesium is usually associated with deficiencies of calcium and potassium.

Hypomagnesemia often occurs with inadequate food intake because of impaired intestinal absorption or as a result of hemodialysis treatment. It may also occur during long-term hyperalimentation or intravenous fluid replacement. Symptoms of hypomagnesemia do not appear until the serum level is very low. Hypomagnesemia together with hypokalemia is associated with a high rate of ventricular dysrhythmias. Patients with a cardiac disorder or an acute myocardial infarction are particularly vulnerable to a depleted magnesium level, and ventricular dysrhythmia or sudden death can occur. Hypomagnesemia is considered more serious than hypermagnesemia.

REFERENCE VALUES

Newborn: 1.5-2.2 mg/dL *or* SI: 0.62-0.9 mmol/L
Infant-child 5 months-6 years: 1.7-2.3 mg/dL *or*
   SI: 0.70-0.95 mmol/L
Child 6-12 years: 1.7-2.1 mg/dL *or* SI: 0.0.70-0.86 mmol/L
12-20 years: 1.7-2.2 mg/dL *or* SI: 0.70-0.91 mmol/L
Adult 21-59 years: 1.6-2.6 mg/dL *or* SI: 0.66-1.07 mmol/L
Adult 60-90 years: 1.6-2.4 mg/dL *or* 0.66-0.99 mmol/L

▽ **Critical Values**

<1.2 mg/dL (SI: <0.5 mmol/L) *or* >4.9 mg/dL (SI: >2.0 mmol/L)

HOW THE TEST IS DONE

Venipuncture is used to obtain a specimen of blood.

SIGNIFICANCE OF TEST RESULTS

Elevated Values

Advanced renal failure
Dehydration
Addison's disease
Multiple myeloma
Hypothyroidism
Tissue trauma
Lupus erythematosus
Magnesium sulfate infusion therapy

Decreased Values

Early renal disease
Chronic glomerulonephritis
Chronic alcoholism
Hypercalcemia
Pancreatitis
Hemodialysis therapy
Prolonged hyperalimentation
Diabetic ketoacidosis
Inadequate dietary intake
Prolonged intravenous therapy
Malabsorption
Hypoparathyroidism
Hyperaldosteronism

INTERFERING FACTORS

- Venous stasis
- Hemolysis

M

NURSING CARE

Nursing measures are similar to those used in other venipuncture procedures (see Chapter 2), with the following additional measures.

Pretest

○ *Patient Teaching.* The nurse instructs the patient to discontinue all food intake for 8 hours before the test.

During the Test

- The blood specimen is obtained without a tourniquet to avoid false-positive results.

Posttest

- The nurse monitors the laboratory test results for early warnings that the patient is developing difficulty related to the magnesium level. When the patient has a low level of magnesium, the serum potassium and serum calcium levels may also be low.

▽ **Nursing Response to Critical Values**

When the serum value of magnesium falls or rises to the critical value, the nurse must notify the physician immediately.

Elevated Critical Value. With severe hypermagnesemia, both cardiac and respiratory systems are slowed markedly. The pulse slows to 60 or less and the respiratory rate and effort are diminished. The patient may experience respiratory failure, unresponsiveness or coma, a loss of deep tendon reflexes, a heart attack or cardiac arrest. To support breathing and oxygenation, the nurse starts oxygen therapy at a low flow rate. If the patient is still somewhat responsive, place the patient in semi-Fowler's position. The nurse takes frequent vital signs and prepares for cardiac monitoring of the patient. Additional specific nursing interventions will depend on the medical cause of the problem and the physician's decisions about treatment.

Decreased Critical Value. Severe hypomagnesemia causes severe neuromuscular changes, as evidenced by tetany, convulsions, and cardiac arrhythmia. The nurse assesses for tetany, the hyperexcitability of nerves, and spasms of muscles. Reflexes are often described as 3 or 4 , brisk or hyperactive. Because of the risk of convulsions, the nurse institutes seizure precautions. Vital signs are taken, noting any irregularity of the pulse or heartbeat. The nurse prepares for cardiac monitoring. Cardiac arrest may occur.

Magnetic Resonance Imaging

Also called: MRI

○ **SPECIMEN OR TYPE OF TEST:** Magnetic field scan

PURPOSE OF THE TEST

Magnetic resonance imaging (MRI) is used to assess anatomic structures, organs, and soft tissue, including visualization of any pathologic condition that is present. It can differentiate between benign and malignant growth and may be used to stage cancer or evaluate the response to treatment of a malignancy.

BASICS THE NURSE NEEDS TO KNOW

MRI is a noninvasive imaging technique that uses large, powerful magnets and a radiofrequency coil to obtain cross-sectional images of body tissues. The images of axial planes are similar to those produced by computed tomography (CT) but MRI has a greater ability to produce images of any plane. This is particularly useful in imaging the head, neck, brain, and spinal cord. MRI can detect anatomic differences among tissues, including the difference between cystic and solid tissues or the differences among muscle, ligament, and tendon. It can also detect pathologic changes, including fluid-filled growths, edema, inflammation, hematoma, and neoplasm.

MRI is based on the biochemical differences among cells. The nuclei of cells contain many atoms that have electric fields. For example, each hydrogen atom has one proton with a positive charge. When in the presence of the strong magnetic field produced by the MRI magnets, the protons spin and move to realign in a new formation. The radio waves stimulate and detect the magnetized protons as they realign and then return to their original position. The different tissues have distinct qualities and patterns of movement. These differences are identified by the radiofrequency coil, and the messages are transmitted to the computer system for number coding and translation into images of the tissue.

Types of Magnetic Resonance Imaging Systems

The conventional MRI uses a *circumferential whole body* scanner. The entire body moves into a narrow chamber that is open at both ends (Figure 66). With an *open configuration* scanner, the patient is not completely enclosed in the cylindrical chamber, but the images may not be as clear as with the conventional scanner and the procedure takes longer. The third type of MRI is the *dedicated extremity* MRI (E-MRI). This system uses a special scanner to image the affected extremity only. The imaging is for the middle and more distal joints of the arm or leg.

M

Safety Concerns

Any ferromagnetic metal implant or other metal fragments within the patient's body are contraindications for this imaging procedure. The magnetic forces of MRI are so great that they will twist, damage, or move the metallic object and cause injury. The metallic items include

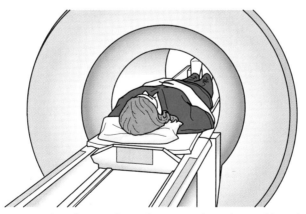

Figure 66. **Magnetic resonance imaging.** As the patient moves into the machine, the scanning process can provide images of neurologic, orthopedic, abdominal, and vascular tissues.

shrapnel, BBs, bullets, or other metal fragments that are imbedded in the body, particularly those located in or near the eyes or brain. Implants that are contraindications for the test include aneurysmal vascular clips, vascular stents, pacemakers, cochlear implants, joint implants, intrauterine devices, surgical screws, clips, staples, and other implanted therapeutic devices.

Dental appliances must be removed, but dental braces and a permanent dental bridge are acceptable. Although they are visible in the MRI images, they are not likely to interfere with the findings. During the imaging, the patient will feel vibration in the fillings of the teeth, but the vibrations will do no damage.

A strong magnetic force also exists around the outside of the scanner. The examination room must be kept clear of all extraneous metal objects such as oxygen tanks, wheelchairs, canes, crutches, and vacuum cleaners. No person can enter the examination room with coins, keys, stethoscopes, pens, credit cards, scissors, or hairpins. If these items are present, they become missiles that will be pulled into the scanner with force. The patient can be seriously injured by these objects.

Magnetic Resonance Angiography (MRA)

Vascular imaging by MRI is done to evaluate blood flow and the structure and location of the major blood vessels. Some studies require no contrast medium. When contrast is used, there is minimal occurrence of side effects and a lower toxicity than iodinated contrast (Frank, Long & Smith, 2007). In the head and neck, this procedure is used for imaging of the circle of Willis and the carotid arteries (Figure 67). In the evaluation of major arteries of the torso, the aorta and the renal, mesenteric, and iliac arteries can demonstrate an aneurysm,

M

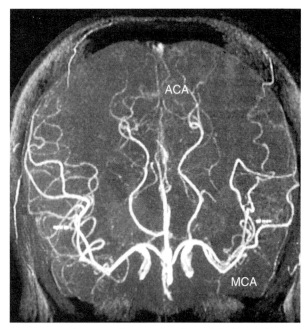

Figure 67. Magnetic resonance angiogram. The anterior view of the head shows the normal intracerebral vessels including the anterior cerebral artery (ACA) and the middle cerebral artery (MCA). No contrast medium was used for the imaging. (From Mettler FA: *Essentials of radiology,* ed 2, Philadelphia, 2005, Saunders.)

dissection, and coarctation. MRA is also used to visualize impaired blood flow in cases of peripheral vascular disease. In vascular applications, the procedure often is done before medical or surgical intervention. The data help to determine whether the problem can be corrected by endovascular stenting, angioplasty, or surgical repair with bypass or graft replacement of the blood vessel.

Brain and Spinal Cord Imaging

MRI is particularly valuable for assessment of the soft tissue of the brain and spinal cord. Although it cannot image the bones of the skull and vertebrae, it provides clear imaging of the organs and tissue contained within these bones. In the study of the brain, MRI provides images of tumors, cerebral edema, ischemia, multiple sclerosis, and other demyelinating diseases. In the study of the spinal cord, MRI provides images of disk degeneration, spinal cord tumor, epidural fat, and postoperative scar tissue that impinge on the cord or its nerve roots (Figure 68).

Musculoskeletal Imaging

The soft tissue structures of the knee, hip, and shoulder joints are most often examined. MRI provides clear images of tears in the menisci, ligaments, tendons, and muscles that provide the structure for the knee or shoulder joint. The procedure can distinguish between an inflammatory problem that will heal with conservative therapy and a tear that will require surgical repair.

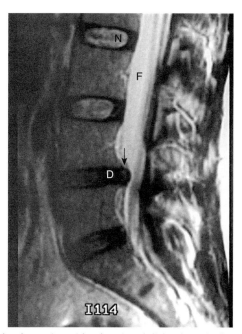

Figure 68. **MRI image of the lumbar spine with a herniated disk.** The spinal canal is filled with cerebrospinal fluid (F), except at the level of the linear nerve roots at the distal end of the spinal cord. Normal disks (N) remain in place between the vertebrae. At L 4-5, note the disk (D) that has herniated and protrudes into the spinal canal, pressing into the nerve roots. A slipped disk will cause acute radiating pain and neurologic symptoms in the lower back and legs. (From Frank ED, Long BW, Smith BJ: *Merrill's atlas of radiographic positioning and procedures,* ed 11, St Louis, 2007, Mosby.)

M

REFERENCE VALUES   No anatomic abnormalities are noted

HOW THE TEST IS DONE
While lying on the MRI table, the patient is moved into the tube of the MRI machine and precise imaging of the tissues is done. With computer systems directions, images of any plane can be produced.

SIGNIFICANCE OF TEST RESULTS
Abnormal Values
Tumor
Stricture
Stenosis
Thrombus
Embolus
Malformation
Abscess
Inflammation
Edema
Fluid collection
Bleeding or hemorrhage
Organ atrophy
Ligament tear

INTERFERING FACTORS
- Jewelry or other metal in the magnetic field
- Metallic implant in the body
- Patient movement during the scanning
- Claustrophobia

NURSING CARE

Pretest
- Although explanations about the test are given by the physician and final instructions are given by the MRI technologist, the nurse can be very helpful by answering the patient's follow-up questions and providing reassurance when the patient is apprehensive. An effective pretest orientation helps the patient be more aware and comfortable with the procedure. A signed consent is required and is placed in the patient's record.
- *Patient Teaching.* The nurse teaches the patient that as he or she moves into the chamber of the MRI machine, the space will be small, with only 3 to 10 inches of extra space around the patient. The chamber is usually lighted and has a fan to help cool the air. During the procedure, the machine's magnets cause loud knocking noises. The patient can wear earplugs or headphones to help lower the level of noise. The technologist and the patient can also communicate during the procedure. The nurse should also tell the patient that the procedure is painless and the imaging time lasts 20 to 90 minutes. The patient must remain still throughout that time so that the imaging will be clear.

○ *Patient Teaching.* Some patients become very anxious and claustrophobic in the narrow, noisy chamber. If the person shows some anxiety, the nurse responds with a calm demeanor. The patient may be able to maintain a calm feeling by using relaxation techniques, guided imagery, or listening to music. The elderly patient can become disoriented in the confusing environment. A friend or family member may be allowed to remain in the room during the procedure.

A sedative is given to the patient who is under the age of 3 or who is older than 3 but apprehensive and unable to remain still. Nursing research shows that based on individual assessments, some children aged 4 to 7 years can cooperate without sedation for brain MRI scans. Teaching coping strategies and diversion techniques to the child and family member is very useful in helping the conscious child to remain still during the scan (Bates, Coumeau, Robertson et al, 2010).

○ *Patient Teaching.* The patient removes all clothing and dons a hospital gown for the procedure. Before entering the room, the patient must remove jewelry, including rings, hair ornaments, hair pins, and body piercing items. These objects interfere with the imaging and would become missiles within the machine. They can also heat up and burn the skin. Patients with tattoos or permanent skin coloring of eyeliner or lip liner will have these areas covered with cool compresses. The tattoos can become red and swollen during the MRI. Some tattoos interfere with the imaging.

- If the patient wears an externally wired device such as a pulse oximeter or EKG leads, it must be detached and removed before the test. If left on, the wires would heat up and burn the patient's skin severely during the imaging process.

During the Test

- The technologist reviews with the patient how to communicate during the time in the chamber. The patient is also instructed to remain motionless on the narrow table during the test. If contrast medium is to be administered, it can cause a mild reaction on rare occasions. If an adverse reaction occurs, it is usually limited to nausea, vomiting, or hives that occur about 15 minutes after the intravenous injection.

Posttest

- If sedatives were administered, the nurse monitors the vital signs on a regular basis until the patient is responsive and awake. If no medication was administered, the patient can be discharged from the radiology unit as soon as the imaging is completed. If intravenous contrast was used, the nurse explains that it will be automatically eliminated in the urine within 24 to 48 hours. No special care measures are needed.

M

Magnetic Resonance Imaging, Pituitary Gland

Also called: Pituitary MRI

SPECIMEN OR TYPE OF TEST: Imaging

PURPOSE OF THE TEST

Magnetic resonance imaging (MRI) of the pituitary gland is performed to identify suspected hypothalamic-pituitary tumors and vascular abnormalities, including aneurysms, infarctions, and malformations.

BASICS THE NURSE NEEDS TO KNOW

MRI has significantly affected endocrine diagnoses because of its ability to identify small lesions of the pituitary gland. In most cases, it has eliminated the need for angiography in patients with suspected aneurysms or vascular malformations. With MRI, the pituitary stalk and gland, as well as the optic chiasm and the intercavernous portion of the carotid artery, are visualized.

REFERENCE VALUES   Normal pituitary size and configuration

HOW THE TEST IS DONE

MRI of the pituitary gland is usually performed once without contrast dye and then again with a contrast agent. Usually, gadolinium diethylenetriaminepentaacetic acid is given intravenously as the contrast medium.

SIGNIFICANCE OF TEST RESULTS

Abnormal Values

Adenomas
Aneurysm
Arachnoid cysts
Craniopharyngiomas
Hemochromatosis
Germinomas
Gliomas
Vascular malformations

INTERFERING FACTORS

• Patient has claustrophobia

NURSING CARE

See p. 440 for the nursing care associated with an MRI.

Mammography

Also called: Mammogram

SPECIMEN OR TYPE OF TEST: Radiography

PURPOSE OF THE TEST

Mammography is used to screen for asymptomatic breast cancer and investigate a symptomatic change in the breast tissue.

BASICS THE NURSE NEEDS TO KNOW

Mammography can identify tumors in the breast that are less than 5 mm in diameter. Because this small size is not palpable on physical examination, mammography can detect cancer at a very early stage of growth. Although this imaging does not detect every malignancy of the breast or those malignancies that are still very small but growing aggressively, it does identify most of the tumors in time to aid in a cure. Because of routine screening by mammography and subsequent early treatment, the rate of death from cancer of the breast has declined dramatically (Kopans, 2010).

In the mammography images, malignancy of the breast appears as a dense mass with irregular margins. The malignancy also may appear as numerous tiny clusters of calcification. Additional abnormalities that may indicate malignancy include a newly developed area of density and asymmetry of the breast. Benign growths also are visible and appear more rounded and have well-defined margins.

REFERENCE VALUES   **The breast tissue is within normal limits.**

HOW THE TEST IS DONE

• X-ray film or digital images of each breast are taken from different angles (Figure 69). The patient is positioned standing or seated in front of the machine, with the breast placed on the platform over the x-ray cassette. The compressor is applied to the top of the tissue. The breast is compressed between the two surfaces to hold the tissue firmly in place. Each breast is imaged separately.

M

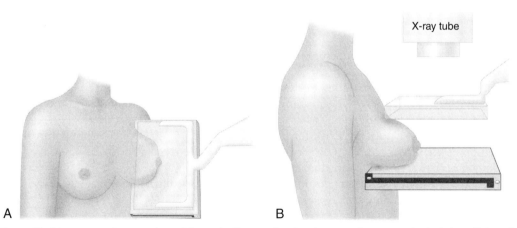

A   B

Figure 69. Mammography procedure. Schematic diagram showing the normal setup to obtain **(A)** mediolateral oblique (MLO) and **(B)** craniocaudal (CC) compression views of the breasts. (From Major NM: *A practical approach to radiology,* Philadelphia, 2006, Saunders.)

SIGNIFICANCE OF TEST RESULTS

Abnormal Values

Benign cyst
Microcalcifications
Fibroadenoma
Malignancy of the breast

INTERFERING FACTORS

- Jewelry and clothing
- Scar tissue from previous surgery
- Body powders, creams, and deodorants
- Silicone breast implants

NURSING CARE

Pretest

○ *Patient Teaching.* The nurse instructs the patient to omit the use of body creams, powders, and deodorants on the day of the test. The metallic elements in these products interfere with visualization of the tissues.

○ *Patient Teaching.* At the imaging center, instruct the patient to remove all jewelry and clothing above the waist. The hospital gown is put on with the opening to the front.

Posttest

Health Promotion

The US Preventive Service Task Force (2009) recommended that at age 50 years, all women begin to have mammograms every 2 years. This method and timing of screening for breast cancer should continue for ages 50 to 74 years. Possibly, women age 75 years and older can discontinue mammography screening. The task force also recommended discontinuance of teaching self-breast examination to patients. These recommendations are meant for women of average risk of developing breast cancer.

These newest guidelines for screening are controversial regarding the age when screening should begin and the frequency of the screening. Some researchers believe that mammography screening should be recommended for the age group 40 to 49 and not started later (ages 50 and above). They also believe that screening should be recommended annually for women ages 50 to 74 years and not every 2 years as is presently stated (Kopans, 2010).

For women who have a high risk for breast cancer, including a positive family history, a mutation of the BRCA gene, or a history of radiation therapy to the chest, the scheduling for mammography screening is individualized. MRI visualization of the breasts may also be used, particularly for high-risk patients. MRI cannot be used for routine screening of the general population, but it is highly sensitive and accurate in the detection of breast cancer.

Measles Antibody

Also called: Rubeola Antibody

SPECIMEN OR TYPE OF TEST: Blood

PURPOSE OF THE TEST

The test of the serum is sometimes used to diagnose the cause of a viral rash, particularly in the pregnant female. A positive immunoglobulin M (IgM) antibody result documents the acute phase of illness. The immunoglobulin G (IgG) antibody is used to document past infection of measles or effective immunization against measles.

The test of the cerebrospinal fluid for measles antibody is used to diagnose the neurologic complications of measles.

BASICS THE NURSE NEEDS TO KNOW

Measles (rubeola) is a viral infection transmitted by droplet and respiratory secretions from an infected person. At the time that the rash appears in acute measles infection, the levels of IgM and IgG antibodies are rising. These values peak in about 10 days. One to three months after the infection, the IgM antibodies disappear. The IgG antibodies decline somewhat, but the value should remain positive for life. There are incidences when the antibody IgG disappears in the late teenage period. If it disappears, the person is vulnerable to infection or reinfection.

Measles can be prevented by administration of a vaccine. Four weeks after vaccination, the antibodies appear in the blood.

REFERENCE VALUES
Antibody IgM: <1:10; negative
Antibody IgG: <1:5; negative

HOW THE TEST IS DONE

Venipuncture is used to collect a specimen of blood.

SIGNIFICANCE OF TEST RESULTS

Elevated Values
Antibody IgM
Measles infection (acute stage)
Multiple sclerosis
Antibody IgG
Past measles infection
Immunity to future measles reinfection
Past vaccination with immunity

INTERFERING FACTORS

• None

| NURSING CARE

Nursing actions are similar to those used in other venipuncture procedures (see Chapter 2), with the following additional measures.
Pretest
• Teach the patient that the elevated or positive value of the IgG antibody indicates immunity to future measles infection. This occurs as a result of immunization or past infection.

Continued

Posttest

◉ *Patient Teaching.* If vaccination has not been done, teach the parents to have their children vaccinated. The vaccine may be a combined measles, mumps, and rubella (MMR) vaccine or measles, mumps, rubella, varicella-zoster (MMRW) vaccine. For children, the recommended schedule is that the vaccine be given at 15 months and again at 4 to 6 years or 11 to 12 years. Despite vaccination programs in the United States, outbreaks of measles infection can occur in population groups that have not been vaccinated, including people who have recently immigrated to this country.

• If the antibody titer is negative after vaccination, encourage the person to be revaccinated.

Mediastinoscopy

SPECIMEN OR TYPE OF TEST: Endoscopy

PURPOSE OF THE TEST

Mediastinoscopy is performed to determine invasion of lung cancer into the mediastinum; this determination can be used to "stage" lung cancer. Staging assists in determining appropriate treatment modalities. Mediastinoscopy also may be performed for diagnosing suspected granulomatous infections and other intrathoracic diseases, including sarcoidosis and lymphoma.

BASICS THE NURSE NEEDS TO KNOW

Mediastinoscopy is a surgical invasive procedure in which the mediastinum is entered to determine whether cancer has invaded the mediastinum or its lymph nodes. The procedure involves the insertion of an endoscope into the mediastinum, permitting visualization of the lymph nodes and biopsy of mediastinal nodes and tissue.

REFERENCE VALUES   No pathologic cells

HOW THE TEST IS DONE

With the patient under general anesthesia, a small incision is made over the suprasternal fossa and a mediastinoscope is inserted gently. The mediastinum, with its lymph nodes, is visualized; it may be photographed and tissue samples removed.

SIGNIFICANCE OF TEST RESULTS

Bronchogenic carcinoma
Esophageal cancer
Granulomatous infections
Lymphomas
Sarcoidosis

INTERFERING FACTORS

- Noncompliance with dietary restrictions
- Phenytoin hypersensitivity (may cause false-positive cytologic findings)

NURSING CARE

The nurse takes actions similar to those for thoracic surgery.

Pretest

- Ensure that an informed consent form has been obtained.
- The nurse supports the patient, who is usually fearful of the outcome.
- ○ *Patient Teaching.* Explain the procedure to the patient.
- ○ *Patient Teaching.* Instruct the patient not to eat or drink after midnight.
- The nurse performs preoperative care according to hospital protocol.

Posttest

- Take vital signs every 15 minutes until they are stable and then every 4 hours for 24 hours.
- The nurse checks the dressing to observe for bleeding or drainage.
- Reassure the patient that chest discomfort is temporary.
- Advise the patient to resume normal activities and diet when he or she has fully recovered from the anesthetic.

◆ **Nursing Response to Complications**

Complications are rare but include accidental puncture of the esophagus, the trachea, or compression of the innominate artery and trachea. The most serious complication is major hemmorrhage requiring emergency thoracotomy. The nurse ensures, before the procedure, preoperative protocols of the hospital have been instituted. Since a pneumothorax is possible, the nurse has equipment available for the insertion of a chest tube.

M

Methacholine Challenge Test

See Pulmonary Function Studies on p. 528.

Metyrapone Stimulation Test

Also called: Metyrapone Test

SPECIMEN OR TYPE OF TEST: Serum

PURPOSE OF THE TEST

Metyrapone testing is performed to diagnose secondary adrenal insufficiency and to assess pituitary-adrenal reserves.

BASICS THE NURSE NEEDS TO KNOW

Review the section on Adrenocorticotrophic Hormone (ACTH), Plasma (p. 44). Metyrapone is given to block cortisol synthesis. A decrease in cortisol will normally stimulate ACTH secretion, which, in turn, will increase the secretion of 11-deoxycortisol. If an increase occurs after the metyrapone is given, ACTH and adrenal function are normal. If an abnormal result occurs, that is, no increase in 11-deoxycortisol occurs, the diagnosis of adrenal insufficiency is established; however, it is unknown whether it is primary or secondary adrenal failure.

Insulin may be used as a stimulant, like metyrapone. The *insulin-induced hypoglycemia test* is similar to the metyrapone test. The hypoglycemia causes a stress response normally resulting in the secretion of corticotropin-releasing hormone (CRH), which causes an increase in ACTH secretion. This test allows the assessment of the hypothalamic-pituitary axis. Timing of the test is important as the results will vary due to circadian variations.

REFERENCE VALUES   11-deoxycortisol level: >7 mcg/dL *or* SI: >202 nmol/L
Serum ACTH: >150 pg/mL *or* SI: >33 pmol/L

HOW THE TEST IS DONE

Metyrapone is given orally at midnight, with milk or a snack. The dose is based on the patient's weight. At 8 AM, a venipuncture is performed.

SIGNIFICANCE OF TEST RESULTS

Abnormal response (no change in value)
Adrenal hyperplasia
Adrenal tumor
Ectopic ACTH syndrome

INTERFERING FACTORS

* Recent radioisotope therapy or testing
* Medication such as chlorpromazine, phenobarbital, corticosteroids

NURSING CARE

Nursing actions are similar to those used in other venipuncture procedures (see Chapter 2), with the following additional measures.
Pretest
* The nurse obtains a medication history and asks the physician if any interfering drugs should be withheld. The medications that are listed as interfering factors all enhance steroid metabolism and would alter the test results.

○ *Patient Teaching.* The nurse explains to the patient the need to take the oral medication on the night before the test and that the specimen of blood will be drawn promptly at 8 am the next morning. Instruct the patient to ingest nothing by mouth for 12 hours before the test.

◇ **Nursing Response to Complications**
For a patient with adrenocorticoid insufficiency, the administration of metyrapone, which inhibits cortisol production, may precipitate an addisonian crisis.

Addisonian Crisis. The nurse should observe for hypotension, muscle weakness, shock, hyponatremia, and hyperkalemia. Report the abnormal assessment findings to the physician immediately. Anticipate need for intravenous access and steroid therapy administration.

Mixed Venous Blood Gases

See Blood Gases, Mixed Venous on p. 145.

Mononucleosis, Infectious

Includes: Monotest; Heterophil Antibody Test

SPECIMEN OR TYPE OF TEST: Blood

PURPOSE OF THE TEST

These serologic tests help to diagnose infectious mononucleosis.

BASICS THE NURSE NEEDS TO KNOW

The Epstein-Barr virus is responsible for most cases of infectious mononucleosis. In this viral infection, the patient's immune response produces heterophil antibodies of the IgM class and Epstein-Barr antibodies. The infection is transmitted from the saliva of infected salivary glands. Once the infection starts, the virus replicates in many organs, including the liver and spleen. Six to 10 days after the symptoms appear, the heterophil antibodies can be detected or measured. The antibody level peaks in 2 to 3 weeks and usually persists for several months.

The monotest is a rapid, simple, and effective test that identifies the presence or absence of infectious mononucleosis antibodies in the patient's serum. The test is most accurate in patients who are in late adolescence and adulthood. It is not an accurate test for younger children. When the infectious mononucleosis antibodies are present, the test result is positive. The heterophil antibody test is used when the titer is to be measured. A heterophil antibody titer of 1:128 or higher means that the test result is positive.

| REFERENCE VALUES | Monotest (rapid heterophil antibody test) : Negative |
| | Heterophil antibody titer: Negative; <1:56 |

HOW THE TEST IS DONE

Venipuncture is used to collect a sample of blood.

SIGNIFICANCE OF TEST RESULTS

Elevated/Positive Values
Infectious mononucleosis

INTERFERING FACTORS

• Hemolysis

M

NURSING CARE

Nursing measures are similar to those used in other venipuncture procedures (see Chapter 2), with the following additional measures.

Pretest

Schedule this test a few days after the onset of illness. Until the antibodies have time to develop, the test results will remain negative. On the laboratory requisition, include the date of the onset of illness. The nurse assesses the patient for manifestations of the infection, including fever, sore throat, lethargy, and lymphadenopathy. Physical assessment findings include an inflamed oropharynx, tonsils, and possible petechiae on the soft palate. On palpation, the liver and spleen may be enlarged.

Posttest

- If the patient is diagnosed with mononucleosis, the virus is in the saliva and is contagious. The patient should refrain from kissing or oral contact with others and not share glasses or food utensils until several weeks after the symptoms disappear. Frequent handwashing is important.
- ○ *Patient Teaching.* If the spleen is enlarged, there is a small risk for possible rupture of the organ. The patient is taught to avoid athletic contact sports until several weeks after the symptoms of active infection disappear. Medical clearance is recommended before a return to athletic sports, such as wrestling, football, soccer, and weight lifting.

Mumps Antibody

Also called: Mumps Serology

SPECIMEN OR TYPE OF TEST: Blood

PURPOSE OF THE TEST

The immunoglobulin M (IgM) antibody test may be used to diagnose a mumps infection in the acute phase. The immunoglobin (IgG) antibody test is used to document long-term immunity after past infection or effective immunization.

BASICS THE NURSE NEEDS TO KNOW

Mumps, or parotitis, is a viral infection, transmitted by droplets from an infected individual to the respiratory tract, gastrointestinal tract, or conjunctiva of a susceptible person. The infection produces classic inflammation of lymph glands, salivary glands, and one or both parotid glands. In the male, the testes may become swollen and inflamed. Immunization with the measles, mumps, rubella (MMR), or measles, mumps, rubella, varicella (MMRV) vaccine usually produces immunity to future infection.

The IgM antibodies become elevated to a titer of 1:10 or higher, indicating the early, acute phase of illness. After 6 weeks, the rise of the IgG antibodies to a titer of 1:5 or higher indicates long-term immunity.

REFERENCE VALUES Mumps antibody IgM: <1-10; negative
Mumps antibody IgG: <1-5; negative

HOW THE TEST IS DONE

Venipuncture is used to obtain a specimen of venous blood.

SIGNIFICANCE OF TEST RESULTS

Elevated Values
Antibody IgM
Acute mumps infection
Antibody IgG
Past mumps infection, with current and future immunity
Mumps vaccination, with current and future immunity

INTERFERING FACTORS

• None

▌ NURSING CARE

Nursing actions are similar to those used in other venipuncture procedures (see Chapter 2), with the following additional measures.
Pretest
◉ *Patient Teaching.* Teach the patient that the positive value of the IgG antibody titer indicates immunity to future mumps infection.
Posttest
• If vaccination has not been done, teach the parents to have their children immunized for MMR or MMRV vaccine at 15 months and again at 4 to 6 years or 11 to 12 years. Despite immunization programs, outbreaks of mumps still occur. Unvaccinated people are usually recent immigrants, but there are others who do not want vaccines for their children or who have limited access to health care.
• With a negative IgG titer, the person has no immunity and is susceptible to mumps infection. The nurse encourages the person to be vaccinated or revaccinated to provide immunity.

M

Myoglobin, Serum

See Cardiac Markers on p. 175.

Myoglobin, Urine

SPECIMEN OR TYPE OF TEST: Urine

PURPOSE OF THE TEST

This test is used to identify the presence of myoglobinuria and to investigate severe muscle damage, ischemia, or inflammation.

BASICS THE NURSE NEEDS TO KNOW

Rhabdomyolysis is the breakdown of striated muscle tissue with a release of myoglobin in the urine. With severe injury or ischemia, skeletal or cardiac muscle tissue releases myoglobin into the blood. The kidneys filter the blood rapidly, and the myoglobin is excreted in the urine.

Myoglobinuria (myoglobin in the urine) in large quantities causes the urine to become a red to dark red and as it stands to a dark brown color similar in appearance to a cola beverage. It is difficult to distinguish by appearance between hemoglobin and myoglobin in the urine because the color change is similar. In addition, myoglobin will cause a false-positive value for hemoglobin or for occult blood when tested by dipstick. Myoglobin is nephrotoxic. Large quantities of this protein can occlude the renal tubules and result in acute tubular necrosis and acute renal failure.

Myoglobinuria has many possible causes. In skeletal muscle damage, the underlying cause may be muscle trauma, such as after a "crushing injury;" strenuous exercise, such as a marathon; or prolonged immobility, such as from muscle compression during prolonged unconsciousness. It may also result from toxic exposure, such as carbon monoxide inhalation or alcohol or cocaine ingestion.

REFERENCE VALUES

Qualitative method: Negative
Quantitative method: <0.5 mg/dL *or* SI: <5 mg/L

HOW THE TEST IS DONE
A random sample of urine is collected in a plastic container.

SIGNIFICANCE OF TEST RESULTS

Elevated Values
Severe muscle trauma
Arterial insufficiency to a large muscle mass
Strenuous exercise
Severe myositis
Myocardial infarction
Prolonged immobility
Dermatomyositis
Drug toxicity (alcohol, cocaine, barbiturates, amphetamine)
Carbon monoxide poisoning
Muscular dystrophy

NURSING CARE

Pretest
- If the patient is conscious, request a urine specimen, collected in a plastic container.
- If the patient is unresponsive or cannot assist, obtain the specimen from the port in the urinary catheter drainage system.

Posttest
- Send the specimen to the laboratory without delay. If the result is very elevated, treatment, including rehydration and restoration of electrolyte balance, must be done quickly to protect and preserve renal function.
- The nurse assesses the color of the urine. As the muscle tissue heals, there will be less myoglobin in the urine and the urine color lightens toward the characteristic yellow color.
- Urinary output is monitored. Urinary myoglobin can cause acute renal failure, which can cause diminished urinary output or anuria.

Neisseria gonorrhoeae

See Gonorrhea tests on p. 351.

Newborn Screening

SPECIMEN OR TYPE OF TEST: Blood

PURPOSE OF THE TEST

The purpose of screening newborn babies is to detect selected genetic disorders at a very early stage of life before devastating illness and damage occurs. The goal is to provide early treatment that would improve the long term prognosis for these children.

BASICS THE NURSE NEEDS TO KNOW

Newborn screening tests began in the 1960s with the development of the Guthrie test to detect the disorder of phenylketonuria (PKU). Since that time, blood tests for numerous other genetic disorders have been developed. Importantly, new laboratory equipment [Tandem Mass Spectrometry (MS/MS)] has been invented to analyze the large numbers of screening specimens in newborns and multiple tests for each baby. Today, there are more than 30 tests available to screen the newborn, using only one blood specimen per baby.

Newborn screening detects disorders that are present at birth but the disorders demonstrate no immediate symptoms. If undetected and untreated, these disorders will result in significant mental retardation, developmental disability, or death. The permanent damage usually occurs within months of birth. One of the selection criteria of a newborn screening test is that the disorder must have effective treatment that can limit the symptoms of illness and prevent disability before it occurs (Gilbert-Barnes, Kapur, Oligny & Siebert, 2007).

In the United States, the decision for mandatory screening and the choices of specific screening tests are controlled by the individual states and their respective legislators. Generally, the individual state health departments and their maternal and child health programs are responsible for implementation of the laws regarding screening in their states. The screening programs and the subsequent treatment for the children with the genetic disorder are funded under title V of the Social Security Act.

Testing for PKU and hypothyroidism are mandatory in all states of this country, but among all the states there is considerable variation regarding other tests that are included in mandatory newborn screening. The diseases that are more commonly assessed by newborn screening are presented in Box 7. In general, the tests include those for cystic fibrosis, selected endocrine tests, selected hemoglobin disorders, and selected disorders of metabolism. In some states, a mandatory screening test for hearing also is done, but since the method is not done by a laboratory test, the topic is beyond the scope of this book.

All screening tests have a somewhat high percentage of false-positive results. A false positive means that the test demonstrated a positive result, but the infant does not have the disease. False-negative results may also occur. False negative means that the infant has the disease, but the laboratory screening test was negative. When there is medical doubt about

BOX 7	Illnesses Commonly Included for Newborn Screening

Cystic fibrosis
Biotinidase deficiency
Sickle cell anemia
Homocystinuria
MCAD deficiency*
Fatty acid oxidation disorders
Phenylketonuria
Congenital adrenal hypoplasia
HB S/ß-thalassemia
Maple syrup urine disease
Tyrosinemia
Congenital hypothyroidism
HB S/C disease
Galactosemia
Organic acid disorders
Other amino acid disorders

*MCAD, Medium- chain acyl-CoA dehydrogenase

the screening test result, a repeat screening test may be done in 7 days. Positive screening tests are always followed up with more specific testing to confirm or exclude the final diagnosis.

REFERENCE VALUES   Negative

HOW THE TEST IS DONE

Capillary puncture of the heel is done to obtain a sample of the newborn's blood. The blood is collected on filter paper and dried before placing the paper in an envelope.

SIGNIFICANCE OF THE TEST RESULTS

Positive values

The conditions that have positive values depend on the tests that are used in the screening. See Box 7 for possible positive test results.

INTERFERING FACTORS

- Oversaturating the filter paper with blood
- Insufficient quantity of blood on the filter paper
- Little to no ingestion of milk [Guthrie test for phenylalanine (PKU) only]
- Antibiotics [Guthrie test for phenylalanine (PKU) only]
- Recent exchange transfusion

NURSING CARE

Nursing actions are similar to those used in capillary puncture procedures (see Chapter 2), with the following additional measures.

Pretest

- The newborn testing will be done between 24 hours after birth and before discharge from the nursery.
- For the infant who is discharged early or who is born at home, the testing is done within 7 days of birth, at the pediatrician's office, laboratory, or designated health care setting.

Neutrophils

See White Blood Cell Differential Count on p. 640.

Norepinephrine

See Catecholamines, Plasma on p. 180.

Nuclear Scan

Also called: Scintigraphy

SPECIMEN OR TYPE OF TEST: Radionuclide study

PURPOSE OF THE TEST

A nuclear scan is used to assess the physiologic function and assist in the localization of abnormality in a designated organ or tissue.

BASICS THE NURSE NEEDS TO KNOW

In most radiologic procedures, the source of the radiation is in a machine that emits radio waves aimed to pass through the patient from the external source. In the nuclear scan, the process is different, because the radiation source is within the patient. Once in the patient's body, the radionuclide is taken up, concentrated, and distributed in the targeted organ or tissue. For a short time, it emits gamma rays in the pattern and concentration that correspond to the physiologic uptake of that tissue. A gamma camera or scintillation scanner detects and records the emission of the gamma rays. The data are converted into a visual image by the computer and its special software.

In a nuclear scan, the source of the radiation is a radionuclide, a radioactive isotope that has a short half-life. This means that the isotope emits gamma rays or photons for a few hours and then loses strength. By the time it is excreted in urine or feces, the radioactivity is greatly reduced or negligible. Technetium (Tc 99m) is one of the most common radionuclides. Others include isotopes of iodine, xenon, gallium, indium, and thallium for scans of specific organs or locations.

In nuclear scanning, the radioisotope that is bound to a specific compound is called a radiopharmaceutical. When administered orally or intravenously to the patient, the radiopharmaceutical is taken up or absorbed by the target tissue or organ. The targeted tissue concentrates the radiopharmaceutical and emits radiation that is detected and imaged by the scanner or camera. Some of these scans, their purposes, and the pertinent patient care information are presented in Table 11.

Abnormal Findings

In a nuclear scan, the pathologic condition that affects the target organ or tissue results in abnormal uptake and distribution of the radionuclide. The abnormality may be a space-occupying lesion or tumor, nonfunctioning tissue such as scar tissue, a loss of structural integrity such as a fracture, or another abnormality. The types of abnormalities include deficiency of uptake, excessive uptake, localization of activity in focal areas of tissue, disseminated activity throughout the organ, and asymmetry when the results should be bilateral and symmetrical.

When the targeted organ or tissue is not visualized, no uptake of the radionuclide has occurred. One possible cause is that vascular or ductal obstruction blocks the radionuclide from reaching the target site. Another possible cause is that the organ is nonfunctional.

Decreased activity in the target organ is called a defect or a cold spot. Areas of tissue are nonfunctional because of the pathologic change in the tissue (Figure 70). For instance, an abnormal liver scan can demonstrate a defect because of a cyst or abscess that has formed a space-occupying lesion. Multiple focal defects are often the result of metastatic disease.

Increased activity in the target organ is called a focal abnormality or hot lesion in otherwise normally functional tissue. The excess activity may also involve the entire organ. For instance, the thyroid scan of the patient with Graves' disease demonstrates increased activity throughout the gland. In this condition, all the thyroid tissue is hyperactive and absorbs a maximum amount of the iodine radionuclide.

N

REFERENCE VALUES   There is normal uptake, distribution, and excretion of the radionuclide by the targeted organ or tissue.

HOW THE TEST IS DONE

An oral or intravenous dose of radiopharmaceutical is administered to the patient and a gamma camera or scintillation scanner records the radioactive emissions (Figure 71). These emissions are then converted to images that correspond to the location, distribution, and concentration of the radionuclide in the targeted organ or tissue.

SIGNIFICANCE OF TEST RESULTS

Abnormal Values

Organ atrophy or fibrosis
Congenital defect
Tumor or cyst
Metastatic lesions
Inflammation or abscess
Hyperactivity of organ function
Hematoma
Traumatic disruption of tissue

TABLE 11 Selected Nuclear Scans		
Name of Scan	**Purpose**	**Special Patient Care Measures**
Brain scan (positron emission tomography [PET] scan)	To evaluate brain tissue metabolism and function, with detection of abnormalities such as dementia, stroke, atherosclerosis, epilepsy, Alzheimer's disease; to identify size and shape of brain, with detection of tumor, hematoma, cyst, atrophy, or edema	Fasting is required for 4-6 hours before the test; water and medications are permitted; Diabetics who take insulin require special pretest measures and should consult the radiology department before the test; Radionuclide is injected intravenously; a computed tomography (CT) scan of the head is usually done at the same time; in the CT/PET scanner, the patient must keep the head motionless
Brain imaging scan (single photon emission computed tomography [SPECT] scan)	To visualize the function of the brain tissue in the evaluation of Alzheimer's disease, cerebrovascular disease, and the location of seizure activity	In the pretest period, the patient must remain in an nonstimulated state, with his or her eyes closed; the room is kept dark, quiet, and without traffic
Cerebrospinal fluid imaging scan (cisternography)	To investigate the passageway and flow of cerebrospinal fluid (CSF) in the ventricles of the brain; To help diagnose hydrocephalus or determine the patency of the CSF shunt; to investigate brain trauma, with the leakage of CSF.	If leakage of CSF from the ears or nose is suspected, packing is placed in these orifices; a lumbar puncture is performed to instill the radiopharmaceutical intrathecally; for adults, images are taken 4-6 hours after administration of the radiopharmaceutical and again after 24 hours. Additional images may be taken at 48 and 72 hours.
Thyroid scan with technetium (Tc 99m) or ^{123}I	To assess thyroid function in different regions within the thyroid gland; To help diagnose causes of hyperthyroidism, hypothyroidism, thyroid nodule(s), and cancer.	Check with patient if they are allergic to iodine or seafood. If patient is allergic to iodine or has been taking propylthiouracil, technetium may be used as the radiopharmaceutical agent. Technetium and iodine may be given intravenously and the image is then taken after 20 minutes. Iodine may be given orally in liquid or capsule form and the scan is then done after 24 hours although some labs do it after 3-4 hours;

N

Continued

TABLE 11	Selected Nuclear Scans—cont'd	
Name of Scan	Purpose	Special Patient Care Measures
		the patient is instructed not to swallow during the imaging; a small pillow is placed under the patient's scapular area and the neck is hyperextended during the procedure; observe for allergic reaction.
Liver-spleen scan	To assess the functional status of the liver and spleen; to identify focal or diffuse areas of deficit caused by tumor, fibrosis, cirrhosis, infection, circulatory abnormality, or trauma	The patient fasts for at least 4 hours before the scanning is done; the radiopharmaceutical is injected intravenously
Hepatobiliary scan	To assess for patency of the hepatic, biliary ducts, and gall bladder; To identify defects, abnormal function and blockage of the flow of bile anywhere in the biliary tract system	The patient takes nothing by mouth for 6-8 hours before the testing (some situations require only fasting for a minimum of 2 hours); Scanning time is up to 4 hours, with possible additional imaging for up to 24 hours
Myocardial perfusion scan with thallium-201, technetium 99m sestamibi or technetium 99m tetrofosmin	To assess the cardiac tissue for damage caused by acute myocardial infarction, particularly when other tests are inconclusive	Studies may be done at rest and/or under exercise or pharmacologic stress. The radionuclide agent is given intravenously. Instruct patient on procedure and the need to remain motionless during the test with their arms over the head. The patient needs to go twice to the nuclear medicine department for imaging. Monitor vital signs and ECG and support patient continuously during the procedure; document and report dysrhythmias. Stress may be induced by use of a treadmill, but more likely with dipyridamole or adenosine.
Gated radionuclide angiography	To evaluate ventricular performance at rest and during stress or exercise; To assess coronary artery disease, cardiomyopathy, valvular disease, and intra-cardiac shunting	The patient has nothing by mouth for 4-6 hours before the test. An ECG is applied to the patient and synchronized with the imaging equipment. Once the radionuclide (usually, technetium 99) is given, multiple images are taken. After a resting gated study, the patient may be assessed with exercise or pharmacologic stress testing.

N

TABLE 11	Selected Nuclear Scans—cont'd	
Name of Scan	**Purpose**	**Special Patient Care Measures**
Pulmonary perfusion scan	To assess the pulmonary vascular circulation and to identify pulmonary emboli	Usually done after a pulmonary ventilation scan. Radio-tagged albumin is given intravenously and imaging is performed immediately.
Pulmonary ventilation scan	To assess lung performance, particularly in chronic obstructive lung disease, restrictive lung disorders, and inflammatory lung disease	If possible maintain patient in an upright position. The radioactive ^{133}xenon gas is inhaled via a mask for 15 seconds. This is followed by rebreathing oxygen for 2-3 minutes and then breathing normal air to clear the lungs of the gas. Another method used is the administration of the radioactive substance by aerosol.
Bone marrow scan	To identify malignancy or abnormal distribution of the bone marrow; to locate active sites for biopsy	The radionuclide is injected intravenously and imaging is done 20 minutes later; the imaging takes 1 hour to perform.
Renal scan	To assess the size, shape, position, and function of the kidneys; To assess for vascular abnormalities and obstructive uropathy To assess for renal function in the patient with hypertension; To evaluate the function of a transplanted kidney and identify any signs of transplant rejection	The patient tells the radiologist if he or she takes non-steroidal antiinflammatory drugs (NSAIDs) or blood pressure medications because they may interfere with the results of the scan. Before the test, extra fluids are often prescribed. The radionuclide is injected intravenously and the scanning is done immediately and for a total scanning time of 20-30 minutes.
Parathyroid scan	To assess patients with symptoms of hyperparathyroidism and to diagnose asymptomatic patients with hypercalcemia	No special preparation is needed. Tc-sestamibi is given intravenously and images are taken at 15 minutes and again at 1-3 hours after the injection.

N

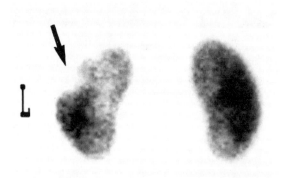

Figure 70. Pyelonephritis in a young child. The posterior view of the renal scan shows defects in the renal cortex in the upper pole of the left kidney *(arrow)* and decreased activity throughout the organ. Diminished activity is the result of acute inflammation and early ischemia, before functional abnormality or tissue damage occurs. In contrast, the right kidney is normal. *(From Mettler FA, Guiberteau MJ [2006]:* Essentials of nuclear medicine imaging, *ed 5, Philadelphia, Saunders.)*

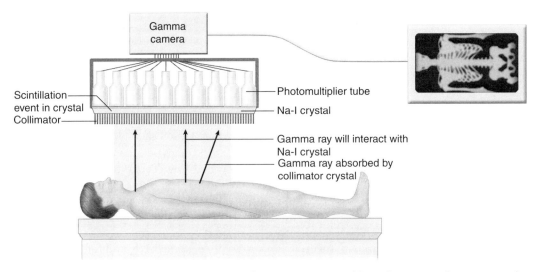

Figure 71. A schematic drawing of the scanner and gamma camera used in nuclear scans. The scanner and camera detect the radioactivity of the isotopes within the body and convert the information to a visible image of the function of the targeted organ. *(From Major, N.M. [2006]:* A practical approach to radiology. *Philadelphia, Saunders.)*

Vascular obstruction
Obstruction of a duct
Ischemia or necrosis of tissue

INTERFERING FACTORS

- Failure to follow specific pretest dietary or medication restrictions
- Recent intake of iodine
- Pregnancy

NURSING CARE

Pretest

- For the patient who is female and of childbearing age, the nurse asks if she is pregnant, the date of the last menstrual period, or if she is breast-feeding. In many radiology departments, a rapid pregnancy urine test (human chorionic gonadotropin [HCG]) is performed before the start of the procedure. Pregnancy is a contraindication because radiation would cause damage to a fetus. If the patient is breast-feeding, she will have to pump her breasts and discard the milk until the radioisotope clears out of her body. Document the patient's responses and inform the physician of any interfering factors. All nuclear scan examinations require a signed consent form. Once the physician has informed the patient about the test and the form is signed, the consent is entered in the patient's record.

- The nurse provides reassurance regarding the scanning process. Other than the venipuncture, the procedure is painless. If the patient is anxious, a family member or friend can be in the room during the scanning procedure. Unlike x-ray imaging, there is no external source of radiation exposure, so that there is no risk to others.

- Sedatives are avoided for the older child or adult. Sedation is sometimes used for the infant or child younger than age 3, particularly when the scan requires an extended period of immobility. A nurse often administers the prescribed sedative and remains readily available to monitor and assist the patient during and after the imaging procedure. The sedative medication is usually chloral hydrate, Nembutal, or phenobarbital.

○ *Patient Teaching.* The nurse provides the pretest patient instructions, which vary for each scan. Some scans have dietary restrictions to prevent an increase in the circulation to the liver or intestines. Many medications interfere with the absorption of the radiopharmaceutical. Often, after consultation with the patient's physician, medications are withheld and the patient remains under medical supervision during the period of the test. If the scan involves the uptake of radioactive iodine, the nurse instructs the patient to avoid the intake of iodine from food (shellfish, kelp preparations) and medication sources (some cough medicines, some multivitamin tablets with minerals, Lugol's solution) for 3 to 5 days before the test.

During the Test

- At the time of the test, the patient removes all clothing, jewelry, and metal objects. A hospital gown is worn.

- If sedatives are administered to young children, the nurse monitors vital signs regularly. This ensures early detection of any untoward response to the medication.

- The technician instructs the patient to remain still while a bolus dose of radionuclide is administered intravenously. In some studies, the scanning process begins immediately after the injection. In others, there is a waiting period before scanning can begin. The radionuclide requires time to be absorbed and concentrated by the target organ.

Posttest

- For the disposal of any urine or feces, the nurse wears gloves and then performs thorough handwashing. The radionuclide is excreted in urine and feces for several days, although the radioactivity level is minimal after a few hours. The body wastes can be disposed of in the toilet.

○ *Patient Teaching.* The nurse instructs the patient to wash his or her hands after voiding or a bowel movement. Parents and others should wash their hands after changing the diapers of an infant who has had a nuclear scan. The patient is reassured that the amount of radioactivity is negligible, but that it can remain on the hands unless they are washed.

N

5′-Nucleotidase

Also called: 5′-NT

SPECIMEN OR TYPE OF TEST: Serum

PURPOSE OF THE TEST

This test is used to help identify diseases of the hepatobiliary system.

BASICS THE NURSE NEEDS TO KNOW

5′-nucleotidase is a liver enzyme found in the plasma membranes of all cells. Its functions are thought to include help with nutrient absorption by cells and cell reproduction. The test level rises dramatically in conditions of extrahepatic or intrahepatic biliary obstruction and cancer of the liver. The test may rise to four to six times the upper limits of the normal value in cases of hepatobiliary obstruction, but demonstrate a normal value or mild elevation in cases of hepatitis. An elevated value of this test will parallel elevations of gamma-glutamyltransferase (GGT) and alkaline phosphatase (ALP) in the presence of hepatobiliary disease.

REFERENCE VALUES   Adults: 2-17 U/L *or* SI: 0.03-0.29 µKat/L

HOW THE TEST IS DONE

Venipuncture is performed to collect a specimen of blood.

SIGNIFICANCE OF TEST RESULTS

Elevated Values
Hepatic cirrhosis
Hepatobiliary disease with hepatic, cystic, or common bile duct obstruction
Metastatic cancer of the liver
Early biliary cirrhosis
Graft versus host disease
Preeclampsia
Rheumatoid arthritis

INTERFERING FACTORS

• Failure to maintain a nothing-by-mouth status

NURSING CARE

Nursing actions are similar to those used in other venipuncture procedures (see Chapter 2).

Occult Blood, Feces

See Fecal Occult Blood on p. 310.

Opiates, Urinary

SPECIMEN OR TYPE OF TEST: Urine

PURPOSE OF THE TEST

The test for urinary opiates is used to identify the presence of drugs of abuse in the opiate classification. When an overdose of an opiate is suspected, urinary testing is performed in emergency room settings.

BASICS THE NURSE NEEDS TO KNOW

Urinary opiate testing includes identification of the presence of the drugs morphine, codeine, opium, heroin, hydrocodone (Hycodan), hydromorphone (Dilaudid), oxycodone (Roxicodone, Percocet, Percodan), and oxymorphone (Numorphan). As prescription medications, these drugs are taken for the relief of pain, but they also have a high potential for abuse, particularly when obtained from illegal sources.

The opiate screen is used medically to obtain a rapid laboratory result when treating a patient who is suspected of a drug overdose. Morphine, heroin, and codeine are the most frequently abused drugs. If the test is positive, confirmatory tests for the specific opiate are performed, particularly when the case is one involving forensics or medico-legal decisions (see also Drugs of Abuse, p 262; Appendix B, p. 658). If the test result will be part of forensic evidence, the established procedure for chain-of-custody must be followed.

Workplace screening for drug abuse is also done. There are different reference values for the urinary screening, as determined by federal regulation (SAMHSA). The reference value is called a cutoff value, meaning that below the cutoff value, the test is negative. Above the cutoff value, the sample is positive.

REFERENCE VALUES   Workplace setting testing: Negative: <2000 ng/mL *or*
SI: <7000 nmol/L
Clinical toxicology: Negative: <300 ng/mL *or* SI: <1050 nmol/L

HOW THE TEST IS DONE

A random sample of 30 to 60 mL of urine is obtained.

SIGNIFICANCE OF TEST RESULTS

Positive Values

Recent use of an opiate drug

INTERFERING FACTORS

• None

Pretest

- The nurse assesses the patient for signs of opiate use. The patient or parent of the affected patient is asked about the use of any drug or medication in the past 24 hours. The patient who has taken a lower amount of the opiate drug may "nod," meaning that he or she alternates between drowsiness and alertness. The patient may also appear restless or experience nausea and vomiting. If the dose of the opiate was large, the patient may be unconscious. The patient's response to the amount of drug taken also varies with the tolerance level. Chronic drug users may have very high levels of the drug in their system, but can tolerate the amount.

  The abnormal assessment findings include constricted pupils and skin that is cold, sweaty, and cyanotic. The patient's rate of breathing is abnormally slow. When a significant amount of the opiate has been taken, the situation is a medical emergency. If the respiratory and central nervous system depression are not reversed, the patient may die of a drug overdose.

Posttest

- Continue to monitor the patient's vital signs, particularly the respirations. With a respiratory rate of less than 8 breaths per minute, the patient becomes hypoxic. The opioid antagonist naloxone (Narcan) may be given intravenously, as prescribed. Respiratory support with an Ambu bag-mask or intubation and ventilator assistance may be needed also.

Osmolality, Plasma

SPECIMEN OR TYPE OF TEST: Plasma, Serum

PURPOSE OF THE TEST

Plasma osmolality is determined to assess the person's fluid status and identify antidiuretic hormone (ADH) abnormalities.

BASICS THE NURSE NEEDS TO KNOW

Osmolality is a measure of the number of particles dissolved in a solution. In the blood, osmolality is created by sodium, chloride, bicarbonate, proteins, glucose, and urea dissolved in the plasma. Osmolality is affected by an increase or decrease in fluid volume or by an increase or decrease in blood particles; therefore, results are interpreted in relation to the urine osmolality and serum electrolytes.

REFERENCE VALUES   Children: 270-290 mOsm/kg H_2O *or* SI: 270-290 mmol/kg
Adults: 285-300 mOsm/kg H_2O *or* SI: 280-300 mmol/kg

▽ **Critical Values**   >320 mOsm/kg *or* SI: >320 mmol/kg
<265 mOsm/kg *or* SI: <265 mmol/kg

HOW THE TEST IS DONE

A venipuncture is performed. Osmolality may also be calculated with the following equation:

$$2(Na^+) + BUN/2.8 + Glu/18$$

SIGNIFICANCE OF TEST RESULTS

Increased Values

Alcoholism
Aldosteronism
Dehydration
Diabetes insipidus
High-protein diet
Hypercalcemia
Hyperglycemia
Hypernatremia
Hyperkalemia

Decreased Values

Addison's disease
Fluid overload
Hyponatremia
Liver failure with ascites
Psychogenic polydipsia
Syndrome of inappropriate antidiuretic hormone

INTERFERING FACTORS

- Hemolysis of specimen
- Medications: diuretics, mineralocorticoids (partial listing)

NURSING CARE

The nursing actions are similar to those of other venipuncture procedures.

▽ **Nursing Response to Critical Values**

Assess patient fluid and electrolyte status. High osmolality will cause fluid to shift out of the cells causing cellular dehydration, and low osmolality will cause fluid to shift into the cells causing cells to swell. Notify the physician, especially if the patient is increasingly stuporous. Initiate seizure precautions for high osmolality levels.

Osmolality, Urine

SPECIMEN OR TYPE OF TEST: Urine

PURPOSE OF THE TEST

Urine osmolality is determined to assess the ability of the kidneys to concentrate or dilute urine and to identify antidiuretic hormone (ADH) abnormalities.

BASICS THE NURSE NEEDS TO KNOW

Osmolality is a measure of the number of particles that are dissolved in a solution. Thus urine osmolality varies based on the person's fluid status and the excretion of metabolic waste products. If the patient is overhydrated, the urinary osmolality decreases as output increases. If the person is dehydrated, the urine osmolality increases as the output decreases. Urine osmolality is based on the concentration ability of the kidneys and the serum levels of sodium, chloride, bicarbonate, proteins, glucose, and urea. Therefore, interpretation of results includes evaluation of serum electrolytes.

REFERENCE VALUES

24-hour Urine Specimen (with Normal Diet and Fluid Intake)
500-800 mOsm/kg H_2O *or* **SI: 500-800 mmol/kg H_2O**

Random Urine Specimen
Neonates: 75-300 mOsm/kg H_2O *or* SI: 75-300 mmol/kg H_2O
Adults and children: 250-1200 mOsm/kg H_2O *or*
SI: 250-1200 mmol/kg H_2O

HOW THE TEST IS DONE

If a random urine specimen is desired, 10 mL of urine is collected in a sterile container and sent to the laboratory. For a 24-hour specimen, all urine voided in a 24-hour period is collected and sent to the laboratory.

SIGNIFICANCE OF TEST RESULTS

Increased Values
Addison's disease
Azotemia
Cirrhosis of the liver
Dehydration
Diabetes mellitus
Diarrhea
Hyperglycemia
Hypernatremia
Syndrome of inappropriate antidiuretic hormone

Decreased Values
Aldosteronism
Diabetes insipidus
Glomerulonephritis
Hypocalcemia

Hyponatremia
Overhydration
Sickle cell anemia

INTERFERING FACTORS

- Noncompliance with nothing-by-mouth status
- Glucosuria
- Recent scans requiring radiopaque dyes
- Medications
- Antibiotics
- Diuretics
- Volume expanders

▌ NURSING CARE

Nursing care is similar to that for other 24-hour urine collection or random sample specimen procedures as described in Chapter 2. For a random specimen, perform the following:

Pretest

◯ *Patient Teaching.* Instruct the patient not to eat or drink overnight before the urine is collected for a random specimen.

During the Test

- Obtain 10 mL of urine in a sterile container.

Posttest

- Send the specimen to the laboratory immediately.
- The results should be interpreted in relation to the serum osmolality.

Ova and Parasites, Feces

Also called: Stool for Ova and Parasites; Stool for O and P

SPECIMEN OR TYPE OF TEST: Feces

PURPOSE OF THE TEST

The microscopic examination of the feces is used to identify the ova of specific parasites in the intestinal tract.

BASICS THE NURSE NEEDS TO KNOW

Numerous parasites can infect individuals and then live in the intestinal tract and other organs during parts of the parasitic life cycle. Many ova, cysts, larvae, or spores from fecal-contaminated soil enter the person via a fecal-oral route (Figure 72). Common methods of transmission are from unwashed hands, eating contaminated raw fruits and vegetables, and drinking from a feces-contaminated water supply. Other parasites invade the body through the skin and then migrate through body tissue to the intestinal lumen (Figure 73) or are transmitted by eating under-cooked meat, raw fish, or plants that are contaminated by the parasite. As these various parasites

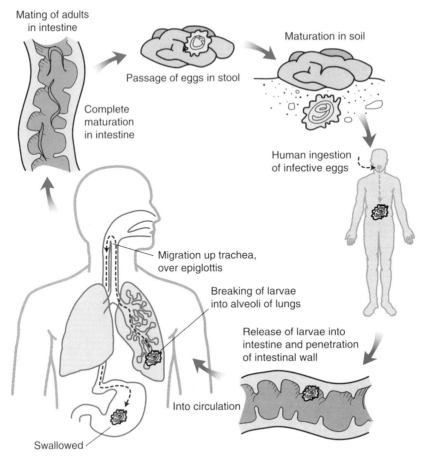

Mating of adults
in intestine

Maturation in soil

Passage of eggs in stool

Complete
maturation
in intestine

Human ingestion
of infective eggs

Migration up trachea,
over epiglottis

Breaking of larvae
into alveoli of lungs

Release of larvae into
intestine and penetration
of intestinal wall

Into circulation

Swallowed

Figure 72. Life cycle of *Ascaris lumbricoides* (roundworm). The transmission is by a fecal-oral route via unwashed hands, eating uncooked fruits and vegetables, or drinking unpurified water contaminated with the ova. *(From Mahon C.R, Lehman D.C, Manuselis G [1996]. Textbook of diagnostic microbiology, ed 4, Philadelphia: Saunders.)*

reach the intestine, they mature to the adult stage of development and deposit ova that can be recovered in stool samples. In the United States, *Ascaris lumbricoides* and *Necator americanus* are the most commonly reported parasitic worm infections (Mahon, Lehman & Mansulis, 2011). A patient may have more than one type of parasite.

REFERENCE VALUES Negative; no parasites or ova are present

HOW THE TEST IS DONE

Stool collection: Collect a small sample of feces directly into a clean, wide-mouthed container and close the lid. A common requirement is to collect three separate specimens over a 10-day period to maximize the identification of infection in at least one of the samples.

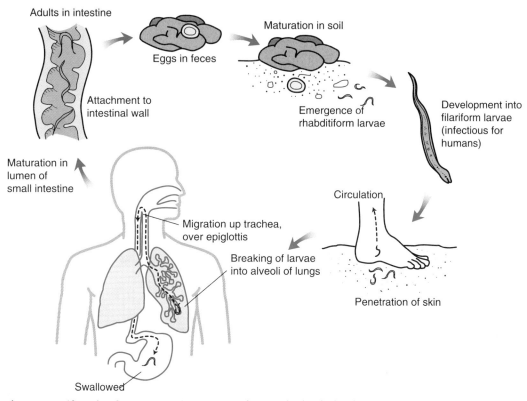

Figure 73. Life cycle of *Necator americanus* or *Ancylostoma duodenale* (hookworm). The hookworm larvae in the soil are transmitted by penetrating the skin of the hands or bare feet of the person. *(From Mahon C.R, Lehman D.C, Manuselis G [2011]. Textbook of diagnostic microbiology, ed 4, Philadelphia: Saunders.)*

O

Perianal swab (for pinworm): Transparent tape is placed on a tongue depressor, sticky side out. Press the tape firmly on the perianal skin. Remove the tape and place it on a glass slide, sticky side down.

SIGNIFICANCE OF TEST RESULTS

Positive Values
Amebiasis
Cryptosporidiosis
Ascariasis
Strongyloidiasis
Pinworm
Whipworm
Giardiasis
Tapeworm
Hookworm

INTERFERING FACTORS
- Antibiotic therapy in the 3- to 4-week pretest period
- Soil, water, or urine contamination of the sample
- Barium sulfate administration in the 2- to 3-week pretest period
- Mineral oil, castor oil, antacids, or antidiarrheal medication in the week before the test

| NURSING CARE

Pretest
- Schedule this test before any barium studies because the barium obscures the microscopic visualization of the ova.
- ◎ *Patient Teaching.* The nurse instructs the patient regarding correct collection procedure. The feces should not be removed from the toilet water. The patient should not use a laxative to assist in evacuation because it would interfere with the microscopic examination of the sample.

Posttest
- The specimen should be delivered to the laboratory as soon as possible.
- If the nurse collects the specimen, he or she wears gloves and, after removing the gloves, washes hands thoroughly. Intestinal parasites are a highly transmissible source of infection via the fecal-oral route or via contact with the skin. The nurse must take precautions to prevent possible self-infection from poor hygiene practices.
- The nurse includes the patient's name, identification number, time and date of the collection on the laboratory requisition and the container label. On the requisition form, pertinent data regarding the patient's clinical history, such as immunosuppression or AIDS, or possible sources of infection, such as backpacking in the mountains or travel to an undeveloped country, are included.
- In rural areas of the southeast United States, and in Central and South America, and the Caribbean Islands, parasitic infection is endemic.

Pancreatic Elastase-1

See Fecal Elastase-1 on p. 309.

Papanicolaou Smear

Also called: PAP Smear
Includes: Human Papilloma Virus testing (HPV DNA)

SPECIMEN OR TYPE OF TEST: Cytology Study

PURPOSE OF THE TEST

The Papanicolaou smear is used to detect inflammation, infection, premalignant changes, and malignancy of the cervix.

BASICS THE NURSE NEEDS TO KNOW

The Papanicolaou (Pap) smear is an inexpensive screening test that examines cervical cell scrapings for abnormality. Most commonly, the reported results are classified according to the Bethesda system. When an abnormality is present, the changes can be of an infectious, inflammatory origin or they can be squamous cell or glandular cell abnormalities. The abnormalities are graded in severity.

The borderline lesion (inconclusive result) is defined as atypical squamous cells of undetermined significance (ASC-US). The squamous intraepithelial lesions (SIL) are graded from low grade to high grade. The low-grade squamous intraepithelial lesion (LSIL) consists of condyloma, mild dysplasia (CIN 1)—a precancerous state—or both. A high-grade squamous intraepithelial lesion (HSIL) ranges from moderate dysplasia (CIN 2) to severe dysplasia (CIN 3), including carcinoma in situ and invasive carcinoma or adenocarcinoma (Box 8).

Human Papilloma Virus

The human papilloma virus is the causative agent for genital warts and almost all cases of carcinoma of the cervix. There are 200 genotypes (genetic subtypes) of this virus, but 15 to 20 of them are capable of causing cancerous cervical mutations (Forbes, Sahm & Weissfeld, 2007). HPV infection is the most common of the sexually transmitted diseases. Diagnosis of the HPV infection and its viral subtype is made by HPV DNA probe assay performed on the cervical cells obtained from the PAP smear. Genotypes 16 and 18 cause 70% of the cases of cervical cancer and the remainder of the cases are caused by various other HPV genotypes (CDC, 2010).

Most women who are sexually active develop an HPV infection. Usually, these infections are cleared spontaneously within a few weeks to months. There are, however, some cases where the virus persists and eventually cancer of the cervix develops. To date, except for those women who

---

BOX 8   The Bethesda System for Reporting Cervical Cytology

- Adequacy of sample
  - Satisfactory
  - Unsatisfactory
- Squamous cell abnormalities
  - Atypical squamous cells
    - ASC of undetermined significance
    - ASC, cannot exclude high-grade lesion
  - Low-grade squamous intraepithelial lesion
  - High-grade squamous intraepithelial lesion
  - Squamous cell carcinoma
- Glandular cell abnormalities
  - Atypical glandular cells, specify site of origin, if possible
  - Atypical glandular cells, favor neoplastic
  - Carcinoma in situ
  - Adenocarcinoma
- Other cancers (e.g., lymphoma, metastatic, sarcoma)

From Katz VL, Lentz GM, Lobo RA et al: *Comprehensive gynecology,* ed 5, St Louis, 2007, Mosby.

P

are immunocompromised, there is no way to predict which women will be unable to eliminate the infection spontaneously.

REFERENCE VALUES   Bethesda system classification: Normal; within normal limits
HPV DNA: Negative

HOW THE TEST IS DONE

Using a vaginal speculum to enhance visibility, the physician or nurse practitioner collects the patient's secretions and cells from the cervix (Figure 74). The fluid and tissue scrapings are placed in the specimen jar with liquid-based/thin prep solution. In the laboratory, the cells of the tissue are examined microscopically. A sample of the cells also can be analyzed for the DNA of the human papilloma virus and its genotype.

SIGNIFICANCE OF TEST RESULTS

Abnormal Values

Cervical dysplasia or cervical intraepithelial neoplasia
Cervicovaginal endometriosis
Condyloma
Human papillomavirus
Genital warts
Carcinoma in situ
Squamous cell carcinoma
Adenocarcinoma

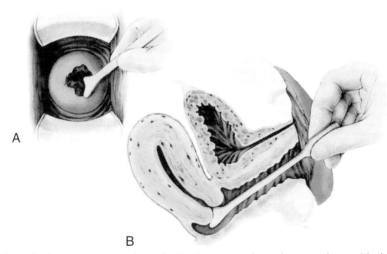

Figure 74. Papanicolaou smear procedure. **A,** Cervix, as seen through a speculum, with the spatula being used to obtain a cell sample. **B,** Longitudinal view at the same point in the procedure. (From Katz VL et al: *Comprehensive gynecology,* ed 5, St Louis, 2007, Mosby.)

INTERFERING FACTORS

- Menstruation
- Recent douching
- Vaginal infection or medication
- Recent sexual intercourse
- Inadequate specimen
- Lubricating jelly on the speculum

NURSING CARE

Pretest

- Schedule the test for when the patient is not menstruating.

○ *Patient Teaching.* The nurse instructs the patient to refrain from sexual intercourse, douching, and vaginal medication for 48 hours before the test. Sexual intercourse can cause inflammation of the tissue. Douching can remove surface cells before the test sample is obtained. Medication obscures the microscopic examination of the cells. If vaginal infection is present, it will be treated and the Papanicolaou test postponed for 2 to 4 weeks.

During the Test

- The nurse assists the patient to lie on the table in the lithotomy position with the legs supported by stirrups. The elderly patient may need extra assistance in positioning because of stiffness and arthritic pain.
- The nurse should wear gloves to avoid contact with the infected tissue.
- After the tissue and fluid samples are obtained, immerse the sample in the Thin-Prep solution. On the specimen container, identify the specimen with the patient's name, identification number, age, physician's name, date of collection, and source of the cells.

Posttest

- Once the gloves are removed, wash hands thoroughly.
- On the requisition form, the same identifying information is written. The physician or nurse practitioner adds any pertinent information, such as the date of last menstrual period, history of an abnormal Pap smear, carcinoma, radiation, chemotherapy, abnormal vaginal bleeding, exposure to diethylstilbestrol, a visible lesion, or recent pregnancy.
- When the woman is informed of abnormal Pap and/or HPV test results, she often requires additional information about the meaning of the results and any follow-up measures that are needed. The nurse recognizes the patient's anxiety or confusion and can help with the emotional stress or lack of knowledge. Additional information and repetition of the instructions may be needed (Montgomery & Bloch, 2010). The nurse can provide help to clarify misconceptions and encourage the patient to complete the follow-up testing.

Health Promotion

The nurse encourages parents to have their daughters routinely vaccinated against HPV infection. The CDC (2010) recommends the vaccination be done between ages 13 to 26 years, but the series can be started as early as 9 years of age. The vaccine is given in a 3-dose series.

- The American College of Obstetricians and Gynecologists guidelines (2009) provide recommendations for the timing and frequency of Pap testing as presented in Box 9. In the roles of health teaching and health promotion, the nurse should encourage women to have the

P

Continued

NURSING CARE—cont'd

Pap test and to return for results and follow-up appointments, as recommended. The nurse can also work in collaboration with community-based health programs because they have been effective in providing breast and cervical screening tests to low-income and uninsured women. For all women, the goal of the Pap smear testing is to detect cervical tissue changes and premalignant conditions before they become advanced or change into malignant tumors. Early detection and treatment greatly reduce the morbidity and mortality of cancer of the cervix.

BOX 9   ACOG 2009 Recommended Guidelines for Timing and Frequency of Pap Testing

- Cervical cytology screening is recommended every 2 years for women between the ages of 21 years and 29 years.
- Women aged 30 years and older who have had three consecutive negative cervical cytology screening test results and who have no history of CIN 2 or CIN 3, are not HIV infected, are not immunocompromised, and were not exposed to diethylstilbestrol in utero may extend the interval between cervical cytology examinations to every three years.
- Co-testing using the combination of cytology plus HPV DNA testing is an appropriate screening test for women older than 30 years. Any low-risk woman aged 30 years or older who receives negative test results on both cervical cytology screening and HPV DNA testing should be screened no sooner than 3 years subsequently.
- In women who have had a total hysterectomy for benign indications and have no prior history of high-grade CIN, routine cytology should be discontinued.
- Because cervical cancer develops slowly and risk factors decrease with age, it is reasonable to discontinue cervical cancer screening between 65 years and 70 years of age in women who have three or more negative cytology test results in a row and no abnormal test results in the past 10 years.

From American College of Obstetricians and Gynecologists. Cervical Cytology Screening. ACOG Practice Bulletin 109. Washington, DC: ACOG, 2009.

Paracentesis and Ascitic Fluid Analysis

 Also called: Abdominal Paracentesis; abdominal tap

SPECIMEN OR TYPE OF TEST: Ascitic Fluid

PURPOSE OF THE TEST

Abdominal paracentesis is used to obtain a sample of the ascitic fluid as part of the investigation of new-onset ascites, suspected malignant source of ascites, and to confirm or exclude infection (peritonitis) in the peritoneal cavity

BASICS THE NURSE NEEDS TO KNOW

A healthy person has less than 50 mL of peritoneal fluid and no distention of the peritoneal (abdominal) cavity. The abnormal condition of accumulated fluid in the peritoneal cavity is called ascites and the fluid is called ascitic fluid. When the ascites is advanced, the fluid volume has dramatically increased. The ascitic fluid can be aspirated by a needle that penetrates into the peritoneal cavity. Laboratory analysis of the fluid specimen includes cytologic study, chemistry analysis, and microbiologic examination, as requested.

As the specimen is collected by the physician, the nurse assesses the quality of the fluid visually. Normal peritoneal fluid should be clear and colorless or pale yellow. Abnormal fluid can appear bright red and bloody, indicating bleeding. Cloudy fluid is often due to infection, a strangulated bowel, or organ rupture. Greenish fluid can result from perforation of the duodenum or gallbladder, causing bile peritonitis. Milky fluid may result from malignancy or blockage of a major lymphatic duct.

Serum-ascites albumin ratio (SAAR) is an important test to begin to determine the cause of the ascites. The calculation is based upon the ratio of the albumin in the serum to albumin in the ascitic fluid. If the SAAR value is 1.1 g/dL or higher (SI: 11 g/L or higher), the value suggests that the ascitic fluid is a transudate and the source is probably hepatic (cirrhosis, portal hypertension). If the SAAR value is <1.1 g/dL (SI: <11 g/L), the value suggests that the ascitic fluid is an exudate and the source is from another cause (possibly malignancy, infection, or inflammation).

REFERENCE VALUES

Ascitic Fluid Analysis
Appearance: Clear, odorless, colorless or pale yellow, scanty
Microbiology: Bacteria and fungi: None present
Cytology: No malignant cells present
Red blood cells: <10^3/μL *or* SI: <1×10^9/L
White blood cells: <500 /μL *or* SI: <0.5×10^9/L
Neutrophils: <250 /μL *or* SI: <0.25×10^9/L (or <50% of the white blood cell count)

HOW THE TEST IS DONE

Paracentesis

Ultrasound may be used to image the pooling of the fluid and locations of the abdominal organs and vascular tissues. This helps to avoid inadvertent puncture of these structures. Under local anesthesia, the physician inserts a long thin needle through the skin and into the peritoneal cavity. The insertion site is usually midline, about 2 inches (5 cm) below the umbilicus. Either a syringe or a three-way stopcock with polyethylene tubing is used to draw off the fluid. The diagnostic paracentesis takes 30 to 45 minutes to complete.

If the physician also wants to drain the peritoneal cavity of a large volume of ascitic fluid for therapeutic purposes, the nurse will assist in connecting sterile IV tubing to the needle or stopcock at one end and a large vacuum container at the other end (Figure 75). Volumes of 4 L or more may be collected.

SIGNIFICANCE OF TEST RESULTS

Malignancy
Pancreatitis
Hepatic cirrhosis
Peritonitis (bacterial, fungal, parasitic, tuberculosis)
Traumatic organ rupture (bowel, liver, spleen)
Ruptured appendix

P

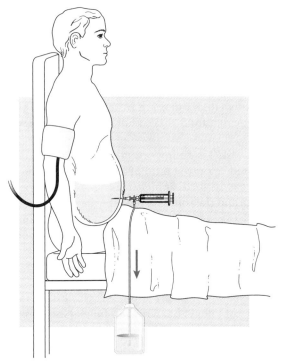

Figure 75. Paracentesis. The three-way stopcock controls the direction of the flow of ascetic fluid into the syringe or the drainage tubing and collection container.

Duodenal ulcer, perforated
Intestine, perforated
Hypoproteinemia
Congestive heart failure

INTERFERING FACTORS

- Coagulation disorder
- Intestinal obstruction
- Abdominal wall infection
- Uncooperative behavior
- History of multiple abdominal surgeries
- Portal hypertension

NURSING CARE

Pretest

- Because of the risk of bleeding, obtain the hematocrit, prothrombin time, partial thromboplastin time, and platelet values within 48 hours of this procedure. The laboratory values are entered into the patient's record and the nurse notifies the physician of abnormal results.

P

- After the physician has informed the patient about the procedure, and its risks and benefits, a signed consent is needed and is placed in the patient's record.
- Before the procedure, the nurse records the patient's baseline vital signs, including temperature. The patient's weight and abdominal girth is also measured.
- Just before the procedure, have the patient void to empty the bladder completely. This helps prevent an inadvertent puncture of the organ during the procedure.
- The nurse positions the patient in full Fowler's, supine, or lateral decubitus position according to the physician's preference. The skin is cleansed, such as with povidone iodine solution, and a sterile drape is put into place.

During the Test

- The nurse stands at the patient's shoulder and provides reassurance to help alleviate fear. Some pain is felt by the patient as the needle penetrates the peritoneum. Encourage the patient to remain immobile.
- The nurse assists with the collection of the fluid. In addition, vital signs are taken and documented every 15 minutes. Because hypovolemic shock can occur when a large volume of fluid is removed, the nurse assesses the patient for signs of impending shock, including pallor, dizziness, diaphoresis (cold, moist skin, sweating), a rising pulse rate, and a falling blood pressure.
- Once the procedure is completed, the physician removes the needle, applies pressure and a small, sterile bandage to the puncture site. One or two sutures may be needed to close the opening.

Posttest

- Vital signs are taken immediately and at intervals thereafter until the patient is stable. The patient's weight and measurement of abdominal girth are taken again, with a comparison to the pretest measurements. All data are recorded in the patient's record. The nurse also documents the time that the paracentesis was done and the name of the physician who performed the procedure. The nurse describes the patient's tolerance of the procedure. Generally, the patient feels better after the removal of excess fluid. Breathing is more comfortable and mobility improves. The nursing documentation includes the amount, color, odor, and characteristics of the fluid that was withdrawn. The amount of peritoneal fluid removed is also entered as output on the record of intake and output.

  All specimens are labeled appropriately, including the patient's name, identification number, date, physician's name, and the identification of the specimen as peritoneal fluid. The collection bottles, specimens, and requisition form are sent to the laboratory, without delay.
- The dressing is checked for excess drainage or bleeding. With the removal of large amounts of fluid from the peritoneal cavity, there may be a rapid shift of fluid, albumin, and potassium from the blood to the peritoneal cavity. The nurse remains alert for hypotension, shock, and a rapid or irregular pulse as indicators of a serious shift of fluid and electrolytes.
- When the patient has the procedure done as an outpatient or in a medical office, he or she is taught to resume normal activities right away, but to restrict physical efforts for a few days. The patient maintains a dry sterile dressing on the puncture site for 5 to 7 days until the next visit with the physician. If the dressing becomes wet with small amounts of fluid leakage at the puncture site, the nurse shows the patient how to replace it with a dry bandage.

Continued

▌ NURSING CARE—cont'd

◆ **Nursing Response to Complications**

The two complications of a paracentesis are hemorrhage and perforation of the intestine. If one of these complications occurs, the symptoms usually become apparent in the posttest period. The nurse would notify the physician immediately of abnormal assessment findings.

Bleeding or hemorrhage. The patient with a hemorrhage into the peritoneal cavity will demonstrate hypotension, tachycardia, dyspnea, diaphoresis, and pallor. The patient may feel abdominal discomfort or acute abdominal pain. Ecchymosis appears on the skin in dependent areas, as toward the back and buttocks.

Peritonitis. The patient is at risk of developing an infection in the peritoneal cavity. The nurse should assess for acute abdominal pain, a boardlike abdomen, abdominal distention, shock, and a fever.

Parathyroid Hormone

Also called: (PTH); Parathormone; Immunoreactive PTH

SPECIMEN OR TYPE OF TEST: Serum, Plasma

PURPOSE OF THE TEST

A parathyroid hormone determination is performed to diagnose suspected parathyroid disorders. It may be performed to differentiate among clinical diagnoses that result in calcium and phosphate abnormalities. PTH is used as a biomarker for bone turnover for patients with kidney disease. High PTH indicates high bone turnover; however, lower levels are not reliable markers. PTH is used to manipulate plasma calcium and phosphate levels in chronic renal failure.

BASICS THE NURSE NEEDS TO KNOW

Parathyroid hormone is produced and secreted by the parathyroid glands. Its role in the body is the regulation of calcium. Its secretion is based on a negative feedback mechanism with calcium (Figure 76).

Parathyroid hormone affects calcium levels by stimulating osteoclast activity and inhibiting osteoblast activity in the bone. This causes bone reabsorption, which shifts calcium and phosphate

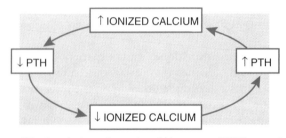

Figure 76. Regulation of parathyroid hormone (PTH) secretion.

out of the bone into the blood. Parathyroid hormone also causes increased reabsorption of calcium at the kidney's distal tubules and decreased reabsorption of phosphate at the proximal tubules. The result of parathyroid hormone activity is an increase in calcium in the blood with a decrease in plasma phosphate levels.

REFERENCE VALUES

(Interpreted in relation to serum calcium and phosphate levels)
Intact parathyroid hormone: 15-75 pg/mL *or* SI: 15-75 ng/L
N-terminal fraction: 50-330 pg/mL *or* SI: 50-330 ng/L
C-terminal fraction: 8-24 pg/mL *or* SI: 8-24 ng/L

HOW THE TEST IS DONE

Parathyroid hormone is measured by radioimmunoassay (RIA), which can measure biologically active intact parathyroid hormone. This fraction represents only a small portion of the total parathyroid hormone. Alternatively, RIA can measure C-terminal or N-terminal portions of the hormone. Two venous samples are needed.

SIGNIFICANCE OF TEST RESULTS

Elevated Values

Hyperparathyroidism
Chronic renal failure
Hypocalcemia

Decreased Values

Hypoparathyroidism
Hypercalcemia
Graves' disease
Lung, kidney, pancreatic, or ovarian cancer

INTERFERING FACTORS

- Noncompliance with fasting requirements
- Elevated lipid levels
- Medications, such as lithium and thiazide diuretics

NURSING CARE

The actions of the nurse are similar to those carried out in other venipuncture procedures (see Chapter 2), with the following additional measures.

Pretest

- Check with the physician if any medications are to be held.
- ○ *Patient Teaching.* The nurse instructs the patient not to eat or drink for 12 hours before the test.

Posttest

- The patient may resume a normal diet.
- Send the specimen to the laboratory on ice.

Parathyroid Scan

SPECIMEN OR TYPE OF TEST: Nuclear Imaging

PURPOSE OF THE TEST

A parathyroid scan may be done to assess the cause of hypercalcemia in patients with recurring kidney stones, low serum phosphate and bone pain, and even in asymptomatic patients.

BASICS THE NURSE NEEDS TO KNOW

See Nuclear Scans on pp. 455.

REFERENCE VALUES   Parathyroid glands are not seen on the scan.

HOW THE TEST IS DONE

A PET or SPECT imaging is done after technetium-99m sestamibi is given intravenously. Images are taken after 15 minutes and again at 1.0 to 3.0 hours.

SIGNIFICANCE OF TEST RESULTS

Adenoma
Hyperplasia

INTERFERING FACTORS

• See Nuclear Scans on pp. 460.

NURSING CARE

See Nuclear Scans on pp. 461.

Patch Test, Skin

SPECIMEN OR TYPE OF TEST: Skin Sensitivity Test

PURPOSE OF THE TEST

This test is used to identify the particular allergen that causes contact dermatitis. It is also used to differentiate contact dermatitis from other causes of eczematous disease.

BASICS THE NURSE NEEDS TO KNOW

Allergic contact dermatitis causes an eczematous skin change. It is an inflammatory skin response that occurs when the skin is in contact with a particular antigen. The person is sensitized to the antigen over time, without the immediate development of a skin reaction. Eventually, reexposure to the antigen induces a vigorous allergic response at the site of contact with the antigen.

Because one part of the treatment of the skin eruption is to remove the antigen from further contact with the patient's skin, the antigen must be identified. In some cases, a patch test is used to identify one or more suspected antigens by evoking a skin reaction to suspected allergens.

The patch test may be carried out by placing the suspected allergen, such as a small piece of clothing, a bit of a cosmetic substance, or a diluted solution of chemical components on the skin. Industrial substances or laboratory chemicals are never used in testing because they can produce an irritant dermatitis or a chemical burn. The most common allergens or sources of contact dermatitis are listed in the section of abnormal results.

The physician grades the results of the skin testing according to severity of the reaction. An erythematous (red), macular (flat), or papular (raised) lesion is labeled as an undecided, doubtful, or weak result. An erythematous, edematous, papular, or vesicular (fluid-filled) area of skin where a particular allergen was placed is identified as a strongly positive reaction. A raised, red, edematous area with large vesicles, bullae (fluid-filled blisters), or possible ulceration is identified as an extreme reaction.

REFERENCE VALUES   Negative; no abnormal skin reactions are noted.

HOW THE TEST IS DONE

Samples of selected allergens used by the patient or of a number of standard allergens are taped to the patient's skin for 48 hours of contact exposure (Figure 77). The readings of the results are performed after 48 hours and again after 72 hours to 7 days, as prescribed.

SIGNIFICANCE OF TEST RESULTS

Abnormal Values

Common Causes of Contact Dermatitis

Nickel (snaps, belt buckles, rings, watchbands, bracelets, earrings)
Formaldehyde (permanent-press clothing, skin and nail products)
Chromates (cement, cutting oil)
Topical medication with neomycin, benzocaine, or ethylenediamine
Epoxy resins (adhesives, glues)
Hair dyes
Lanolin
Chemicals in sunscreen creams
Permanent-wave solutions
Fragrances in perfumes and soaps

INTERFERING FACTORS

- Concurrent dermatitis from another source
- Exposure of the patch site to water or excessive perspiration
- Inaccurate interpretation of the results
- Inaccurate timing for reading of the results

P

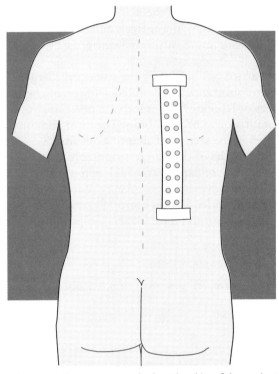

Figure 77. Patch test, skin. Various allergens are applied to the skin of the patient's back. Those substances that cause an allergic skin response are identified as sources of contact dermatitis.

NURSING CARE

Pretest
- Schedule this test after an episode of acute dermatitis has subsided and after treatment with corticosteroids has ceased. After the physician has informed the patient about the test, a written consent from the patient is needed. The consent is entered in the patient's chart.
- If particular products that the patient uses are to be tested, instruct the patient to bring them in beforehand. The patch test must be prepared, and a detailed list of the ingredients must be written.

During the Test
- The nurse or physician tapes the allergen patch to the patient's upper back between the scapula and the spinal column. A diagram on paper is made to identify the location of each allergen.

Posttest
◉ *Patient Teaching.* The nurse instructs the patient to refrain from showers and physical exercise during the following 48 hours. This is because water and perspiration will loosen the tape of the patch. The patient is also told that if itching, irritation, or pain occurs under one of the discs of allergen, it should be removed immediately.

○ *Patient Teaching.* The patient is instructed to return in 48 hours for the first evaluation of the results. The patch is removed at that time. After a 30-minute to 1-hour wait, the skin is assessed for any reaction in the area of the allergens. The nurse instructs the patient to return for the second appointment to reevaluate the skin because a delayed reaction can occur. This second reading is done at 96 hours (4 days) after the patch is applied. The patient is advised that exercise and showers are permitted while waiting for the second evaluation, but that soap must not be used, and that the patient must not scrub, scratch, or rub the skin in the test area.

Percutaneous Umbilical Blood Sampling

Also called: PUBS; Cordocentesis

SPECIMEN OR TYPE OF TEST: Blood

PURPOSE OF THE TEST

This procedure primarily is used to obtain a specimen of fetal blood for the assessment of Rh isoimmunization, a fetal anemia. It may also be used to identify chromosomal abnormality, detect fetal infection, measure acid-base balance, and to detect other hematologic abnormalities.

A small amount of the fetal blood is reserved for a complete blood count.

BASICS THE NURSE NEEDS TO KNOW

The percutaneous umbilical blood sampling can be performed in the second or third trimester. The normal values of fetal cord blood vary based on the gestational age of the fetus. Because of the risk of fetal death that can occur after the PUBS procedure, the test is reserved for conditions that require rapid diagnosis or to obtain data about the fetus' condition that cannot be obtained in any other way.

Fetal Blood Analysis

Red Cell Isoimmunization

This occurs when the fetus has Rh-positive red blood cell antigens and the mother has Rh-negative erythrocytes. The maternal antibodies are transmitted to the fetus and cause fetal hemolysis of erythrocytes. If the erythrocyte incompatibility is not prevented or controlled, the fetus experiences a hemolytic anemia called erythroblastosis fetalis or Rh disease. The fetal cord blood is tested for blood type, the presence of Rh antigens, the hematocrit level, and the reticulocyte count. The treatment is individualized, but an intrauterine blood transfusion can be given to the fetus.

Prenatal Chromosomal Analysis

The karyotype consists of the characteristics of the chromosomes, their number, form, size, structure, and grouping. Chromosomal abnormality in the fetus is identified by analysis of the fetal blood cells using chromosomal-specific DNA probes.

P

Congenital Infection

Infection in the pregnant woman can cross the placental barrier and infect the fetus. The fetal blood analysis for infection includes measurement of fetal antibodies, white blood cells, eosinophils, liver enzymes, and platelets. Viral culture of the fetal blood and the amniotic fluid may be performed to identify the infectious organism. Because fetal antibodies do not develop until the 22nd week of gestation, fetal cord blood samples cannot verify the infection before this time.

Thrombocytopenia

This is a low platelet count, which can cause fetal intracranial bleeding during pregnancy, labor, or the neonatal period. In most cases, the mother has immune thrombocytopenia and passively transmits the maternal antiplatelet antibodies to the fetus. If the fetus is affected severely, the fetus can receive an intrauterine platelet transfusion, administered via the umbilical vein.

REFERENCE VALUES

Hematologic evaluation: Within normal limits for gestational age
Chromosomal analysis: Normal karyotype
Biochemistry analysis: Within normal limits for gestational age
Immunoglobulin G (IgG) antibodies: Within normal limits
IgM antibodies: Within normal limits

Hemoglobin
Fetus of 18-20 weeks 11.47 ± 0.78 g/dL *or* SI: 115 ± 7.8 g/L
Fetus of 21-22 weeks 12.28 ± 0.89 g/dL *or* SI:123 ± 8.9 g/L
Fetus of 23-25 weeks 12.40 ± 0.77 g/dL *or* SI: 124 ± 7.7 g/L
Fetus of 26-30 weeks 13.35 ± 1.17 g/dL *or* SI: 134 ± 11.7 g/L

RBC
Fetus of 18-20 weeks 2.66 ± 0.29 × 10^6 cells/µL *or* SI: 2.66 ± 0.29 ×^{12} cells/L
Fetus of 21-22 weeks 2.96 ± 0.26 × 10^6 cells/µL *or* SI: 2.96 ± 0.26 ×^{12} cells/L
Fetus of 23-25 weeks 3.06 ± 0.26 × 10^6 cells/µL *or* SI: 3.06 ± 0.26 ×^{12} cells/L
Fetus of 26-30 weeks 3.52 ± 0.32 × 10^6 cells/µL *or* SI: 3.52 ± 0.32 ×^{12} cells/L

Hematocrit
Fetus of 18-20 weeks 35.86 ± 3.29% *or* SI: .036 ± 0.03 volume fraction
Fetus of 21-22 weeks 38.53 ± 3.21% *or* SI: 0.39 ± 0.03 volume fraction
Fetus of 23-25 weeks 38.59 ± 2.41% *or* SI: 0.39 ± 0.03 volume fraction
Fetus of 26-30 weeks 41.54 ± 3.31% *or* SI: 0.42 ± 0.03 volume fraction

HOW THE TEST IS DONE

Guided by ultrasound imaging, the physician inserts a sterile 20- to 22-gauge spinal needle through the maternal abdomen and uterus. The needle is then advanced into the umbilical cord until it is placed in one of the umbilical veins (Figure 78). Once the needle placement is verified,

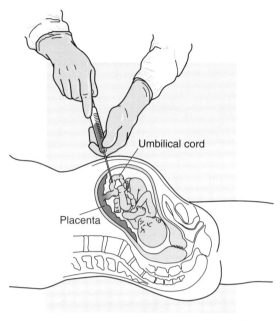

Figure 78. Percutaneous umbilical blood sampling. Under ultrasound guidance, the needle is advanced through the skin and into the uterus. Once the needle punctures the umbilical cord and one of the umbilical veins, a small amount of cord blood is aspirated into the syringe.

a syringe is used to aspirate 0.5 to 3 mL of venous blood. The blood is then transferred to microtubes for specific laboratory analyses.

SIGNIFICANCE OF TEST RESULTS

Hemolytic Anemia
Rh disease
Minor antigen disorders

Chromosome Disorder
Cystic fibrosis
Sickle cell anemia
Muscular dystrophy
Hemophilia A, B
Inborn errors of metabolism
Down syndrome
Retinoblastoma
Wilms' tumor
Thalassemias
Phenylketonuria
Enzyme G-6-PD deficiency

Infection
Toxoplasmosis
Rubella
Varicella
Cytomegalovirus
Human parvovirus B19

Platelet Disorder
Thrombocytopenia

INTERFERING FACTORS
- Maternal obesity
- Uncooperative behavior
- Severe polyhydramnios
- Unfavorable fetal position
- Specimen contamination

NURSING CARE

Pretest
- Once the woman has been informed of the procedure by her physician, obtain her written consent for the procedure and the genetic testing. The signed form is placed in the patient's record.
- Assist the patient in removing all clothes and putting on a hospital gown.
- Place the patient in a lateral position on the examining table.
- Assess and record the mother's vital signs and the fetal heart rate.
- The nurse provides emotional support. The patient's anxiety level is often high because of concern for the safety of the fetus, fear of the procedure, or concern about the potential for abnormal test results.

During the Test
- The nurse cleanses the woman's abdomen with the appropriate povidone-iodine or surgical soap solution, and then places the surgical drape. As the physician administers the local anesthetic, the nurse provides reassurance to the patient. The injection causes a slight stinging sensation in the abdominal area.
- The nurse begins the frequent assessment and recording of the fetal heart rate. The fetal cardiac contractions can be counted during the imaging of the fetus on the ultrasound monitor.
- Prepare any additional medications, as prescribed. If the fetus moves excessively, the mother may receive intravenous sedation to limit fetal movement. As an alternative, the fetus may receive an intravenous sedative or muscle relaxant via the umbilical vein.
- Once the blood is obtained, the nurse assists with depositing it in the microtubes. Ensure that all blood samples are properly labeled with the patient's name, identification number, age, physician's name, date and that the specimen is fetal blood (cord blood). The requisition form with its identifying information also states that the specimen is fetal blood (cord blood) obtained by percutaneous umbilical cord sampling. The gestation of the pregnancy is included.

P

Posttest
- Once the needle is removed, the nurse begins to monitor the fetal heart rate and takes the mother's vital signs. In the recovery area, external fetal monitoring of the fetal heart rate and uterine contractions continues. It is common for the mother to have mild uterine cramping for a short while. The fetal monitoring is discontinued when the fetal heart rate remains stable in a normal range and the uterine contractions cease.
- At regular intervals, the nurse observes the abdomen for signs of bleeding. The small sterile dressing that covers the puncture site should remain dry and intact.
- Prophylactic antibiotics are administered, as prescribed. If indicated, the nurse also administers prescribed $Rh_o(D)$ immune globulin (RhoGAM) to the Rh-negative mother. This will help prevent Rh disease of the newborn in a future pregnancy.

○ *Patient Teaching.* In preparation for discharge, the nurse instructs the patient to rest for the remainder of the day. The patient should take her temperature at least two times per day. She should report a fever to her physician without delay. She is instructed to return to the physician for a follow-up evaluation and to learn the test results.

○ *Patient Teaching.* When serious or severe chromosomal abnormality exists, the parents experience emotional distress. Genetic counseling is an essential component of care before testing and after the test results are known. This helps the parents make an informed choice about the continuation of the pregnancy. In obstetric management, the alternatives include continuation or termination of the pregnancy. If the pregnancy is continued, plans are made for intensive antepartal monitoring, for possible cesarean section for fetal distress during labor, and for the special postdelivery needs of the newborn.

◇ **Nursing Response to Complications**

The PUBS procedure is a potential risk for the fetus, with a fetal death rate of 1.6%. Continued bleeding from the puncture of the umbilical vein is the probable cause. Many patients do have minimal bleeding that ceases a few minutes after the needle is removed, but more severe bleeding can occur. Other complications include fetal bradycardia, maternal or fetal infection, and premature labor. The nurse assesses for complications and notifies the physician of abnormal findings.

Bleeding. Prolonged bleeding from the umbilical cord is identified by continued staining or wetness from amniotic fluid on the mother's abdominal dressing. The drainage is pink. Fetal movements may be hyperactive or lethargic.

Fetal bradycardia. Fetal bradycardia can be observed on the fetal monitor. Bradycardia is identified by a fetal heart rate less than 120. In addition, the fetus is lethargic, with fewer than normal movements.

Maternal infection. If the mother develops infection, she experiences chills and fever. She also may have uterine cramping. The nurse monitors the patient's temperature and examines the abdomen for signs of redness, swelling, or purulent drainage. If the fetus develops an infection, it is lethargic, with fewer than normal movements.

Premature labor. Premature labor may develop, as characterized by uterine contractions recorded on the fetal monitor. The mother may complain of backache, uterine cramping, or rhythmic contractions. There may be leakage of amniotic fluid from the vagina because of premature rupture of the membranes.

P

Perfusion Studies, Cardiac

Also called: Nuclear myocardial scans, perfusion imaging, thallium scan, myocardial perfusion imaging

SPECIMEN OR TYPE OF TEST: Nuclear Imaging

PURPOSE OF THE TEST

Nuclear scanning or radionuclide imaging of the heart is done to determine the severity and location of coronary stenosis, the viability of the myocardium, to identify those at risk for an infarction and to determine treatment options for patients with coronary artery disease (CAD).

BASICS THE NURSE NEEDS TO KNOW

Varying techniques may be used to noninvasively assess the ability of the coronary arteries to maintain perfusion to the heart. These include single-proton emission computed tomography (SPECT) and positron emission tomography (PET). The procedure may be done at rest (no physiologic demand) or at stress (induced physiologic demand)

SPECT involves the use of a gamma camera, which produces a 3-dimensional image of the heart. The camera rotates around the patient and multiple images are obtained. It can accurately stratify patients at risk. It can locate sites of perfusion abnormalities. PET scans permit assessment of coronary artery disease, especially metabolic and chemical changes, which result in perfusion problems. While it has higher specificity than SPECT images, PET scans are more costly and have greater radiation exposure.

Commonly used radionuclides for these scans are thallium 201, Tc-99m sestamibi, and Tc-99m tetrofosmin. Thallium was the first agent used in myocardial perfusion studies, but Tc-99m (sestamibi or tetrofosmin) provide better gamma camera imaging.

Dual isotope imaging may also be done. While patient is at rest, thallium is given. Then exercise is done and sestamibi is given followed by a second set of images. The timing of the rest and poststress imaging varies with hospital protocols.

REFERENCE VALUES	Normal myocardial perfusion; no "cold" spots

HOW THE TEST IS DONE

SPECT scanning is performed with an Anger gamma camera combined with a computer. Continuous counts of emitted photons are made during the cardiac cycle. The scan identifies "cold" spots, areas of decreased uptake. Cold spots identify areas of ischemia and infarction. The radioisotope can be given under a state of no physical demand, which is known as a *resting study,* or it can be done after inducing stress on the heart, which is called *stress imaging*.

Stress on the heart may be induced by exercise or by pharmacologic agents. Stress imaging is done because blood flow abnormalities may not be evident at rest. Stress imaging distinguishes ischemic sites from infarcted areas.

SIGNIFICANCE OF TEST RESULTS

Abnormal Values

Cold spots indicate and distinguish areas of infarction and ischemia.

INTERFERING FACTORS

- Cardiomyopathies
- Coronary anomaly
- Coronary spasms
- Patient movement
- Obesity
- Conduction defects

NURSING CARE

When a SPECT study is done:

Pretest

- Usually, long-acting nitrates are held for 8 to 12 hours before the test.
- Calcium channel blockers and β-blockers are held
- The patient fasts for 4 to 6 hours before the test but may drink water.
- ○ *Patient Teaching.* Instruct patient to avoid caffeinated drinks for 24 hours.
- ○ *Patient Teaching.* Explain procedure to the patient, including the need to remain motionless and that the camera will rotate.
- Intravenous access is established.
- The nurse informs the patient of the need to go to the nuclear medicine department twice.
- With the single photon emission computed tomography (SPECT) scan, the nurse assesses the patient for claustrophobia.
- If dipyridamole (Persantine) is to be given, hold xanthine-containing medications; such as theophylline.
- If adenosine is to be given, hold dipyridamole for 12 to 24 hours.

During the Test

- The patient is placed supine on the table with arms over the head.
- The radiopharmaceutical agent is give intravenously and multiple scintigraphic images are taken.
- Stress is induced by exercise or a pharmacologic agent. A treadmill is preferred over a bicycle. Bruce or a modified Bruce protocol is used. The Bruce protocols are multistage maximal treadmill programs broken into 3-minute intervals. Between stages there is an increase in the grade (incline) of the treadmill. The radiopharmaceutical agent is given intravenously at peak stress. Exercise is continued for 30 to 60 seconds.
- If the patient is unable to perform an exercise stress test, pharmacologic stress may be induced with the intravenous administration of dipyridamole, adenosine, or dobutamine. Dobutamine is only used if the others are contraindicated.
- Dipyridamole may be given orally or intravenously, although intravenous is preferred. Imaging agent is given 3 to 4 minutes after the dipyridamole infusion is complete. Observe patient response. If pain, headache, dizziness, flushing, or nausea occurs, aminophylline may be ordered to relieve symptoms.
- Adenosine is given intravenously. The imaging agent is given halfway through the adenosine infusion. Common patient responses include flushing, shortness of breath, and chest pain. Reassure patients that these symptoms are transient. Heart block may also occur and is relieved when the infusion is stopped.

Continued

P

NURSING CARE—cont'd

- If dobutamine is given, it is administered intravenously. The imaging agent is given during the infusion. The patient may complain of palpitations, chest pain, and flushing. Premature ventricular contractures may be observed. Less common is the incidence of ventricular tachycardia and atrial fibrillation.
- After the completion of the stress test, the patient is placed supine on the table and multiple scintigraphic images are taken.

Posttest
- Assess the patient's response.
- Three to 4 hours later, the patient may return for a repeat scan.

Pericardiocentesis

Also called: Pericardial fluid analysis

SPECIMEN OR TYPE OF TEST: Pathology

PURPOSE OF THE TEST

Analysis of pericardial fluid is performed to determine the cause of and appropriate therapy for acute pericarditis, subacute effusive-constrictive pericarditis, neoplastic pericardial disease, and pericardial effusion of unknown cause.

BASICS THE NURSE NEEDS TO KNOW

Pericardiocentesis is a diagnostic and therapeutic procedure in which the pericardial space is accessed with a needle or cannula, and fluid is aspirated (Figure 79). For diagnostic purposes, the fluid is then analyzed. For therapeutic purposes, either fluid is drained on a one-time basis or a catheter is inserted and left in place for 1 to 48 hours (rarely, it may be kept in for 72 hours).

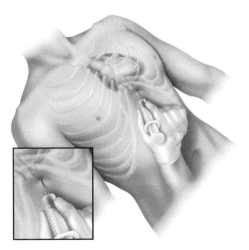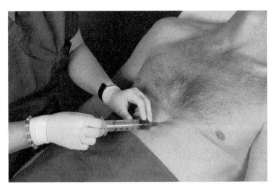

Figure 79. Pericardiocentesis. (From Custalow CB: *Color atlas of emergency department procedures,* Philadelphia, 2005, Saunders.)

Normally, the pericardial space between the visceral and parietal pericardium contains approximately 20 to 50 mL of clear serous fluid. If the pericardium becomes inflamed, diseased, or is disrupted, a pericardial effusion may occur. As fluid builds up in the pericardial space, cardiac tamponade may result. Cardiac tamponade will eventually lead to a decrease in cardiac output, with an increase in right atrial pressure, pulsus paradoxus, and hypotension. If progressive and untreated, cardiac tamponade will result in death.

REFERENCE VALUES   Pericardial fluid is sterile, clear, and colorless or straw-colored.

HOW THE TEST IS DONE

Pericardiocentesis for diagnostic purposes is not an emergency situation and can be performed in the controlled environment of an operating room or special procedure room. The procedure begins after skin preparation and infiltration of a local anesthetic, usually 1% lidocaine without epinephrine. A small incision is made in the skin, the site being determined by the desired approach.

The physician inserts a needle and approximately 20 mL of fluid is removed for analysis. Echocardiography is used to guide the needle into the pericardial sac. See Echocardiography, pp. 270. If cytologic studies are performed, a heparinized container is necessary. The fluid is usually analyzed for color; hemoglobin concentration; hematocrit value; red blood cell, white blood cell, and differential counts; and protein and glucose determinations. In addition, Gram stains and culture, fungal stains and culture, and cytologic studies are performed. Additional fluid is removed if viral and parasite studies, immunologic and serologic screens, or lipoelectrophoresis are planned.

If therapeutic pericardiocentesis is desired after the specimens are obtained, a catheter is inserted and positioned to allow drainage.

SIGNIFICANCE OF TEST RESULTS

Bacterial, viral, or fungal infection
Malignancy

INTERFERING FACTORS

- A patient who is uncooperative and unable to lie still during the procedure.
- Those receiving anticoagulant therapy, with bleeding disorders or thrombocytopenia, are not appropriate candidates.
- If cultures of the fluid are planned, administration of antibiotics will affect the results.

NURSING CARE

Pretest
- Ensure that an informed consent form has been signed.
- Check laboratory work for bleeding problems. Take medication history to check for anticoagulant use.
- Obtain a baseline ECG if ordered.

Continued

NURSING CARE—cont'd

- The nurse documents baseline vital signs and heart sounds.
- Sedation is often given because of the risk of movement during the procedure.

○ *Patient Teaching.* The nurse explains the procedure to the patient. Instruct the patient to remain motionless during the procedure. Warn the patient they may feel pressure as the needle is inserted.

○ *Patient Teaching.* If the procedure is elective, the nurse instructs the patient to maintain a nothing-by-mouth status for 4 to 6 hours before the test.

- Administer sedation as prescribed.
- Clip site of excess hair if necessary.

○ *Patient Teaching.* Inform patient and family that the procedure takes 20 to 60 minutes.

During the Test

- Position the patient. Usually a semi-Fowler's position is used with the head of the bed elevated to 30 to 60 degrees.
- Ensure that an intravenous infusion is present and patent.
- Give oxygen via nasal cannula.
- The nurse maintains telemetric or cardiac monitoring and reports any abnormality immediately. Vital signs are taken frequently. Have a defibrillator and emergency drugs on hand.
- The nurse continuously reassures and supports the patient, who will feel the local anesthetic being infiltrated and may experience a sharp pain when the pericardium is infiltrated.

Posttest

- Exert pressure on site for approximately 5 minutes
- Apply small dressing or bandage to site
- The patient may return to pretest activities gradually if vital signs are stable.

○ *Patient Teaching.* On discharge, instruct patient to check site for bleeding or signs of infection.

◇ **Nursing Response to Complications**

Complications from pericardiocentesis include puncture or laceration of the cardiac chamber, laceration of a coronary artery, ventricular fibrillation, pneumothorax, and peritoneal puncture. Puncture or laceration of the cardiac chamber and laceration of the coronary artery will cause cardiac tamponade.

Cardiac tamponade. A feared complication of a pericardiocentesis is cardiac tamponade, which is due to bleeding into the pericardial sac. As blood accumulates into the pericardial sac, the heart is restricted. The nurse will observe a decrease in cardiac output, muffled heart sounds, increase in right atrial pressure, and pulsus paradoxus. Notify the physician immediately. If the size of the pericardial effusion is significant, emergency surgery may be necessary.

Ventricular fibrillation. The mechanical trauma of a pericardiocentesis may cause ventricular fibrillation during the procedure. The nurse observes the cardiac monitor and informs the physician if this lethal dysrhythmia occurs. The nurse anticipates this response to the procedure by having a code cart available with its emergency medications.

Pneumothorax. Anxiety, restlessness, dyspnea, tachypnea, pallor, and decreased breath sounds are indications of a pneumothorax. Notify the physician immediately and anticipate an order for a chest radiograph to evaluate the size of the pneumothorax.

Persantine Scan

See Stress Test, Cardiac on pp. 558.

Peripheral Blood Smear

See Red Blood Cell Morphology on pp. 535-538.

PET Scan

See Positron Emissions Tomography on pp. 506-510.

Phenylalanine, Blood

Also called: PKU Test; Phenylketonuria Test; Phenylalanine Screening Test; Guthrie Screening Test

SPECIMEN OR TYPE OF TEST: Serum, Plasma

PURPOSE OF THE TEST

The blood phenylalanine test is performed to screen for phenylketonuria (PKU) and other causes of hyperphenylalaninemia. It is also used to monitor patients who have PKU and are treated by dietary modification.

BASICS THE NURSE NEEDS TO KNOW

In normal amino acid metabolism, the enzyme phenylhydroxylase is needed to convert phenylalanine to tyrosine. When this enzyme or its cofactor BH_4 is absent, the levels of phenylalanine and its metabolite phenylpyruvic acid are elevated in the blood and urine.

Phenylketonuria (PKU) is an inherited autosomal recessive disorder. Unless early detection and proper dietary intervention occur, the elevated blood level of phenylalanine will cause permanent central nervous system damage and mental retardation. The severity of PKU varies from mild to severe, based on the degree of enzyme deficiency that exists.

The phenylalanine level is not elevated at birth because no dietary intake of protein has occurred. In the infant with this defect in amino acid metabolism, the serum level begins to rise within 24 hours, usually after starting to feed with breast milk or formula. The ideal time to screen the blood for phenylalanine is 48 hours after birth. Laws in every state require PKU testing of all newborns within a specified period. If the Guthrie test is performed in the first 24 hours of life, the test should be repeated within 2 weeks. The repeat test greatly reduces the chance of a false-negative result.

The Guthrie test is a screening tool that identifies only hyperphenylalaninemia. If an elevated result occurs, the test is repeated in 24 hours to ensure accuracy. If both results are positive, further testing with a different test methodology is needed to verify the cause of the elevated blood level. The serum phenylalanine value of greater than 20 mg/dL (SI: >1200 μmol/L) is

P

diagnostic of PKU. When the neonate has PKU and is untreated, the serum phenylalanine level can rise to 15 to 30 mg/dL (SI: 907-1815 μmol/L) by the 10th day of life.

Premature or low-birth-weight infants have higher serum values than do full-term infants of normal weight. This false-positive serum elevation is caused by immaturity of the liver. Antibiotics also interfere with the Guthrie method of analysis and cause a false-positive result.

When positive blood results are verified, DNA testing is done to confirm the PKU diagnosis in the neonate. DNA testing also is offered to the parents and family members to determine their carrier status and to provide genetic counseling, if desired.

REFERENCE VALUES

Guthrie Test
<4 mg/day/L *or* SI: 242 μmol/L

Fluorometry Method
Full-term newborn: 1.2-3.4 mg/dL *or* SI: 73-206 μmol/L
Premature newborn: 2-7.5 mg/dL *or* SI: 121-454 μmol/L
Adult: 0.8-1.8 mg/dL *or* SI: 48-109 μmol/L

▽ Critical Values

Guthrie test: >4 mg/day/L *or* SI: >242 μmol/L

HOW THE TEST IS DONE

For either test method, a heelstick puncture is used to obtain two to three drops of blood. The blood sample is collected by capillary tube or PKU card or filter paper.

SIGNIFICANCE OF TEST RESULTS

Elevated Values

Phenylketonuria
Severe burns
Hyperphenylalaninemia
Liver disease
Sepsis

INTERFERING FACTORS

- Oversaturating the filter paper with blood
- Insufficient quantity of blood on the filter paper
- Little to no ingestion of milk (PKU testing only)
- Antibiotics (PKU testing only)
- Recent exchange transfusion

NURSING CARE

Health Promotion
When the mother and baby are to be discharged early, the nurse reminds her to have a repeat PKU test for the child within 2 weeks. All states in the United States, and many other countries worldwide, mandate phenylalanine testing of all newborns within 28 days. The goal is to

identify PKU at a very early stage and provide effective dietary treatment so that mental retardation does not occur.

Pretest

- Nursing actions are similar to those used in other capillary puncture procedures (see Chapter 2), with the following additional measures.
- The nurse needs to state when the baby started on milk or breast-feeding.
- Ensure that the laboratory requisition slip includes the name, date, time of the test, date of birth, and time of the first milk feeding. Note the administration of any antibiotics or blood transfusion.

During the Test

- With the filter paper or card, only one side of the paper is blotted to fill the circles. The paper should not be turned over to soak the other side. Cord blood cannot be used for this test.

▽ **Nursing Response to Critical Values**

After the elevated phenylalanine test value is verified and the diagnosis is made, nutritional guidance and knowledge will help the parents' effectiveness in providing for the health of their baby. The nurse can provide information about a phenylalanine-restricted diet, with synthetic protein and a tyrosine supplement. The nurse can also provide the parents with opportunities to ask questions or receive guidance about the ongoing needs of their child.

Phosphorus

Also called: HPO_4^-; Phosphate, Blood

SPECIMEN OR TYPE OF TEST: Blood

PURPOSE OF THE TEST

Serum phosphorus helps diagnose kidney disorders and acid-base imbalance. It is also used to detect disorders of calcium, bone, or endocrine origin.

BASICS THE NURSE NEEDS TO KNOW

Phosphorus is a mineral element present in bone cells and extracellular fluid, including serum. Phosphorus from dietary intake provides for necessary replacement of the mineral. The homeostatic balance of the mineral in the extracellular fluid is maintained, and excess phosphorus is excreted in the feces and urine.

An inverse relationship exists between the serum levels of phosphorus and calcium. If the serum level of either mineral falls, the serum level of the other mineral rises. Serum phosphorus concentrations have a diurnal rhythm. The level is highest in the morning and lowest in the evening. The normal values also vary over a lifespan, with the highest serum values occurring in infants and children and the lowest values occurring in elderly individuals.

Elevated Value

An elevated level of serum phosphorus is called *hyperphosphatemia*. In the adult, the lab value is greater than 4.7 mg/dL (SI: >1.5 mmol/L). Severe hyperphosphatemia produces no symptoms but does cause hypocalcemia. With a rapid elevation of serum phosphorus to a level of greater than 6 mg/dL (SI: >1.94 mmol/L), the serum calcium level declines and causes symptoms of

P

hypotension and tetany from calcium depletion. The most common cause of hyperphosphatemia is severe renal insufficiency.

Decreased Value

A decreased value of the serum phosphorus level is called *hypophosphatemia*. In the adult, the laboratory value is less than 2.7 mg/dL (SI: 0.87 mmol/L). The patients who are most commonly affected by hypophosphatemia are the elderly and postoperative patients, as well as patients who undergo long-term hemodialysis treatment. Hypophosphatemia is a serious problem because it will affect neuromuscular, neuropsychiatric, skeletal, gastrointestinal, and cardiopulmonary function.

REFERENCE VALUES	Neonate: 4.5-9.0 mg/dL *or* SI: 1.45-2.91 mmol/L Child: 4.0-7.0 mg/dL *or* SI: 1.29-2.26 mmol/L Adult: 2.8-4.5 mg/dL *or* SI: 0.89-1.45 mmol/L
▽ Critical Values	<1 mg/dL (SI: <0.32 mmol/L)

HOW THE TEST IS DONE

Venipuncture or capillary puncture is used to collect a specimen of blood

SIGNIFICANCE OF TEST RESULTS

Elevated Values

Renal failure
Milk-alkali syndrome
Osteolytic metastatic bone cancer
Myelogenous leukemia
Postanesthesia hyperthermia
Cirrhosis of the liver
Pulmonary embolism
Diabetic ketoacidosis
Vitamin D toxicity
Respiratory acidosis
Sarcoidosis
Acidosis, respiratory, lactic
Pseudohypoparathyroidism

Decreased Values

Osteomalacia
Osteoblastic bone cancer
Acute gout
Vitamin D deficiency
Renal tubular disease
Hyperparathyroidism
Hypercalcemia
Vomiting, diarrhea
Sepsis

Acute respiratory infection
Prolonged nasogastric drainage
Severe malabsorption
Starvation
Respiratory alkalosis

INTERFERING FACTORS

• Carbohydrate-rich meals

NURSING CARE

Nursing actions are similar to those used in other venipuncture procedures (see Chapter 2), with the following additional measures.

Pretest

• Schedule the test for early morning to avoid diurnal fluctuations.

○ *Patient Teaching.* The nurse instructs the patient to discontinue all food and fluids for 8 hours before the test because carbohydrate intake and recent food intake tend to decrease the serum phosphate level.

Posttest

• The nurse monitors the laboratory results for abnormal values. Severe depletion of phosphate can cause many physical changes in physiologic functions. A rising serum calcium level may accompany a low phosphorus level and respiratory alkalosis may cause hypophosphatemia.

▽ **Nursing Response to Critical Values**

The physician must be notified immediately when the phosphorus level is decreased to the critical value level. There may be resultant cardiac, respiratory, musculoskeletal, and central nervous system dysfunction. This includes decreased cardiac contractility and cardiac output, respiratory failure, tremor, weakness, convulsions, slurred speech, coma, and myopathy. About 20% of patients with a critical low level of hypophosphatemia will die.

The nurse takes vital signs. The respiratory assessment findings often include dyspnea, adventitious sounds, and weak respiratory effort. The nurse also assesses for neurologic changes, including tremors, slurred speech, ataxia, stupor, or coma. As an initial intervention, the nurse maintains the patient on bedrest with side rails, in semi-Fowler's to full Fowler's position to enhance breathing and cardiac output. The nurse also initiates seizure precautions and prepares for cardiac monitoring.

Platelet Aggregation

Also called: Aggregometer Test; Platelet Function Studies

SPECIMEN OR TYPE OF TEST: Blood

PURPOSE OF THE TEST

The platelet aggregation test is used to evaluate platelet function and to detect a hereditary or acquired platelet bleeding disorder.

BASICS THE NURSE NEEDS TO KNOW

After an injury to a blood vessel, platelets are the first component of clotting to respond. The platelets adhere to the blood vessel wall at the site of injury and form a plug that prevents additional blood loss. The platelets change shape, become sticky, and are capable of binding plasma proteins, including fibrinogen. The platelets then adhere to each other in platelet aggregation (Figure 80).

With abnormal platelet function, the patient has deficient clotting ability and a tendency to bleed. There are inherited and acquired causes of platelet dysfunction, but the most common cause is medication that interferes with platelet function. Aspirin or aspirin-containing compounds, penicillins, and numerous other medications can result in decreased or absent platelet function.

REFERENCE VALUES   More than 60% of platelets aggregate in response to each chemical testing substance that stimulates platelet aggregation

HOW THE TEST IS DONE

Venipuncture is used to obtain a sample of venous blood.

SIGNIFICANCE OF TEST RESULTS

Decreased Values

Aspirin, nonsteroidal antiinflammatory drugs and other medications
Uremia
Liver disease
Bernard-Soulier syndrome
Wiskott-Aldrich syndrome
von Willebrand's disease
Disseminated intravascular coagulation (DIC)

INTERFERING FACTORS

- Lipemia
- Caffeine
- Nicotine
- Thrombocytopenia

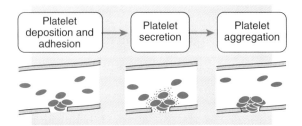

Figure 80. Platelet response to vascular injury.

NURSING CARE

Nursing actions are similar to those used in other venipuncture procedures (see Chapter 2), with the following additional measures.

Pretest

- The nurse should make a list of all prescribed and over-the-counter medications the patient is taking. Aspirin, antihistamines, nonsteroidal antiinflammatory agents, penicillin, antimicrobials, psychotropic drugs, and many others interfere with platelet aggregation and can cause a bleeding disorder. Schedule this test for 7 to 10 days after discontinuing medications that disrupt platelet function.

○ *Patient Teaching.* The nurse instructs the patient to fast from food or to eat only low-fat foods for 8 hours before the test. Caffeine intake and smoking must be avoided on the day of the test. The patient is instructed to discontinue taking aspirin, aspirin-containing medications, and nonsteroidal antiinflammatory medications for 7 to 10 days before the test.

Posttest

- Ensure that the venipuncture site has sealed and that the patient is not bleeding. The nurse uses sterile gauze to apply pressure to the puncture site. Keeping pressure on the site, the patient can also raise his or her arm overhead. The combination of pressure and elevation should help the process of coagulation and stop the bleeding.
- If the platelet aggregation results are lower than normal, the nurse should observe for characteristic bleeding in the patient. This can include spontaneous bruising, epistaxis, and bleeding from mucous membranes, particularly the gingiva of the oral cavity, intestine, or bladder. With trauma or surgery, the patient may bleed profusely. Some general anesthetics can also decrease platelet aggregation ability.

Platelet Count

Also called: Thrombocyte Count

SPECIMEN OR TYPE OF TEST: Blood

PURPOSE OF THE TEST

The platelet count is used to assess the ability of the bone marrow to produce platelets and to identify the destruction or loss of platelets in the circulation. It is also used to evaluate the untoward effects of chemotherapy or radiation treatment.

BASICS THE NURSE NEEDS TO KNOW

Platelets function to initiate the process of coagulation. When there is a nick or opening in a blood vessel, platelets quickly aggregate, adhere to the endothelial surface of the blood vessel, and plug the opening. As additional platelets and clotting factors arrive, the clot becomes firm and seals off the opening effectively.

Variation in Normal Values

In laboratory testing, considerable variation exists in the normal platelet count reference range. The normal value is slightly decreased during menstruation and pregnancy. The platelet count is also reduced relative to the excess fluid in the blood. This dilution effect occurs with the administration of fluids, including intravenous fluids and packed red cell transfusions. When

P

the platelets are counted, variation exists between the reference range performed by manual counting and that carried out by an automated counter. The nurse should use the reference value of the laboratory that performs the cell count.

Elevated Values

Thrombocytosis is an excess number of platelets (>400,000 cells/μL or SI: >400 × 10^9/L) in the blood. The condition may be reactive in response to acute inflammatory disease, blood loss, or trauma. This condition rarely causes symptoms and is self-limiting. The elevated level of platelets returns to a normal value as the underlying condition is corrected. Thrombocytosis also may be a symptom of myeloproliferative disease, such as chronic myelocytic leukemia. When the platelet count rises severely, there is potential for a hemorrhage or thrombosis. The hemorrhage probably results from defects in the platelets and the inability to form a clot. Thrombosis in either veins or arteries can occur as platelets aggregate and trap erythrocytes in the microcirculation. Common sites of vascular occlusion include the splenic, hepatic, and pulmonary veins; the mesenteric and axillary arteries; and the fingers and toes.

Decreased Values

Thrombocytopenia is a decreased number of platelets (<100,000 cells/μL or SI: <100 × 10^9/L) in the blood. This condition causes a prolonged bleeding time because the patient's clotting ability is seriously compromised. The decrease in platelets is caused by three possible categories of pathophysiologic change: (1) deficient platelet production, (2) rapid platelet destruction, and (3) abnormal pooling of the platelets (Table 12). The most common cause is the accelerated destruction of platelets. The bone marrow responds with accelerated production of new cells, but when the platelet destruction is rapid and extensive, the response of the marrow is inadequate. With inadequate numbers of platelets, the patient is vulnerable to bleeding, particularly into the skin.

REFERENCE VALUES	150,000-450,000 cells/μL *or* SI: 150-450 × 10^9/L
▽ Critical Values	<50,000 cells/μL *or* SI: <50 × 10^9/L >1,000,000 cells/μL *or* SI: >100 × 10^9/L

HOW THE TEST IS DONE

Venipuncture or capillary puncture is done to collect a sample of blood

SIGNIFICANCE OF TEST RESULTS

Elevated Values

Polycythemia vera
Myelofibrosis
Chronic myelocytic leukemia
Thrombocythemia
Posthemorrhage regeneration
Iron deficiency anemia
Multiple myeloma

TABLE 12	Pathophysiologic Causes of Thrombocytopenia	
Category	**Pathophysiology**	**Cause**
Deficient platelet production	Impairment of bone marrow with reduced numbers of stem cells or megakaryocytes	Drugs, aplastic anemia, radiation, chemotherapy, malignancy of the bone marrow
	Ineffective thrombopoiesis	Deficiency of iron, vitamin B_{12}, folic acid
	Defective production or regulation of thrombopoietin	Inherited genetic disorder
Platelet destruction	*Intracorpuscular destruction* Defects in platelet structure with short platelet life span	Inherited genetic disorder
	Extracorpuscular destruction	Autoimmune processes
	Immunologic destruction of platelets by immunoglobulin G antibodies	Infection
	Excess clotting or mechanical damage to platelets	DIC Infection Cardiac valve replacement Microvascular clotting disorder
Abnormal distribution or pooling	Splenic disorder with hypersplenism	Malignancy, infection infiltrates, congestion

Postsplenectomy response
Acute or chronic infection
Inflammatory diseases
Hodgkin's disease
Lymphoma
Chronic renal disease
Renal cysts

Decreased Values
Idiopathic thrombocytopenic purpura
Megaloblastic anemia
Liver disease
Infection
Massive blood transfusion
Malignancy of the spleen
Radiation-chemotherapy
Leukemia
Fanconi syndrome
Wiskott-Aldrich syndrome
Uremia

P

Systemic lupus erythematosus
Aplastic anemia
Severe iron deficiency anemia
Parasitic diseases (malaria, toxoplasmosis, histoplasmosis)
Disseminated intravascular coagulation (DIC)
Thyroid disease
Eclampsia

INTERFERING FACTORS
- Platelet clumping
- Multiple transfusions

NURSING CARE

Nursing actions are similar to those used in other venipuncture procedures (see Chapter 2), with the following additional measures.

Pretest
- The nurse instructs the patient to avoid strenuous exercise before the test because exertion and stress elevate the test results temporarily.

Posttest
- Assess the venipuncture site for signs of bleeding or ecchymosis. If the patient has a low platelet count, the venipuncture site can leak blood because of a failure to form a clot. To promote clotting, use sterile gauze to apply pressure to the site, or raise the arm above the head while maintaining pressure on the site.

○ *Patient Teaching.* When the platelet count is decreased, institute measures to protect the patient from trauma, bruising, or cuts. The nurse teaches the patient to avoid bruising or bleeding. Suggested measures include using an electric razor to avoid shaving nicks in the skin, using a soft toothbrush to avoid scratching the gingiva, and walking carefully near tables and other wooden furniture to avoid bumping into a corner or hard surface. The nurse also teaches the patient to avoid the use of aspirin because this medication interferes with the platelets' ability to form a clot. The patient must learn to read the labeled ingredients on over-the-counter medications to avoid anything containing acetylsalicylic acid. This compound is commonly present in medications to relieve flulike symptoms, colds, and headaches. If the patient us unsure, he or she can ask the pharmacist for assistance.

▽ **Nursing Response to Critical Values**
If the lab results indicate a critical value in either a lack or an excess of platelets, the nurse should notify the physician immediately. When the platelet count is at or below the critical value on the low side, there is a high risk of spontaneous hemorrhage. The nurse takes baseline vital signs and begins to assess at regular intervals for signs of bleeding. Superficial bleeding in the skin is evidenced by petechiae, purpura, or ecchymosis. Epistaxis or bleeding from the gingiva in the mouth may occur. Hematuria may occur. If the patient recently delivered a baby, she may exhibit vaginal bleeding or bleeding from the incision of a caesarean section. Hemorrhage into the brain will cause a stroke. If the platelet count is at or above the critical value on the high side, thrombosis can occur. The clot can develop anywhere throughout the body, including the brain, abdominal organs, and heart. The nurse takes baseline vital signs and begins to observe for symptoms of sudden onset, including acute pain, neurologic symptoms, or a change in the level of consciousness.

Plethysmography, Arterial

Also called: Pulse Cuff Recording (PCR)

SPECIMEN OR TYPE OF TEST: Pressure Measurements

PURPOSE OF THE TEST

Plethysmography is a noninvasive test that evaluates the arterial blood flow in the extremities. It detects the presence of peripheral arterial vascular disease and the presence of partial obstruction in the arterial circulation in the upper or lower extremity.

BASICS THE NURSE NEEDS TO KNOW

Peripheral artery disease (PAD) is a relatively common problem in people older than 70 years and in people older than 50 years who have diabetes or who smoke. The atherosclerotic plaque in the arteries of one or both legs can cause one or more segmental locations of partial obstruction of arterial circulation to the distal extremity. In plethysmography testing, the location of the restricted blood flow is identified by lower systolic pressure readings.

Ankle-Brachial Index (ABI)

When the legs are evaluated, a baseline systolic pressure measurement of the brachial artery is obtained first. The pressure readings of the legs are then taken in segmented locations. The ABI result is calculated by dividing the ankle pressure reading by the brachial pressure reading. In the normal patient with no obstruction of the arterial circulation, the systolic readings in the various leg segments are all approximately the same as the baseline brachial systolic pressure, with an ABI index of 1.

With partial obstruction of one or more segments of the arterial circulation, the systolic pressure will be lower in that segment of measurement. An ABI value of less than 1 means there is lower pressure in a distal segment of the artery because of less blood flow. An ABI of 0.95 is abnormal. An ABI of 0.50 means that there is severely compromised arterial circulation at a particular segment location. For comparison, the examination is done on both extremities. Since this test serves as a screening test, abnormal results are followed up with more precise testing by Doppler ultrasound imaging or contrast angiography and CT or MRI imaging.

REFERENCE VALUES	No evidence of arterial peripheral vascular disease; normal systolic measurements; ABI = 1

HOW THE TEST IS DONE

Plethysmographic cuffs are inflated at different levels on the extremities, and the plethysmograph machine records the systolic measurement of each cuff location (Figure 81). A Doppler ultrasound probe at an arterial location in the ankle identifies when blood flow is cut off during insufflation and provides the systolic pressure measurement when the pulse returns during deflation. The test takes about 30 minutes to complete.

P

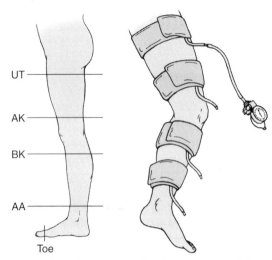

Figure 81. Arterial plethysmography of lower extremity. Segmental arterial pressure measurements are taken at the various cuff positions. *AA,* above ankle; *BK,* below knee; *AK,* above knee; *UT,* upper thigh. (From Pfenninger JL, Fowler GC: *Pfenninger and Fowler's procedures for primary care*, ed 3, St Louis, 2011, Mosby.)

SIGNIFICANCE OF TEST RESULTS

Abnormal Values
Peripheral vascular disease
Arterial occlusive disease
Arterial thrombus or embolus
Arterial trauma

INTERFERING FACTORS
• Smoking

NURSING CARE

Pretest
• After the physician explains the procedure to the patient, obtain written consent from the patient and place it in the patient's record.
○ *Patient Teaching.*
• The nurse instructs the patient to refrain from smoking for 30 minutes before the test. Nicotine is a vasoconstrictive substance that will alter the results.
• The nurse assists the patient in removing all clothing and putting on a hospital gown. Restrictive clothing can alter the circulatory flow to the extremities.
• Place the patient in a supine position with a pillow under the head. Reassure the patient that there is no pain with the test. The patient will only feel the pressure as each cuff is inflated.
Posttest
• Deflate and remove the cuffs.

Plethysmography, Venous

Also called: Impedance Plethysmography, Venous

SPECIMEN OR TYPE OF TEST: Pressure Measurements

PURPOSE OF THE TEST

Venous plethysmography is used to help detect deep vein thrombosis and to screen patients who are at high risk for the development of venous thrombosis.

BASICS THE NURSE NEEDS TO KNOW

Using blood pressure cuffs and electrodes, venous plethysmography measures the change in blood volume of the extremities. The electrodes and the recorder produce a linear waveform pattern (a line tracing) that is recorded on a graph paper strip. The test is safe and noninvasive, with a high degree of accuracy in the detection of a thrombus in the leg. However, it may not be able to detect a thrombus in the calf, when the clot does not occlude the vein.

In normal venous circulation, the blood moves toward the heart from the distal extremities. If a vein is compressed temporarily by a blood pressure cuff, the venous flow is interrupted. Distal to that compression point, the veins become engorged. On deflation of the cuff and release of the compression, the vein quickly empties excess blood and resumes normal venous outflow.

As the compression is applied to a normal vein, the venous plethysmographic waveform pattern shows a gradual rise in height from the baseline. This phase is called *venous capacitance* and represents the filling of the distal vein to its fullest capacity. On release of the compression, the waveform drops rapidly and returns to baseline

Abnormal Results

When a deep vein is obstructed by a thrombus, there is a backup of the venous blood and engorgement of the distal part of the vein. In plethysmography, once the vein is compressed temporarily by the blood pressure cuff, the blood flow is further interrupted. Increased engorgement of the distal vein cannot occur because the vein has already filled to capacity. On deflation of the cuff and release of the compression, only minimal venous blood flow resumes because the thrombus continues to obstruct the lumen. Correspondingly, the waveform demonstrates a limited, slow return to the baseline. With an abnormal result of this screening test, follow-up vascular imaging is done by Doppler ultrasound or contrast angiography with CT or MRI.

REFERENCE VALUES	Normal waveform patterns with adequate venous capacity and maximum venous outflow; no evidence of deep vein thrombosis

HOW THE TEST IS DONE

Plethysmographic cuffs and electrodes are applied to the thigh and calf to control and monitor venous blood flow (Figure 82). The cuffs are inflated, and the recorded waveforms demonstrate the filling of the vein to maximal capacity. On rapid release of the cuffs, the waveform demonstrates the venous outflow of the distal vein. The total time required to complete the test is 30 to 45 minutes.

P

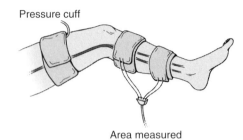

Pressure cuff

Area measured

Figure 82. For venous plethysmography testing, elevate the leg 25 to 30 degrees with the knee flexed and the hip rotated externally. (From Pfenninger JL, Fowler GC: *Pfenninger and Fowler's procedures for primary care*, ed 3, St Louis, 2011, Mosby.)

SIGNIFICANCE OF TEST RESULTS

Abnormal Values

Venous thrombosis
Thrombophlebitis
Venous obstruction (partial or complete)

INTERFERING FACTORS

- Muscle tension in the leg
- Compression of pelvic veins
- Low cardiac output
- Shock
- Arterial occlusive disease

NURSING CARE

Pretest
- After the physician has informed the patient about the procedure, obtain written consent from the patient and place it in the patient's record.
- Help the patient remove all clothing and put on a hospital gown. Any compression from restrictive clothing alters the venous circulation from the extremities. Place the patient in the supine position with the legs elevated above the heart and supported by pillows. The affected leg and hip are externally rotated, and the knee is flexed.

○ *Patient Teaching.* Advise the patient to refrain from movement and talking during the test.

Posttest
- Remove the deflated cuffs and electrodes.
- Wipe the conductive gel off the skin.

Positron Emission Tomography

Also called: PET Scan

SPECIMEN OR TYPE OF TEST: Nuclear Scan

P

Patient Handout–Brain PET Scan

PURPOSE OF THE TEST

The positron emission tomography (PET) scan is used to provide images of brain function and function of other specific target organs in the body. It detects areas of metabolic change in the tissue at a very early stage of disease. It also is used to guide or manage treatment of disease, monitor the tissue response to treatment, and in cancer staging.

BASICS THE NURSE NEEDS TO KNOW

The PET scan is a nuclear scan that uses radioactive isotopes to emit energy signals. Once the radioisotope is linked to a particular substance it is called a radiopharmaceutical. The intravenous radiopharmaceutical will move through the circulation of the body until it is taken up by the designated tissues that are to be scanned. The most commonly used radiopharmaceutical is 18FDG, an isotope linked to glucose.

Cells that grow and multiply rapidly, such as cancer cells, will demand nourishment in the form of glucose in greater amounts than normal tissue. These highly active, abnormal cells will demonstrate increased uptake of 18FDG. In tissue, the radioactive isotopes decay quickly releasing energy in concentrated amounts that correspond to the metabolism that is occurring in the tissue. Conversely, tissues that have minimal metabolic function or nonfunction demonstrate decreased uptake and concentration of the radiopharmaceutical. These visible abnormal changes in metabolism are distinctly different from those of normal tissue.

PET/CT

The positron emission tomography scan of today is a combination of the PET scan combined with computed tomography (CT) in a process of seamless imaging. The patient moves on a gantry table through the CT scanner first and continues directly through the PET scanner behind the CT. The combination scan provides more precise orientation, location, and detail of the abnormalities. Depending on the purpose of the test, the PET/CT may be done as a brain scan or a total body scan that includes head to toe imaging.

Abnormal Results

In imaging of the brain, the PET/CT is helpful in providing information associated with Alzheimer's disease when the patient only has mild impairment. In early Alzheimer's disease, the PET scan shows hypometabolism in the parietal and temporal lobes bilaterally. As the disease progresses, the frontal lobes also demonstrate hypometabolism. Although the PET/CT scan cannot make a definitive diagnosis of Alzheimer's disease, it can clearly identify and diagnose the other causes of dementia, including multiinfarct dementia and frontotemporal dementia. These other dementias have different metabolic patterns that are distinct and recognizable. The PET scan can also identify a brain tumor and differentiate benign from malignant growth. In addition, the PET scan is used for location of abnormal brain tissue that causes epileptic seizures, usually as a part of presurgical assessment.

In the PET/CT scanning of the body, the purpose is usually to search for cancer metastases. It helps in the staging of cancer by detection of tumor metastasis and nodal involvement in any locations beyond the site of the primary tumor (Figure 83). The PET component is able to detect metastasis in the tissue before a tumor develops. Conversely, the metastatic site may be known and the PET/CT is used to locate the primary site. The scan is also used to evaluate the results of cancer treatment or restage when cancer reappears after initial surgery has been done. With PET/CT scan results, treatment decisions are made or modified to select the best

P

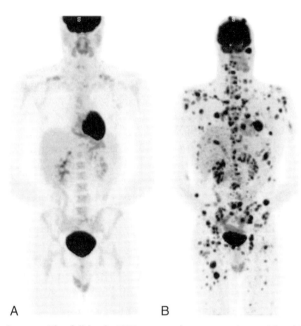

A   B

Figure 83. PET scan images. The full body PET scan evaluates a patient with a history of melanoma on the scalp. **A,** The scan shows no definite evidence of cancer recurrence. **B,** Six months later the scan shows profound and widely disseminated metastases throughout the body. (From Frank ED, Long BW, Smith BJ: *Merrill's atlas of radiographic positioning and procedures*, ed 12, St Louis, 2012, Mosby.)

therapy for the patient and to avoid surgery when the result would be "futile" because of metastasis.

Before coronary angiography or coronary artery bypass surgery, the PET/CT may be used to assess fatty acid metabolism or assess myocardial viability. When glucose uptake demonstrates viable myocardial tissue, the patient can benefit from coronary revascularization. However, when the PET/CT scan shows no adequate uptake of the 18FDG, the myocardial tissue is nonviable and the patient's heart will not benefit from improved coronary artery blood flow.

The whole body scan also may be used to detect the location of infection or inflammation. In infection, the 18FDG radiopharmaceutical will be accumulated by the granulocytes and macrophages at the infection site. These cells require glucose for their metabolism and function in clearing the infection. In inflammation, the radiopharmaceutical will accumulate in inflamed tissues, even when there is no infection.

REFERENCE VALUES   The imaged organs and tissues demonstrate normal perfusion, uptake, and metabolism

HOW THE TEST IS DONE

For the PET scan, a special radiopharmaceutical is injected intravenously. Once the radioactive substance enters the targeted tissue(s) by perfusion and metabolism, the emitted radioactive emissions are received by detectors within the PET scanner. The signals are then converted by computer hardware and software functions to provide images of the metabolism and function of the tissue. For the CT component, contrast medium may or may not be used. The CT scan provides the imaging of the anatomy of the body from x-ray imaging that moves forward in a spiral direction around the body. Detectors within the CT scanner receive the data as the x-rays pass through the body. The computer hardware and software convert the data to images of the patient's anatomy. Once the PET images are superimposed or fused on the CT images, the combined information of anatomy and function of the tissue is very useful for diagnosis.

SIGNIFICANCE OF TEST RESULTS

Abnormal Findings
Tumor, benign or malignant
Metastatic cancer
Epilepsy
Alzheimer's disease
Dementia
Cardiac ischemia
Inflammation
Infection

INTERFERING FACTORS

- Failure to follow the dietary restrictions in the pretest period.
- Claustrophobia
- Obesity
- Diabetes
- Body movement during scanning
- Metallic objects on the body

NURSING CARE

P

Pretest

- If the patient has a history of cancer diagnosis or treatment, schedule this test according to the time-delay protocol of the nuclear medicine institution and in consultation with the physician and radiologist. If the scan is done too soon after biopsy or surgery, a false-positive result can occur. If the scan is done too soon after radiation therapy or chemotherapy, a false-negative result can occur.

○ *Patient Teaching.* The nurse visits the hospitalized patient, or phones the patient who lives at home, to interview the patient and teach about the PET scan procedure and the pretest instructions. The purpose of the nurse's call is also meant to establish personal contact, to answer the patient's questions, and allay anxiety. Patients who know they have cancer or suspect a brain disorder or heart disease are likely to worry about this test and its potential findings. The nurse works with the patient to promote cooperation and trust. Another purpose is to identify any patient problems such as obesity, diabetes, or a history of claustrophobia or anxiety because these factors will require pretest modifications (Nguyen, Akdoman & Osmar, 2008).

Continued

NURSING CARE—cont'd

○ *Patient Teaching.* The nurse instructs the patient to limit the intake of caffeine and sugar in the 24 hours before the test. The patient then discontinues food intake for 4 to 6 hours before the scan, but water and medications are permitted.

- On the morning of the scan, the nurse measures and records vital signs, height, weight, and blood glucose level. The patient must change into a hospital gown, remove any metallic objects as jewelry, and void before the test. An intravenous line is established so the nuclear technologist can administer the radiopharmaceutical. A blanket is provided so that the patient maintains body warmth. The warmth enhances the uptake of the radiopharmaceutical in desired body tissues and limits the uptake in body fat. Once the radionuclide is injected, the patient is instructed to sit or lie down for about 1 hour. This time is needed for the uptake and concentration of the radiopharmaceutical in various tissues.

During the Test

- The patient is assisted to lie on the scanning table. If the brain is to be scanned, the patient's head will be placed inside the scanner. The patient is reminded to remain still. He or she may be asked to perform certain activities inside the scanner, such as speaking, reasoning, or listening to music at particular times during the scanning process.
- If the whole body is to be scanned, the patient lies on the scanning table and the table moves slowly through the ring of the CT/PET scanners. The patient is given a call light to summon help if needed. Music in the room helps to promote relaxation. The patient is reminded to refrain from movement or speaking during the test.
- The time needed for the scanning process is 15 to 60 minutes, depending on the type of scan and the scanning equipment used.

Posttest

- The patient can go home or return to the hospital room as soon as the scan is finished. For this scan, there is a small amount of patient exposure to radiation. However, the 18FDG has a half life of 109 minutes. By the time the scan is finished, much of the radionuclide has already decomposed. The remainder will be eliminated in the urine during the next 24 hours.

○ *Patient Teaching.* The nurse instructs the patient to drink extra fluids, to help eliminate the radiopharmaceutical in the urine. The patient should wash his or her hands after each voiding to rid the skin of any possible radioactive contamination.

Potassium, Serum

Also called: K^+

SPECIMEN OR TYPE OF TEST: Blood

PURPOSE OF THE TEST

Serum potassium is used to evaluate electrolyte balance, acid-base balance, hypertension, renal disease or renal failure, and endocrine disease. It is used to monitor patients receiving treatment for ketoacidosis, as well as those receiving hyperalimentation, dialysis, diuretic therapy, or intravenous fluid and electrolyte replacement.

BASICS THE NURSE NEEDS TO KNOW

Potassium is a major electrolyte that is present in all body fluids. Most of the potassium is concentrated in the intracellular fluids, with only a very small amount of the total potassium in the extracellular fluids, including the blood. The renewable source of potassium is the daily food intake. The extracellular potassium level remains within a relatively narrow range. The regulation of the extracellular potassium concentration is performed by the kidneys, with excretion of excess potassium in urine and feces (Figure 84).

Considerable danger is associated with either depletion or excess of potassium. Abnormal potassium concentration causes disturbances in the membrane potential and altered function of neuromuscular tissue, including the loss of cardiac contractility. With depletion or excess of this cation, the patient is at risk for the development of shock, respiratory failure, or cardiac dysrhythmias (Figure 85), including ventricular fibrillation.

Elevated Value

An elevated level of potassium in the extracellular fluid and blood is called *hyperkalemia*. The most common source of hyperkalemia is renal disease. The potassium value also rises with mineralocorticoid deficiency or metabolic acidosis. Additionally, damage to tissue and cells causes a release of intracellular potassium into the extracellular fluids.

In renal disease, the glomeruli may be unable to filter the blood, causing a rise in the serum value and a decrease in the excretion of potassium in the urine. In acute renal failure, the potassium level begins to rise with the onset of oliguria (scanty urinary output). In chronic renal failure, the potassium level does not begin to rise until there is a 75% reduction in the glomerular filtration rate.

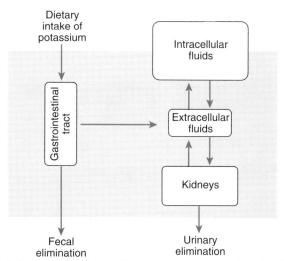

Figure 84. Homeostatic balance of potassium. Once the potassium is absorbed from the small intestine, most of it is stored in cells and a small amount remains in the extracellular fluids, including blood. Excess potassium is excreted from the body in feces and urine. The kidneys are the best regulators of potassium homeostasis.

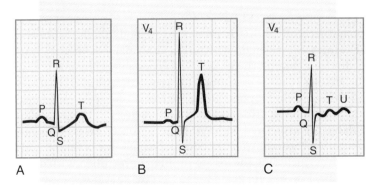

Figure 85. ECG changes in potassium imbalance. **A,** Normal ECG pattern; **B,** Moderate hyperkalemia with tall peaked T waves; **C,** Moderate hypokalemia with T wave and elevation of the U wave.

Decreased Value

A decreased amount of potassium in the extracellular fluid is called *hypokalemia*. It can occur with fluid losses from the gastrointestinal tract, skin, or kidneys. The most common cause of urinary potassium loss is from diuretic therapy. Hypokalemia can also result from a decreased dietary intake or from alkalosis. In alkalosis, the potassium has increased entry into the cells, and the intracellular concentration of potassium increases.

REFERENCE VALUES	Newborn: 3.7-5.9 mEq/L *or* SI: 3.7-5.9 mmol/L
	Infant: 4.1-5.9 mEq/L *or* SI: 4.1-5.9 mmol/L
	Child: 3.4-4.7 mEq/L *or* SI: 3.4-4.7 mmol/L
	Adult: 3.5-5.1 mEq/L *or* SI: 3.5-5.1 mmol/L

▽ Critical Values   Newborn: <2.7 mEq/L (SI 2.7 mmol/L) *or* >6.5 mEq/L
          (SI: >6.5 mmol/L)
       Adult: 2.5 mEq/L or less (SI: 2.5 mmol/L or less)
          or >6.0 mEq/L (SI: >6.0 mmol/L)

HOW THE TEST IS DONE

Venipuncture or arterial puncture is done to obtain a specimen of blood.

SIGNIFICANCE OF TEST RESULTS

Elevated Values

Rapid or excessive intravenous potassium replacement
Dehydration
Renal failure
Addison's disease
Massive hemolysis

Acidosis
Diabetic ketoacidosis
Traumatic crush injury
Severe burns

Decreased Values
Diuretic therapy
Intravenous fluid therapy without potassium replacement
Vomiting or diarrhea
Severe burns
Renal tubular acidosis
Excessive sweating
Fistula drainage
Bartter syndrome
Alkalosis
Aldosteronism

INTERFERING FACTORS

- Hemolysis

NURSING CARE

Nursing actions are similar to those used in other venipuncture or arterial puncture procedures (see Chapter 2), with the following additional measures.

During the Test

- The blood sample should be drawn from the arm that does not have an intravenous fluid administration. The fluid and possible electrolyte concentration would alter the test results.

Posttest

- Monitor the test results and notify the physician of any abnormal value. Untreated hyperkalemia or hypokalemia can cause changes in the myocardium and the neuromuscular system, including very serious cardiac arrhythmias (Table 13). For patients who are at risk for potassium imbalance, vital signs should be monitored routinely. The nurse also monitors the heartbeat to detect any changes in rate or rhythm.
- The nurse monitors and documents intake and output because fluid losses from intestinal drainage, vomiting, diarrhea, fistula drainage, burned skin, and urinary diuresis all can cause loss of potassium. Impaired renal function and diminished urinary output cause a rise in the serum potassium level.

▽ **Nursing Response to Critical Values**

Once the values reach a critical level (high or low value), the patient is in a life-threatening situation, with danger of severe cardiac dysrhythmia, cardiac arrest, and death. The nurse immediately notifies the physician of the abnormal test value.

The nurse assesses the patient for manifestations of potassium imbalance. With hyperkalemia, the manifestations include restlessness, hyperactivity of the gastrointestinal tract with nausea, abdominal cramping, and diarrhea, skeletal muscle weakness, and flaccidity. The ECG reading shows peaked T waves. In hypokalemia, the manifestations include muscle weakness,

Continued

| NURSING CARE—cont'd

hyporeflexia, leg cramps, and paresthesia, The ECG changes include dysrhythmias and there is an irregular pulse. The patient in severe crisis will hypoventilate and respiratory failure can occur.

The nurse prepares for an electrocardiogram (ECG) or for cardiac monitoring. In addition, the nurse prepares for the administration of oxygen and delivery of prescribed medication or intravenous therapy to correct the potassium imbalance. Specific treatment will depend on the type and severity of the imbalance and its cause.

TABLE 13   ECG* Changes Associated with Critical Values of Serum Potassium

Serum Potassium Level	ECG Manifestations
Hyperkalemia	
>6.5 mEq/L (SI: >6.5 mmol/L)	Peaked T waves
7-8 mEq/L (SI: 7-8 mmol/L)	Prolonged P–R interval
	Loss of P waves
	Widening of the QRS complexes
>8-10 mEq/L (SI: >8-10 mmol/L)	Sine wave pattern
	Cardiac standstill; asystole
Hypokalemia	
2-2.5 mEq/L (SI: 2-2.5 mmol/L)	Sagging of the ST segment
	Flattened or depressed T wave
	Elevation of the U wave
<2 mEq/L (SI: <2 mmol/L)	Smaller T waves
	Increased height (amplitude) of U waves

*ECG, Electrocardiogram.

Pregnancy-Associated Plasma Protein A

Also called: PAPP-A

PURPOSE OF THE TEST

The PAPP-A test is one of several first-trimester tests used to screen for Down syndrome of the fetus.

SPECIMEN OR TYPE OF TEST: Blood

BASICS THE NURSE NEEDS TO KNOW

In pregnancy, plasma protein A is made by the placenta. The protein appears in the maternal blood and in the amniotic fluid early in the first trimester. The normal value increases with the gestational age. After delivery, the level declines rapidly and may be undetectable after a few days to a few weeks. In testing for Down syndrome, the window for accuracy of this laboratory test is during the 9- to 14-week gestational period (Bahado-Singh & Argoti, 2010). When Down syndrome affects the fetus, the PAPP-A test result will show a lower than normal value.

Pregnant women are offered testing for fetal Down syndrome in the first or early in the second trimester. The combined first-trimester screen consists of human chorionic gonadotrophin (pp. 193-195), pregnancy-associated plasma protein -A (PAPP-A), and nuchal translucency measurement (pp. 328-329). The results are not interpreted singly, but in combination to provide greater accuracy. Because these tests are for screening purposes and false-positive results do exist, follow-up testing with amniocentesis or chorionic villus sampling and fetal genetic testing is indicated.

REFERENCE VALUES

Pregnancy, serum
8 weeks gestation: 90-7000 mU/L
10 weeks gestation: 140-7000 mU/L
12 weeks gestation: 900-9000 mU/L
14 weeks gestation: 2200-39, 500 mU/L

Pregnancy, amniotic fluid
8 weeks gestation: <10-64 mU/L
10 weeks gestation: <10-210 mU/L
12 weeks gestation: <10-16.5 mU/L
14 weeks gestation: < 10-110 mU/L
17 weeks gestation: <10-2135 mU/L
Adults, male and nonpregnant females: 3.8-10.4 mU/L

HOW THE TEST IS DONE

Venipuncture is used to obtain a specimen of maternal blood.
When amniocentesis is done, a sample of amniotic fluid can be analyzed for the PAPP-A value.

SIGNIFICANCE OF THE TEST RESULTS

Elevated Values
Pregnancy

Decreased Values
Possible Down syndrome of the fetus

INTERFERING FACTORS

• Lipemia

NURSING CARE

Nursing actions are similar to those used in other venipuncture procedures (see Chapter 2), with the following additional measures.

Pretest
The patient should discontinue food intake for 6 hours before the test because lipemia can alter the test results. Water is permitted.

Continued

Posttest

The patient will consult with her obstetrician or a genetic counselor regarding the results of the first-trimester multiple marker pregnancy screening tests. Lower than normal PAPP-A test results are an indicator of Down syndrome. However, by itself, the PAPP-A result is not sufficient to make a diagnosis. All three results of the triple marker screening will be considered together. A follow-up with either amniocentesis or chorionic villus sampling may be indicated.

Progesterone

SPECIMEN OR TYPE OF TEST: Blood

PURPOSE OF THE TEST

Serum progesterone levels are used to determine ovulation and to assess the function of the corpus luteum, particularly in cases of habitual abortion, first-trimester bleeding, and infertility.

BASICS THE NURSE NEEDS TO KNOW

In the menstruating female, progesterone is produced by the ovaries. Progesterone functions to help prepare the endometrium of the uterus for the implantation of the fertilized ovum. The corpus luteum of the ovary produces a small but steady supply during the preovulatory or follicular phase of the menstrual cycle. After ovulation, the progesterone level rises over a 4- to 5-day period in the luteal phase of the menstrual cycle. The serum level reaches and maintains its peak for about 1 week and then falls rapidly before the start of menstruation. A normal value in the luteal phase indicates that the patient is ovulating normally. In testing for the cause of infertility in the female, serial blood samples are obtained during the menstrual cycle to determine the day of ovulation.

During pregnancy, progesterone is synthesized in great quantity by the placenta, and the serum level rises progressively throughout the term of the pregnancy. Serial testing may also be done throughout a pregnancy to monitor for abnormal gestational development of the fetus, such as inevitable abortion. If the patient is in her first trimester and is bleeding, a serum progesterone value greater than 250 ng/dL (SI: >7.95 nmol/L) indicates a viable intrauterine pregnancy.

P

REFERENCE VALUES Child, prepuberty 7-52 ng/dL *or* SI: 0.2-1.7 nmol/L

Menstruating Female
Follicular phase: 15-70 ng/dL *or* SI: 0.5-2.2 nmol/L
Luteal phase: 200-2500 ng/dL *or* SI: 6.4-79.5 nmol/L

Pregnant Female
First trimester: 1025-4400 ng/dL *or* SI: 32.6-139.9 nmol/L
Second trimester: 1950-8250 ng/dL *or* SI: 62.0-262.4 nmol/L
Third trimester: 6500-22,900 ng/dL *or* SI: 206.7-728.2 nmol/L

HOW THE TEST IS DONE
Venipuncture is used to collect a specimen of blood.

SIGNIFICANCE OF TEST RESULTS

Elevated Values
Congenital adrenal hyperplasia
Molar pregnancy
Ovarian tumor

Decreased Values
Threatened abortion
Short luteal phase syndrome
Ectopic pregnancy
Hypogonadism

INTERFERING FACTORS

- Recent radioactive isotope scan

NURSING CARE

Nursing actions are similar to those used in other venipuncture procedures (see Chapter 2), with the following additional measures.

Pretest
- Schedule this test before or at least 7 days after a nuclear scan. The measurement of progesterone is performed by the radioimmunoassay method of analysis. The radioisotopes of a nuclear scan would interfere with the analysis and results of the progesterone test.
- When a series of blood tests throughout the menstrual cycle is required, make sure that the patient understands the testing plan and schedule of test dates.

Posttest
- On the requisition form, the physician writes the pertinent data, including the patient's sex, the date of the patient's last menstrual period, and the trimester of pregnancy. These data are used to help determine whether the results are within normal limits.
- In the pregnant female who is bleeding in the first trimester, a progesterone level that is below 150 ng/dL (SI 4.77 mmol/L) indicates a failing intrauterine pregnancy or an ectopic pregnancy. The nurse alerts the physician of this very low result.
- The nurse uses effective listening skills to help support the patient who has a history of miscarriage or who is pregnant and has intrauterine bleeding. The patient may express apprehension or anxiety about a possible loss of this pregnancy.

Progesterone Receptor (PR)

See Biopsy, Breast on p. 118.

Prostate-Specific Antigen

Also called: PSA

SPECIMEN OR TYPE OF TEST: Serum

PURPOSE OF THE TEST

The tumor marker prostate-specific antigen, combined with a digital rectal examination, is a screening test to detect cancer of the prostate gland. After treatment of cancer of the prostate gland, it is used to detect recurrence of the cancer.

BASICS THE NURSE NEEDS TO KNOW

Prostate-specific antigen is produced by the cells of the prostate gland. Some of this protein is secreted into the blood, where the amount is measurable. Men have a normally low level of PSA in the blood, but the amount rises abnormally with benign or malignant changes in the prostate gland. As a screening test, it can detect the serum elevation before there are symptoms of disease, but it cannot distinguish between a benign or malignant cause. When the screening test is positive, the follow-up testing plan is individualized because of several variables.

The recommendations about routine screening with PSA are subject to some debate. The PSA test has a more than 20% false-negative result, meaning that the test result is negative, but the patient actually has cancer of the prostate. It also has false-positive results, meaning that when the PSA test results are in the 4 to 10 ng/mL range, only 20% of those men actually have cancer of the prostate. It is also noted that in evidence-based practice terms, PSA screening for prostate cancer has not been proven to save lives (Ferri, 2011)

When the PSA test results are moderately positive, repeat testing several weeks later or serial testing several times over the next 18 months may be recommended in a "watch and wait" approach. However, rising PSA test results over time, PSA "velocity" (a rise of 0.79 ng/mL within 1 year) or a very high PSA value are considered as serious and a follow-up prostate gland biopsy is usually indicated.

P

REFERENCE VALUES   Male: 40-59 years old: 4 ng/mL or less *or* SI:<4 mcg/L or less

HOW THE TEST IS DONE

Venipuncture is used to collect a specimen of blood.

SIGNIFICANCE OF TEST RESULTS

Elevated Values
Adenocarcinoma of the prostate
Benign prostatic hypertrophy
Prostatitis

INTERFERING FACTORS

- Prostate gland manipulation
- Recent urethral instrumentation

Nursing actions are similar to those used in other venipuncture procedures (see Chapter 2 for additional information).

Health Promotion

The American Cancer Society recommends offering a PSA test annually to all men age 50 and older and who have a life expectancy of at least 10 years. Men who are at risk (African Americans and those with a family history of prostatic cancer) may begin annual PSA testing at age 45 years. In addition, a digital rectal examination (DRE) is offered annually to improve chances of prostate cancer detection (Ferri, 2011).

Pretest

- The PSA blood test is done before the digital rectal examination. A false-positive PSA result would occur if the prostate manipulation is done within 48 hours before the blood work.
- Schedule the PSA blood test before or at least 2 to 4 weeks after any urethral instrumentation procedure, such as a transurethral resection, prostatic biopsy, or cystoscopy. The tissue manipulation from these procedures would cause a release of the prostate-specific antigen and falsely elevate the result of the blood test.

Posttest

- Although an elevated PSA value is suggestive of cancer, the result is not conclusive; the diagnosis can only be confirmed by biopsy of the prostate gland. The nurse listens to the patient's feelings of apprehension and provides support. The nurse can encourage his decision to continue with additional diagnostic testing to obtain additional information.

Protein C and Protein S

See Coagulation Inhibitors on pp. 119.

Protein Electrophoresis, Serum

P

SPECIMEN OR TYPE OF TEST: Serum

PURPOSE OF THE TEST

Serum protein electrophoresis is used in the detection of hepatobiliary disease and monoclonal gammopathy, and in the evaluation of nutritional status.

BASICS THE NURSE NEEDS TO KNOW

In the blood, total protein consists of albumin and globulins. They are plasma proteins manufactured in the liver. The process of electrophoresis uses an electric field to separate these fractional components in greater detail and measure the amount of each component. Different diseases cause alterations in the concentration of the plasma proteins and in the characteristic patterns of protein electrophoresis. The pattern of monoclonal proteins demonstrates a tall narrow spike in the M protein of gamma globulin. It is an abnormality that is characteristic of plasma cell dyscrasias and lymphoproliferative disorders, including multiple myeloma, lymphoma, chronic lymphocytic leukemia, and several other diseases. Asymptomatic multiple myeloma will demonstrate a serum M protein level of 3 g/dL or more (SI: 30 g/L or more).

Albumin

This is the largest component and makes up two thirds of the total plasma proteins. The functions of albumin are to (1) maintain the oncotic pressure (the pressure that holds water in the blood vessels), (2) maintain a reserve nitrogen pool for tissue growth and repair, and (3) serve as a carrier protein for numerous substances, such as medications, lipids, bilirubin, hormones, minerals, and fat-soluble vitamins.

Globulins

The three main subgroups of globulins are α-, β-, and γ-globulins. α_1-*Globulin* primarily consists of α_1-antitrypsin, a protease inhibitor that inactivates trypsin in the blood. α_2-*Globulin* consists of two important plasma proteins: haptoglobulin and α_2-globulin. Haptoglobulin binds the hemoglobin that has been released from the lysis of erythrocytes. α_2-Macroglobulin is a protease inhibitor. Because of its large size relative to other globulins, it cannot pass through the glomeruli and enter into glomerular filtrate. In nephrotic syndrome, when other smaller globulins are lost via glomerular filtrate, the concentration of α_2-macroglobulin increases dramatically.

β_1-*Globulin* consists mainly of transferrin, the iron-transporting protein. It carries ferric ions from intracellular storage to the bone marrow. β_2-*Globulin* consists primarily of the low-density lipoprotein that transports cholesterol to the cells. Other β-globulins are fibrinogen and complement factors.

γ-*Globulins* consist of the immunoglobulins G, A, D, E, and M. They are usually identified as IgG, IgA, IgD, IgE, and IgM. Each of these plasma proteins is designed to carry out antibody activity by binding with and neutralizing specific antigens.

REFERENCE VALUES

Adult
Albumin: 3.5-5.0 g/d/L *or* SI: 35-50 g/L
α_1-globulin: 0.1-0.3 g/d/L *or* SI: 1-3 g/L
α_2-globulin: 0.6-1.0 g/d/L *or* SI: 6-10g/L
β-globulins: 0.7-1.1 g/d/L *or* SI: 7-11 g/L
γ-globulins: 0.8-1.6 g/d/L *or* SI: 8-16 g/L
No monoclonal proteins detected

HOW THE TEST IS DONE

A venipuncture is performed to collect a specimen of blood.

SIGNIFICANCE OF TEST RESULTS

Elevated Values
Albumin
Dehydration
α_1-*Globulins*
Inflammatory disease

Malignancy
Infection
Trauma
Hepatic disorders
α₂-Globulins
Nephrotic syndrome
Tumor
Inflammatory disease, subacute or chronic
β-Globulins
Hyperlipoproteinemia
Monoclonal gammopathies
γ-Globulins
Polyclonal gammopathies:
  Chronic liver diseases (hepatitis, cirrhosis)
  Collagen diseases (systemic lupus erythematosus, rheumatoid arthritis)
  Infection, chronic
  Inflammatory disease, chronic (sarcoidosis)
Monoclonal gammopathies: (multiple myeloma, Waldenström's macroglobulinemia, chronic lymphocytic leukemia, amyloidosis, lymphoma)

Decreased Values
Albumin
Metastatic cancer
Heart failure
Malnutrition
Thermal injury
Nephrotic syndrome
Protein-losing enteropathies (Crohn's disease, ulcerative colitis, intestinal fistula)
α₁-Globulins
Hereditary α₁-antitrypsin deficiency
α₂-Globulins
Hemolysis
Pancreatitis
Hepatocellular damage
β-Globulins
Hypo β-lipoproteinemia
γ-Globulins
Response to cancer chemotherapy or immunosuppressive medications
Lymphocytic leukemia
Lymphosarcoma
Multiple myeloma
Immune deficiency

INTERFERING FACTORS

• Lipemia

NURSING CARE

Nursing actions are similar to those used in other venipuncture procedures (see Chapter 2 for additional information).

Pretest

- It is preferred that the patient fast from food for 6 to 8 hours because lipemia interferes with the analysis of the specimen.

Protein, Total, Serum

Also called: Total Serum Proteins

SPECIMEN OR TYPE OF TEST: Serum

PURPOSE OF THE TEST

Total serum protein is a nonspecific test that provides general information about the patient's nutritional status and the severity of diseases of the liver, bone marrow, and kidneys. The test is also used to investigate the cause of edema.

BASICS THE NURSE NEEDS TO KNOW

Liver tissue manufactures the serum proteins including albumin, fibrinogen, other coagulation factors, and most of the α- and β-globulins. The various plasma proteins function to (1) maintain oncotic pressure in the blood vessels; (2) provide a reserve source of protein for tissue growth and repair; (3) provide transport for lipids, lipid-soluble substances, iron, copper, magnesium, and calcium; (4) act as immunologic agents; (5) provide factors for coagulation; (6) provide numerous enzymes for a variety of activities.

Total serum protein measures the amounts of albumin and globulins combined. Albumin is the most abundant protein, consisting of up to two thirds of the total amount of serum protein. When the value of total protein and albumin are decreased, edema of the tissue occurs. Decreased values of total protein can occur because of poor nutritional intake, intestinal malabsorption, malignancy, failure of the liver to manufacture proteins, or from losses via the urinary tract or skin.

During sleep overnight, the normal serum protein decreases 1.1 to 1.3 g/dL (SI: 1.0-1.3 g/L). With prolonged bed rest, the value will decline even further. In a normal pregnancy, the maternal value declines in the third trimester. When the individual is erect, walking or exercising, the value rises.

REFERENCE VALUES

Premature infant: 3.6-6.0 g/dL *or* 36-60 g/L
Newborn: 4.6-7.0 g/dL *or* 46-70 g/L
7 months-1 year: 5.1-7.3 g/dL *or* 51-73 g/L
1-2 years: 5.6-7.5 g/dL *or* 56-75 g/L
3 years and older: 6.0-8.0 g/dL *or* 60-80 g/L
Adult, ambulatory: 6.4-8.3 g/dL *or* 64-83 g/L
Adult, bed rest: 6.0- 7.8 g/dL *or* 60-78 g/L

HOW THE TEST IS DONE

Venipuncture is performed to collect a specimen of blood.

For premature infants and newborns, a capillary tube is used to collect blood from a heelstick puncture.

SIGNIFICANCE OF TEST RESULTS

Elevated Values

Total Protein

Dehydration

Multiple myeloma

Cancer

Decreased Values

Prolonged intravenous fluids

Protein-losing enteropathies (Crohn's disease, ulcerative colitis, intestinal fistula)

Acute burns of the skin

Nephrotic syndrome

Severe protein deficiency

Chronic liver disease

Cirrhosis

Malabsorption syndrome

Agammaglobulinemia

INTERFERING FACTORS

- Prolonged bed rest
- Massive intravenous transfusion
- Lipemia

NURSING CARE

Nursing actions are similar to those used in other venipuncture and capillary puncture procedures (see Chapter 2), with the following additional measures.

Pretest

- The nurse instructs the patient to fast from food and fluid for 6 to 8 hours before the test. The fats in food intake would elevate the test results.

During the Test

- The blood sample should be drawn from the arm that does not have intravenous fluid administration because intravenous fluids will dilute the blood and falsely lower the test values.

Protein, Urine, 24-Hour

SPECIMEN OR TYPE OF TEST: Urine

PURPOSE OF THE TEST

The urine protein test is used to measure the protein loss in the urine and to help confirm the presence of renal disease.

BASICS THE NURSE NEEDS TO KNOW

Protein is minimally present in the urine of individuals with normal renal function. The urinary proteins consist of albumin and many small globulins. In normal renal anatomy and physiology, the albumin molecules are large and most cannot be filtered through healthy glomerular membrane tissues. The smaller globulins are filtered by the glomeruli, but most are resorbed by the proximal tubules. Additional glycoproteins are secreted by cells in the distal tubules and the ascending Henle's loop. These minimal losses of protein into the urine are considered normal. A value greater than 150 mg/24 hr is called *proteinuria*.

When proteinuria occurs, measurement is done to determine the daily amount of protein that is lost in the urine. A value of less than 1.0 g/24 hr is considered a minimal proteinuria. A value of 1.0 to 4.0 g/24 hr is considered as moderate proteinuria and a value of greater than 4 g/24 hr is considered as heavy proteinuria. In addition, there will be diagnostic follow-up testing to determine the underlying cause of the protein loss. In renal disease, glomerular damage can cause a loss of large proteins into the urine. Tubular damage prevents resorption of the proteins. The damage may also be in the lower urinary tract where proteins are deposited directly into the urine.

Urinary protein levels can increase after strenuous exercise, with salt depletion, or during a period of dehydration, infection, or inflammation. These events cause a higher level of proteinuria but are not considered indications of renal or urinary tract disease.

REFERENCE VALUES   40-150 mg/dL *or* SI: 400-1500 µmol/L

HOW THE TEST IS DONE

A 24-hour urine specimen is collected in a large, clear, glass or plastic container.

SIGNIFICANCE OF TEST RESULTS

Elevated (Abnormal) Values
Glomerulonephritis
Nephrotic syndrome
Diabetic nephropathy
Renal failure
Renal transplant rejection
Sarcoidosis
Toxic agents
Heavy metal poisoning
Cancer
Urinary infection
Preeclampsia
Toxemia of pregnancy
Multiple myeloma

P

INTERFERING FACTORS

- Contamination of the specimen with mucus, vaginal or prostate secretions, or white blood cells
- Dilute urine from excessive fluid intake
- Failure to collect all urine
- Warming of the specimen

NURSING CARE

Nursing actions related to timed urine collection procedures are presented in Chapter 2, with the following additional measures.

Pretest

○ *Patient Teaching.* Instruct the patient to collect a 24-hour urine specimen. Remind the patient that all urine is to be collected in the container. Keep the urine refrigerated or on ice during the collection period.

○ *Patient Teaching.* Instruct female patients to collect the urine at a time when no menstrual flow occurs. Advise all patients to drink a regular amount of fluids during the collection period.

During the Test

- Have the patient void at 8 AM and discard the urine.
- The test period starts at this time, and all urine is collected for 24 hours, including the 8 AM specimen of the following morning.
- Ensure that the patient's name, identification number, and the time and date of the start and finish of the test are written on the specimen label and requisition form.

Posttest

- Keep the specimen refrigerated until it is transported to the laboratory.

Prothrombin Time

Also called: Pro Time
Includes: International Normalized Ratio (INR)

SPECIMEN OR TYPE OF TEST: Serum

PURPOSE OF THE TEST

The prothrombin time test is used to evaluate the extrinsic coagulation system; to help screen for coagulation deficiency of factors I, II, V, VII, and X; and to monitor oral anticoagulant therapy. It also is used to investigate the effects of liver failure, identify disseminated intravascular coagulation (DIC), and screen for vitamin K deficiency.

BASICS THE NURSE NEEDS TO KNOW

The prothrombin time test measures the amount of time needed to form a clot. The clot formation is dependent on the functional integrity of coagulation factors II, V, VII, and X. A deficiency of any of these factors prolongs the prothrombin time. Each test includes the control time in the report of the patient's value. The control time is the normal reference value to be used in the evaluation of the patient's test result.

One use of the prothrombin time and the internationalized normalized ratio (INR) is to monitor the effect of anticoagulant warfarin (Coumadin) therapy. This anticoagulant prolongs the prothrombin time and prevents deep vein thrombosis, pulmonary embolism, myocardial infarction, and other conditions with potential for clot formation. If an excessive level of warfarin is given, there is a risk for hemorrhage. The response to oral anticoagulation varies widely among individuals because of their genetic makeup. Genetic testing can now identify the patient's response to warfarin and recommend an individualized, more accurate dosage of the drug.

International Normalized Ratio

The INR is a special mathematical calculation of the prothrombin time, used to monitor the effect of an oral anticoagulant. For the patient receiving oral anticoagulant therapy with warfarin (Coumadin), the therapeutic range of the INR is 2.0 to 3.0. For the patient with a mechanical heart valve, the therapeutic range of the INR is 2.5 to 3.5.

There are now many anticoagulated patients living at home, maintained on warfarin. There is frequent need to monitor their INR values and verify that results are in the therapeutic range. Thus the patients have many visits to the laboratory, physician, or anticoagulation clinic. After receiving training, some of the patients are able to use the point-of-care INR monitor to perform self-testing at home. Studies show that many patients are able to perform the monitoring accurately and effectively. The evidence-based results show they can maximize the time interval in maintaining the therapeutic range of anticoagulation. When monitoring is done correctly, these patients have few episodes of complication, such as developing a clot or hemorrhage. Ongoing patient education and support is essential for the patient's success (Bockwoldt, 2010; Ng, 2009; Bradbury, 2008).

Elevated Values of Prothrombin Time

Some diseases cause an increased value of the prothrombin time. Severe liver disease and injured liver cells are unable to use fat-soluble vitamin K to manufacture clotting factors. Additionally, an elevated prothrombin time value will occur when fat-soluble vitamin K cannot be absorbed from the intestine because of hepatobiliary or pancreatic obstruction. When vitamin K cannot reach the liver, it is unavailable for the manufacture of clotting factors. DIC is an acute disorder of coagulation that results in formation of microthrombi and bleeding. As part of a DIC panel of tests, the prothrombin time is severely elevated in this disease (see also Disseminated Intravascular Coagulation Screen, p. 259).

REFERENCE VALUES	PT: 10-14 seconds INR: 1.00-1.30
▽ Critical Values	PT: >46 seconds INR: 5 or higher

HOW THE TEST IS DONE
Venipuncture or capillary puncture is used to collect a sample of blood

SIGNIFICANCE OF TEST RESULTS

Elevated Values

Excess anticoagulant therapy
DIC
Fibrinogen deficiency
Prothrombin deficiency
Deficiency of vitamin K
Liver disease
Hepatobiliary or pancreatic obstruction

INTERFERING FACTORS

- Lipemia

NURSING CARE

Nursing actions are similar to those used in other venipuncture procedures (see Chapter 2), with the following additional measures.

Pretest

- If the patient receives intermittent doses of heparin, the nurse ensures that the blood is drawn at least 2 hours after the last dose. Recent heparin administration prolongs the prothrombin time excessively.

○ *Patient Teaching.* The nurse instructs the patient to discontinue intake of alcohol and caffeine for 24 hours before the test. Lipemia from these substances interferes with the accuracy of the test.

During the Test

- If the patient receives intravenous heparin, the blood should be drawn from a vein in the opposite arm from that which has the intravenous infusion or heparin lock device.

Posttest

- Ensure that the venipuncture site has sealed and that the patient is not bleeding. The nurse uses sterile gauze to apply pressure to the puncture site as needed. Keeping pressure on the site, the patient can also raise his or her arm overhead. The combination of pressure and elevation should help promote coagulation.
- As warfarin (Coumadin) therapy is started, the PT and INR measurements are generally done once a day. While the dosage is being increased, the nurse monitors the laboratory results for an excess anticoagulation effect. After the therapeutic range has been reached and is stable, the PT and INR testing is done about once a month.

○ *Patient Teaching.* The nurse instructs the patient to maintain a routine, prescribed schedule of blood testing to monitor the anticoagulant effect. The nurse also teaches the patient to recognize early signs of bleeding that could indicate excessive anticoagulation. If bleeding occurs, the patient should notify the physician of the problem immediately.

▽ **Nursing Response to Critical Values**

The physician should be notified immediately of a severe elevation of the PT or INR result, because a high risk of hemorrhage exists. The nurse assesses the patient for signs of spontaneous bleeding, including petechiae (small red hemorrhagic spots on the skin), ecchymosis

Continued

(bruising), hematoma, blood in the urine, feces, or gastric secretions, and bleeding in the mucous membranes, particularly the gingiva (gums) in the oral cavity. Vital signs are taken and monitored frequently thereafter, until the risk of bleeding has diminished.

If the patient receives warfarin (Coumadin) anticoagulant medication and the INR value is severely elevated, the nurse withholds the next dose until the physician responds to the notification. The physician may reduce or discontinue the medication temporarily. When the INR is >5 without bleeding, the nurse also prepares to give the antidote of vitamin K, as prescribed. If this is not successful or the patient is still bleeding, the physician may prescribe fresh frozen plasma, to be given intravenously. This infusion provides replacement of coagulation factors that will help stop the bleeding.

Pulmonary Function Studies

SPECIMEN OR TYPE OF TEST: Spirometry

PURPOSE OF THE TEST

Pulmonary function studies are performed to evaluate the patient's respiratory status, especially those experiencing shortness of breath or other breathing difficulty. These studies may be used to evaluate the therapy for, or progression of, obstructive and restrictive lung disease. Portions of the test are used as parameters for weaning patients from mechanical ventilation and as part of preoperative evaluations.

A challenge or provocation test is included as part of the pulmonary function studies in patients with suspected hypersensitivity of the airways. *Bronchial provocation tests* or *bronchial challenge tests* are performed for patients who have symptoms suggestive of asthma but who do not show evidence of air flow limitations. They may be used to assess airway function over time and to evaluate various therapeutic interventions.

BASICS THE NURSE NEEDS TO KNOW

Spirometry is a method of measuring the volume of gas that moves into and out of the lungs. The patient breathes through a tube connected to the spirograph, which records on a moving sheet of paper the volume of gas displaced in the spirometer. Two or more volumes form a pulmonary capacity (Figure 86).

The pulmonary volumes consist of the tidal volume (Vt), inspiratory reserve volume (IRV), expiratory reserve volume (ERV), and residual volume (RV). The Vt, the normal volume of air inhaled or exhaled during a single breath in a resting state, is normally 5 to 7 mL/kg of body weight. Minute volume (MV) is obtained by multiplying the Vt by the respiratory rate.

The IRV is the amount of air that can be inspired over and above the inspired Vt. The ERV is the air remaining in the lungs, which can be expelled after a normal exhalation. The RV is the amount of air remaining in the lungs that cannot be forcibly expelled.

Pulmonary capacities consist of vital capacity (VC), inspiratory capacity (IC), functional residual capacity (FRC), and total lung capacity (TLC).

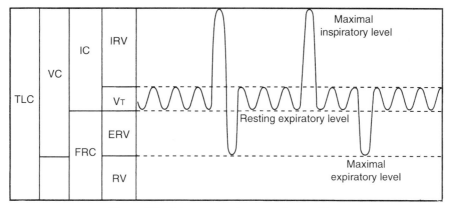

Figure 86. Pulmonary volumes and capacities.

The VC is the amount of air that can be expelled from the lungs after a maximum inspiration: VC = Vt + IRV + ERV. A timed VC expresses the volume of air expelled forcibly over a certain amount of time. This forced expiratory volume (FEV) provides an index of pulmonary function. It is the amount of gas exhaled over a given period. It is reported with a subscript to indicate time in seconds. The FEV_1 is the amount of air expelled in the first second of forced exhalation after a maximal inspiration. FEV_2 refers to the amount of air expelled in the first 2 seconds, and FEV_3 is the amount of air expelled in 3 seconds. FEV is reported as a percentage of the forced vital capacity (FVC).

In cases of obstructive and restrictive lung disease, FEV_1 decreases. With obstructive lung disease, this decrease in FEV_1 is the result of increased resistance to outflow. With restrictive lung disease, the decrease in FEV_1 is the result of a decreased ability to inhale an adequate volume of air. Therefore, with restrictive lung disease, an FEV_1 to FVC ratio is a more accurate parameter for evaluating patient status and treatment.

In addition to FEV, the average rate of flow for a specific segment of the FVC may be measured while the FVC is being assessed. The segment measured is usually between 25% and 75% of the FVC. Previously called the maximum midexpiratory flow rate (MMEF), it is now called forced expiratory flow ($FEF_{25\%-75\%}$). The $FEF_{25\%-75\%}$ is the mean rate of expiratory air flow between 25% and 75% of the FVC.

The IC is the maximal amount of air that can be inspired: IC = Vt + IRV. The FRC is the amount of air left in the lungs after a normal resting exhalation: FRC = ERV + RV. The TLC is the amount of air in the lungs after a maximal inspiration: TLC Vt + IRV + ERV + RV.

In addition to the volumes and capacities, maximum voluntary ventilation (MVV) may or may not be determined. The MVV is the total amount of air that is moved into and out of the respiratory tract over 12 seconds with the patient's maximum effort to breathe quickly and deeply. The result is multiplied by 5 and expressed in liters per minute. It is sometimes called maximum breathing capacity.

An estimated volume of pulmonary function is called dead space volume (Vds). The Vds is that portion of inhaled air or gas that does not take part in gas exchange. It is made up of the anatomic dead space (area from the nose and mouth to the terminal bronchioles) and alveolar dead space (areas of the lungs that are not perfused). Physiologic Vd consists of the anatomic

P

Vd and the alveolar Vd. Normally, no measurable alveolar Vd exists. However, anatomic Vd usually is 1 mL of Vd per pound of body weight or 2 mL of Vd per kilogram of ideal body weight. The alveolar Vd increases with pathologic states that decrease blood flow to the lungs.

Pulmonary volumes may also be used to assess alveolar ventilation. *Alveolar ventilation* is estimated by taking the Vt and subtracting the Vds (Vt −Vds).

A challenge or provocation test is included as part of the pulmonary function studies in patients with suspected hypersensitivities of the airways. *Bronchial provocation tests* or *bronchial challenge tests* are performed as part of the pulmonary function studies for patients who have symptoms suggestive of asthma but who do not show evidence of air flow limitations. They also may be used to assess airway function over time and to evaluate various therapeutic interventions. The provocation tests are contraindicated for anyone whose baseline FEV is less than 1.5 L, who has a history of severe responses to identifiable antigens, or who has had a viral infection of the upper airway within 8 weeks before the test.

Various substances can be used in the provocation test. Inhalation challenges are performed with methacholine or histamine. The *methacholine challenge test* and the *histamine challenge test* use nonspecific agents, which are usually administered with a nebulizer. Specific agents may also be given by inhalation. These specific antigens are given in varying concentrations. When indicated, the patient may be exposed to occupational inhalants.

Instead of inhalational stimulants, oral challenges may be given, but these take several hours or days. Substances ingested are acetylsalicylic acid (aspirin), tartrazine, sodium salicylate, metabisulfite, and monosodium glutamate.

An *exercise challenge* may be used to induce bronchospasms, which are characteristic of hyperresponsive airways when they occur after short-term exercise. Before the test is performed, a baseline FEV_1 is obtained. The exercise challenge is accomplished with either a treadmill or an exercise bike under controlled environmental temperature and humidity. With 5 to 10 minutes of exercise, the heart rate usually reaches at least 80% of the predicted maximum heart rate. The exercise is stopped, and the FEV_1 is measured.

The provocation tests are considered abnormal if there is a 20% or greater fall in FEV_1. At the end of the provocation test, a bronchodilator may be given by inhalation, and postbronchodilator pulmonary function may be evaluated.

P

REFERENCE VALUES*   **Adults (70-kg man; values are 20% to 25% lower in women)**
Tidal volume (Vt): 500 mL
Inspiratory reserve volume (IRV): 3100 mL
Expiratory reserve volume (ERV): 1200 mL
Residual volume (RV): 1200 mL
Vital capacity (VC): 4800 mL
Inspiratory capacity (IC): 3600 mL
Functional residual capacity (FRC): 2400 mL
Total lung capacity (TLC): 6000 mL
FEV_1: 84%
FEV_2: 94%
FEV_3: 97%

*Reference values vary with age, gender, height, and ethnicity. Lungs volumes peak around age 25, then gradually decrease with age. Volumes are 20% to 25% lower in females. Since height affects the size of the thorax, the taller the person, the larger their lung volumes. Likewise, ethnicity may affect the size of one's thorax and, therefore, lung volumes.

HOW THE TEST IS DONE

Pulmonary function studies are usually performed in the respiratory therapy department or in a physician's office. To establish a closed system with the spirometer, a nose clip is placed over the patient's nose, and the spirometer's mouthpiece is held in the mouth with the patient's lips maintaining an airtight seal. The patient is then instructed when to breathe normally, inhale maximally, and exhale maximally. This procedure is repeated several times. If the patient is unable to cooperate fully, a one-way valve may be inserted to obtain a *stacked* vital capacity.

Simple spirometry can be done at the bedside or at home. For example, patients with asthma may be taught to monitor their peak expiratory flow (PEF).

SIGNIFICANCE OF TEST RESULTS

Elevated Values

FRC

Chronic obstructive pulmonary disease

FEV

Chronic obstructive pulmonary disease

Decreased Values

VT

Atelectasis

Fatigue

Pneumothorax

Pulmonary congestion

Restrictive lung disease

Tumors

IRV

Asthma

Exercise

Obstructive pulmonary disease

ERV

Ascites

Kyphosis

Obesity

Pleural effusion

Pneumothorax

Pregnancy

Scoliosis

RV

Advanced age

Obstructive pulmonary disease

FEV

Restrictive pulmonary disease

P

FRC
Adult respiratory distress syndrome
IC
Restrictive pulmonary disease
VC
Diaphragm restriction
Drug overdose with hypoventilation
Neuromuscular diseases
Restrictive or depressed thoracic movement

INTERFERING FACTORS

- Fatigue
- Lack of patient cooperation
- Smoking
- Abdominal distention or pregnancy
- Poor seal around mouthpiece (or tube)
- Medications
- Analgesics, bronchodilators, sedatives

NURSING CARE

Pretest

- Assess the patient's cardiac status. Hold the test and notify the physician if the patient has a history of angina or recent myocardial infarction.
- ○ *Patient Teaching.* The nurse can maximize patient cooperation by explaining the procedure and the need for full participation. Demonstrate the nose clip and mouthpiece. The patient should wear dentures if necessary for a proper mouth seal. Instruct the patient not to smoke for 6 hours before the test.
- The nurse checks with the physician about administering a bronchodilator and intermittent positive-pressure breathing therapy before the test.
- Ensure that no constricting clothes are worn.
- Ensure that oral intake is light to prevent stomach distention.
- The nurse instructs the patient to void immediately before the test.
- Schedule the test before any other tests or procedures that may fatigue the patient.

During the Test

- If an abnormal response to a specific substance occurs during a provocation test, a placebo substance should be given to ensure that the bronchospasms were not induced by the spirometry.

Posttest

- Advise the patient to resume normal diet and activity. The patient can resume taking medications and therapies as prescribed.

Red Blood Cell Count

Also called: RBC; Red Cell Count; Erythrocyte Count

SPECIMEN OR TYPE OF TEST: Blood

PURPOSE OF THE TEST

The red blood cell count may be part of a routine complete blood count, or it may be repeated as a single test when the patient's health condition includes an abnormal altered red cell count. The red cell count also is used to evaluate anemia and polycythemia.

BASICS THE NURSE NEEDS TO KNOW

The maintenance of a normal number of erythrocytes in the blood is dependent on the ability of the bone marrow to replace continuously the erythrocytes that are lost or destroyed. Because of the fragility of the cell membrane, the life span of the RBC is approximately 120 days. The bone marrow must produce approximately 1 million new erythrocytes per second to maintain adequate replacement.

The stimulus for additional production of erythrocytes is cellular oxygen deficiency that triggers the flow of erythropoietin by the kidneys. Erythropoietin stimulates the manufacture of new red blood cells by the bone marrow.

Numerous factors can create an imbalance between erythrocyte production and destruction. With excess production and a normal rate of destruction, the red blood cell count is elevated. With either diminished production or excess destruction of red cells in the blood, their number is decreased.

Variation in Normal Values

The normal red cell count is higher in men than in women, and it is higher in individuals who live at high altitudes. The normal value is lower in men older than age 65. The red cell count is 5% to 6% lower when the blood is drawn from a recumbent patient than from one in an upright position.

Elevated Values

Increases in the red cell count may be a result of hyperactivity of the bone marrow cells or of an increase in erythropoietin from renal disease. Relative polycythemia may also produce an increased red cell count. When this problem is caused by dehydration, there are a normal number of erythrocytes, but they are more concentrated in the diminished fluid volume of the plasma.

Decreased Values

Decreases in the red blood cell count can occur from an excessive loss of cells, such as with a hemorrhage. It can also occur because of rapid or accelerated hemolysis of the red blood cells. When the bone marrow tissue is damaged, or when a lack of erythropoietin from renal disease exists, too few red cells are produced, and the blood count is low.

REFERENCE VALUES   Male: $4.6 - 6.0 \times 10^6/\mu L$ *or* SI: $4.6 - 6.0 \times 10^{12}/L$
Female: $4.0 - 5.4 \times 10^6/\mu L$ *or* SI: $4.0 - 5.4 \times 10^{12}/L$

R

HOW THE TEST IS DONE

Venipuncture or capillary puncture is used to obtain a sample of blood.

SIGNIFICANCE OF TEST RESULTS

Elevated Values

Polycythemia
Renal tumor
Dehydration

Decreased Values

Hemorrhage
Fluid overload
Anemia
Aplastic anemia
Bone marrow depression
Hemolysis of erythrocytes
Sickle cell anemia
Glucose-6-phosphate dehydrogenase deficiency
Leukemia
Hodgkin's disease

INTERFERING FACTORS

- Hemolysis
- Coagulation of the specimen
- Multiple blood transfusions
- Hemodilution

NURSING CARE

Nursing measures include care of the venipuncture or capillary puncture site as described in Chapter 2, with the following additional measures.

Pretest

- Plan to obtain the specimen when the patient is calm and rested. Exercise, exertion, and fear all increase the red blood cell count.

During the Test

- Ensure that the arm or hand that has an intravenous line or saline lock is not used to obtain the specimen. Intravenous fluid dilutes the blood and falsely decreases the cell count.

Posttest

- When value of the red cell count is lower than normal, the patient is anemic. The nurse also monitors the laboratory results of the hemoglobin and hematocrit because these values will also be lower than normal. In some conditions, such as glucose-6-phosphate dehydrogenase deficiency, sickle cell anemia, or other hemoglobinopathy, the patient must contend with a chronic, life-long anemia problem. In other cases, such as during treatment with chemotherapy or radiation, the effect of bone marrow suppression, or after a hemorrhage, the anemia is a more recent development. Medical intervention depends on the origin of the red blood cell or bone marrow problem.

- With a low red cell count, the nurse assesses for signs of anemia, including pallor, fatigue, dyspnea on exertion, palpitations, and dizziness. The patient's main problems are activity intolerance and fatigue. The problems occur because there are too few red blood cells to supply sufficient oxygen to the cells. The heart must work harder to increase the circulation and use the red cells that are available.

Red Blood Cell Morphology

Also called: Peripheral Blood Smear; Blood Smear Morphology

SPECIMEN OR TYPE OF TEST: Whole blood

PURPOSE OF THE TEST

The cells of the blood are examined to help identify causes of anemia and to evaluate the function of the bone marrow.

BASICS THE NURSE NEEDS TO KNOW

Morphology refers to the shape and structure of cells. Red blood cell morphology is a microscopic or automated analyzer examination of stained red blood cells to identify any altered shapes or structures. In most hematologic diseases, specific characteristic changes can be seen in the blood cells. Changes in the size, structure, and shape of the cells or changes in the number and distribution of the cells may occur, or a combination of these changes may be seen. The microscopic visualization of these changes helps diagnose or confirm the hematologic diagnosis. In addition to red cell morphology, the peripheral smear can be used to examine white blood cell and platelet morphology.

The Shape and Structure of Red Blood Cells

Normal erythrocytes are circular discs of uniform size, color, shape, and appearance. The red cells should be paler in the center than on the periphery. They are described as *normocytic* (normal in size) and *normochromic* (normal in color). The patient can be anemic despite these normal characteristics. A normocytic, normochromic anemia is one that is caused by hemolysis of erythrocytes or severe blood loss. The cells are normal, but too few of them remain in the blood.

Abnormal erythrocytes vary in size, color, hemoglobin content, shape, staining properties, and structure. The altered size is caused by a defect in erythropoiesis. The bone marrow can be adversely affected by genetics, poor nutrition or changes in either bone marrow cells or bone marrow function.

Abnormal color is the result of an alteration in hemoglobin content. Too little hemoglobin results in a pale color of the erythrocytes. The problem may be the result of iron deficiency or abnormal hemoglobin synthesis.

Poikilocytosis refers to abnormally shaped red cells. Abnormal erythrocyte structure includes the presence of a nucleus that identifies these cells as normoblasts, basophilic stippling, Howell-Jolly bodies, or Heinz bodies. The variations of some of the characteristics of erythrocytes, and their relationships to hematologic disease, are presented in Table 14.

R

TABLE 14	Characteristics of Erythrocytes: Relationships to Hematologic Diseases		
Characteristics	Interpretation	Pathophysiology	Disorders
Size			
Normocytic	Normal cell size	Adequate response by the bone marrow	None
		Shortened life span of the erythrocytes—increased hemolysis	Acute blood loss Hemolytic anemia
		Impaired release of iron from the reticuloendothelial system	Anemia of chronic disease
Macrocytic or megalocytic	Larger than normal cell size	Marrow disorder with defective DNA that affects cell development during erythropoiesis	Deficiency of vitamin B_{12} or folic acid Megaloblastic anemias
		Uptake of cholesterol and bile salts by the erythrocyte membranes	Liver disease and obstructive jaundice
Microcytic	Smaller than normal cell size	Deficiency of heme, a lack of iron, or impaired hemoglobin synthesis	Iron deficiency anemia, thalassemia, sideroblastic anemia, lead poisoning, vitamin B_6 deficiency
Schistocyte	Red cell fragments	Partial splitting or phagocytosis of the cell, without loss of hemoglobin	Hemolytic anemia, disseminated intravascular coagulation, malignant hypertension, cancer, cardiac valve prosthesis, burns, uremia
Color			
Normochromic	Normal hemoglobin content	Normal iron stores, normal hemoglobin synthesis	Anemia caused by hemorrhage, with loss of erythrocytes
Hyperchromic	Erythrocyte saturated with hemoglobin	A relative increase of hemoglobin within the erythrocyte that has a small diameter and small cell membrane; the cell is spherical	Spherocytosis

R

TABLE 14	Characteristics of Erythrocytes: Relationships to Hematologic Diseases—cont'd		
Characteristics	Interpretation	Pathophysiology	Disorders
Hypochromic	Erythrocyte with diminished hemoglobin	Iron deficiency in proportion to erythropoiesis	Iron deficiency anemia
		Defective hemoglobin synthesis	Thalassemia, lead poisoning, sideroblastic anemia
Shape			
Elliptocyte	Elliptical or oval shape	Cytoplasm and cholesterol in the cell membrane are polarized in areas of convexity; increased hemolysis can occur	Hereditary elliptocytosis, thalassemia, iron deficiency anemia, sickle cell disease, other hemolytic diseases
Spherocyte	Sphere-shaped cell	Genetic disease of the bone marrow; the abnormal cells have a shorter life span	Hereditary spherocytosis, immune disease, and other hemolytic anemias
Target cell	Hemoglobin is distributed on the perimeter and in the center, giving a "target" appearance	Deficient hemoglobin for the normal cell size	Hemoglobin C, D, S diseases, thalassemia, iron deficiency anemia
		Too large a cell membrane and cell size for a normal amount of hemoglobin	Obstructive jaundice, liver disease
Sickle cell	Crescent-shaped cells	In conditions of deoxygenation, the hemoglobin S becomes elongated and rigid; cell membranes also become sickle shaped	Sickle cell trait, sickle cell disease, other sickling hemoglobinopathies
Poikilocytosis	Varied, irregular shapes of cells (teardrop, tennis racket, horned, and helmet shapes)	Irreversible alteration of cell membrane from rapid erythropoiesis or extramedullary erythropoiesis	Megaloblastic anemia, hemolytic anemia, uremia, liver disease, metastatic cancer, toxicity, idiopathic myelofibrosis

R

Continued

TABLE 14	Characteristics of Erythrocytes: Relationships to Hematologic Diseases—cont'd		
Characteristics	**Interpretation**	**Pathophysiology**	**Disorders**
Structure			
Nucleated	Normoblasts are immature red cells with nuclei	Normal in fetus or infant, but not in adults; extreme demand on bone marrow to produce cells rapidly	Erythroblastosis fetalis, thalassemia major
		Extramedullary erythropoiesis	Idiopathic myelofibrosis
		With neutrophilia, the bone marrow cells are altered	Leukemia, metastatic cancer of the bone marrow, multiple myeloma, Gaucher's disease
Basophilic stippling	Basophilic granules in cells	Abnormal hemoglobin synthesis and increased erythropoiesis	Lead poisoning, megaloblastic anemia
Howell-Jolly bodies	Remnants of nuclear material in cells	Abnormal erythropoiesis	Postsplenectomy, megaloblastic anemia, hemolytic anemia
Heinz bodies	Irregular patches of hemoglobin in cells	Genetic abnormality of hemoglobin formation; hemoglobin is oxidized and nonfunctional	Cell injury, hemoglobinopathy hemolytic anemia

REFERENCE VALUES   Normal cell shape and structure

HOW THE TEST IS DONE

Venipuncture or capillary puncture is done to obtain the specimen of blood. For the peripheral smear, two slides are prepared immediately using drops of venous or capillary blood.

SIGNIFICANCE OF TEST RESULTS

See Table 14 for abnormal values.

INTERFERING FACTORS

• Hemolysis
• Coagulated specimen

NURSING CARE

Nursing measures include care of the venipuncture or capillary puncture site as described in Chapter 2. No other special nursing measures are required.

Red Cell Indices

See Complete Blood Cell Count on p. 208.

Renin

Also called: Plasma renin activity (PRA)

SPECIMEN OR TYPE OF TEST: Plasma

PURPOSE OF THE TEST

Plasma renin levels are determined as part of hypertension screening and to diagnose primary aldosteronism.

BASICS THE NURSE NEEDS TO KNOW

Renin is a proteolytic enzyme produced and secreted by the juxtaglomerular cells of the kidneys. Renin is secreted whenever a reduction of blood pressure to the kidneys occurs. Renin in the circulation acts on angiotensinogen to form angiotensin I, which is converted to angiotensin II—a powerful vasoconstrictor and stimulant for aldosterone secretion. This action is called the renin-angiotensin-aldosterone system or axis (see Figure 11 on p. 52).

Because renin is a powerful vasoconstrictor, its role in hypertension has been studied. Most patients with hypertension have normal renin levels. Some hypertensive patients with excessive fluid retention have low renin levels, and other hypertensive patients have high renin levels.

It has been difficult to correlate renin levels with clinical states because renin levels vary between individuals and laboratory techniques vary in the measurement of these levels. In addition, many factors will influence secretion rates of renin, including dietary ingestion of sodium. For this reason, some clinicians correlate renin levels with the sodium content of the patient's diet. The sodium content of the diet is measured by a 24-hour urine sodium level test.

Another method to evaluate renin is to perform a *sodium-depleted renin test*, during which a diuretic (usually furosemide) is given.

REFERENCE VALUES*   **Adult**
With normal sodium:
    Supine position: 0.5-1.6 ng/mL/hr *or* SI: 8.3-26.6 ng/L/sec
    Upright position: 1.9-3.6 ng/mL/hr *or* SI: 31.7-60 ng/L/sec
With low sodium:
    Supine position: 2.2-4.4 ng/mL/hr *or* SI: 36.6-73.3 ng/L/sec
    Upright position: 4.0-8.1 ng/mL/hr *or* SI: 66.7-135 ng/L/sec
After furosemide:
    Upright position: 6.8-15.0 ng/mL/hr *or* SI: 113-250 ng/L/sec

*Varies depending on the method of analysis.

R

HOW THE TEST IS DONE

The procedures vary. A random renin test simply requires a venipuncture preferably in the morning. The specimen is placed on ice and immediately sent to the laboratory. If the renin level is to be correlated with sodium intake, a 24-hour urine specimen for sodium and creatinine is required.

   If a renin determination from a renal vein is planned, it is carried out under fluoroscopy; a catheter is inserted into the renal vein via the femoral vein access.

SIGNIFICANCE OF TEST RESULTS

Elevated Values

Hypertension, severe
Cirrhosis
Hypovolemia
Hypokalemia
Secondary Addison's disease
Chronic renal failure
Hepatitis

Decreased Values

Fluid retention with high-sodium diet
Primary aldosteronism
Excessive licorice intake
Hypertension with fluid retention
Cushing's syndrome

INTERFERING FACTORS

- Noncompliance with dietary and medication restrictions
- Improper positioning during the test
- Medications such as antihypertensives, clonidine, diuretics, estrogen, minoxidil, nitroprusside, propranolol, reserpine, and vasodilators

R

NURSING CARE

The actions of the nurse vary depending on the technique used.

Pretest

- Instruct the patient on the procedure.
- Take a medication history because so many medications will influence the result.
- Check with the prescriber on whether any medications should be held.
- If a random sampling is ordered, instruct the patient to maintain a prone position or an upright position for 2 hours before the test. The position is based on physician preference.
- If a renal vein level determination is ordered, the nurse explains the need to go to the radiology department for fluoroscopy. Explain equipment, groin preparation, and local anesthetic.

○ *Patient Teaching.* If a sodium depletion renin test is ordered, instruct the patient to maintain a low-sodium diet for 3 days.

- If a sodium depletion renin test is ordered, assess the patient's cardiovascular status before the diuretic is given.
- If the renal vein is accessed, monitor the patient's vital signs and distal pulse according to hospital protocol. Hospital protocol will determine how long to maintain pressure on the femoral site.

Posttest

- If the femoral approach to the renal vein is used, assess the site for hematoma and bleeding.

Reticulocyte Count

Also called: Retic Count

SPECIMEN OR TYPE OF TEST: Blood

PURPOSE OF THE TEST

The reticulocyte count is used to evaluate erythropoiesis, distinguish among different types of anemia, assess the severity of blood loss, and evaluate the bone marrow response to treatment of anemia.

BASICS THE NURSE NEEDS TO KNOW

Reticulocytes are immature erythrocytes. The cells are formed by the bone marrow and one day later, they are released into the peripheral blood circulation where they mature into erythrocytes (red blood cells) with a full complement of hemoglobin in each red blood cell. The values may be reported as a number count of the cells or as the percentage of reticulocytes compared to mature erythrocytes. Most times, the laboratories use automated cell counters to determine the results. When manual examination and counting is done, the reference values for manual counting are used and these values are lower than the automated count values.

Elevated Values

An increase in reticulocytes indicates the ability of the bone marrow to produce erythrocytes. The elevated value is considered a healthy response to a loss of erythrocytes from hemorrhage or hemolysis. It is also a healthy response to anemia or to a reduced amount of hemoglobin in the red blood cells. The reticulocyte count also may rise after effective treatment of anemia. When the demand for erythrocytes is high, the marrow releases very immature reticulocytes into the blood rather than allow these blood cells to mature for the full time in the marrow. The rise in the reticulocyte is a very positive finding for the patient who has recently received a bone marrow transplant. The rising reticulocyte count means that the transplanted marrow is beginning to function.

R

Decreased Values

The reduced number of reticulocytes indicates that erythropoiesis is decreased in the bone marrow. The cause may be a lack of stimulation by erythropoietin, a disease that affects the bone marrow cells, or a faulty maturation process in the bone marrow. Additional testing will be needed to determine the cause of a low reticulocyte count.

REFERENCE VALUES

Manual count, Adult: 24,000-84,000 cells/μL *or* SI: 24-84 × 10⁹/L

Manual count, Adult: 0.5%-1.5% (percentage of reticulocytes)

Automated count, 12 yr-Adult: 58,600-146,200 cells/μL
    or SI: 56.8-146.2 ×10⁹/L

Automated count, 12 yr-Adult: 1.32%-4.91% (percentage of reticulocytes)

HOW THE TEST IS DONE

Venipuncture or capillary puncture is done to obtain a blood sample.

SIGNIFICANCE OF TEST RESULTS

Elevated Values

Hemolytic anemia

Hemorrhage/acute blood loss

Chronic blood loss

Decreased Values

Aplastic anemia

Iron deficiency anemia

Anemia of chronic disease

Sideroblastic anemia

Megaloblastic anemia

Pernicious anemia

Impaired bone marrow function

INTERFERING FACTORS

- Multiple blood transfusions
- Coagulation of the specimen
- Hemolysis

NURSING CARE

Nursing measures include care of the venipuncture or capillary puncture site as described in Chapter 2, with the following additional measures.

Pretest

- If possible, the nurse schedules this test before a blood transfusion is started. Once blood is administered, dilution of the cells occurs, and the reticulocyte count decreases in proportion to the fluid volume. If multiple transfusions were already given, the results of this test are invalid. The reticulocytes are from the transfused blood and do not indicate the current status of the patient's bone marrow function.

During the Test

- The blood sample should not be taken from the arm in which there is intravenous tubing. The fluid administration dilutes the blood and causes a low cell count.

Rheumatoid RF Factor

Also called:

SPECIMEN OR TYPE OF TEST: Serum, Synovial Fluid

PURPOSE OF THE TEST

The test for rheumatoid factor is used in the diagnosis and prognosis of rheumatoid arthritis.

BASICS THE NURSE NEEDS TO KNOW

Rheumatoid factor is a group of immunoglobulins that are directed against other immunoglobins to form complexes. These immune complexes are found in the blood and synovial fluid. When the immune complexes are at high levels within joints, they may contribute to tissue injury.

At a level of 80 IU/mL or higher, rheumatoid factor is present or positive in the serum of the majority of patients with rheumatoid arthritis and some other rheumatic conditions. A high correlation exists between the presence of rheumatoid factor and rheumatoid arthritis; however, the exact nature of the relationship is unknown. Synovial fluid also can be analyzed for rheumatoid factor, using the patient's joint fluid instead of serum. The test results are comparable.

In rheumatoid arthritis, the highest serum values occur in patients who have severe active disease. The test is not specific to rheumatoid arthritis, however, as patients with Sjögren syndrome also have high serum values of rheumatoid factor. Additionally, positive results at low levels (80 IU/mL or lower) occur in some normal elderly individuals and in those with chronic infection or inflammation from another cause.

REFERENCE VALUES	Negative
	Nephelometric method: <30 U/mL *or* <30 kU/mL
	Sheep cell agglutination method: <1:17

HOW THE TEST IS DONE

Venipuncture is used to obtain a sample of blood.

R

SIGNIFICANCE OF TEST RESULTS

Positive Values

Rheumatoid arthritis
Sjögren syndrome
Systemic lupus erythematosus
Dermatomyositis
Scleroderma
Polymyositis
Waldenström's disease
Sarcoidosis

INTERFERING FACTORS

• Severe lipemia

NURSING CARE

Nursing measures include care of the venipuncture site as described in Chapter 2.

Pretest

• The patient should fast from food for 6 to 8 hours before the blood is drawn. Lipemia will interfere with the accuracy of test results

Rubella Antibody

Also called: German Measles Antibody

SPECIMEN OR TYPE OF TEST: Blood

PURPOSE OF THE TEST

Antibody testing is used to detect the presence of rubella antibodies in the acute or convalescent phase of illness or to identify immunity, postvaccination. The presence of immunoglobulin M (IgM) antibody in the amniotic fluid, or umbilical cord blood identifies the transmission of the rubella virus to the fetus.

BASICS THE NURSE NEEDS TO KNOW

Rubella is a viral infection that is transmitted by droplet infection from the nasopharynx of the infected person to the susceptible individual. The virus also can cross the placental barrier of the infected pregnant woman. Rubella infection in the fetus has devastating consequences, particularly if it occurs in the first trimester of pregnancy.

When the rubella IgM and IgG antibodies are negative, the person has not been infected with the rubella virus. It also means that no immunity exists and that the person is susceptible to infection. A positive value of IgM antibody is an indicator of acute infection. In rubella infection, this antibody titer stays positive for 4 to 5 weeks and then disappears. The IgG antibody also rises during the convalescent phase of the infection and remains elevated for life. The positive value of the IgG antibodies indicates immunity to future rubella infection.

If the pregnant woman contracts rubella infection, the fetus could become infected if the virus passes through the placenta. The genetic material (RNA) of the rubella virus can be detected in the amniotic fluid and in the WBCs of fetal blood. If the fetus or newborn infant is suspected of congenital rubella, rubella titers are performed. The presence of IgM antibodies is a strong indicator of the congenital infection.

REFERENCE VALUES
IgM antibody: Negative
IgG antibody: Negative
RNA-PCR testing: negative for rubella virus

HOW THE TEST IS DONE

Venipuncture is used to obtain a specimen of venous blood.

Amniocentesis (p. 66) or Percutaneous Umbilical Blood Sampling (p. 483) may be needed to identify congenital rubella infection in the fetus

SIGNIFICANCE OF TEST RESULTS

Positive Values
IgM Antibody
Rubella, acute infection
IgG Antibody
Immunity to future rubella infection
Congenital rubella infection in the fetus or newborn

INTERFERING FACTORS

• None

NURSING CARE

Nursing measures include care of the venipuncture site as described in Chapter 2, with the following additional measures.

Pretest

○ *Patient Teaching.* The nurse teaches that when IgG antibodies are elevated and positive, the person need not worry about future exposure to rubella infection because he or she has immunity.

Posttest

• If the pregnant woman did not have previous immunity and now tests positive for IgM or IgG antibodies, the fetus has been exposed to rubella infection. The expectant parents will be advised of the risks for many malformations to the fetus. The nurse provides emotional support to the parents during this stressful time as they learn of the potential harm to the fetus.

Health Promotion

If vaccination has not been done, the nurse teaches parents to have their children immunized with the measles, mumps, and rubella (MMR) or measles, mumps, rubella and varicella-zoster (MMRV) vaccine at 15 months and again at 4 to 6 or 11 to 12 years of age.

• The nurse also recommends health screening for rubella antibodies to determine susceptibility or immunity in female patients who are of childbearing age. If the young nonpregnant

Continued

female is negative for rubella IgG antibodies, she should be vaccinated, but then she must avoid pregnancy for 1 month after the vaccine is administered. The vaccine will provide her with protection from the infection and will protect the fetus during a future pregnancy. If the unvaccinated patient is already pregnant, she must avoid contact with any person who possibly has rubella. She can be vaccinated following her delivery.

Rubeola Antibody

See Measles Antibody on p. 444.

Severe Acute Respiratory Syndrome Tests

Also called: SARS Tests

SPECIMEN OR TYPE OF TEST: Blood, Nasal, and Throat Secretions; Stool

PURPOSE OF THE TEST

The various specimens are collected to identify the RNA of the SARS virus as the cause of the acute respiratory infection or to identify the immunoglobulins specific to the SARS virus. The tests help to distinguish this source of infection from other infectious organisms that cause respiratory illness or pneumonia.

BASICS THE NURSE NEEDS TO KNOW

SARS is a newly discovered corona virus that causes severe and sometimes fatal respiratory illness. The infected person transmits the virus to others via respiratory droplets and person-to-person contact. Additional modes of transmission include aerosol transmission and fomites in the environment. Most cases are transmitted to those who are in close contact with the infected person, such as members of the patient's household, professionals who care for the infected patient, and research laboratory personnel who work with the virus.

S

REFERENCE VALUES   Serology
Immunoglobulin M (IgM) antibodies against the SARS associated corona virus: Negative
Immunoglobulin G (IgG) antibodies against the SARS associated corona virus: Negative

Reverse Transcriptase Polymerase Chain Reaction (RT-PCR):
Negative for the RNA of the SARS-related corona virus

HOW THE TEST IS DONE

Samples will be collected from various sources in the body where the virus is known to locate.

Serology: Venipuncture is used to collect a specimen of blood.

Nasopharyngeal, swab, or aspirate: For the aspirate specimen, 1 to 2 mL of sodium chloride is sprayed into both nasal passages and the aspirated solution is placed in a sterile container with a special leak-proof, sealed top. For the swab specimen, an individual culture swab is placed in each side of the nasal passage for a few seconds to absorb the secretions. The swabs are then placed in the culture tube that contains a viral transport medium.

Throat (oropharyngeal) swab: With a culture swab, the posterior pharynx and tonsillar areas are swabbed and the applicator with secretions is placed in a culture tube that contains a viral transport medium.

Sputum: The patient rinses the mouth and then performs deep coughing to produce sputum. If the specimen must be obtained by suction, the procedure involves increased risk of transmission from the aerosolization associated with the procedure. The physician collects the specimen during bronchoalveolar lavage, tracheal aspiration, or a bronchoscopy. Any sputum specimens are placed in a sterile cup with a screw-topped and tightly sealed lid.

Feces: A culture swab is inserted in the rectum and rotated. After a short interval, it should have fecal material on it. The swab is placed in the culture tube with viral transport medium and the top of the tube is closed firmly.

SIGNIFICANCE OF TEST RESULTS

Abnormal Values

Severe acute respiratory syndrome (SARS)

Influenza

Respiratory syncytial virus (RSV)

Legionella pneumonia

Mycoplasma pneumonia

Pneumococcal pneumonia

INTERFERING FACTORS

- Inadequate specimen

NURSING CARE

Pretest

- All specimens are potentially hazardous and are collected under conditions of strict precautions. The laboratory and the epidemiology departments are contacted before the specimens are collected.
- Because of the high risk of nosocomial spread of the virus, the nurse implements precautions for aerosol droplet and person-to-person contact including gown, double gloves, goggles, and face mask (N-95 respirator). Handwashing is essential. Guided by the department of epidemiology, the nurse ensures that all personnel follow correct infection control procedures at all times.

S

Continued

NURSING CARE—cont'd

During the Test

- When tracheal suctioning, endotracheal tube insertion or suctioning, or bronchoscopy is used to obtain sputum, the risks increase of transmission by aerosolization. To do the test, the patient must be placed in a negative-pressure room and any health care personnel in the room must wear the protective equipment identified previously.

Posttest

- The specimens are labeled with correct patient identification, the date, time, name of the physician, and the source of the specimen. The specimens are bagged and packed in ice, according to infection control procedures and procedures for biohazards. Usually, the hospital laboratory works with the Centers for Disease Control and Prevention (CDC) regarding analysis of the specimens. On completion of the collection procedures, all personnel in the room must wash their hands before exiting the room.

Sickle Cell Tests

Includes: High Performance Liquid Chromatography (HPLC), Hemoglobin electrophoresis, Sickle cell solubility test (Sickledex)

SPECIMEN OR TYPE OF TEST: Blood

PURPOSE OF THE TEST

The sickle cell tests of high performance liquid chromatography or hemoglobin electrophoresis are methods of analysis to detect *variant* (abnormal) hemoglobin S (HbS) of the newborn and to confirm the diagnosis of sickle cell disease or trait. The sickle cell solubility test (Sickledex) is used to screen for the presence of hemoglobin S in the blood, but it cannot differentiate between sickle cell disease and sickle cell trait.

BASICS THE NURSE NEEDS TO KNOW

Sickle cell hemoglobin (HbS) is the most common of the variant hemoglobins. The term *sickled* is used because when there is low level of oxygen in the blood, HbS converts the erythrocytes into sickle or crescent shapes (Figure 87). In sickle cell disease, these damaged erythrocytes carry less oxygen to cells and tissues. Ongoing hemolysis of the damaged erythrocytes also occurs and causes chronic hemolytic anemia throughout life. In a sickle cell crisis, the many sickled cells become trapped in small blood vessels, causing obstruction, infarction, thrombus, or embolus in the circulation, with acute or chronic damage to organs and tissues.

   Sickle cell trait or disease is an autosomal recessive genetic disorder. The homozygous (pure) form of HbS causes the disease of sickle cell anemia (HbSS). Abnormal chromosomes that produce hemoglobin S were inherited from both parents. The heterozygous (mixed) form of HbS produces sickle cell trait. The person with sickle cell trait inherited the HbS chromosome from one parent but not the other. The person with the trait condition does not have sickle cell

S

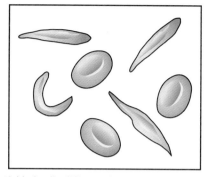

Figure 87. Sickled cells differ in shape from normal erythrocytes.

anemia and under normal physiologic conditions will not develop a vaso-occlusive crisis (Pack-Maybien & Haynes, 2009).

Newborn testing to diagnose sickle cell anemia is done by high performance liquid chromatography or hemoglobin electrophoresis. Both have a very high rate of accuracy in detection of hemoglobin S. In the United States, the required testing is mandated within the first 1 to 3 days after birth, before the neonate leaves the birth setting. Follow-up verification testing is done when the infant has the first visit to the health care provider, but no later than 2 months after birth. If the infant is diagnosed with sickle cell disease, this schedule allows time for early treatment of the baby with prophylactic penicillin and pneumococcal pneumonia vaccination. Follow-up DNA testing may also be used to confirm or exclude sickle cell disease.

The sickle cell solubility test (Sickledex) is an additional screening test that may be used. This test cannot differentiate between sickle cell trait and sickle cell anemia, but with a positive result, follow-up testing with one of the other methods described above will provide the definitive diagnosis. The Sickledex test cannot be used with the neonate but is effective at ages 3 to 6 months and on older children or adults who were not screened at birth.

REFERENCE VALUES   Negative; No hemoglobin S is present

HOW THE TEST IS DONE

Heelstick capillary puncture is used to obtain a specimen of blood from the heel of the neonate.

Capillary puncture in the finger is used for older children and adults.

SIGNIFICANCE OF TEST RESULTS

Positive Values

Sickle cell anemia

Sickle cell trait

INTERFERING FACTORS

• Blood transfusion within the past 3 to 4 months

S

NURSING CARE

Nursing measures include care of the capillary puncture site as described in Chapter 2, with the following additional measures.

Pretest

• No special nursing intervention is needed.

Posttest

Health Promotion

In all states of the United States and its territories, all newborns now have mandated screening for sickle cell disease, regardless of ethnicity (U.S. Preventive Services Task Force, 2007).

• The health care provider and the genetics counselor inform the parents about the test results, and when the results are positive, provide time for the parents to discuss and understand the results.

• The nurse provides support and clarification to the parents who have an infant who tested positive for sickle cell disease or trait. The parents often have feelings of concern, guilt, and fear about the well-being of their infant. In discharge planning, the nurse encourages the parents to keep all appointments with the health care provider for follow-up care for their infant. With sickle cell disease, early preventive measures and comprehensive disease management will greatly reduce the incidence of vaso-occlusive crises and effectively prolong the patient's life.

• When one child of the family tests positive for the trait or disease, the nurse encourages testing of all members of the family. If the individual knows his or her genetic status regarding this mutation, he or she can make informed decisions regarding health and reproduction.

Sigmoidoscopy and Anoscopy

SPECIMEN OR TYPE OF TEST: Endoscopy

PURPOSE OF THE TEST

Sigmoidoscopy is used as a screening test for cancer of the colon. It also is used to investigate the source of unexplained rectal bleeding or infection in the lower colon, to evaluate the postoperative anastomosis of the lower colon, and to diagnose or monitor inflammatory bowel disease. Anoscopy is used to investigate anal and rectal symptoms, such as bleeding, pain, discomfort, or prolapse. Sigmoidoscopy is often performed with anoscopy.

BASICS THE NURSE NEEDS TO KNOW

Sigmoidoscopy uses a flexible, fiberoptic endoscope (sigmoidoscope) to examine the sigmoid colon and rectum. About 50% of colon cancer and polyps of the colon are located in the left colon between the anus and the splenic flexure. During a sigmoidoscopy procedure, the polyps can be removed and suspicious tissue can be biopsied or cultures taken. The examination can be done in the physician's office, without conscious sedation or pain medication. One of the drawbacks of sigmoidoscopy is that the other 50% of the polyps and cancerous tumors are located between the right colon and transverse colon, beyond the view of the sigmoidoscope.

In addition, if a polyp or tumor is encountered by sigmoidoscopy, the patient will need a follow-up colonoscopy to view the remainder of the colon.

Anoscopy uses a short tubular instrument with a light to examine the rectum and anal canal. The anoscopy examination allows for visualization of the mucosa, with identification of problems of bleeding, fistula, infection, inflammation, or other abnormality.

There is a low prevalence of anal cancer in the general population. However, there is a rising incidence of anal cancer in HIV-infected men who have sex with men. Testing for the human papilloma virus (HPV) may be done during the anoscopy examination. When indicated, the anal examination can include a male PAP smear and the cell brushings can be examined microscopically for abnormal cytology. The Bethesda system is used to grade the anal cytologic changes (see Box 8, p. 471). A biopsy will be taken of anal cells that are graded as high-grade dysplasia (precancerous) or cancerous for a definitive diagnosis.

REFERENCE VALUES No tissue abnormalities are seen in the sigmoid colon, rectum, or anus

HOW THE TEST IS DONE

The patient is placed in a lateral position on the examination table (Figure 88). The well-lubricated instrument is inserted into the anus and advanced to the desired depth. A tissue biopsy, PAP smear, or culture specimen may be obtained during the procedure. The time needed for the examination is 5 to 10 minutes.

SIGNIFICANCE OF TEST RESULTS

Abnormal Values
Sigmoidoscopy
Colitis
Polyps
Colorectal cancer
Gay bowel syndrome

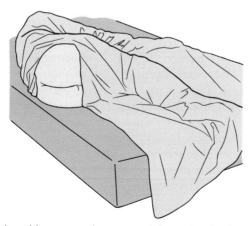

Figure 88. Positioning for sigmoidoscopy and anoscopy. The patient is placed in left lateral decubitus (SIMS) position. The draping minimizes the exposure and helps reduce the patient's feelings of embarrassment. (Modified from Pfenninger JL, Fowler GC: *Pfenninger and Fowler's procedures for primary care*, ed 3, St Louis, 2011, Mosby.)

S

Irritable bowel syndrome
Sigmoid volvulus
Crohn's disease
Intestinal ischemia
Parasitic disease
Anoscopy
Hemorrhoids
Rectal fissure
Fistula in ano
Crohn's disease
Pilonidal sinus with abscess
Abscess
Polyps
Anal herpes
Human papilloma virus infection
Colorectal or anal carcinoma
Perianal hematoma
Prolapsed rectum
Foreign body

INTERFERING FACTORS

- Uncooperative patient behavior
- Severe bleeding
- Suspected bowel perforation
- Peritonitis
- Acute diverticulitis
- Paralytic ileus

NURSING CARE

Health Promotion
The US Preventive Task Force (2008) recommends that colorectal screening can be done by fecal occult blood test, flexible sigmoidoscopy, or colonoscopy. For the average-risk individual, the recommended routine screening schedule for adults should begin at age 50 and continue to age 75. They also recommend against routine screening for colorectal cancer for asymptomatic people aged 76 to 85 because the net benefits are small, and against routine colorectal screening of asymptomatic adults older than 85 because the benefits of screening do not outweigh the harm. The American Cancer Society recommends that asymptomatic adults have colorectal cancer screenings starting at age 50. The screening options are flexible sigmoidoscopy, double-contrast barium enema, or computed tomography colonography every 5 years or colonoscopy every 10 years (Wilkins & Reynolds, 2008).

Health Promotion
The nurse can help teach people of the importance of colorectal cancer screening. The onset of this disease is usually after age 50 and the risk of developing colorectal cancer increases with each decade thereafter. Screening offers prevention by removal of polyps before they become

cancerous and early detection of a tumor before symptoms occur. Prevention and early intervention for colorectal cancer has a higher rate of cure.

Health Promotion

There is a need for education of the public as to the benefits of regular screening tests. For many years, people were taught to observe for symptoms of disease and then seek medical advice and diagnosis. Today, the emphasis is on screening to detect abnormality before the problem is advanced enough to cause symptoms. The educational focus should include "unlearning" old information, as well as learning the new and greatly improved methods of detection.

Pretest

- Once the physician has explained the test to the patient, the patient signs a consent form. The nurse ensures that the form is entered in the patient's record.

○ *Patient Teaching.* For sigmoidoscopy, the nurse explains how the patient will cleanse the bowel before the procedure. Because the protocol for bowel preparation varies, the nurse will teach according to the protocol that the examining physician uses. The preparation usually consists of administering a combination of a laxative and one or two Fleet enemas. The goal is to empty the lower colon of fecal matter. For most anoscopy examinations, no bowel preparation is used, but some physicians require an enema beforehand.

During the Test

- Assist the patient into a side-lying position on the examining table and drape the patient.
- The nurse provides reassurance and helps promote patient relaxation during the procedure. The patient may be instructed to take a few deep breaths to help relax the sphincter muscles as the instrument is inserted. During the passage of the sigmoidoscope, the patient may feel cramping pain as air is instilled. During the anoscopic examination, there is small discomfort, but little to no pain. The nurse can help distract the patient from temporary discomfort.
- The nurse also assists the physician with the collection of tissue or other specimens.

Posttest

- Label any tissue specimen containers with the appropriate patient identification, the procedure, tissue source, and time/date of the procedure. Send specimens and the requisition form to the laboratory without delay.

○ *Patient Teaching.* The nurse instructs the patient who had a sigmoidoscopy that flatulence and mild gas discomfort may be experienced from the air that was put into the colon during the examination. When a biopsy is performed during either a sigmoidoscopy or an anoscopy, it is normal to see a small amount of blood in the stool. These aftereffects are temporary. The nurse advises the patient to contact the physician for problems with severe pain, nausea, vomiting, or heavy bleeding.

Single Photon Emission Computed Tomography Scan, Brain

Also called: SPECT Scan

SPECIMEN OR TYPE OF TEST: Radionuclide Scan

PURPOSE OF THE TEST

The cerebral single photon emission computed tomography (SPECT) scan of the brain is often used to investigate cerebrovascular diseases, dementia, epilepsy, and head trauma. It may be used to assess and diagnose a disorder, as well as to evaluate the brain's response to treatment. It also is used to evaluate suspected brain death.

BASICS THE NURSE NEEDS TO KNOW

Because of brain physiology, many substances in the cerebral vascular circulation cannot cross the *blood- brain barrier* to perfuse functioning brain tissues. SPECT imaging of the brain uses an intravenously injected radionuclide that circulates and rapidly exits from the cerebral capillary circulation, crossing the blood-brain barrier. There is a rapid uptake of the radionuclide by functioning brain tissues proportionate to the cerebral blood flow. Once it is in functioning brain tissue, the radionuclide emits gamma rays and a multidetector rotary camera and computer software produces corresponding images of the brain.

The images can identify deficits in areas of brain tissue that show minimal function or nonfunction, such as occurs with ischemia following a transient ischemic attack. It can also provide images of excess activity in a particular area, such as the abnormal tissue that triggers epilepsy. In the study of dementia, this nuclear scan can help identify the cause of dementia and distinguish among Alzheimer's disease, multiinfarct dementia, and frontal lobe dementia. In cases of head trauma, SPECT can identify mild brain tissue injury that is not visible on the CT scan.

REFERENCE VALUES   **No abnormalities of brain tissue and brain function are noted.**

HOW THE TEST IS DONE

After the radiopharmaceutical is injected intravenously, a gamma camera records the radioactive emissions. The emissions are then converted to images that correspond to the location, distribution, and concentration of the radionuclide in the brain. The imaging is performed about 1 to 2 hours after the radiopharmaceutical is introduced. The normal imaging time is 20 to 30 minutes.

SIGNIFICANCE OF TEST RESULTS

Abnormal Values

Stroke
Transient ischemic attack
Multiinfarct dementia
Alzheimer's disease
Epilepsy
Hypertensive encephalopathy
Human immunodeficiency virus encephalopathy
Intracranial trauma

INTERFERING FACTORS

- Movement of the head during imaging
- Failure to remove metal objects from the imaging field

NURSING CARE

Pretest

- After the physician explains the procedure, the nurse ensures that written consent is obtained from the patient. The form is then entered in the patient's record.
- The nurse instructs the patient to avoid caffeine intake (e.g., coffee, tea, and cola) for 24 hours before the test.
- The nurse or technician assists the patient in removing all clothes and putting on a hospital gown. All jewelry and metal objects are removed from the head, hair, and neck. The patient is placed in supine position on the scanning table.
- The person who needs a SPECT scan is usually elderly and suffering from dementia or has residual trauma to the brain. The unfamiliar room and the procedure may be confusing or frightening to this type of patient. Instructions may be difficult to follow. If these conditions exist, the patient will need simple instructions and close guidance. Because there is no radiation hazard to people in the room, a member of the family or a familiar person can assist and help calm the patient during the test.
- Remind the patient to keep the head still during the injection of the radiopharmaceutical and during the imaging procedure. Explain that the room will be kept calm for 10 minutes before and after the radiopharmaceutical is administered. During this quiet time, the patient should keep his or her eyes open. Blinking is allowed. Earplugs are unnecessary.
- The quiet, stimulus-free environment promotes a resting basal state of brain activity. The patient keeps his or her eyes open during administration of the radionuclide so that the occipital lobes are more clearly visible.

During the Test

- The patient's head is positioned in alignment with the body. An intravenous line is established for the administration of the radiopharmaceutical. To maintain a quiet environment, dim the lights in the room, keep noise to a minimum, and prevent traffic in the room. During the scanning process, the patient will hear the quiet sounds of the scanner, but no pain or discomfort is experienced.

Posttest

- The intravenous line is removed and a small bandage is applied to the venipuncture site.

○ *Patient Teaching.* Because the kidneys will remove the radionuclide from the blood and excrete it in the urine, the nurse instructs the patient to wash his or her hands after voiding. This prevents radioisotopes from remaining on the skin. By 6 hours after the test, the radioactivity level of the isotope is minimal to none.

Single Photon Emission Computed Tomography Scan, Heart

See Perfusion Scan, Cardiac on pp. 488.

Sodium-Depleted Renin Test

See Renin on pp. 539.

Sodium, Serum

Also called: Na⁺

SPECIMEN OR TYPE OF TEST: Blood

PURPOSE OF THE TEST

The serum sodium level is used to monitor electrolyte balance, water balance, and acid-base balance. It also is used in the evaluation of disorders of the central nervous system, musculoskeletal disorders, or diseases of the kidneys or adrenal glands.

BASICS THE NURSE NEEDS TO KNOW

Sodium is a major electrolyte found in all body fluids and is responsible for osmolarity and intravascular osmotic pressure.

With the change of sodium concentration in the blood, resultant changes occur in the water content into or out of cells. Thus the alteration of sodium content is responsible for dehydration or overhydration within cells or in extracellular fluids. The daily intake of sodium is balanced by an equivalent amount of sodium excretion in urine.

Elevated Values

An elevation of serum sodium that is caused by sodium retention or an excessive loss of water is called *hypernatremia*. When a loss of water occurs, the concentration of sodium and the osmolarity of the blood increase. In nonrenal causes of hypernatremia, a loss of body fluid occurs without adequate replacement. This can occur in diuresis, profuse sweating, diarrhea, burns, and respiratory infection. Renal losses of fluid may result from advanced renal failure.

Decreased Values

A low level of serum sodium is called *hyponatremia*. The cause is usually an excessive loss of sodium or excessive water retention. The origin of the problem is frequently due to a renal problem. Metabolic alkalosis, ketonuria, or endocrine deficiency may also cause hyponatremia. In all these conditions, excessive loss of sodium or excessive resorption of water by the kidneys occurs. Nonrenal causes of sodium loss include fluid and electrolyte losses from the gastrointestinal tract, "third space" losses, and severe thermal injury.

REFERENCE VALUES | Infant (0-7 days): 133-146 mEq/L *or* SI: 133-146 mmol/L
Child (1 year or older): 138-145 mEq/L *or* SI: 138-145 mmol/L
Adult: 136-145 mEq/L *or* SI: 136-145 mmol/L

▽ Critical Values | <125 mEq/L (SI: <125 mmol/L) *or* >160 mEq/L (SI: >160 mmol/L)

HOW THE TEST IS DONE

Venipuncture or capillary puncture is used to obtain a specimen of blood.

SIGNIFICANCE OF TEST RESULTS

Elevated Values

Dehydration
Cushing's syndrome
Aldosteronism
Inadequate thirst
Diabetic acidosis
Azotemia
Excessive saline infusion
Profuse sweating
Advanced cancer

Decreased Values

Diuretic therapy
Acute or chronic renal failure
Nephrotic syndrome
Salt-wasting nephritis
Chronic pyelonephritis
Addison's disease
Diabetic ketoacidosis
Burns
Acute water intoxication
Cirrhosis/ascites
Heart failure
Central nervous system disturbance (trauma, tumor)
Hypothyroidism
Hypopituitarism
Vomiting/diarrhea

INTERFERING FACTORS

• Hemolysis

NURSING CARE

Nursing measures include care of the venipuncture or capillary puncture site as described in Chapter 2, with the following additional measures.

Pretest

• The blood sample should be collected without use of a tourniquet to avoid clotting or hemolysis. The arm that has an intravenous infusion should not be used, to avoid hemodilution and false results.

• No fasting is required for this test. The test for sodium is usually part of the electrolyte panel of sodium, chloride, potassium, and carbon dioxide.

Continued

S

| NURSING CARE—cont'd

Posttest

- For the patient with disturbances in sodium values, the nurse should measure daily input and output of fluids. These measurements include recording all oral and intravenous intake and all fluid output as from urine, drainage, vomiting, diarrhea, and fistula drainage.

▽ **Nursing Response to Critical Values**

Once the values reach either critical level, the patient can have significant dysfunction of the brain and nervous system. The nurse immediately notifies the physician of the abnormal test value. Specific treatment will depend on the type and severity of the imbalance and its cause.

The nurse assesses the patient for manifestations of severe sodium imbalance. With severe hypernatremia, the manifestations include somnolence, confusion, coma, and respiratory paralysis. When the sodium value reaches the elevated critical level in less than 24 hours, the mortality rate is greater than 70%.

With moderate hyponatremia, the patient is asymptomatic. Once the sodium value declines to the critical level or lower, the manifestations include lethargy, weakness, somnolence, seizures, and coma. Death can occur from severe hyponatremia.

Stress Testing, Cardiac

Also called: Graded Exercise Testing (GEX); Graded Exercise Stress Testing (GEST); Exercise Stress Testing (EST); Exercise Tolerance Testing (ETT), Exercise Electrocardiography

SPECIMEN OR TYPE OF TEST: Electrophysiology, Echocardiography, Nuclear Scans

PURPOSE OF THE TEST

Stress testing is an invaluable technique for (1) assessing the at-risk population, (2) diagnosing chest pain syndromes and dysrhythmias associated with ischemia, (3) evaluating the effectiveness of therapy (surgical or pharmacologic), and (4) identifying the initial level of function in cardiac rehabilitation programs and evaluating the results.

For patients presenting to the emergency room with chest pain, especially nonradiating pain, who have normal repeated ECGs and biomarkers, stress testing may be done after 6 to 8 hours of observation. Another option is a stress test, which can be done on an outpatient basis 72 hours after the chest pain, if the patient is at low risk for a cardiac event. The purpose of these stress tests is risk stratification and therapeutic planning of interventions.

BASICS THE NURSE NEEDS TO KNOW

Stress testing is an important noninvasive procedure for evaluating the cardiovascular status of patients who are known to have cardiac disease or are at risk for cardiac disease. The test increases the demand placed on the heart by increasing physical activity or using pharmacologic agents. Rarely, if a pacemaker is in place, pacing will be used to increase the heart rate.

There are a variety of cardiac stress tests to determine whether the heart is able to meet increased oxygen demands. Stress testing can be incorporated into electrocardiography testing, into an echocardiography study, and into cardiac nuclear scans (perfusion or gated studies).

REFERENCE VALUES   **ECG Stress Testing**
Increased heart rate
No ST segment changes
No dysrhythmias

HOW THE TEST IS DONE

Stress testing requires the use of a bicycle ergometer (Figure 89) or a treadmill with continuous electrocardiac recording. The test is performed in a series of stages in which the patient exercises for 3 minutes. A variety of protocols are used in stress testing. The Bruce protocol involves a gradual

S

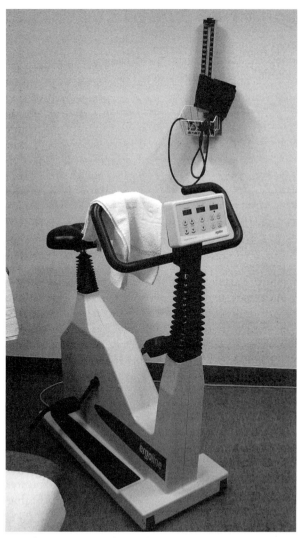

Figure 89. Cycle ergometer for cardiac exercise testing. (From Walsh D, et al.: *Palliative medicine*, Philadelphia, 2008, Saunders.)

increase in speed and incline of the treadmill. The Ellestad protocol involves increasing speeds and intervals of shorter duration. At the end of each stage, a 12-lead electrocardiograph (ECG) is recorded. After each stage, the workload or "graded load" is increased. This is accomplished by increasing the speed or resistance of the bicycle or treadmill. The stress testing continues until the patient reaches 85% of the maximum heart rate, becomes symptomatic, or displays electrocardiographic changes consistent with ischemia. The maximum heart rate is usually determined by normograms. A gross estimate of the maximum heart rate is 220 beats per minute minus the patient's age.

If a patient is physically unable to exercise to the point of 85% of the maximum heart rate, medication may be used to reach the desired heart rate. These medications include dipyridamole (Persantine), adenosine, and dobutamine. Dipyridamole may be given intravenously or by mouth. It causes coronary artery dilation similar to the response of the coronary arteries to exercise. After peak effect is reached (85% maximum heart rate), an echocardiogram or a nuclear scan may performed (see pp. 270 and pp. 455). With a perfusion nuclear scan, a follow-up scan is usually performed 4 hours later.

The use of adenosine is similar to dipyridamole stress testing. Adenosine also has a vasodilating effect, but has a much shorter half-life then dipyridamole. Adenosine and dobutamine may also be used with cardiac nuclear scans.

SIGNIFICANCE OF TEST RESULTS

A 1-mm depression of the ST segment is a positive stress test, indicating myocardial ischemia.

INTERFERING FACTORS

- Severe anxiety may interfere with the patient's ability to participate fully in the stress testing.
- False-positive results may be due to bundle branch block, ventricular hypertrophy, or digitalization. False-negative results may be due to the use of β-blockers.
- Medical/orthopedic conditions, which impede mobility: lung disease, joint pain, muscle weakness.

NURSING CARE

Pretest
- Inform the patient about the purpose and procedure of the test.
- Routine cardiac medications are usually continued.
- Assess for the following contraindications to stress testing: chest pain; hypertension; thrombophlebitis; second- or third-degree heart block; serious dysrhythmias; severe congestive heart failure; and neurologic, musculoskeletal, or vascular problems that would impede mobility on the bicycle or treadmill.
- Obtain baseline vital signs.

○ *Patient Teaching.* Instruct the patient not to eat, smoke, or drink alcohol for 3 to 4 hours before the test.

○ *Patient Teaching.* If the adenosine stress test is being done, the nurse explains to patient the need to avoid theophylline-based drugs, dipyridamole, over-the-counter drugs, and caffeine for 24 hours. The nurse also instructs the patient to wear comfortable clothes and rubber-soled walking shoes. Warn the patient that during the exercise, he or she will feel his or her heart racing. The nurse instructs the patient to report chest pain during the procedure.

During the Test
- Have emergency equipment and drugs available (code cart).
- The patient is attached to electrodes for recording a 12-lead ECG.
- A blood pressure cuff is put in place for quick access. A baseline blood pressure reading is obtained.
- As the graded exercises begin, a multichanneled ECG is recorded. A 12-lead ECG is recorded, and the blood pressure is checked at each workload stage (usually every 3-minute increment).
- Observe for signs to stop the stress testing, for example, falling blood pressure, severe hypertension, persistent SVT (supraventricular tachycardia), three consecutive premature ventricular contractions, chest pain, leg cramps, or exhaustion. The stressing may or may not be discontinued if ST segment depressions occur, blood pressure does not rise, or frequent or coupled premature ventricular contractions or bundle branch block occurs.
- If dipyridamole or adenosine is used, assess for the following side effects: myocardial infarction, dysrhythmias, bronchospasm, chest pain, nausea, headache, flushing hypotension, and dizziness. Have aminophylline available to treat serious side effects.

Posttest
- Cardiac monitoring is continued for 5 to 10 minutes after the testing to evaluate the patient's physiologic response.
- Blood pressure is checked.
- Remove conduction jelly and assist in dressing the patient if necessary. The nurse evaluates the patient's physical and emotional response to the testing.
- Instruct the patient to rest and not take hot showers or baths for 2 to 4 hours.

◇ **Nursing Response to Complications**

Stress testing is performed in a controlled environment; however, dysrhythmias and myocardial ischemia may occur.

Dysrhythmias. During the stress test the nurse in the stress laboratory will continuously observe the cardiac monitor for dysrhythmias and inform the physician of their presence. The nurse anticipates this complication by having antiarrhythmia medications on hand.

Myocardial ischemia. Myocardial ischemia may be evident by electrocardiographic changes and by patient complaint of chest pain. Stress testing is immediately stopped if chest pain occurs.

Sweat Test

Also called: Chloride, Sweat; Cystic Fibrosis Sweat Test; Iontophoresis Sweat Test

SPECIMEN OR TYPE OF TEST: Sweat

PURPOSE OF THE TEST

The chloride sweat test is used to diagnose cystic fibrosis in children.

BASICS THE NURSE NEEDS TO KNOW

Cystic fibrosis is a genetic disorder that causes abnormal secretion by the exocrine glands of the pancreas and other distinct exocrine glands of the body. In cystic fibrosis, increased sodium and chloride content exists in the sweat gland secretions. Because the chloride ion concentration on the skin can be measured, the chloride sweat test is the preferred method to diagnose cystic fibrosis in infants and children.

In children up to age 20, an elevated sweat chloride value greater than 60 to 200 mEq/L (SI: >60 to 200 mmol/L) is abnormal and confirms the diagnosis of cystic fibrosis. A value of 41 to 60 mEq/L (SI: 41 to 60 mmol/L) is considered borderline and the test must be repeated. Because other disorders can cause elevation of the sweat chloride concentration, the family history and clinical manifestations of cystic fibrosis disease are included in the interpretation of the test results. In most cases of cystic fibrosis, the test becomes positive within 3 to 5 weeks after birth.

Cystic fibrosis DNA detection may be performed by other methodologies. To evaluate the genetic makeup of the fetus, a sample of amniotic fluid that contains fetal cells can be analyzed for DNA mutations, including those of cystic fibrosis (see Amniocentesis and Amniotic Fluid Analysis, pp. 66-72). To test the child or adult, including the pregnant woman for the abnormal genetic changes of cystic fibrosis, a sample of cells from the mucosal surface of the inner cheek can be analyzed (see Genetic Testing for Cystic Fibrosis, pp. 331-333).

REFERENCE VALUES   Infants and children: 5-35 mEq/L *or* SI: 5-35 mmol/L

HOW THE TEST IS DONE

A sample of sweat is obtained by stimulating skin sweat production with pilocarpine and low-voltage electric current in a process called *iontophoresis*. The electric current introduces small amounts of pilocarpine into the skin. The pilocarpine drug stimulates a sweat response. On removal of the electrodes, the sweat is collected on filter paper, weighed, and then analyzed for chloride content.

SIGNIFICANCE OF TEST RESULTS

Elevated Values
Cystic fibrosis
Hypothyroidism
Adrenal insufficiency
Malnutrition
Renal insufficiency
Glucose-6-phosphate deficiency

INTERFERING FACTORS

- Dermatitis or skin lesion
- Improper placement of the electrodes
- Inadequate sweat collection
- Salt depletion in the body
- Excessive sweating with fever or exercise before the test

NURSING CARE

Pretest

○ *Patient Teaching.* The nurse explains the test procedure to the parents and the child who is old enough to understand. The electrodes will be applied to the skin on the inner aspect of the forearm or, for the infant, on the back. Reassure them that the electrodes do not cause a shock or pain. The patient will feel a mild, tingling sensation.

- Encourage the parents to accompany the child during the test and to bring a book or favorite toy for the child. These distractions will help to pass the time and ease the child's apprehension.
- This test must not be performed on the child who is receiving oxygen or who is in a mist tent. Danger of explosion exists when electric current mixes with oxygen.

Posttest

- The nurse assesses the skin. It may appear reddened at the site of the electrode placement, but is not considered a serious problem.

Syphilis Tests

Includes: Venereal Disease Research Laboratory Test (VDRL), Rapid Plasma Reagin Test (RPR), Fluorescent Treponemal Antibody Absorption Test (FTA-ABS), Treponema pallidum passive particle agglutination (TP-PA)

SPECIMEN OR TYPE OF TEST: Blood, Cerebrospinal Fluid

PURPOSE OF THE TEST

These blood tests are used to screen for or confirm the diagnosis of syphilis. The VDRL is used to monitor the response to therapy and to test the cerebrospinal fluid for late-stage syphilis.

BASICS THE NURSE NEEDS TO KNOW

Treponema pallidum is the spirochete that causes syphilis. The spirochete is transmitted as the result of sexual contact with an infected partner. In addition, a pregnant woman with primary or secondary stage syphilis can transmit the spirochete to her fetus.

Two of these tests (VDRL and RPR) are used as screening tests and two (FTA-ABS and TP-PA are syphilis antibody tests used to confirm positive screening test results. The results are reported as reactive, weakly reactive, or nonreactive or they may be reported as measurable titers. Each blood test has distinct advantages and disadvantages at the various phases of the disease.

Screening tests for syphilis are used for testing large numbers of people, such as in the military or screening blood donors. These tests are very sensitive (accurate) to detect syphilis, but they are not totally specific, meaning that they also react positively to other conditions. Thus, the VDRL and RPR have a false-positive rate of 10% to 30%. False positive means that the person has a positive test result but does not have syphilis. Common factors and conditions that cause a false-positive screening test result include connective tissue disorders, infections including mononucleosis, chickenpox, and hepatitis, cardiovascular disease, drug addition, and nonillness conditions

S

that include aging, pregnancy, and recent vaccination (Mahon, Lehman & Manuselis, 2011). Follow-up antibody testing is used to verify or exclude a diagnosis of syphilis.

The Venereal Disease Research Laboratory (VDRL) test is an effective screening test for syphilis. In most cases, the blood becomes reactive 1 to 3 weeks after a chancre—the first symptom—appears. It is 100% reactive in the secondary phase and remains reactive in most cases of latent syphilis. After effective treatment has eradicated the spirochete, the VDRL results become negative or nonreactive. This is the only test used on cerebrospinal fluid to assess for neurosyphilis.

Rapid plasma reagin test (RPR) is used to screen for the disease. A positive test result should be followed up with one of the specific treponemal antibody tests to confirm the diagnosis.

Fluorescent treponemal antibody absorption test (FTA-ABS) identifies the specific antibodies to *T. pallidum* that are present in the serum. This test is the most sensitive for all stages of syphilis. It is used to confirm positive test results with the VDRL or RPR, but it cannot be used as a screening test. This test also cannot be used to monitor treatment because once the results are reactive, they remain reactive for life.

Treponema pallidum passive particle agglutination (TP-PA) detects the treponemal antibodies in the blood. It is used to confirm or refute a positive screening test. It is used only to detect late-stage syphilis.

REFERENCE VALUES   Negative; nonreactive

HOW THE TEST IS DONE

Serum: Venipuncture is used to collect a specimen of blood.
Cerebrospinal fluid: A sterile tube is used to collect a sample of cerebrospinal fluid during a lumbar puncture.

SIGNIFICANCE OF TEST RESULTS

Positive Values
Syphilis

INTERFERING FACTORS
- Lipemia
- Alcohol

NURSING CARE

Nursing measures include care of the venipuncture or capillary puncture site as described in Chapter 2, with the following additional measures.

Pretest

○ *Patient Teaching.* The nurse instructs the patient to avoid alcohol intake for 24 hours before the test. Fasting from food for 8 hours is also recommended, but water is permitted. The alcohol and food restrictions help to reduce the serum lipid content that interferes with test results.

Posttest
- When the antibody test result is positive for this sexually transmitted disease, the patient should inform all sexual partners of the test results. Sexual partners are advised to undergo testing. Syphilis, a communicable disease, is reported to the state health department.
- The nurse administers the medication to treat the infection. Penicillin is the antibiotic of choice, given intramuscularly or intravenously, as prescribed. Instruct the patient to refrain from sexual contact for at least 1 month after treatment. Cure of the infection is verified by VDRL testing.

Health Promotion

The nurse should educate the patient about how this infection is transmitted, and how to protect from reinfection by using safe sex practices. It is imperative that the patient receive the antibiotic medication, to avoid or limit the devastating complications of this infection. The patient should understand how to recognize the symptoms and the importance of following through with the prescribed treatment until the infection is cured.

Tau, Phosphorylated (p-Tau)

See Lumbar Puncture and Spinal Fluid Analysis on pp. 423-424.

Testosterone, Total, Free

Also called:

SPECIMEN OR TYPE OF TEST: Serum, Plasma

PURPOSE OF THE TEST

The measurement of serum testosterone is used to diagnose precocious sexual development in the boy who is younger than age 10. It helps diagnose deficient activity of the testes or ovaries. It is part of the testing that determines the cause of male infertility or sexual dysfunction. In the female, it helps determine the cause of hirsutism or virilization.

BASICS THE NURSE NEEDS TO KNOW

Total testosterone consists of the measurement of testosterone that is free, loosely bound to albumin, and the part that is strongly bound to sex-hormone-binding globulin. Free testosterone is the amount of the total hormone that is unbound in the serum. Total testosterone is usually the test used when measurement of testosterone is needed.

In the male, almost all the testosterone is synthesized by the testes. In the female, small amounts are synthesized by the ovaries and adrenal glands. Testosterone is the dominant androgen and, in the male, is responsible for spermatogenesis. Androgens affect many other organs and tissues, resulting in increased total body mass and *hirsutism*, the distribution of body hair. When hirsutism is excessive, it is caused by excessive testosterone or its hormonal precursor, androstenedione. In the female, the testosterone level is one of the tests to investigate hirsutism.

T

REFERENCE VALUES*   **Total Testosterone**
Male child (1-5 years): 0.3-30.0 ng/dL *or* SI: 0.01-1.04 nmol/L
Female child (1-5 years): 2-20 ng/dL *or* SI: 0.07-0.69 nmol/L
Adult male: 280-1100 ng/dL *or* SI: 9.72-38.17 nmol/L
Adult female: 15-70 ng/dL *or* SI: 0.52-2.43 nmol/L

Free Testosterone
Male child (6-9 years): 0.1-3.2 pg/mL *or* SI: 0.3-11.1 pmol/L
Female child (6-9 years): 0.1-0.9 pg/mL *or* SI: 0.3-3.1 pmol/L
Adult male: 50-210 pg/mL *or* SI: 174-729 pmol/L
Adult female: 1.0-8.5 pg/mL *or* SI: 3.5-29.5 pmol/L

*Varies significantly from lab to lab.

HOW THE TEST IS DONE

A venous blood sample is obtained.

SIGNIFICANCE OF TEST RESULTS

Elevated Values

Ovarian tumor
Adrenal tumor
Hyperthyroidism
Congenital adrenal hyperplasia
Testicular tumor
Idiopathic precocious puberty
Central nervous system lesion

Decreased Values

Hypogonadism

INTERFERING FACTORS

• Recent radioactive isotope scan

NURSING CARE

Nursing measures include care of the venipuncture or capillary puncture site as described in Chapter 2, with the following additional measures.

Pretest

• The nurse schedules this test before or 7 days after any radioisotope scan because radioisotopes can interfere with the laboratory method of analysis.

Posttest

• The patient often has symptoms that he or she may find embarrassing or difficult to accept because they involve changes in the physical appearance and a disturbance in body image. For the female, manifestations may include male pattern baldness, acne, and hirsutism.

T

For the male, infertility may exist. For the child with precocious puberty, both physical and sexual organs are developed beyond the age-related norms. The nurse can help the patient by using an open and calm approach in interactions and using listening skills if the patient verbalizes his or her feelings.

Thoracentesis, Pleural Fluid Analysis, and Pleural Biopsy

Also called: Pleural tap, Pleural fluid aspiration

SPECIMEN OR TYPE OF TEST: Pleural Fluid; Possible Pleural Biopsy Tissue

PURPOSE OF THE TEST

Thoracentesis is performed to remove fluid from the pleural space for diagnostic or therapeutic reasons. Examination of pleural fluid identifies or confirms diagnoses of cancer, infection, or severe fluid overload (congestive heart failure, liver failure, and systemic or pulmonary hypertension). The biopsy tissue and/or fluid is used to identify cancer or other pathologic change in the pleural tissue.

BASICS THE NURSE NEEDS TO KNOW

An accumulation of fluid in the pleural space is abnormal. Thoracentesis is an invasive procedure used to remove fluid from the pleural space. It is indicated for new or large effusions. It may be performed for diagnostic or therapeutic reasons, or both. During thoracentesis, pleural fluid is removed. In addition, a percutaneous needle biopsy of the pleura may be performed.

Pleural Fluid Analysis

Pleural effusions (accumulation of fluid in the pleural space) may be a result of neoplastic or infectious processes or of leakage of fluid from the vascular system. If the effusion is due to neoplasm or infection, the fluid is usually called an *exudate*. If the fluid is due to leakage from the blood vessels, it is called a *transudate*. To distinguish between exudates and transudates, pleural fluid is evaluated for protein, specific gravity, glucose, and a blood cell count with differential. Pleural fluid is also obtained for cultures to identify tuberculosis, fungal, and various bacterial infections. Cytologic examination of the pleural fluid is performed to rule out malignancy. For a diagnostic thoracentesis usually 5 to 100 mL of fluid are removed.

Pleural Biopsy

If tissue samples are removed from the pleura during the thoracentesis, they will be examined microscopically to identify the cell types. Malignancy of the pleura can be detected.

REFERENCE VALUES | Normal pleural fluid
No pathogens or malignant cells are present

T

HOW THE TEST IS DONE

Thoracentesis and Pleural Fluid Collection

After the patient is positioned in a seated, upright position with arms folded and their head resting on a pillow on the overhead table, the lower posterior chest is exposed and prepared, and a local anesthetic is given. A needle is inserted into the pleural space guided by ultrasound and the fluid is aspirated. The fluid is placed in a sterile container. The nurse affixes the label containing the patient's identification data, date, and the type of fluid. The container is sent to the laboratory immediately. If pleural fluid is to be drained, a catheter is inserted using the needle as guide.

If the patient is on a mechanical ventilator or is unable to sit up, they can be placed in supine or recumbent position with the head of the bed elevated to 30 to 40 degrees on their unaffected side. The arm of the affected side is raised above the patient's head.

Pleural Biopsy

A pleural biopsy may be performed at this time. If a *pleural biopsy* is planned, a special biopsy needle is used with a hooked biopsy trocar. Usually, three tissue specimens are obtained from three pleural sites. Specimens are placed in a sterile container with fixative and labeled with the patient's identification data, date, and the source of the tissue specimen. The container is sent to the lab immediately.

SIGNIFICANCE OF TEST RESULTS

Bacterial, viral, or fungal infection
Malignancy
Collagen disease
Lymphoma
Systemic lupus erythematosus
Liver failure
Nephrotic syndrome
Myxedema
Pancreatitis

INTERFERING FACTORS

- Uncooperative patient

NURSING CARE

Pretest

- Explain the procedure and the purpose of the test to the patient. Inform patient the procedure usually takes about 30 minutes. If a catheter is inserted to maintain drainage, explain the purpose to the patient and the need not to pull on it.
- No food or fluid restrictions are necessary.
- Ensure that a signed consent form has been obtained.
- Perform and document a baseline assessment. A blood pressure cuff is left in place to permit easy monitoring of the blood pressure during the procedure.

- Check the patient's recent laboratory values of the prothrombin time (PT), partial thrombo-plastin time (PTT), and platelet count to identify the potential for bleeding problems.
- Observe for any local cutaneous infection.
- Check for allergy to local anesthetic.
- If prescribed, initiate supplemental O_2.
- A pulse oximeter is attached.
- ○ *Patient Teaching.* Warn the patient not to cough or move during the procedure.
- Obtain a thoracentesis tray and place at the bedside.

During the Test

- The nurse continuously monitors the patient's response to the procedure.
- The nurse monitors the pulse oximeter readings for changes in O_2 sat.
- If the patient is mildly anxious, a mild sedative may be ordered. The nurse may also use guided imagery to comfort the patient.
- The patient is positioned in an upright position, seated on the side of the bed with the legs resting on a footstool. The patient's arms should be supported on a padded overbed table (Figure 90). If the patient is on a mechanical ventilator or is unable to sit up, he or she may lie on the unaffected side with the back flush with the edge of the bed. The head of the bed may be elevated 30 to 40 degrees.
- The nurse provides emotional support to the patient because pressure pain may be experienced even though local anesthetic is given.
- After the physician inserts a thoracentesis needle with a stopcock attached, fluid is drawn off for analysis. Be sure the stopcock is turned to prevent opening to the atmosphere. A catheter may be inserted at this point if a large amount of fluid is to be drained.
- Pleural fluid is drained slowly and limited to 1.5 L/24 hr to prevent reexpansion pulmonary edema and hypotension.
- When the physician performs a biopsy, the nurse instructs the patient to exhale fully and perform the Valsalva maneuver. This prevents air from entering the pleural space when the tissue sample is taken.
- Procedure may be stopped if the patient experiences chest pain, shortness of breath, or coughing. Pleuritic pain may occur. Listen for a pleural friction rub.
- The needle/catheter is removed on exhalation.

Posttest

- The nurse checks vital signs every 15 minutes until they are stable and assesses bilateral breath sounds.
- Pressure is applied to the insertion site for 5 minutes to control bleeding.
- Apply dry sterile dressing to site.
- The nurse documents the amount, color, and character of the fluid obtained and a notation of how the patient tolerated the procedure. Normal pericardial fluid is clear and colorless to straw color.
- If it is ordered, the nurse schedules a chest x-ray that would assess for potential pneumothorax.
- The nurse encourages the patient to lie on the uninvolved side for 1 hour to improve oxygenation.
- The nurse continues assessments by observation of the small dressing over the site for bleeding or drainage and palpates around the site for subcutaneous emphysema.
- As the lungs reexpand, the patient may develop a cough. Reassure patient this is normal.

Continued

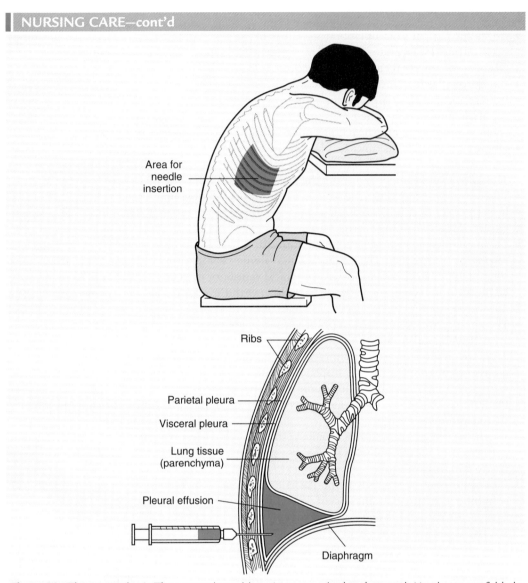

Figure 90. Thoracentesis. **A,** Thoracentesis position. Arms are raised and crossed. Head rests on folded arms. This position allows the chest wall to be pulled outward in an expanded position. If an overbed table is not available, the arms may be left down but positioned forward of the hips or crossed in front of the chest. **B,** The usual site for the insertion of a thoracentesis needle for a right-sided effusion. The actual site varies with each patient, depending on the location and volume of the effusion. The physician tries to keep the needle as far away from the diaphragm as possible, while at the same time inserting the needle close to the base of the effusion so that gravity can help with drainage.

○ *Patient Teaching.* Nurse instructs the patient and family that the dressing may be removed after 24 hours. The nurse instructs the patient and family to check the site for bleeding and signs of infection (redness, swelling, and drainage).
• If the procedure is done as an outpatient, ensure the patient has another person drive them home.

◆ **Nursing Response to Complications**

The major complication after thoracentesis is a pneumothorax. Another complication the nurse needs to observe for is reexpansion pulmonary edema. It occurs when large amounts of pleural fluid are removed, causing an increase in negative intrapleural pressure. If the lungs do not reexpand to fill the space, edema can result. Bleeding is a rare complication. Because thoracentesis is an invasive procedure, infection is possible, but extremely rare because thoracentesis is performed using sterile technique. Another rare complication is the accidental puncture of the liver or spleen.

Pulmonary edema. The nurse will assess for pulmonary edema by checking bilateral breath sounds and observing for indications of hypoxia. The nurse will report crackles and hypoxia immediately. The nurse will anticipate the physician's orders for oxygen, diuresis, intubation, and mechanical ventilation.

Bleeding. The nurse assesses for indications of bleeding: tachycardia, restlessness, hypotension, and bloody drainage. The nurse reports indications of bleeding immediately.

Pneumothorax. Anxiety, restlessness, dyspnea, tachypnea, pallor, and decreased breath sounds are indications of a pneumothorax. If a tension pneumothorax has occurred, there will be a mediastinal shift to the unaffected side. Notify the physician immediately and anticipate an order for a chest radiograph to evaluate the size of the pneumothorax. If a tension pneumothorax is present, the nurse needs to assess the patency of any chest tube that has been inserted.

Thyrocalcitonin

See Calcitonin on pp. 157.

Thyroglobulin Autoantibodies

Also called: Antithyroid Antibodies

SPECIMEN OR TYPE OF TEST: Serum

PURPOSE OF THE TEST

Thyroglobulin antibodies are evaluated to detect autoimmune-based thyroid disease.

BASICS THE NURSE NEEDS TO KNOW

Some thyroid disorders may be autoimmune in origin. To evaluate this potential cause, antithyroid antibodies are measured. One of these antibodies is thyroglobulin autoantibody. The thyroglobulin autoantibodies act on the antigen *thyroglobulin*, the storage form of thyroid hormones. The presence of these antibodies helps confirm the diagnosis of autoimmune disease; however, their absence does not rule out the potential diagnosis.

REFERENCE VALUES   Immunofluorescence method: Titer less than 1:100
Hemagglutination method: Negative

HOW THE TEST IS DONE
Venipuncture is performed.

SIGNIFICANCE OF TEST RESULTS
Elevated Values
Graves' disease
Hashimoto's thyroiditis
Hyperthyroidism
Hypothyroidism
Nontoxic nodular goiter
Pernicious anemia
Rheumatoid arthritis
Systemic lupus erythematosus
Thyroid cancer

INTERFERING FACTORS
• Oral contraceptives

NURSING CARE

The nursing actions are similar to those of other venipuncture techniques presented in Chapter 2.

Thyroid Scan

Also called: Radionuclide Thyroid Scanning

SPECIMEN OR TYPE OF TEST: Nuclear Imaging

PURPOSE OF THE TEST
A thyroid scan is done to differentiate causes of hyperthyroidism, to locate ectopic tissue, evaluate whether a nodule is functional, and to assess for congenital hypothyroidism.

A thyroid scan may be done with ^{131}I or ^{123}I to determine the ability of the gland to take up iodine. This is called a radioactive iodine uptake study (RAIU). This may be ordered before initiating iodine therapy for thyroid cancer.

A whole body scan may be performed to assess for metastasis of thyroid cancer after therapy with radioactive iodine.

BASICS THE NURSE NEEDS TO KNOW
To produce its hormones, the thyroid gland must extract iodide from the extracellular fluid. Once it has taken up enough iodide to meet its needs, the iodide left in the extracellular fluid is excreted in urine. The thyroid gland cannot distinguish between dietary iodine and radioactive iodine. Thus it will take up the radioactive iodine, which can be scanned by a gamma camera. The functioning of the thyroid gland can be evaluated by the amount of radioactive iodine it

takes up. In thyrotoxic states, more iodide is needed and the uptake is increased, whereas in hypothyroid states, less than normal amounts of iodide are needed, thus less is taken up by the thyroid gland.

In addition to an increase or decrease in uptake by the thyroid gland, scanning may also identify "hot" or "cold" spots. Cold nodules are areas of the gland that take up less or no radio-active iodine. Hot nodules are areas that take up more radioactive iodine than does the surrounding tissue. Cold spots may indicate cancer, whereas hot spots are usually not malignant. An echogram (sonogram) may be obtained to distinguish if the cold spot is a solid or semicystic lesion or a pure cyst. Pure cysts are rarely cancerous.

Additional information on nuclear scans is presented on p. 455.

REFERENCE VALUES   Normal anatomic position and size, with homogenous (equally distributed) uptake of the isotopes throughout the glandular tissue (Figure 91)

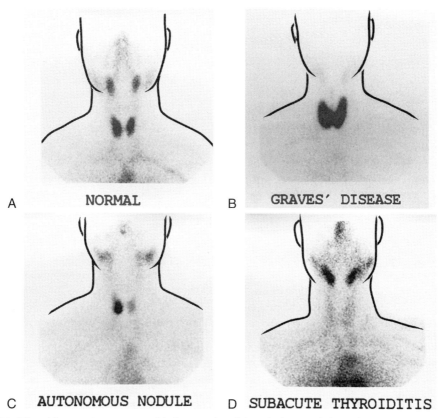

A NORMAL   **B** GRAVES' DISEASE

C AUTONOMOUS NODULE   **D** SUBACUTE THYROIDITIS

Figure 91. Thyroid scan. Appearance of **(A)** normal and **(B-D)** abnormal thyroid scans following an injection of technetiuim-99m. (From Mettler FA, Guiberteau MJ: *Essentials of nuclear medicine imaging*, ed 5, Philadelphia, 2006, Saunders.)

HOW THE TEST IS DONE

Radionuclide agents used in a thyroid scan are ^{123}I and technetium (Tc 99m). These agents are given intravenously, which allows scanning to be done by the gamma camera within 20 minutes. ^{123}I may also be given orally and the thyroid is scanned after 24 hours.

SIGNIFICANCE OF TEST RESULTS

Elevated Values

Early Hashimoto's thyroiditis
Hyperthyroidism (Graves' disease, toxic nodular goiter)
Hypoalbuminemia
Iodine-deficient goiter
Lithium ingestion

Decreased Values

Cretinism
Excessive iodide intake
Hypothyroidism (primary or secondary)
Thyrotoxicosis as a result of ectopic thyroid metastasis, subacute thyroiditis, or thyrotoxicosis factitia

INTERFERING FACTORS

- Dietary intake of iodized foods (e.g., salt, bread)
- Iodine-deficient diet
- Previous radiographic studies with iodine-based dye
- Severe diarrhea
- Renal failure
- Noncompliance with dietary restrictions
- Medications such as anticoagulants, antihistamines, antithyroid medications, corticosteroids, lithium, multivitamins, penicillin, phenothiazines, phenylbutazone, salicylates, and thyroid hormones

NURSING CARE

Pretest

- The nurse obtains a medication history to determine if any interfering drugs were taken.
- Assess for allergy to iodine and seafood.
- Schedule any x-ray studies requiring dyes after the radioactive iodine uptake study.
- Check patient's renal status. Report elevations in patient's BUN and serum creatinine.
- ○ *Patient Teaching.* Instruct the patient not to eat or drink for 4 hours before the test.
- ○ *Patient Teaching.* Describe the scanning equipment to the patient. The probe is placed over the anterior portion of the neck. Emphasize that no discomfort is involved but that the patient must lie absolutely still while the scan is performed. The nurse informs the patient that the oral radioactive iodine, if being used, has little or no taste. It comes in capsule or liquid form. Explain to the patient the need for two scans because the uptake of the radioactive

iodine is usually maximized at 24 hours but some thyroid conditions may cause the peak uptake to occur earlier.

- Remove all metal objects and jewelry from the neck.
- Transport the patient to the nuclear medicine laboratory when scheduled.

During the Test

- Patient is placed in supine position with a small pillow under the shoulder blades with the neck hyperextended.
- Patient is asked not to swallow during the scanning.
- Two hours after oral ingestion of the radioactive iodine, a light meal may be consumed.

Posttest

- The patient resumes a normal diet.
- The nurse monitors the patient for allergic response.
- Wear gloves for 24 hours after the test when handling the patient's bedpan or urinal. Wash hands with soap and water after removing gloves.
- Wear gloves when handling soiled linens. Follow hospital protocol for disposing of soiled linens in special containers.

O *Patient Teaching.* Instruct the patient to wash hands with soap and water after voiding for 24 hours and to flush the toilet 2 to 3 times after each use. This is done because a small amount of the radioactive iodine will be excreted in the urine.

Thyroid-Stimulating Hormone

Also called: TSH; Thyrotropin

SPECIMEN OR TYPE OF TEST: Serum

PURPOSE OF THE TEST

Thyrotropin (thyroid-stimulating hormone [TSH]) levels are obtained to (1) diagnose hypothyroidism, (2) distinguish between primary and secondary hypothyroidism, and (3) monitor patient response to thyroid replacement therapy.

BASICS THE NURSE NEEDS TO KNOW

TSH is secreted by the anterior pituitary gland by a negative feedback mechanism (Figure 92). Thyrotropin causes the thyroid gland to increase its production and secretion of thyroid hormones.

Because of the thyrotropin regulatory mechanism with the thyroid hormones, its level will be affected by primary thyroid abnormalities. If the patient has hyperthyroidism, thyrotropin will be suppressed. If the patient has primary hypothyroidism, thyrotropin secretion will become significantly elevated. This elevation may create a compensatory euthyroid state. Exogenous thyroid hormones will also suppress thyrotropin secretion. TSH varies very little with age. Patients with upper reference range values are at increased risk of developing hypothyroidism.

T

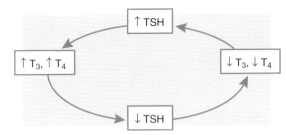

Figure 92. Thyroid hormone regulation. Thyroid hormone production and secretion are based on a negative feedback mechanism, with thyroid-stimulating hormone (TSH) secreted by the anterior pituitary gland. T_3, triiodothyronine; T_4, thyroxine.

REFERENCE VALUES   Adult: 0.4-4.2 µU/L *or* SI: 0.4-4.2 mU/L
Newborn (<5d) 1.0-39 µU/L *or* SI: 0.7-27 mU/L

HOW THE TEST IS DONE

Venipuncture is performed. If the test is required on a newborn, a heelstick is performed and the blood is collected on filter paper.

SIGNIFICANCE OF TEST RESULTS

Elevated Values

Addison's disease
Goiter (some forms)
Hyperpituitarism
Pituitary adenoma
Primary hypothyroidism
Thyroid cancer

Decreased Values

Hyperthyroidism
Overdose of exogenous thyroid replacement
Secondary hypothyroidism
Tertiary hypothyroidism
Thyroiditis

INTERFERING FACTORS

- Radioisotope administration within 1 week
- Extreme stress
- Medications: antithyroid medication, aspirin, corticosteroids, dopamine, heparin, lithium, potassium iodide, and thyroid replacement therapy
- If newborn is tested too soon after birth, false positive results can occur. There is a sharp and significant increase in thyrotropin with birth. It returns to normal after 3 days.

NURSING CARE

Health Promotion

The nurse encourages all women older than age 65 to have their TSH level checked every 3 to 5 years. If a woman complains of fatigue and has loss of hair or a husky voice, the nurse would encourage medical follow-up including a TSH level. Screening with a capillary blood collection and special filter paper is done on all newborn babies to assess for congenital hypothyroidism. In the newborn, early detection of hypothyroidism allows for early medical treatment and prevention of the onset of mental retardation and physical deformities.

Nursing actions related to venipuncture and capillary puncture are presented in Chapter 2, with the following additional measures.

Pretest

- The nurse assesses for and reports any clinical states that would increase the patient's endogenous glucocorticoid levels.
- Check with the physician regarding withholding medications that may interfere with test results.

Thyrotropin-Releasing Hormone Test

Also called: TRH Test; TSH-Releasing Hormone

SPECIMEN OR TYPE OF TEST: Serum

PURPOSE OF THE TEST

Thyrotropin-releasing hormone (TRH) determinations are rarely performed today because the thyrotropin (TSH) test is usually adequate to support the diagnosis. TRH testing is performed when clinical manifestations of thyroid dysfunction are evident, but other tests are not clear.

BASICS THE NURSE NEEDS TO KNOW

TRH is produced and secreted by the hypothalamus. It acts as a moderator of the thyroid hormone-thyrotropin negative feedback mechanism. In response to synthetic TRH being given intravenously, the anterior pituitary gland will normally increase its secretion of thyrotropin within 5 minutes. The thyrotropin levels peak in 20 to 30 minutes and will return to baseline within 2 to 4 hours.

REFERENCE VALUES	After TRH is given, TSH increases. Male: 14-24 µU/mL *or* SI: 14-24 mU/L Female: 16-26 µU/mL *or* SI: 16-26 mU/L

HOW THE TEST IS DONE

TRH determinations may be performed in a number of ways, with the dose and route of the TRH varying. The most common method is the bolus intravenous administration of synthetic TRH after blood is drawn for a baseline thyrotropin level. After 30 minutes (and sometimes again after

60 minutes), when the thyrotropin response is normally peaking, a second specimen is drawn for a thyrotropin determination.

SIGNIFICANCE OF TEST RESULTS

Elevated Values
Normal response
Hypothyroidism

Decreased Values
Cushing's syndrome
Depression
Hyperthyroidism
Multinodular goiter
Pituitary lesions
Renal failure

INTERFERING FACTORS

- Corticosteroids
- Levodopa
- Salicylates (high dose)

NURSING CARE

The nursing implementation for this test is similar to that for Thyroid-Stimulating Hormone (see pp. 577), with the following additional measure.

Pretest
- Inform the patient of the need for multiple venipuncture procedures.

Thyroxine, Total

Also called: T_4; Total T_4; Total Thyroxine

SPECIMEN OR TYPE OF TEST: Serum

PURPOSE OF THE TEST

Thyroxine levels are obtained to evaluate thyroid function, confirm the diagnosis of hyperthyroidism or hypothyroidism, and evaluate therapy for hyperthyroidism or hypothyroidism.

BASICS THE NURSE NEEDS TO KNOW

The thyroid gland produces and secretes the hormones *thyroxine* (T_4) and *triiodothyronine* (T_3). This gland takes up iodide from the extracellular fluid and uses it to produce thyroglobulin, the precursor of all thyroid hormones. The thyroglobulin is stored in the thyroid gland until thyroxine and triiodothyronine are processed before secretion from the gland. Secretion of triiodothyronine and thyroxine is primarily regulated by a negative feedback mechanism with thyrotropin (see Figure 92). Thyrotropin is secreted by the anterior pituitary gland.

Once secreted by the thyroid gland, triiodothyronine and thyroxine are bound primarily to thyroid-binding globulin and to a lesser degree to albumin and prealbumin. The small amount of the hormones not bound to protein is called *free thyroxine* and *free triiodothyronine*. It is the free hormones that are biologically active. The bound hormones are released from the protein as the hormones are needed. In the peripheral circulation, thyroxine will lose one of its iodide molecules and become triiodothyronine, the more potent of the thyroid hormones.

Because the majority of the thyroid hormones are bound to protein, the evaluation of thyroid hormone levels should include the person's protein levels. If the patient has decreased proteins to carry the hormone, a greater amount of the hormone will be in the free state or active form. Radioimmunoassay (RIA) measures both bound and unbound thyroxine.

REFERENCE VALUES	Newborn: 6.4-23.2 µg/dL *or* SI: 82.4-298.6 nmol/L
	Children:
	    2-10 months: 7.8-16.5 µg/dL *or* SI: 100.4-212.4 nmol/L
	    1-10 years: 6.4-15 µg/dL *or* SI: 82.41-193.1 nmol/L
	    10-20 years: 4.2-11.8 µg/dL *or* SI: 54.11-151.9 nmol/L
	Adult: 5-12 µg/dL *or* SI: 64.4-154.4 nmol/L

▽ Critical Values	<2.0 µg/dL (SI: <26 nmol/L) and >20 µg/dL (SI: >257 nmol/L)

HOW THE TEST IS DONE

Venipuncture is performed.

If a thyroxine determination is ordered on a newborn, umbilical cord blood may be used or a heelstick can be performed. With the heelstick method, special filter paper is used to blot the blood, and the filter paper is sent to the laboratory in a container that protects against light.

SIGNIFICANCE OF TEST RESULTS

Elevated Values

Hyperthyroidism
Acute or subacute thyroiditis
Toxic multinodular goiter

Decreased Values

Hypothyroidism
Chronic or subacute thyroiditis
Myxedema
Cretinism
Severe illness

INTERFERING FACTORS

- Liver disorders, which affect blood protein levels.
- Protein-wasting diseases such as chronic renal failure.
- Medications: androgens, aspirin, chlorpropamide, chlorpromazine, estrogen, heparin, iodides, thyroid replacement medications, lithium, methadone, phenothiazines, phenytoin, reserpine, steroids, sulfonamides, sulfonylureas, and tolbutamide.

T

NURSING CARE

Nursing actions are similar to those used in other venipuncture or capillary puncture procedures (see Chapter 2), with the following additional measures.

During the Test

- If a heelstick is performed, the heel is first cleansed with antiseptic and the skin is pierced with a sterile lancet. Completely saturate the circles on the filter paper.
- Because pregnancy will normally cause an increase in thyroxine levels, indicate the pregnancy on the requisition slip, as applicable.

Posttest

- Send the filter paper to the laboratory in a container that protects against light.

▽ **Nursing Response to Critical Values**

For very low thyroxine levels, assess the patient for myxedema coma. For very high thyroxine levels, assess the patient for thyroid storm. Assessments for both extremes of thyroxine levels include careful evaluation of the patient's mental status. Report change in mentation to the physician immediately.

Thyroxine-Binding Globulin

Also called: TBG; T_4-Binding Globulin

SPECIMEN OR TYPE OF TEST: Serum

PURPOSE OF THE TEST

Thyroxine-binding globulin (TBG) is evaluated when clinical manifestations of thyroid dysfunction and thyroid hormone levels do not correlate.

BASICS THE NURSE NEEDS TO KNOW

TBG is the primary protein carrier of thyroxine and triiodothyronine. The thyroid hormones bound to TBG provide a storehouse of the hormones, which are released from the protein as needed. Because TBG carries approximately 70% of the total amount of thyroid hormones in the circulation, TBG levels significantly affect total hormone concentrations. TBG levels will affect the free forms of triiodothyronine and thyroxine.

REFERENCE VALUES   Infant: 1.6-4.2 mg/dL *or* SI: 16-42 mg/L
Child: 2.9-5.0 mg/dL *or* SI: 29-50 mg/L
Adult: 1.2-3.0 mg/dL *or* SI: 12-30 mg/L

HOW THE TEST IS DONE

Venipuncture is performed.

SIGNIFICANCE OF TEST RESULTS

Elevated Values
Congenital abnormality
Estrogen therapy
Hepatitis, acute
Hypothyroidism
Pregnancy

Decreased Values
Androgens
Cirrhosis of the liver
Congenital abnormality
Glucocorticoids
Hyperthyroidism
Recent surgery
Renal failure
Starvation

INTERFERING FACTORS

- Heparin
- Phenylbutazone
- Phenytoin
- Salicylates

NURSING CARE

Nursing actions related to venipuncture are presented in Chapter 2, with the following additional measures.

Pretest

- Obtain a medication history to determine if any drug is being taken that affects normal thyroid binding.

Tilt Table

Also called: Head Up Tilt (HUT)

SPECIMEN OR TYPE OF TEST: Physiologic

PURPOSE OF THE TEST

The tilt table test is done to determine if a patient's fainting or loss of consciousness is due to vasovagal or neurocardiogenic syncope.

T

BASICS THE NURSE NEEDS TO KNOW

Vasovagal or neurocardiogenic syncope is due to a nervous system reflux, which causes the heart rate to decrease and the blood vessels to dilate. This causes a decrease in blood to the brain and the patient faints. While not lethal, it can cause injuries due to falling. If the tilt table test is negative (the patient does not faint), other causes of syncope must be investigated.

REFERENCE VALUES	If the patient faints during the test, it is considered positive for vasovagal syncope.

HOW THE TEST IS DONE

Patient is placed on the tilt table, which has a foot rest. Safety belts are applied to prevent falls. The table is tilted upright to 60 to 80 degrees for approximately 45 minutes. If no response occurs, medication may be given to increase the heart rate and the table would remain tilted for another 45 minutes or until there is a response.

SIGNIFICANCE OF TEST RESULTS

Positive Values
Vasovagal syncope

INTERFERING FACTORS

* Anxiety

NURSING CARE

Pretest
* Reassure the patient of the presence of someone with them throughout the procedure.
* Check with the prescriber on whether any medications are to be held
* ○ *Patient Teaching.* Instruct the patient not to eat or drink for 4 to 6 hours before the test.
* ○ *Patient Teaching.* Inform patient they may experience nausea, sweating, dizziness and/or fainting.

During the Test
* Position patient on tilt table and apply safety belts.
* Apply blood pressure cuff and start an intravenous access.
* Take base line vital signs.
* Apply electrodes and monitor ECG.
* ○ *Patient Teaching.* Instruct patient not to shift weight and to keep their feet on the foot rest during the test.
* ○ *Patient Teaching.* Ask patient to report any symptoms they may be experiencing.
* Record vital signs periodically and when patient complains of light-headedness or near fainting.
* If the patient faints, lower the table until it is flat and monitor until fully recovered. Recovery is usually immediate.

Posttest
* Take and record vital signs.
* Assist patient off the table and observe their response.

T

Tolbutamide Stimulation Test

SPECIMEN OR TYPE OF TEST: Serum

PURPOSE OF THE TEST

The tolbutamide stimulation test is performed to identify insulin-producing tumors of the pancreas.

BASICS THE NURSE NEEDS TO KNOW

Tolbutamide (Orinase) is an oral hypoglycemic agent. Its duration of action is short, being rapidly inactivated by the liver. For this reason, tolbutamide is used in stimulation tests to evaluate exaggerated and prolonged insulin secretion. This condition may occur with insulinoma, which is an insulin-secreting tumor of the pancreatic islets of Langerhans. It presents with spontaneous fasting hypoglycemia.

The goal in giving tolbutamide is to create a hypoglycemic state and see the insulin response to the induced hypoglycemia. Normally, insulin secretion decreases with hypoglycemia. If the insulin secretion stays at high levels and is prolonged, the test result is positive.

REFERENCE VALUES | Serum insulin level: <195 µU/mL *or* SI: <1354 pmol/L

HOW THE TEST IS DONE

The tolbutamide stimulation test is performed by administering tolbutamide intravenously over a 2-minute period. Serum insulin levels are obtained every 5 minutes for 15 minutes. Each specimen is obtained by venipuncture or an intravenous catheter will be inserted to prevent multiple needle insertions.

SIGNIFICANCE OF TEST RESULTS

If the insulin level is maintained or prolonged, the test confirms the diagnosis of insulinoma.

INTERFERING FACTORS

- Liver disorders
- Renal failure
- Medications such as chloramphenicol, dicumarol, MAO inhibitors, phenylbutazone, salicylates, and sulfonamides

T

NURSING CARE

Nursing actions related to venipuncture are presented in Chapter 2, with the following additional measures.

Pretest

- Explain to the patient the need for several venipuncture procedures or explain the purpose of the intravenous catheter.

Continued

> ▌ NURSING CARE—cont'd

During the Test
- Observe the patient for a reaction to tolbutamide, which is most commonly a skin rash.

Posttest
- Observe the patient for prolonged hypoglycemia, especially in elderly individuals.

◈ **Nursing Response to Complications**

Prolonged hypoglycemia may occur with the administration of tolbutamide.

Hypoglycemia. The nurse needs to assess for hypoglycemia: hunger, diaphoresis, palpitations, anxiety, tremulousness, vagueness and, if extreme, convulsions and coma. The physician should be notified immediately. If the patient is awake and able to swallow, oral glucose may be given.

Total Iron Binding Capacity

See Iron Studies on pp. 400-406.

Total Triiodothyronine

See Triiodothyronine on pp. 589.

Toxoplasmosis Serology

Also called: Toxoplasmosis Titer

SPECIMEN OR TYPE OF TEST: Blood; Umbilical Cord Blood

PURPOSE OF THE TEST

The antibody tests help in the diagnosis of toxoplasmosis, a parasitic infection.

BASICS THE NURSE NEEDS TO KNOW

Toxoplasma gondii is a protozoan parasite that infects household cats as well as domestic food animals (e.g., sheep, pigs). Oocysts in the feces of the infected animal are deposited in the environment. The infection is transmitted to people by the fecal-oral route. This includes ingestion of contaminated water or food, or having the oocysts on the hands after casual contact with contaminated soil or kitty litter. The individual also may become infected after eating undercooked meat of an infected animal. In pregnancy, maternal infection can be transmitted to the fetus via placental blood (Figure 93).

In acute toxoplasmosis, immunoglobulin (IgM) antibodies appear in 1 to 2 weeks, and the titer peaks at 6 to 8 weeks. Testing for IgM antibodies is very useful in the diagnosis of acute infection and congenital infection. Many individuals already have IgG antibodies from a previous asymptomatic infection, and the low or insignificant elevations persist for months to years.

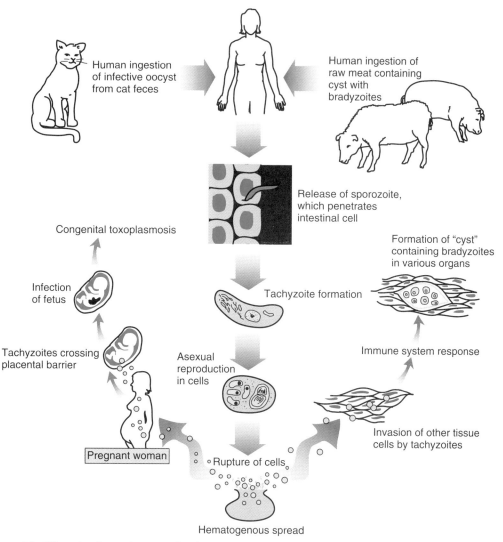

Figure 93. Life cycle of *Toxoplasma gondii*. The person ingests the infective stage of the parasite from infected feline fecal contamination on the hands or by eating raw or undercooked meat of an infected animal. In the person, the parasite passes through several maturation stages and infects cells and organs of the body. If the person is pregnant, the infection passes from the mother to the fetus. (From Mahon CR, Lehman DC, Manuselis G: *Textbook of diagnostic microbiology,* ed 4, Philadelphia, 2011, Saunders.)

A rising IgG titer, however, may be evidence of recovery from acute infection. The specific laboratory titers are dependent on the methodology used.

When the woman develops acute toxoplasmosis within the first 4 or 5 months of her pregnancy, the tachyzoites travel from her blood, through the placenta, and into the fetus via the umbilical cord. Congenital infection of the fetus can result in intrauterine death or cause fetal brain damage, central nervous system disturbance, or chorioretinitis. Testing is performed on the cord blood, obtained by sampling blood from the umbilical vein (see also Percutaneous Umbilical Cord Blood Sampling pp. 483). An elevated IgM antibody in the cord blood is considered diagnostic for congenital toxoplasmosis.

REFERENCE VALUES   IgM antibodies: Negative
IgG antibodies: Negative; <1:4

HOW THE TEST IS DONE

Venipuncture is done to obtain a sample of blood.

SIGNIFICANCE OF TEST RESULTS

Positive Values

Toxoplasmosis infection

INTERFERING FACTORS

• None

NURSING CARE

Nursing measures include care of the venipuncture or capillary puncture site as described in Chapter 2, with the following additional measures.

Pretest

• Schedule the test to be performed at the onset of illness and 2 to 3 weeks later during the convalescent phase.

Posttest

Health Promotion

The nurse can teach people the importance of cooking meat thoroughly to eliminate this source of potential infection. The parasite can remain on the hands after touching contaminated soil or cleaning a kitty litter box used by an infected cat. Therefore, people should be reminded of the importance of hand-washing, particularly before preparing or eating food. Pregnant women should not clean the kitty litter box.

Transbronchial Biopsy

See Bronchoscopy on pp. 153.

Transcatheter Bronchial Brushing

See Bronchoscopy on pp. 153.

Transesophageal Echocardiography

Also called: TEE, Transesophageal Ultrasound

SPECIMEN OR TYPE OF TEST: Ultrasonography

PURPOSE OF THE TEST

Indications for transesophageal echocardiography include diagnosis of (1) a thoracic aortic pathologic condition, including suspected aneurysms; (2) mitral valve disease; (3) suspected endocarditis; (4) congenital heart disease, for example, atrial septal defect; (5) left atrial intracardiac thrombi; and (6) cardiac tumors. It also is used to assess cardiac function during minimally invasive cardiac surgery (MICS) and to assess prosthetic valves.

BASICS THE NURSE NEEDS TO KNOW

A transesophageal echocardiogram is an invasive procedure that uses ultrasound techniques to detect enlargement of cardiac chambers and variations in chamber size during the cardiac cycle. It also assesses valvular function, septal defects, and pericardial effusion. Although these functions can be accomplished with a transthoracic echocardiogram, transesophageal echocardiography permits a better view of the posterior atrium and aorta. Transesophageal echocardiography also is indicated when a transthoracic approach is inadequate, such as when the patient is obese or has chest wall structure abnormalities.

REFERENCE VALUES   No anatomic *or* functional abnormalities

HOW THE TEST IS DONE

Transesophageal echocardiography is similar to transthoracic echocardiography (see pp. 270), except that the ultrasound probe is fitted into the end of a flexible gastroscopy tube and advanced down the esophagus behind the heart.

SIGNIFICANCE OF TEST RESULTS

Abnormal Values
Abnormal heart valves
Aneurysm
Cardiomyopathy
Congenital heart disorders
Congestive heart failure
Idiopathic hypertrophic subaortic stenosis
Mural thrombi
Myocardial infarction
Pericardial effusion
Restrictive pericarditis
Tumor of the heart

INTERFERING FACTORS

- Transesophageal echocardiography should not be performed if the patient has a history of irradiation of the mediastinum, esophageal dysphagia, or structural abnormalities

T

NURSING CARE

Pretest

- Ensure that a signed informed consent has been obtained.
- The nurse questions the patient about any disorder of the esophagus, stomach, throat, or vocal cords. The nurse also inquires if the patient has dentures, bridges, or plates.
- The nurse reports to the physician any history of arthritis of the neck, respiratory problems, or anticoagulation therapy.
- Maintain the patient on a nothing-by-mouth status for 6 to 8 hours.
- The nurse describes the procedure to the patient, especially the need for a mouthguard, positioning, and the need to swallow when asked.
- If the patient has prosthetic heart valves, the nurse administers prophylactic antibiotics, as prescribed.
- Report any indications of infection in the mouth or throat.
- The nurse administers antianxiety medication, as prescribed.

During the Test

- Administer medication to decrease secretions, as ordered.
- Place patient on a cardiac monitor.
- A topical anesthetic is sprayed into the throat to prevent gagging.
- The nurse instructs the patient to gargle with viscous lidocaine and then to swallow it. Warn the patient that it will make the tongue and throat feel "swollen."
- A mouthguard is placed to prevent the patient from biting down on the endoscope.
- The patient is positioned on the left side in the chin-chest position. The head may be supported with a small pillow.
- The probe is lubricated with lidocaine jelly and the physician slowly inserts it as the patient swallows.
- Have a Yankauer device available for suctioning.
- The nurse monitors the patient for a vasovagal response from the medication given to dry up secretions. The patient also is assessed for gagging. The nurse observes the oximeter for oxygen saturation readings.

Posttest

- Assess the patient for return of the gag reflex before resuming oral intake.
- The nurse instructs the patient to avoid hot liquids or foods for 2 hours.
- If in an outpatient setting, the nurse ensures the patient is accompanied home by another person.
- Give lozenges for relief of throat discomfort.

◇ **Nursing Response to Complications**

Transesophageal echocardiography has several complications that are related to the placement of the probe in the esophagus, including esophageal perforation, transient hypoxia, dysrhythmias, and a vasovagal response.

Esophageal perforation. An esophageal perforation will be evident during the procedure. Bleeding and pain will occur. The nurse will assist the physician as directed.

Transient hypoxia. Transient hypoxia may be noted with the insertion of the ultrasound probe. The nurse maintains the patient on a pulse oximeter and administers oxygen as ordered.

Dysrhythmias. During the procedure the patient is kept on a cardiac monitor. The nurse needs to monitor for dysrhythmias and response to possible lethal dysrhythmias. Dysrhythmias may also occur because of a vasovagal response (stimulation of the vagus nerve causes lowering of the heart rate). Notify the physician and anticipate treatment based on established protocols.

Transferrin and Transferrin Saturation

See Iron Studies on pp. 400-406.

Transthoracic Needle Biopsy

See Biopsy of the Lung, Percutaneous, Needle on pp. 127.

Triglycerides, Serum

See Lipid Profile on pp. 417.

Triiodothyronine

Also called: T_3; T_3 Total; Total T_3

SPECIMEN OR TYPE OF TEST: Serum

PURPOSE OF THE TEST

Triiodothyronine levels are obtained as part of the diagnostic process to determine hyperthyroidism or hypothyroidism and to diagnose triiodothyronine toxicosis.

BASICS THE NURSE NEEDS TO KNOW

The thyroid gland produces and secretes the hormones thyroxine and triiodothyronine. This gland takes up iodine from the extracellular fluid and uses the iodine to produce thyroglobulin, the precursor of all thyroid hormones. The thyroglobulin is stored in the thyroid gland until thyroxine and triiodothyronine are processed before secretion from the gland. Secretion of triiodothyronine and thyroxine is primarily regulated by a negative feedback mechanism with thyrotropin (see Figure 92). Thyrotropin is secreted by the anterior pituitary gland.

Once secreted by the thyroid gland, triiodothyronine and thyroxine are bound primarily to thyroid-binding globulin and, to a lesser degree, to albumin and prealbumin. The small amount of the hormones not bound to protein is called *free thyroxine* and *free triiodothyronine*. It is the free hormones that are biologically active. The bound hormones are released from the protein as the hormones are needed. In the peripheral circulation, thyroxine will lose one of its iodine molecules and become triiodothyronine, the more potent of the thyroid hormones.

Because the majority of the thyroid hormones are bound to protein, the evaluation of thyroid hormone levels should include the person's protein levels. If the patient has decreased proteins to carry the hormone, a greater amount of the hormone will be in the free state or active form.

Low T_3 levels are common in severe illness, especially in the elderly. This is called euthyroid syndrome or nonthyroidal illness syndrome.

T

REFERENCE VALUES*   Newborn: 100-740 ng/dL *or* SI: 1.5-11.4 nmol/L
Children:
    1-12 months: 105-245 ng/dL *or* SI: 1.6-3.7 nmol/L
    1-10 years: 105-269 ng/dL *or* SI: 1.6-4.1 nmol/L
    10-20 years: 80-213 ng/dL *or* SI: 1.2-3.3 nmol/L
Adult: 40-204 ng/dL *or* SI: 0.6-3.1 nmol/L

*Range varies among different laboratories.

HOW THE TEST IS DONE

Venipuncture is performed. In infants and small children, a heelstick may be done.

SIGNIFICANCE OF TEST RESULTS

Elevated Values
Hyperthyroidism
Pregnancy
Toxic adenoma of the thyroid gland
Toxic nodular goiter

Decreased Values
Hypothyroidism
Liver disease
Recent surgery
Renal disease
Sick euthyroid syndrome

INTERFERING FACTORS

- Significant increase or decrease in thyroxine-binding globulins
- Medications such as estrogen, heparin, iodides, triiodothyronine replacement therapy, lithium, methadone, methimazole, methylthiouracil, phenylbutazone, phenytoin, progestins, propranolol, propylthiouracil, reserpine, salicylates, steroids, and sulfonamides

| NURSING CARE

Nursing actions are similar to those for other venipuncture procedures, as presented in Chapter 2.

Pretest
- Check if any medications are to be held.
- Assess for liver disease and pregnancy, which causes elevation in the hormone.

Troponin, Serum

See Cardiac Markers on pp. 175.

Type and Crossmatch

Also called: Blood Compatibility Testing

SPECIMEN OR TYPE OF TEST: Blood

PURPOSE OF THE TEST

In preparation for transfusion, testing is performed to determine the major blood groups, to screen for antibodies, and to determine the compatibility of the blood of the recipient and that of the potential donor.

BASICS THE NURSE NEEDS TO KNOW

Human blood is typed by group, based on the presence or absence of A, B, AB, O, and Rh antigens. Blood group A has A antigens on the erythrocytes and anti-B antibodies in the serum. Blood group B has B antigens on the erythrocytes and anti-A antibodies in the serum. Blood group AB (universal receiver) has a double set of antigens on the erythrocytes and no antibodies in the serum, whereas blood group O (universal donor) has no antigens on the erythrocytes and a double set of antibodies in the serum (Table 15). When Rh antigens also are present on the erythrocytes, the person is classified as Rh positive. With no Rh antigens on the erythrocytes, the person is classified as Rh negative.

In preparation for blood transfusion, the intended recipient's blood is tested for ABO/Rh$_O$(D) type and red cell antibody screening. If antibodies are detected, additional testing is done to identify the antibodies. In the crossmatch part of the test, the donor's blood type is determined and the blood is screened to identify antibodies. In selecting a donor's blood that matches that of the recipient, a compatibility of antigens and antibodies must exist so that the transfusion is safe for the recipient. Incompatibility results in agglutination (clumping) and hemolysis of the erythrocytes. Incompatible donor blood must not be administered to the recipient.

The process of typing and crossmatching the blood determines a probable ABO compatibility between the blood of the donor and that of the recipient. A specialized computer software system is used to determine that the donor and recipient bloods are ABO compatible. Despite careful work, some incidence of transfusion reaction occurs. The process of typing and crossmatching cannot detect all possible antibodies, nor can it detect reactions to components other than erythrocytes. Most cases of severe transfusion reaction, however, are a result of clerical error, including administration of the wrong unit of blood to the patient or identification of the wrong patient. Complications of a severe transfusion reaction include a shortened life span or hemolysis of the erythrocytes. The patient who has a severe reaction develops anaphylaxis and rapid death may occur.

TABLE 15	Erythrocyte Antigens and Antibodies: ABO System	
Blood Group	**Erythrocyte Antigens**	**Serum Antibodies**
A	A	Anti-B
B	B	Anti-A
AB	AB	None
O	None	Anti-A, anti-B

T

REFERENCE VALUES Not applicable

HOW THE TEST IS DONE

Intended recipient's blood: Venipuncture is used to obtain a specimen of blood. When transfusion is planned, the blood must be collected within 3 days before the transfusion is administered.

SIGNIFICANCE OF TEST RESULTS

Positive Crossmatch

Incompatibility between the donor's blood and the recipient's blood

Negative Crossmatch

Probable compatibility between the donor's blood and the recipient's blood
The donor unit of blood is considered safe for transfusion to the recipient

INTERFERING FACTORS

- Hemolysis
- Improper identification procedure

NURSING CARE

Nursing measures include care of the venipuncture or capillary puncture site as described in Chapter 2, with the following additional measures.

Pretest

- Ask the intended recipient about a history of blood transfusion in the past 3 months because antibodies from a previous transfusion may be present. Additional laboratory testing is needed when the antibody screen is positive.

During the Test

Every hospital or facility that performs blood transfusions must have a written complete protocol for identification. Every staff member involved in obtaining the recipient's blood specimen, the type and crossmatch testing, and the administration of the transfusion must follow the identification protocol, exactly as written. An example of this protocol is described as follows:

- When blood is to be drawn, the intended recipient must be identified with absolute certainty by the person who draws the blood using the following steps: the intended recipient states his or her name, and the hospital wristband is compared with the verbal identification.
- A transfusion wristband is also applied to the recipient's wrist. This wristband contains the recipient's name and hospital identification number and the date and initials of the phlebotomist. The specimen tubes and the requisition form also are labeled with the same identification information.
- The requisition form is signed by the phlebotomist, indicating that all identification information has been verified on the two wristbands and by the intended recipient.

Posttest

- Once the type and crossmatch is completed, the donor blood units are available for the recipient. Donor blood that has been crossmatched is usually held for no more than 24 hours.
- The same careful identification procedure is used when the blood is to be administered. The consequences of an error in identification are profound. When identification error occurs, it can result in the death of the patient.

Ultrasound

Also called: Sonogram

SPECIMEN OR TYPE OF TEST: Sound Wave Imaging

PURPOSE OF THE TEST

Ultrasound examines organs, blood vessels, and structures of the body to identify malposition, malformation, malfunction, or the presence of a foreign body. It also may be used as a visual guide for accurate placement of a needle in a biopsy or aspiration procedure. In pregnancy ultrasound, the test is used to determine the age of the fetus and gestation of the pregnancy, as well as to assess for possible congenital or genetic malformation.

BASICS THE NURSE NEEDS TO KNOW

Ultrasound is a scanning procedure that transmits sound waves in a directed path through the skin and into body tissues. The sound waves quickly bounce back or "echo" when they encounter a solid structure or tissue of different density (Figure 94). The sound waves are converted to a visual image that can be analyzed for abnormality.

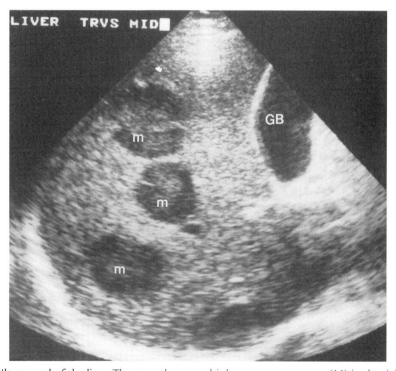

Figure 94. Ultrasound of the liver. The scan shows multiple cancer metastases (M) in the right lobe of the liver. In the ultrasound image, the gallbladder (GB) is seen along the upper right border of the liver. In this patient, the primary site of the cancer was in the colon. (From Frank ED, Long BW, Smith BJ: *Merrill's atlas of radiographic positioning and procedures*, ed 11, St Louis, 2007, Mosby.)

U

The ultrasound pulsations transmit through fluid and body tissue, but do not transmit through air, bone, or barium. When the sound wave signals pass through tissues of varying densities, the most common images are in varying shades of white, gray, and black that correspond to the tissue size, shape, structure, and density.

Doppler ultrasound is a different method of ultrasound. It detects the presence, direction, speed, and character of arterial or venous blood flow within the vascular lumen. The Doppler pulses echo off the moving erythrocytes in the blood in patterns that correlate with the flow of the blood. The echoes are converted to an audio signal, a linear graphic reading, or color images that demonstrate the flow of blood in a designated area of an artery or vein. The audio signal changes according to the character of the blood flow. The blood flow may be characterized as normal; disturbed, as at the bifurcation of a blood vessel; or turbulent, as encountered beyond the point of a partial obstruction. Severely obstructed circulation produces a weak signal or silence. This type of ultrasound is very helpful in assessing the circulation in a vascular graft after bypass or transplant surgery has been performed (see also Ultrasound, Doppler, Vascular, pp. 597-601).

Transducer

The transducer, in the form of a scan head or probe, is the instrument used to generate and transmit the ultrasound energy and then receive the echo sound waves that bounce back from the tissue within. The returning sound waves are converted to audio signals or visual images. When the transducer is used externally, the scan head is moved over the skin in defined patterns, according to the anatomic location of the target tissue and the viewing plane that is desired. Other transducers are specialized probes used within the body. These probes can be used in the esophagus, vagina, rectum, or lumen of a blood vessel. The internal application is useful because the sound waves are placed near the particular organ or tissue. The procedure reduces or eliminates the interference of other tissues and of the air of the lungs or bowel.

Many different ultrasound scans are used to examine organs, tissues, lymph nodes, and the vascular circulation. The more common scans are listed in Box 10.

Abdominal Ultrasound

Ultrasound is a major diagnostic tool for the examination of the liver, hepatobiliary tract, spleen, and pancreas. In the liver, it can detect a cyst, abscess, hematoma, primary neoplasm, and metastatic tumor. It is the best diagnostic tool to detect gallstones (Figure 95). It also may

BOX 10 Ultrasound Procedures	
Popliteal artery scan	Pelvic scans
Inferior vena cava scan	Female pelvic scan
Abdominal aorta scan	Obstetric scan
Carotid artery scan	Endovaginal scan
Abdominal scan	Male pelvic scan
Liver scan	Thyroid scan
Gallbladder, biliary tract scan	Scrotum scan
Pancreas scan	Breast scan
Renal scan	Transesophageal echocardiography
Spleen scan	Echocardiography

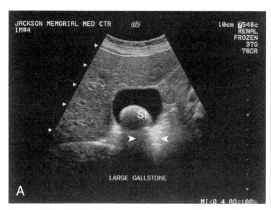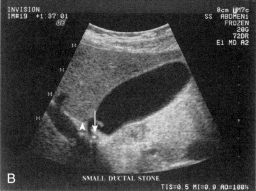

Figure 95. Gallbladder ultrasound. **A,** A large gallstone (ST) within the gall bladder; **B,** A distended gallbladder because of a small gallstone *(long arrow)* lodged in the distal cystic duct *(short arrowhead)*. (From Frank ED, Long BW, Smith BJ: *Merrill's atlas of radiographic positioning and procedures,* ed 11, St Louis, 2007, Mosby.)

show thickening of the gallbladder walls associated with acute cholecystitis or dilation of the biliary tract associated with obstruction. An enlarged or edematous pancreas is measurable by ultrasound. Pancreatic abscesses, pseudocysts, and pancreatic tumors are readily identified. Ultrasound identifies a congenital absence of the spleen or the existence of multiple spleens. It can also identify the presence and size of space-occupying lesions, such as cysts or tumors, and is accurate in the measurement of the size of the spleen.

Cardiac Ultrasound

Two cardiac ultrasound procedures are covered separately in detail in this text: Transesophageal Echocardiography (pp. 587-590) and Echocardiogram (pp. 270-271).

Renal Ultrasound

Renal ultrasound clearly defines the kidneys, including their size, shape, position, collecting systems, and surrounding tissues. Renal masses that are greater than 2 cm are readily detected, and renal cysts are a frequent finding. Ultrasound can identify the location and severity of obstruction. Renal ultrasound may be used as a guide for needle placement in renal biopsy, for drainage of a renal abscess, or for placement of a nephrostomy tube.

Pelvic Ultrasound

In the diagnosis of gynecologic problems in the female, one use of ultrasound is to identify an ovarian malignancy at an early stage. In the case of abnormal uterine bleeding, ultrasound will identify submucous leiomyomas and evaluate the thickness of the uterine wall. Pelvic ultrasound often precedes any invasive gynecologic diagnostic test, such as dilation and curettage. The procedure may also be used to monitor ovulation in the diagnosis and treatment of infertility and in follow-up after treatment for pelvic inflammatory disease. For the female, the examination consists of imaging from both transabdominal and transvaginal approaches to obtain complete visualization.

Ultrasonography in the male is used to assess the texture, size, and condition of the prostate gland, prostatic urethra, seminal vesicles, vas deferens, and testes. It is also used to guide the

U

placement of the needle during biopsy of the prostate gland. Ultrasound is part of the diagnostic workup to detect and stage prostate cancer.

Pregnancy Ultrasound

In conditions related to pregnancy, ultrasound identifies an early ectopic pregnancy, a multiple pregnancy, possible fetal abnormality, and assessment of fetal growth (see also Genetic Sonogram, pp. 328-331). It is also used to guide aspiration procedures including amniocentesis, cordocentesis, periumbilical cord sampling, and the aspiration of multiple oocytes for in vitro fertilization.

Thyroid Ultrasound

An ultrasound of the thyroid gland is usually done to investigate *goiter* (enlargement of the thyroid gland), a palpable nodule or cyst, and to identify tumors. The patient lies flat with a rolled towel under the posterior neck, which causes hyperextension of the neck

REFERENCE VALUES   No anatomic or functional abnormalities exist. The organs are normal in size, shape, contour, and position. The internal structures of the organs and nearby tissues are within normal limits.

HOW THE TEST IS DONE

High-frequency sound waves from the transducer are directed into an area of the body in a specific pattern. The echoes of the ultrasound are converted to visual images, linear tracings, or audible sounds.

SIGNIFICANCE OF TEST RESULTS

Abnormal Values

Cyst
Tumor
Hypertrophy
Obstruction or stricture
Calculus
Aneurysm
Foreign body
Vascular occlusion
Venous thrombosis
Atherosclerotic plaque
Abscess
Congenital anomaly
Hematoma, bleeding
Pregnancy, fetal development

INTERFERING FACTORS

- Air
- Overlying bones
- Bowel gas
- Barium
- Obesity

NURSING CARE

Pretest

- Obtain the patient's signed consent, particularly for any ultrasound procedure that involves insertion of a transducer into a body cavity or blood vessel.
- The nurse schedules the ultrasound examination before or several days after any barium studies. Barium is an opaque substance that would block the transmission of ultrasound impulses. Residual barium causes an ultrasound problem for about 24 hours after a barium x-ray examination.

○ *Patient Teaching.* The nurse or ultrasound technician instructs the patient about any dietary restrictions or modifications. Any abdominal ultrasound examination requires fasting from food for 12 hours. If the patient has a tendency toward bowel gas, a low-residue diet is implemented for 24 to 36 hours, followed by a 12-hour fast from all foods. Some abdominal ultrasound protocols require an enema before the examination because intestinal gas and feces must be removed from the colon. Gynecologic ultrasound procedures often require drinking 40 oz of water without voiding before the test. This fills the urinary bladder and moves it upward and away from the uterus.

- The nurse also reassures the patient that the examination is safe and painless. To alleviate anxiety, the examiner provides reassurance before and during the test.
- A small child or an agitated, anxious adult patient may be accompanied by a calming parent or other adult.

During the Test

- Inform the patient to remove all clothes, jewelry, and metallic objects. A hospital gown is worn. The patient is positioned on the examining table and is instructed to remain still during the examination. Neonates and infants are kept warm during the examination. The dark room, a pacifier, and gentle touch help keep the infant calm.
- The examiner applies the acoustic gel to the skin surface in the area to be examined. The gel serves as a conducting agent and eliminates the thin layer of air that would cause a barrier to the transmission of impulses. As the sound waves are transmitted, the image appears on a video screen.

Posttest

- Remove the acoustic gel from the skin. This prevents soiling of the patient's clothes.

Ultrasound, Doppler, Vascular

Also called: Doppler Flow Studies

SPECIMEN OR TYPE OF TEST: Ultrasound

PURPOSE OF THE TEST

In vascular studies, Doppler ultrasound detects stenosis or occlusion in an artery (Figure 96) or vein, assists with the diagnosis of peripheral vascular or cerebrovascular disease, evaluates the results of arterial reconstruction or vascular bypass surgery, and assesses for possible trauma to an artery.

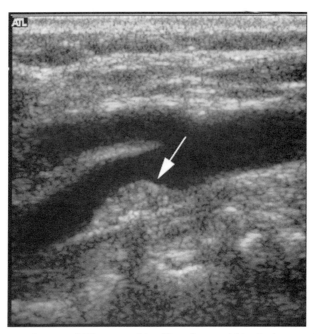

Figure 96. Carotid artery ultrasound. The arrow identifies plaque within the lumen of the internal carotid artery. The lumen is partially occluded. (From Rumack C, Wilson SR, Charboneau JW: *Diagnostic ultrasound,* ed 3, St Louis, 2005, Mosby.)

BASICS THE NURSE NEEDS TO KNOW

The Doppler ultrasound transducer transmits low-intensity sound waves that are directed at a specific blood vessel. The transmitted sound waves strike moving red blood cells and bounce back to the transducer-receiver. The received impulses are translated into an audible signal, a visual image, or a waveform recording. Additionally, the systolic pressure in the upper and lower extremities can be measured.

Using the *audible signal,* changes in the pitch and volume of the blood flow can be heard. When the blood flow is normal, the sound is loud and of higher pitch. Conversely, when blood flow is constricted or partially obstructed, the sound is softer or fainter and the pitch is low. Total obstruction in a blood vessel produces no sound at all.

Waveform recordings are used to evaluate the circulation in lower extremities. The waveform recordings are Doppler signals that are transformed into a linear image. The waveforms are recorded on a graph paper and appear on the monitor (Figure 97). In abnormal venous flow, as in partial or total venous occlusion, the augmentation signal of an upward spike is absent. Reflux flow, such as that caused by incompetent venous valves, is also evident on the waveform. The normal arterial waveform is characterized by three phases called the systolic, diastolic, and wall rebound phases. When the artery is stenosed, the waveform pattern diminishes in height. In severe obstruction, the diastolic phase and wall rebound phase are absent.

Color-flow Doppler imaging demonstrates the change in blood flow in various colors. Blood flow that moves toward the transducer is imaged as a shade of red. Blood flow that moves away from the transducer is imaged as a shade of blue. When blood flow within the artery or vein is

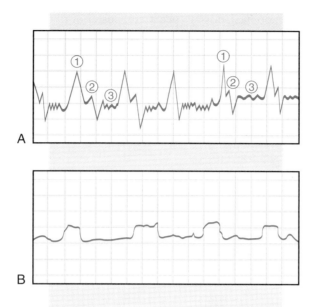

Figure 97. Normal versus abnormal Doppler arterial waveform patterns. A, Normal waveform with triphasic pattern of sharp upstroke and downstroke and good amplitude. *1*, systolic component; *2*, diastolic component; and *3*, elastic wall rebound. B, Abnormal waveform pattern with monophasic pattern of low amplitude and flat waves. This pattern indicates severe arterial obstruction.

normal, the color is intense, and the lumen of the blood vessel should be filled with color. With obstruction of the blood flow, such as with deep vein thrombosis, the color fades from red to orange or yellow or from blue to aqua or white. This method may be used to assess cranial neck vessels and is also used to assess the abdominal aorta and the peripheral vascular system. The technique can detect an embolus, stenosis, a thrombus, an aneurysm, and venous insufficiency.

REFERENCE VALUES   **Arterial or venous examination:** Normal frequency and volume of audio signal, normal waveform pattern, and normal color for blood flow velocity. There is no evidence of vascular stenosis or obstruction from a thrombus or embolus.

HOW THE TEST IS DONE

Venous and Arterial Doppler Tests

Acoustic gel and the Doppler probe are placed on the skin at the desired vascular sites. Audible signals are heard and interpreted. Three to five waveforms are recorded at each vascular site. The specific vascular sites and sides of the body (right or left) are identified to avoid confusion and error.

Venous sites of the lower extremities are the posterior tibial, greater saphenous, common femoral, superficial femoral, and popliteal veins. Venous sites of the upper extremities and neck are the brachial, axillary, subclavian, and jugular veins. Arterial pulse sites of the lower extremities are the common femoral, popliteal, dorsalis pedis, and posterior tibial pulses. Arterial pulse sites in the upper extremities and neck are the brachial, radial, ulnar, and carotid pulses.

Segmented Pressures

Blood pressure cuffs are applied to both upper thighs, above and below the knees, and above the ankles. Gel is applied to the skin. The pressure cuffs are inflated one at a time. On deflation of each, the Doppler probe identifies the systolic pressure by audio signal, and the numeric value is recorded. The ABI is calculated from the ankle and brachial pressures.

SIGNIFICANCE OF TEST RESULTS

Abnormal Values

Arterial stenosis or occlusion
Venous thrombosis
Incompetent venous valves
Atherosclerotic plaque

INTERFERING FACTORS

- Nicotine, alcohol, and caffeine
- Anxiety
- Uncooperative patient behavior

NURSING CARE

Pretest

- After the physician has informed the patient about the test, obtain a written consent from the patient.
- ○ *Patient Teaching.* The nurse instructs the patient to avoid nicotine, alcohol, caffeine, and other stimulants and depressants that will cause vasoconstriction. To help control the patient's anxiety, the nurse reassures the patient that the test is painless.
- In most cases, vascular testing will be done in a radiology setting or a vascular laboratory. The room lighting should be reduced to promote relaxation. The patient will put on a hospital gown. For arterial tests, the patient is in the supine position. For venous tests of the lower extremities, the patient is placed in the supine position with two pillows under the legs to elevate them above the heart. The leg and hip are externally rotated, and the knee is flexed (Figure 98).

During the Test

- The procedure is to locate the pulse points on the upper or lower extremities and apply acoustic gel. At each pulse point, apply the transducer head to the skin and listen to the blowing sounds produced by the audio mode of the Doppler instrument.

Posttest

- Remove the acoustic gel from the skin. Record the findings in the patient's record.
- At the bedside, the nurse may perform ongoing audio Doppler assessments of pulses, particularly on the patient who has lower limb ischemia and pulses that are too faint to be palpated. The assessments may also be done to check the distal blood flow after a vascular graft or bypass graft is in place.

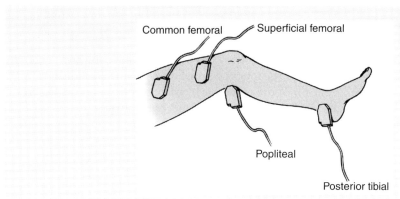

Figure 98. Doppler ultrasound of venous circulation in the legs. The patient is supine with the head of the bed slightly elevated. The Doppler transducer is placed over locations on the various veins where the circulation can be detected ultrasonically. (From Pfenninger JL, Fowler GC: *Pfenninger and Fowler's procedures for primary care*, ed 3, St Louis, 2011, Mosby.)

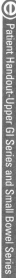

Upper Gastrointestinal Series

Also called: Upper GI Series
Includes: Esophagography, Small Bowel Series

SPECIMEN OR TYPE OF TEST: Radiography

PURPOSE OF THE TEST

The upper GI series detects disorders of structure or function of the esophagus, stomach, and duodenum. One week postoperatively, it is used to evaluate the results of gastric surgery. As an extension of the upper GI series, the small bowel series detects disorders of the jejunum and ileum.

BASICS THE NURSE NEEDS TO KNOW

The upper GI series involves a radiologic examination from the oral part of the pharynx to the duodenojejunal junction. When the small bowel requires examination, the small bowel series often follows the upper GI series directly, but it can be performed as a single procedure. The common sources of abnormality in the upper GI tract are stricture, inflammation, swelling, ulcers, tumors, motility disorders, or structural changes in the wall of the intestine.

The barium liquid is a radiopaque contrast medium that outlines the size, shape, and contour of the intestinal lumen. Air may be instilled to provide double contrast and better visualization of the lumen of the esophagus, stomach, and duodenum. Fluoroscopy and x-ray films are used at intermittent intervals to obtain the gastrointestinal images.

REFERENCE VALUES   No structural or functional abnormalities are found.

U

HOW THE TEST IS DONE

Upper Gastrointestinal Series

The patient drinks a barium solution to provide contrast views during swallowing and peristaltic action in the esophagus. As the barium coats the mucosal lining of the stomach, additional films are taken to outline the shape and contour of the organ. The patient's positional changes (vertical, supine, prone, and lateral) help coat the mucosa throughout the stomach. With positional changes, the barium will flow into an ulcer and fill the crater (Figure 99).

Small Bowel Series

When a small bowel series is included in this radiologic study, the transit time of the barium can be from 30 minutes to 6 hours before it reaches the colon. At the start of the small bowel series, additional barium is taken orally. The transit time can be shortened by having the patient drink 200 mL of iced water or eat a light meal after all the additional barium has left the stomach. Fluoroscopic views are taken three times in the first hour and every 30 minutes thereafter. Radiographic films are taken of any abnormality.

Enteroclysis Method

When the small bowel series is performed separately, enteroclysis may be used to instill the barium. A radiopaque catheter is passed through the nose or mouth and advanced past the pylorus and into the duodenum. Barium, followed by methylcellulose solution, is instilled by

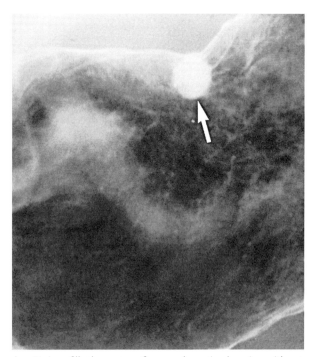

Figure 99. Upper GI series. Barium fills the crater of a round peptic ulcer *(arrow)* located near the lesser curvature of the stomach. (From Gore RM, Levine MS: *Textbook of gastrointestinal radiology,* ed 3, Philadelphia, 2008, Saunders.)

U

the catheter route directly into the small bowel. Views of the total small bowel can be completed in 20 to 30 minutes.

SIGNIFICANCE OF TEST RESULTS

Abnormal Values

Esophagus
Reflux esophagitis
Esophageal scarring or stricture
Barrett's esophagus
Infectious esophagitis

Stomach-Duodenum
Peptic ulcer (gastric, duodenal)
Cancer (stomach, duodenum)
Pyloric obstruction
Benign tumor
Gastric inflammatory disease
Perforation
Diverticula

Small Bowel
Malabsorption
Crohn's disease
Chronic appendicitis
Stricture
Hodgkin's disease
Cancer
Diffuse sclerosis
Surgical resection
Congenital abnormality
Intussusception
Perforation

INTERFERING FACTORS

- Failure to maintain nothing-by-mouth status
- Excess air in the small bowel

NURSING CARE

Pretest
- After the physician explains the test to the patient, a patient consent form must be signed. The nurse ensures that the signed form is entered into the patient's record.
- *Patient Teaching.* The nurse instructs the patient to fast from all food for 8 hours and all liquids for 4 hours before the test. In addition, most oral medications are withheld in the 8 hours before the test. Narcotics and anticholinergics are withheld for 24 hours before the test because they slow the motility of the intestinal tract.

Continued

| **NURSING CARE—cont'd**

During the Test
- The hospitalized patient may return to the nursing unit for an interval before the small bowel filming begins. The nurse obtains instructions from the radiology department about the nothing-by-mouth status or about a prescribed meal.

Posttest
- A laxative is given to the patient to help evacuate the barium promptly. Retained barium can cause constipation, obstruction, or fecal impaction.

○ *Patient Teaching.* The nurse informs the patient that the feces will be gray or whitish for 24 to 72 hours until all barium has been evacuated. The patient is advised to rest for the remainder of the day because the test is tiring.

Urea Nitrogen, Blood

Also called: BUN; Blood Urea Nitrogen

SPECIMEN OR TYPE OF TEST: Serum

PURPOSE OF THE TEST

The blood urea nitrogen (BUN) level is used to evaluate renal function. With the serum creatinine level, it is used to monitor patients in renal failure or the patients receiving dialysis therapy. Increasingly, BUN is being used as a marker to assess renal response to heart failure.

BASICS THE NURSE NEEDS TO KNOW

BUN is the major nitrogenous end product of protein and amino acid catabolism. It is produced in the liver and distributed throughout intracellular and extracellular fluid. Urea nitrogen is excreted from the body primarily by the kidneys; lesser amounts are excreted in sweat or degraded by intestinal bacteria.

In the kidneys, almost all urea is filtered out of the blood by glomerular function. Some urea is resorbed with water in the renal tubules, but most is removed from the body in urine. The amount of urea excreted is dependent on the state of hydration and renal perfusion. If the patient is dehydrated, low tubular flow of urinary filtrate occurs, and more urea is absorbed. If overhydration and a high tubular flow rate exist, less urea is resorbed, resulting in a lower serum level.

Urea nitrogen level can rise from renal and nonrenal factors. Nonrenal factors include increased urea production associated with increased dietary protein intake and increased catabolism, such as occurs with corticosteroid therapy or muscle-wasting diseases. When excess urea is produced, the serum level rarely rises above 40 mg/dL (SI: >14.2 mmol/L). Some medications will cause a slight increase in the BUN level.

Renal causes of an elevated BUN level may result from prerenal, intrarenal, or postrenal problems. Prerenal disease includes poor renal blood flow, as in shock or renal artery stenosis with a resulting decrease in the glomerular filtration rate. Intrarenal disease includes damage to the renal parenchyma. Renal causes of azotemia result in a dramatic rise in the BUN level. Postrenal problems are related to obstruction in the kidney or in the urinary tract.

U

REFERENCE VALUES

Infant (birth-1 year): 4-19 mg/dL *or* SI: 1.4-6.8 mmol/L
Child to adult (1-60 years): 5-20 mg/dL *or* SI: 1.8-7.1 mmol/L
Older adult (>60 years): 8-23 mg/dL *or* SI: 2.9-8.2 mmol/L

▽ Critical Value

100 mg/dL *or* higher (SI: 35.7 mmol/L or higher)

HOW THE TEST IS DONE

Venipuncture is used to obtain a specimen of blood.

SIGNIFICANCE OF TEST RESULTS

Elevated Values

Acute or chronic renal failure
Shock
Renal artery stenosis
Hemorrhage
Postrenal syndrome
Stress
Congestive heart failure
Burns
Increased protein intake
Dehydration
Hyperalimentation
Ketoacidosis
Long-term steroid therapy
Diabetes mellitus

Decreased Values

• Overhydration
• Starvation
• Intravenous therapy
• Low-protein diet
• Acromegaly
• Severe liver damage

INTERFERING FACTORS

• None

NURSING CARE

Care of the patient is similar to that for other venipunctures, as described in Chapter 2.
▽ **Nursing Response to Critical Values**
Any BUN over 100 is extremely elevated and defines the condition of uremia and the nurse must notify the physician of the test result. The patient will be stuporous or comatose. Usually, renal failure is identified at much lower levels. A patient with values at this level needs dialysis to remove the waste products of metabolism.

U

Uric Acid

SPECIMEN OR TYPE OF TEST: Serum

PURPOSE OF THE TEST

The elevated level of uric acid is used to confirm the diagnosis of gout and helps detect renal impairment that causes prerenal azotemia and renal failure.

BASICS THE NURSE NEEDS TO KNOW

Uric acid is the end product of protein metabolism and is excreted from the body by the kidneys and intestinal tract. The production of uric acid comes from a combination of dietary intake of protein and purine foods, purine biosynthesis, and catabolism of body tissues. The normal excretion of uric acid by the kidneys should eliminate two thirds of the uric acid from the blood daily. The remaining one third is in the bile and intestinal secretions. The level of uric acid in the blood is maintained by a balance between the amount that is produced and the amount that is excreted (Figure 100).

Elevated Values

Hyperuricemia is an elevated level of uric acid in the blood. It may occur from excessive production of uric acid but more frequently, it occurs because of impaired excretion. The conditions of abnormal overproduction include abnormal metabolism of purines and amino acids, excessive catabolism of body tissues, such as in cancer before and after chemotherapy or radiation, some hemolytic disorders, and conditions that cause acidosis or lactic acidosis. Impaired excretion or urate retention is usually a result of renal disease that affects tubular secretion and reabsorption. It may also be caused by reduced renal blood flow and decreased renal filtration of the blood. Hyperuricemia exists when the serum urate level is greater than 8.0 mg/dL (SI: >452 µmol/L).

Gout produces an elevated level of uric acid in the blood. The condition may be asymptomatic or may cause acute gouty arthritis, often affecting the metatarsal joint of the big toe (Figure 101). The condition can cause acute attacks of pain, redness, and swelling, with quiet periods in between acute episodes. The urate crystals can form tophi, or nodular deposits of urate crystals in the joints, cartilage, bones, bursae, and subcutaneous tissue. The urate crystals also can accumulate in the renal pelvis and cause uric acid kidney stones to form. Some patients develop gout with lower elevations of serum uric acid and some have high levels of serum uric acid and do not acquire this inflammatory disease.

Decreased Values

Hypouricemia is an abnormally low level of uric acid in the blood. It usually results from defects in renal tubular absorption. The disorder can be congenital or acquired, but an increased urinary loss of urate and, therefore, a low level of uric acid in the blood occurs.

REFERENCE VALUES	**Adult**
	Male: 3.4-8.0 mg/dL *or* SI: 202-476 µmol/L
	Female: 2.4-6.6 mg/dL *or* SI: 143-393 µmol/L

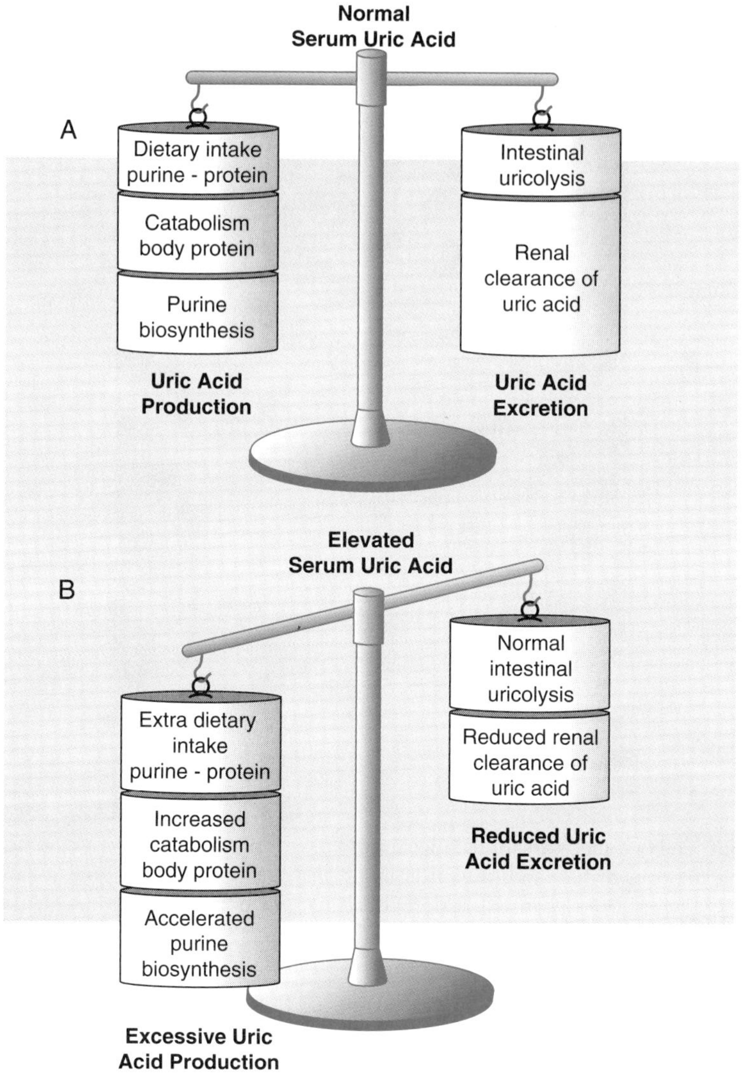

Figure 100. Uric acid production and excretion. **A,** Normal physiology. **B,** Pathophysiology of hyperuricemia.

HOW THE TEST IS DONE

Venipuncture is used to obtain a specimen of blood.

SIGNIFICANCE OF TEST RESULTS

Elevated Values

Gout

Renal failure

Polycystic kidney disease

Leukemia

U

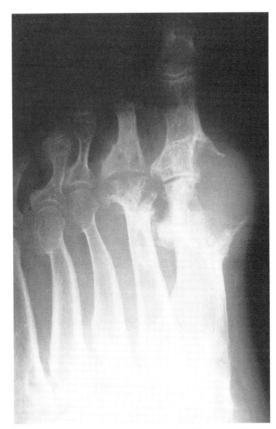

Figure 101. Gout. The first metatarsal-phalangeal joint of the big toe is the most commonly affected by gout. The chronic deposits of sodium urate result in a *tophus*, a painful foreign body inflammation. On a radiograph, this large tophus has caused erosion at the margins of the joints. (From Mettler FA: *Essentials of radiology*, ed 2, Philadelphia, 2005, Saunders.)

Tumor lysis during chemotherapy or radiation therapy
Lymphoma
Multiple myeloma
Hemolytic anemia
Lead toxicity
Polycythemia vera
Pernicious anemia
Acute alcohol ingestion

Decreased Values
Fanconi syndrome
Wilson's disease
Hodgkin's disease
Multiple myeloma
Bronchogenic carcinoma

INTERFERING FACTORS

- Starvation
- High purine diet
- Stress
- Alcohol ingestion

NURSING CARE

Nursing measures include care of the venipuncture site, as described in Chapter 2.

Pretest

- On the requisition form, list all medications taken by the patient. Many medications cause either a false-positive or a false-negative result.

○ *Patient Teaching.* Instruct the patient to discontinue all food and fluids for 8 hours. Alcohol also should be discontinued before the test, because it will elevate the uric acid blood level.

Posttest

○ *Patient Teaching.* When gout has been diagnosed, the nurse teaches the patient to drink adequate fluids daily. This will help flush urate crystals from the kidneys The patient is also instructed to reduce the intake of high purine foods, including liver, kidneys, sweetbreads, and legumes, because high purine foods increase the level of uric acid. The intake of alcohol should be avoided because alcohol will increase the production of uric acid and alter the excretion of urate from the kidneys.

- If the serum level rises to 12 mg/dL (SI: 714 μmol/L) or higher, urate crystals can accumulate in the renal tubules and ureters, resulting in obstruction and renal failure. This crisis can occur after administration of cytotoxic drugs, after a malignancy is irradiated, as a result of acute alcohol ingestion, or with adult respiratory distress syndrome. The nurse should notify the physician of this severe elevation that is a marker of cell injury crisis. Specific interventions will depend on the cause of the problem.

Uric Acid, Urine

SPECIMEN OR TYPE OF TEST: Urine

PURPOSE OF THE TEST

The urinary uric acid test measures the urinary excretion of uric acid in patients with renal calculi or in those at risk for the development of a calculus. The test also is used to assess the effect of enzyme deficiency or metabolic abnormality that results in the overproduction of uric acid.

BASICS THE NURSE NEEDS TO KNOW

As an end product of protein metabolism, uric acid and urate crystals are excreted by the kidneys and bowel. *Hyperuricosuria*, a high level of uric acid in the urine, may be caused by excess secretion or excess production of uric acid.

When leukemia is treated with cytotoxic drugs or when malignant tumors are irradiated, tumor necrosis and a metabolic breakdown of cellular material occur. This causes a massive amount of uric acid and urate crystal production that can result in elevation of the urine uric acid level. The urate crystals can block the renal tubules and ureters, resulting in renal failure.

U

REFERENCE VALUES   Average diet: 250-750 mg/24 hr *or* SI: 1.48-4.43 mmol/24 hr
Purine-free diet: <420 mg/24 hr *or* SI: <2.48 mmol/24 hr
High purine diet (adult): <1000 mg/24 hr *or* SI: <5.9 mmol/24 hr

HOW THE TEST IS DONE

A 24-hour urine collection is used to measure the amount of daily uric acid that is excreted. The laboratory will provide a collection container with sodium hydroxide, which keeps the pH of the urine in an alkaline state. This prevents precipitation of urate crystals.

SIGNIFICANCE OF TEST RESULTS

Elevated Values
Uric acid nephrolithiasis
Viral hepatitis
Gout
Leukemia
Lesch-Nyhan syndrome
Radiation therapy
Chemotherapy
Wilson's disease
Cystinosis
Sickle cell anemia
Polycythemia vera

Decreased Values
Glomerulonephritis
Lead toxicity
Folic acid deficiency
Renal failure

INTERFERING FACTORS

- Failure to collect all urine during the test period
- High- or low-purine diet
- Many medications (including aspirin, antiinflammatory drugs, diuretics, vitamin C, and x-ray contrast medium)

NURSING CARE

Nursing actions related to the timed urine collection procedure are presented in Chapter 2, with the following additional measures.
Pretest
- Instruct the patient to collect all urine of the 24-hour test period and store it in a large container. Ice or refrigeration is not required.

During the Test
- The nurse asks the patient to void at 8 AM. Discard the 8 AM specimen. All urine is collected for 24 hours thereafter, including the 8 AM specimen of the following morning.
- Ensure that the label and requisition slip contain the patient's complete identification and the time and date of the start and finish of the test.

Posttest
- List all medications taken by the patient on the requisition slip.
- Arrange for transport of the specimen to the laboratory on ice if required.

Urinalysis

Also called: UA

SPECIMEN OR TYPE OF TEST: Urine

PURPOSE OF THE TEST

Urinalysis is performed to screen for urinary tract disorders, kidney disorders, urinary neoplasm, and other medical conditions that produce changes in the urine. This test also is used to monitor the effects of treatment of known renal or urinary conditions.

BASICS THE NURSE NEEDS TO KNOW

Urinalysis produces a large amount of information about possible diseases of the kidneys and lower urinary tract, as well as systemic diseases that alter the composition of the urine. Analysis of the urine consists of two parts: the chemical analysis and the microscopic analysis. The chemical analysis is usually performed by the dipstick method (Figure 102). Microscopic analysis may

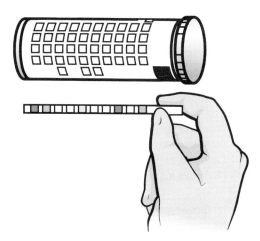

Figure 102. Urinalysis: Dipstick method of testing. A reagent strip is used for urine chemistry analysis, with a color chart to identify results. (See Box 11, p. 618 for the procedure).

U

be done routinely, but also is done in response to a specific request or as a follow-up to abnormal results of the chemical analysis.

Color and Clarity

There are many possible causes of changes of the color or clarity of urine, some of which are presented in Table 16. In addition, some medications and chemicals are responsible for changes in urine color.

Specific Gravity

The specific gravity is a measurement of the ability of the kidneys to concentrate and excrete the urine. Water has no urinary components and has a specific gravity of 1.000. Concentrated urine has a higher than normal specific gravity because the proportion of urinary components is greater. Diluted urine has a lower than normal specific gravity because it contains fewer components. A specific gravity of urine that remains fixed (unvarying over time) at the low value of 1.010 indicates severe renal damage. The cause is often due to renal tubules that cannot resorb water and effectively concentrate the urine.

pH

As part of the acid-base balance, the kidneys remove excess hydrogen ions from the blood and excrete them in the urine. In abnormal physiology, a urine pH greater than 6.5 indicates the presence of bicarbonate in the urine. Alkaline urine may occur because of systemic alkalosis (respiratory or metabolic) or because of a renal tubular disorder. If the renal tubules are damaged, metabolic acidosis and an inability to regulate acid-base balance will occur. A urinary pH less than 5.5 indicates the absence of bicarbonate ions in the urine. The cause of the problem

TABLE 16	Causes of Change in Urine Color and Clarity
Characteristic	Cause
Clarity	
Cloudy, smoky, hazy	Pyuria
	Bacteriuria
	Phosphates in the urine
Color	
Colorless	Overhydration
	Diuretic therapy
	Diabetes mellitus
	Diabetes insipidus
Dark red or pink	Acute intermittent porphyria
	Hematuria
	Ingestion of beets, berries, fava beans, red food coloring, rhubarb
Dark yellow or orange	Bile
Green	*Pseudomonas* bacteriuria
	Urinary bile pigments

may be systemic acidosis (respiratory or metabolic), with the excess hydrogen ions of the extracellular fluids spilling into the urine.

Protein

The presence of excess urinary albumin is an indicator of glomerular disease. The nephrotic syndrome produces a heavy loss of albumin in the urine. The renal loss also may be associated with systemic disease that causes glomerular damage.

Bilirubin

Bilirubinuria (bilirubin in the urine) is an abnormal finding that results from an increase in the serum conjugated (direct) bilirubin. The level of urine bilirubin rises in some conditions of hepatocellular jaundice and liver disease and in jaundice from conditions that result in biliary obstruction.

Glucose

Glycosuria (glucose in the urine) is usually an indicator of significant hyperglycemia and diabetes mellitus. When a fasting specimen is obtained, it is highly specific and accurate in the detection of glucose in the urine. The nonfasting random sample is much less specific.

Ketones

In children, *ketonuria* (ketones in the urine) can occur during febrile illness or as the result of severe diarrhea and vomiting.

In starvation or abnormal carbohydrate metabolism, large quantities of ketone bodies appear in the urine before the serum levels of ketones are elevated. Urinalysis is useful in monitoring known diabetics, particularly when the patient has an infection, hyperglycemia, or is pregnant.

Occult Blood

A positive result for occult blood in the urine occurs when intact erythrocytes, hemoglobin, or myoglobin are present. Hematuria is caused by diseases of the kidney or lower urinary tract or by a nonurinary problem of medical origin. When the occult blood test result is positive, a microscopic examination of the urine is performed to identify red blood cells (RBCs) and RBC casts. Additional laboratory or diagnostic tests are also indicated to diagnose and locate the cause of the bleeding.

Red Blood Cells

Normal urine may exhibit a few RBCs without any significant pathologic cause. The presence of a few cells is considered acceptable under high power field (HPF) microscopic visualization. Significant hematuria is indicated by one episode of gross hematuria or one episode of high-grade microhematuria, with an RBC count greater than 100 cells per HPF. Significant hematuria is an indicator for further diagnostic evaluation.

White Blood Cells

An elevated white blood cell (WBC) count in the urine is called pyuria (pus in the urine). The microscopic urinalysis finding of 5 to 10 WBCs per HPF (5 to 10 WBCs/mm^3) is a significant elevation that indicates the presence of urinary tract infection. Neutrophils are the predominant type of white blood cells that appear in the urine.

U

Bacteria

Most urinary tract infections are characterized by a significant number of bacteria in the urine. The bacteria are visualized during high-power microscopic examination of the specimen. The finding of a bacteria count greater than 10^5 bacteria per milliliter is considered diagnostic of urinary tract infection. Bacteria also can be detected with the nitrite dipstick method. In the presence of most urinary bacteria, the dipstick turns pink (positive result) within 60 seconds. This method does not measure the severity of infection or identify the type of bacteria, but it is an effective method to screen for asymptomatic bacteriuria.

Leukocyte Esterase

The leukocyte esterase test is an indirect method used to detect bacteria in the urine. The dipstick method identifies lysed or intact WBCs. When these cells are present, the bacteria must also be present.

Casts

Casts are globulin protein structures that are precipitated in the renal tubules. They are found in the urine sediment, and the different types are identified during microscopic examination. The presence of a great number of casts is an indicator of renal parenchymal disease. Granular casts are associated with glomerulonephritis and renal pathologic conditions. Fatty casts are produced in nephrotic syndrome. Cellular casts can have RBCs, WBCs, renal tubular cells, or a mix of these different cells. They are indicators of inflammation or infection of glomeruli, renal tubules, or renal interstitial tissue. Hyaline casts are the most common type of cast, but their presence may or may not be significant. Hyaline casts can appear after strenuous exercise, with fever, or in congestive heart failure. Persistent large numbers of hyaline casts are an indication of renal disease.

Crystals

Crystals are the end products of food metabolism and, when present, are found in urinary sediment. Crystals can be found in healthy urine, although most individuals have few or none present in urine. Crystals are seen commonly in patients with urolithiasis (kidney stones), toxic damage to the kidneys, or chronic renal failure. The presence of cellular elements or crystals, or both, causes the urine to become cloudy.

REFERENCE VALUES

Color and clarity: Yellow, clear
Specific gravity: 1.016-1.022 with normal fluid intake
pH range: 4.6-6.8 (average value: 6)
Protein: Negative; average concentration: 2-10 ng/dL
Bilirubin: Negative
Glucose: Negative
Ketones: Negative
Occult blood: Negative
RBCs: 0-2 per HPF
WBCs: 0-5 per HPF
Bacteria: Negative
Leukocyte esterase: Negative
Casts: 0-4 hyaline casts per low power field (LPF)
Crystals: Few

HOW THE TEST IS DONE

A clean container with a lid is used to collect 15 mL or more of urine. A random sample may be used, but the first-voided specimen of the morning is preferred. The urine is collected using the midstream clean-catch procedure.

SIGNIFICANCE OF TEST RESULTS

Elevated/Positive Values

Specific Gravity
Dehydration
Fever
Profuse sweating
Vomiting, diarrhea, or both
Glycosuria
Proteinuria
Heart failure
Adrenal insufficiency
Altered secretion of antidiuretic hormone

pH
Metabolic alkalosis
Respiratory alkalosis
Bacteriuria (*Proteus* spp., *Pseudomonas*)
Vegetarian diet
Nasogastric suctioning
Fanconi syndrome

Protein
Nephrotic syndrome
Renal disorders associated with hypertension, diabetes mellitus, systemic lupus erythematosus, or amyloidosis

Bilirubin
Hepatitis
Biliary obstruction

Glucose
Hyperglycemia
Diabetes mellitus

Ketones
Acidosis
Alcoholic ketoacidosis
Diabetic ketoacidosis
Fasting or starvation
Increased protein intake

Occult Blood
Glomerulonephritis
Urolithiasis
Urinary tract infection

U

Tumor, benign or malignant
Polycystic kidney
Renal infarct
Lupus nephritis
Benign prostatic hypertrophy
Blood dyscrasia, hemolysis of RBCs
Endocarditis
Leukemia
Poison (snake or spider bite)
Parasitic disease
Thermal or crush injury
Trauma
Severe exercise, jogging
Red Blood Cells
Benign tumor
Cancer: renal, bladder
Urinary calculi
Glomerulonephritis
Lupus nephritis
Sclerosis
Urinary tract infection
Trauma from exercise
White Blood Cells
Urinary tract infection
Pyelonephritis
Cystitis
Prostatitis
Urethritis
Bacteria
Chronic urinary tract infection
Pyelonephritis
Cystitis, acute or chronic
Leukocyte Esterase
White blood cells in urine
Casts
Glomerulonephritis
Chronic renal disease
Nephrotic syndrome
Bacterial pyelonephritis
Renal failure
Crystals
Uric Acid Crystals
Gout
Rapid nucleic acid turnover
Urolithiasis

Calcium Oxalate Crystals
Chronic renal failure
Ethylene glycol ingestion
Urolithiasis
Triple Phosphate Crystals
Obstructive uropathy
Urinary tract infection
Urolithiasis

Decreased Values
Specific Gravity
Overhydration
Diuresis
Hypotension
Pyelonephritis
Glomerulonephritis
Renal tubular dysfunction
Severe renal damage
Diabetes insipidus
pH
Metabolic acidosis
Respiratory acidosis
Diabetes mellitus
Diarrhea
Starvation
Renal failure

INTERFERING FACTORS

- Insufficient quantity of urine
- Contamination of the specimen
- Warming of the specimen

NURSING CARE

Pretest

○ *Patient Teaching.* The nurse instructs the patient to collect a sample of urine, preferably on arising in the morning. The specimen must not be contaminated by toilet paper, toilet water, feces, or secretions. Women should not collect urine during menstruation to prevent contamination with bloody discharge. The patient also needs instruction on how to cleanse the urinary meatus and how to collect the urine. The information on the midstream clean-catch procedure is presented Chapter 2, pp. 33.

During the Test

- If the patient has an indwelling urinary catheter, the nurse collects the urine specimen from the port in the drainage tubing that is connected to the Foley catheter. The nurse cleanses the port with an alcohol swab and then uses a syringe with a 22- or 25-gauge needle to enter

Continued

the port and aspirate the urine. If there is no visible urine in the tubing, a clamp may first be applied to the tubing just below the port. The urine is aspirated from the port after a few minutes. The specimen is placed in the specimen container and the clamp is then opened to reestablish drainage. Specimens are never removed from the collecting bag because the urine is not fresh. In addition, the collection tube is never separated (opened) from the Foley catheter to collect urine directly from the catheter. If the drainage system is opened, bacteria can enter and cause a urinary tract infection.

Posttest

- Label the container with the patient's name and identifying information, the time, and the date of the voiding.
- Arrange for transport of the specimen to the laboratory as soon as possible because the most accurate results are obtained from warm, fresh specimens. If there is delay, refrigeration of the specimen will preserve the elements in the urine, but crystals will precipitate. Allowing the specimen to stand at room temperature will cause decomposition of the bacteria and WBCs.
- The nurse can perform dipstick testing of the specimen (Box 11).

BOX 11   Accuracy in the Performance of Urinary Dipstick Testing

- Keep the container of test strips tightly closed when it is not in use. To prevent deterioration of the chemicals, protect the strips from exposure to light, heat, and moisture.
- Perform the test on a fresh sample of urine without delay.
- As the reagent strip is removed from the urine, tap the strip gently on the specimen container to remove excess urine.
- For each test, wait the required time before reading the results.
- Read the test results in a setting that has good lighting. Hold the strip in a horizontal position to prevent the mixing of chemicals from one pad to another.
- In comparing the test pad to the manufacturer's color chart, align the squares and tests accurately. Do not allow the moist strip to touch the chart and discolor the squares.

Urinary Glucose/Sugar

See Glucose, Urinary on pp. 347.

Urobilinogen, Urinary

Also called: Urinary Urobilinogen; 2-Hour Urine Urobilinogen

SPECIMEN OR TYPE OF TEST: Urine

PURPOSE OF THE TEST

This test is used to help detect hemolytic anemia and early detection of liver disease, including hepatitis and cirrhosis

BASICS THE NURSE NEEDS TO KNOW

Conjugated bilirubin exits from the liver as a component of bile. It flows through the biliary system and enters the intestine at the duodenum. In the small intestine, bilirubin is converted to urobilinogen by the bacterial flora of the intestine. About half the urobilinogen is excreted in fecal material and the remainder enters the portal vein circulation. Most of this circulatory portion of urobilinogen will return to the liver via the enterohepatic (portal vein) circulation and will be recycled into bile. The remainder of the circulatory portion is filtered out of the blood by the kidneys and is excreted in urine (Figure 103).

Urinary urobilinogen increases when there is excessive hemolysis of red blood cells that produces excess bilirubin formation by the liver and when there is liver disease that interferes with the enterohepatic circulation. Urinary urobilinogen decreases when there is obstruction in the flow of bile to the intestine and poor kidney function that impairs the filtration and removal of urobilinogen and bilirubin.

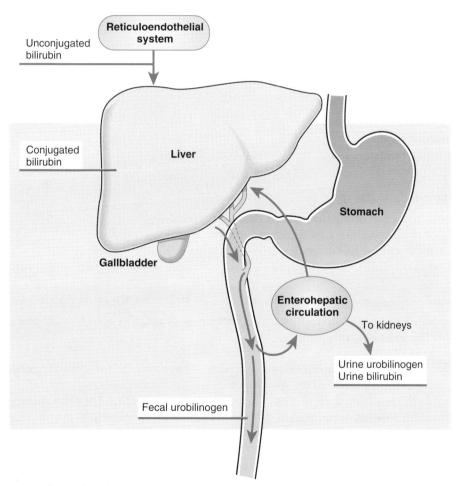

Figure 103. Pathways for bilirubin metabolism. Several organs and organ systems make different forms and amounts of bilirubin and urobilinogen. These substances are ultimately eliminated in the feces and urine.

REFERENCE VALUES   0.3-1.0 Ehrlich units/2 hr *or* SI: 0.5-1.7 μmol/2 hr
0.05-2.5 ng/24 hours *or* SI: 0.05-2.5 mg/24 hr

HOW THE TEST IS DONE

The 2-hour urine collection is scheduled for the afternoon, between 2 PM and 4 PM. This timing coordinates with the body's pattern for excretion of urine urobilinogen.

Alternatively a 24-hour collection may be required.

SIGNIFICANCE OF TEST RESULTS

Elevated Values

Moderate hepatocellular damage
Hepatitis
Hepatotoxicity from drugs or toxins
Hepatic anoxia
Portal vein cirrhosis
Hemolysis of erythrocytes
Intravascular hemolysis
Hemolytic anemia
Pernicious anemia

Decreased Values

Biliary tract obstruction
Massive hepatocellular damage
Renal insufficiency

INTERFERING FACTORS

- Failure to collect all of the urine in the collection period
- Exposure of the specimen to warmth or sunlight
- Recent or current use of antibiotics

NURSING CARE

Nursing actions are similar to those used in other timed urine collections (see Chapter 2), with the following additional measures.

Pretest

○ *Patient Teaching.* The nurse explains the procedure to the patient to maximize the cooperation and accuracy in the collection of the specimen.

Schedule the test from 2 PM to 4 PM. The patient voids just before 2 PM, and this specimen is discarded because urine has been in the bladder for an unknown period.

Give the patient 500 mL of water to drink, all at once.

During the Test

- From 2 PM to 4 PM, the nurse collects all voided urine and places it in a dark-colored, sterile urine container. As an alternative, a clear container can be covered with aluminum foil to protect the urine from light. Keep the urine in the refrigerator. The reason for these measures is that urobilinogen is unstable and will convert to urobilin in the presence of sunlight, fluorescent light, or warmth.

- If a 24-hour collection is required, the container is larger and also dark colored or covered with foil. The 24-hour urine collection procedure is described in Chapter 2, pp. 36-37.

Posttest

- On completion of the collection, the specimen label is applied to the container. It includes the patient's name, identification number or bar code, the physician's name, and date and time of the collection. The requisition form contains the same information. The specimen is sent to the lab promptly.

Uroflowmetry

Also called: Simple Uroflowmetry; Urodynamic Studies (UDS)

SPECIMEN OR TYPE OF TEST: Urine; Voiding Measurements

PURPOSE OF THE TEST

Uroflowmetry is used to help evaluate lower urinary tract (bladder, urethra) dysfunction, including voiding abnormality.

BASICS THE NURSE NEEDS TO KNOW

The broad category of urodynamic studies evaluates voiding and lower urinary tract function. Uroflowmetry is the initial test that is performed to assess bladder and sphincter function. This test is generally ordered for patients with complaints of incontinence or retention of urine.

Urinary incontinence is the involuntary leakage of urine through the urethral meatus. When incontinence is defined by its symptoms, the problem is identified as urge incontinence, stress incontinence, or total incontinence. When the incontinence is defined by its cause, the problem is one of bladder storage, bladder emptying, or urinary sphincter dysfunction. *Urinary retention* or obstruction may be classified as bladder or urethral dysfunction.

Determination of the urinary flow rate is a noninvasive procedure that provides measurable baseline data about the patient's ability to void urine. The data measure the volume of urine voided, the pattern of micturition, and the time or rate of voiding. The patient's data are compared with normal micturition patterns and numeric values of the flow rate. When the patient's values are higher than normal, the problem is one of incontinence. When the patient's values are lower than normal, the problem is one of impaired urinary flow.

In any person, the urinary flow rate varies with the volume of urine that is voided. The patient's results are compared with normal values based on the volume voided. The flow rate of any individual also varies from one voiding episode to another. The uroflowmetry test is repeated several times to obtain reliable data. Additionally, normal voiding rates vary between males and females and among different age groups across the life span. The interpretation of the patient's values is age and gender specific.

U

REFERENCE VALUES   Average Volume and flow rate: 200 mL in 15-20 sec
Flow Rate: Age and gender specific
Male <40 years: 22 mL/sec
    40-60 years: 18 mL/sec
    >60 years: 13 mL/sec
Female <50 years: >25 mL/sec
    >50 years: >18 mL/sec

HOW THE TEST IS DONE

The patient urinates into a toilet that is equipped with a funnel and uroflowmeter. As voiding activates the uroflowmeter and its transducer, electronic data are received, transmitted, analyzed, and recorded. Specific variations in the procedure are based on differences in the manufacturers' equipment and protocol. The total time for completion of the test is 10 to 15 minutes.

SIGNIFICANCE OF TEST RESULTS

Elevated Values
Conditions that cause reduced urethral resistance
Incontinence (stress, urge, or total)

Decreased Values
Urethral or bladder neck obstruction
Poor muscular contraction of the bladder

INTERFERING FACTORS

- Body movement during voiding
- Toilet tissue in the apparatus
- Straining during urination

NURSING CARE

Pretest
○ *Patient Teaching.* The nurse instructs the patient to drink fluids and refrain from voiding for several hours before the test. The bladder must be full when starting the test.
During the Test
- Ensure the patient's privacy for the test. The bathroom contains a toilet with the uroflowmeter installed in it.
○ *Patient Teaching.* Instruct the patient to void into the urometer funnel without straining or body movement. The nurse also informs the patient not to dispose of the toilet tissue in the funnel or collection container.
Posttest
- No specific patient instruction or intervention is needed.

Urography, Intravenous

See Computed Tomography, Kidneys, Ureters and Bladder on pp. 218-219.

Vanillylmandelic Acid

See Catecholamines, Urinary on pp. 182.

Varicella-Zoster Antibody

Also called: VZV Antibody

SPECIMEN OR TYPE OF TEST: Blood

PURPOSE OF THE TEST

The immunoglobulin IgM antibody test occasionally is used to identify the current infection with the varicella-zoster virus. The immunoglobulin IgG antibody test is used to confirm past infection or vaccination that provides immunity from future chickenpox infection.

BASICS THE NURSE NEEDS TO KNOW

The varicella-zoster virus is a herpesvirus that causes the primary infection of varicella (chickenpox) and years later can cause the reactivated infection of shingles (herpes zoster infection). A negative result for varicella-zoster antibodies means that the person has no immunity from chickenpox and is susceptible to acquire this infection. If a person has positive IgG antibodies or a high IgG titer, it means there is immunity to future chickenpox infection, but there may not be immunity to shingles.

In the acute illness phase, the IgM antibody test becomes positive 1 to 3 days after the skin eruption occurs. In the convalescent phase, the IgG antibody becomes positive 9 to 10 days after the skin eruption occurs. If the pregnant woman contracts this infection in the last 3 weeks of pregnancy, the fetus may develop chickenpox. Positive IgM antibodies in the amniotic fluid or cord blood means that the fetus has a varicella infection.

Antibody testing is done in the pretransplant patient. If there is no immunity to varicella-zoster, vaccination will be considered before the transplant occurs.

REFERENCE VALUES   IgM: Negative
IgG: Negative; titer 1:4

HOW THE TEST IS DONE

Venipuncture is performed to obtain a sample of the blood.

If the pregnant female has varicella infection, amniotic fluid analysis from amniocentesis or blood from a percutaneous umbilical blood sampling may be obtained to identify infection in the fetus.

SIGNIFICANCE OF TEST RESULTS

Positive Values

Past or present varicella-zoster infection
Immunity to future varicella infection

V

INTERFERING FACTORS

• Infection with another type of herpesvirus

NURSING CARE

Nursing actions are similar to those used in venipuncture procedures (see Chapter 2), with the following additional measures.

Pretest

• Inform the adult patient that a positive IgG antibody titer indicates immunity from future chickenpox infection.

Posttest

• If the newborn has a recent exposure to the varicella-zoster virus, the nurse maintains the infant in isolation in the newborn nursery. To determine the presence of perinatal infection, the physician may have the infant's blood tested for IgM antibodies. To reduce the severity of the infection in this newborn, the nurse prepares to administer varicella immunoglobulin to the baby, as prescribed by the physician.

Health Promotion

To prevent chickenpox, the recommended time for infant child vaccination with measles, mumps, rubella, varicella-zoster (MMRV) is between 12 and 15 months old. If the varicella vaccination is given separately, it is given no earlier than 12 months old. A second dose is given between 4 and 6 years old.

The vaccine is also recommended for people who are frequently in settings where infection rates are higher, including hospitals, day care centers, schools, prisons, military settings, and colleges. The nonpregnant female also should be vaccinated to prevent severe illness during a future pregnancy and avoid potential risk to the fetus.

Health Teaching

The nurse can teach individuals and community groups about the importance of early vaccination of their infants and young children, encouraging them to have their children vaccinated to prevent this infection.

Vasopressin

Also called: Antidiuretic Hormone (ADH), Arginine-Vasopressin (AVP)

SPECIMEN OR TYPE OF TEST: Plasma

PURPOSE OF THE TEST

A serum antidiuretic hormone (ADH) determination is obtained to diagnose diabetes insipidus and syndrome of inappropriate antidiuretic hormone (SIADH).

BASICS THE NURSE NEEDS TO KNOW

Vasopressin (ADH) is produced by the hypothalamus and stored in the posterior pituitary gland. Its major function in the body is to act on the cells in the collecting ducts of the kidney, making them more permeable to water. The result is an increased reabsorption of water. This action is independent of electrolyte levels, and electrolytes are not reabsorbed with the water. The purpose of this action is to maintain normal plasma osmolality. ADH also has a vasopressor effect. It causes arteriole smooth muscles to constrict, thus elevating the blood pressure.

ADH is released from the posterior pituitary gland in response to several stimuli. The major stimulus is an increase in plasma osmolality. Whenever the osmoreceptors in the anterior hypothalamus sense even minor changes in plasma osmolality, neural stimulation of the pituitary gland will result in an increased secretion of ADH, which will result in an increased reabsorption of water at the renal collecting ducts. With the increase in water in the extracellular fluid, blood tonicity will decrease. Because the increase in water results in decreased blood osmolality, the osmoreceptors will cease the neural stimulation necessary for ADH secretion (Figure 104).

Another stimulant for ADH release is the extracellular fluid volume. A drop in blood volume is sensed by stretcher receptors primarily in the vena cava and right atrium. By way of the brainstem, these receptors tell the hypothalamus to stimulate the release of ADH from the posterior pituitary gland. The resultant increase in fluid volume from water retention results in a decrease in stretcher receptor stimulation. In addition, as arterial blood pressure drops, pressor receptors found in the aorta and coronary sinuses will stimulate the release of ADH to increase extracellular fluid volume and thus the patient's blood pressure.

ADH secretion may be increased by drugs (e.g., nicotine, opiates, barbiturates, chlorpropamide) and severe pain, stress, and hyperthermia. Decreased sensitivity of the kidneys to ADH occurs with the intake of lithium carbonate and demeclocycline.

REFERENCE VALUES | If serum osmolality is >290 mOsm/kg: 2-12 pg/mL *or*
SI: 1.85-11.1 pmol/L
If serum osmolality is <290 mOsm/kg: <2 pg/mL *or*
SI: <1.85 pmol/L

HOW THE TEST IS DONE
Venipuncture is performed and specimen sent to the lab immediately.

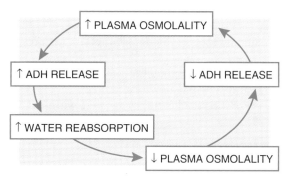

Figure 104. **Vasopressin (ADH) regulation.** ADH is secreted by the posterior pituitary gland primarily in response to an increase in plasma osmolality.

SIGNIFICANCE OF TEST RESULTS

Elevated Values

Syndrome of inappropriate antidiuretic hormone
Guillain-Barre syndrome
Tuberculosis

Decreased Values

Diabetes insipidus
Nephrotic syndrome
Psychogenic polydipsia

INTERFERING FACTORS

• Noncompliance with diet, activity, and medication restrictions
• Pain
• Stress
• Mechanical ventilation
• Alcohol
• Medications such as anesthetics, antipsychotics, carbamazepine, chlorothiazide, cyclophos-
  phamide, estrogen, lithium, oxytocin, phenytoin, and vincristine

NURSING CARE

Nursing actions related to venipuncture are presented in Chapter 2, with the following additional
measures.

Pretest

○ *Patient Teaching.* The nurse instructs the patient not to eat or drink for 12 hours before
the test.

○ *Patient Teaching.* The nurse also instructs the patient to avoid substances that increase ADH
secretion, such as nicotine, alcohol, caffeine, and diuretics. Instruct the patient to limit physical
activity for 12 hours before the test. The patient should lie down and rest for 30 minutes before
the blood is drawn.

• Obtain a medication history to determine if any interfering drugs are being taken. In the
  pretest period, the nurse checks with the physician to determine if these drugs are to be
  withheld or continued.
• Assess the patient for pain and stress, which may interfere with results.

Posttest

• Send specimen to the laboratory immediately.
• Instruct the patient to resume normal activity and diet.
• The nurse administers prescribed medications that were withheld for the test.

Vectorcardiogram

Also called: VCG

SPECIMEN OR TYPE OF TEST: Electrophysiology

PURPOSE OF THE TEST

A vectorcardiogram is used to assess ischemia, conduction defects, and chamber enlargement (hypertrophy or dilation).

BASICS THE NURSE NEEDS TO KNOW

A vectorcardiogram is a graphic recording of electric forces of the heart. It is a noninvasive procedure that graphically records the direction and magnitude of the heart's electric forces by means of a continuous series of vector loops. Three planes of the heart are recorded (frontal, sagittal, and horizontal).

REFERENCE VALUES   Normal cardiac axis

SIGNIFICANCE OF TEST RESULTS

Abnormal Values

Myocardial ischemia

Conduction defects

Atrial and/or ventricular hypertrophy

Atrial and/or ventricular dilation

Cardiomyopathy

INTERFERING FACTORS

• Patient who is unable to lie still

NURSING CARE

See section on electrocardiogram for nursing care (pp. 277).

Venography

Also called: Phlebography

SPECIMEN OR TYPE OF TEST: Radiography

PURPOSE OF THE TEST

Venography is used to investigate venous function, suspected obstruction, venous insufficiency, postphlebitic syndrome, and the source of pulmonary embolism. It also evaluates veins before and after bypass surgery, reconstructive surgery, or thrombolytic therapy to determine the effectiveness of treatment. Venography is the best method to identify a deep vein thrombosis below the knee.

BASICS THE NURSE NEEDS TO KNOW

Venography is an invasive technique that provides visualization of the venous system, particularly in the lower extremities. *Thrombosis* (the formation of a blood clot) is the most common venous pathologic condition. Deep vein thrombosis and thromboembolism are caused by three general pathologic conditions: damage to the vein, venous stasis, and decreased fibrinolytic activity. As the thrombus enlarges, it occludes the lumen of the vein and ultimately destroys the venous valve or valves. In the early stage of formation, the thrombus is soft and friable. When located in a vein of the leg, a piece of the thrombus can break off, travel, and lodge as a pulmonary embolus in the arterial vasculature of the lungs.

Examination of the veins by venography can be carried out by different procedures. *Ascending venography* is used to identify the presence and location of deep vein thrombosis and to assess the patency of the deep venous system in the lower extremity. *Descending venography* is used to assess valve competency. *Venography of the upper extremities* evaluates occlusion, lesions, or thrombosis in the subclavian or axillary veins. *Venacavography* evaluates the superior or inferior vena cava for obstruction, malformation, traumatic injury, and placement of the inferior vena cava filter.

REFERENCE VALUES   No evidence of intraluminal filling defects, obstruction, incompetent venous valves, calcifications, or dilated collateral veins

HOW THE TEST IS DONE

Contrast medium is injected into the vein via an intravenous catheter. With the assistance of a tilt table and guidance imaging by fluoroscopy, the contrast medium illustrates the flow patterns of the venous circulation and identifies the site of occlusion in the vein.

In venography of the lower extremities, either ascending or descending venography may be used. Ascending venography uses an intravenous catheter that has been placed in a small vein on the dorsum of the foot. In descending venography, a catheter is placed in the common femoral vein. Upper extremity venography uses intravenous catheter placement in a vein of the wrist or at the elbow. Central venography or venography of specific organs uses various selected venous sites for the physician's insertion of the intravenous catheter and delivery of the contrast medium.

Imaging will be done by x-rays, computed tomography (CT), or magnetic resonance (MR).

SIGNIFICANCE OF TEST RESULTS

Abnormal Values
Deep vein thrombosis
Tumor
Vascular tumor
Venous compression syndrome
Venous insufficiency
Varicose veins
Congenital malformation
Traumatic injury to the vein

INTERFERING FACTORS

- Allergy or sensitivity to contrast medium
- Renal failure
- Heart failure
- Severe pulmonary hypertension

NURSING CARE

Pretest

- After the physician explains the procedure, obtain a written consent from the patient and place it in the patient's record.
- Identify any sensitivity reaction that occurred during a previous radiograph study that used contrast medium.
- Ensure that the pretest blood urea nitrogen and creatinine determinations are performed and that the results are posted in the patient's chart. The kidneys must clear the contrast material from the blood, and these tests verify that renal function is adequate. Notify the physician of abnormal elevations of these test results. Record the patient's baseline vital signs.

○ *Patient Teaching.* Instruct the patient regarding the pretest preparation. Solid foods are omitted for 4 hours before the test, but water and clear liquids are permitted. The patient will be asked to remove all jewelry and clothing, wearing a hospital gown for the procedure.

During the Test

- The patient is positioned according to the views required. Lower extremity views are done with the patient in supine position or tilted upward to a semierect position.
- Provide emotional support during the period of discomfort. The injection of contrast material is painful.
- On completion of the test, an intravenous solution of 200 to 300 mL of heparinized saline is administered. This flushes the contrast medium from the veins.

Posttest

- The nurse takes vital signs and assesses the catheter site for swelling, pain, redness, ecchymosis, and hematoma. All findings are recorded.
- The nurse keeps the patient on bed rest for 2 hours. Food intake may be resumed. The patient is encouraged to drink extra fluids for 24 hours to help flush the remaining contrast medium from the veins and kidneys. Frequent urination is expected until the *diuresis* (increased excretion of urine) is complete.

◆ **Nursing Response to Complications**

The complications that can occur are related to the contrast medium that was used in the test. Although the incidence is not frequent, the nurse monitors the patient for potential problems and notifies the physician if they occur.

Cellulitis. During the test, if more than 5 to 10 mL of contrast material infiltrates the tissue, chemical cellulitis will result in the posttest period. The nurse assesses the tissue near the injection site for tenderness, pain, redness, and swelling.

Thrombophlebitis. The contrast medium can be irritating to the vein and cause phlebitis or thrombophlebitis. Along the path of the vein that received the injection of contrast, the nurse observes for redness, swelling, and pain. Like cellulitis, the manifestations often begin 2 to 12 hours posttest and usually subside in a few days.

Mild sensitivity reaction. Sensitivity reactions can range from mild to very severe. The mild reaction may begin during the test or shortly afterward. The patient develops a histamine response, including urticaria, itching, edema, and redness of the skin. When the reaction remains mild, the nurse prepares to administer the antihistamine diphenhydramine hydrochloride (Benadryl), as prescribed. The nurse monitors the respirations of the patient because of the potential for a more severe allergic reaction.

V

Continued

Severe allergic reaction. If the allergic reaction is severe, it can progress toward anaphylaxis in a very rapid manner. An anaphylactic response may occur during the test, very soon after injection of the contrast medium. The patient develops respiratory distress, wheezing, or stridor. Cyanosis develops as the airway becomes swollen, edematous, and increasingly obstructed. The patient develops tachycardia, hypotension, and chest pain. Cardiac arrest may occur.

As the respiratory problems begin, the physician must be notified immediately. At the onset of the reaction, the nurse calls for the crash cart to be brought to the patient's bedside. The nurse prepares to administer oxygen and prescribed medications that will help reverse the anaphylaxis and acute respiratory distress. These medications include epinephrine (Adrenaline) subcutaneously, and aminophylline intravenously. Benadryl may also be prescribed intravenously.

Ventilation-Perfusion Scan

See Lung Scans on pp. 428.

Vitamin B$_{12}$

Also called: Cobalamin

SPECIMEN OR TYPE OF TEST: Serum

PURPOSE OF THE TEST

This test is used to identify vitamin B$_{12}$ deficiency or to investigate the cause of hematologic and neurologic symptoms that suggest a deficiency.

BASICS THE NURSE NEEDS TO KNOW

Vitamin B$_{12}$ is an essential vitamin and coenzyme needed for the formation of normal erythrocytes and other bone marrow functions. In terms of dietary intake, this vitamin is present in meat, milk, butter, cheese, fish, and eggs. The absorption of the vitamin occurs in stages. Initially, it is bound to intrinsic factor, manufactured by the gastric parietal cells. In the ileum, it is absorbed into the portal vein system, aided by intrinsic factor and pancreatic enzymes. Some vitamin B$_{12}$ will be used by the bone marrow for hematopoiesis and the remainder is stored by the liver.

Elevated Level

The vitamin B$_{12}$ level is elevated in the blood when a disorder increases the manufacture of transport substances or increases hematopoiesis. Various hematologic malignancies and severe liver disorders are possible causes for elevated vitamin B$_{12}$ levels.

Decreased Level

Several possible causes exist for a decreased amount of vitamin B$_{12}$ in the blood. The most common cause is a problem with the production and function of intrinsic factor. It is estimated that 10% to 25% of the elderly have unrecognized and untreated vitamin B$_{12}$ deficiency, probably due to hypochlorhydria, achlorhydria, or atrophic gastritis that interferes with vitamin B$_{12}$ absorption. These individuals tend to ignore the manifestations of pernicious anemia until they experience cognitive impairment or peripheral neuropathy. Without intrinsic factor, the available vitamin B$_{12}$ cannot enter the circulation from the intestinal tract. Impaired absorption from the ilium may also lower the vitamin B$_{12}$ level. A lack of dietary intake of the vitamin may be the cause, but it is not a very common occurrence. Persons who are strict vegetarians are the most vulnerable to a deficit of this vitamin.

Without sufficient vitamin B$_{12}$ in the blood and a depletion of the vitamin reserves that were stored in the liver, the patient develops megaloblastic anemia, with erythrocytes that are too large. Because of their size, the erythrocytes have difficulty passing through the microcirculation, and they become damaged. The short life span of these erythrocytes is 27 to 35 days before hemolysis occurs. In addition, the lack of this vitamin impairs the bone marrow production of white blood cells and platelets, causing *thrombocytopenia* (a low platelet count) and *leukopenia* (a low white blood count).

REFERENCE VALUES	Newborn: 160-1300 pg/mL *or* SI: 118-959 pmol/L
	Adult: 200-835 pg/mL *or* SI: 148-616 pmol/L
	Adult (60-90 years): 110-770 pg/mL *or* SI: 81-568 pmol/L

HOW THE TEST IS DONE
Venipuncture is performed to obtain a sample of venous blood.

SIGNIFICANCE OF TEST RESULTS
Elevated Values
Chronic myelogenous leukemia, acute or chronic
Chronic renal failure
Polycythemia vera
Liver disease (cirrhosis, hepatitis)
Liver metastases

Decreased Values
Pernicious anemia
Intrinsic factor antibodies
Postgastrectomy
Atrophic gastritis
Achlorhydria
Malabsorption in the ileum
Dietary deficiency

INTERFERING FACTORS
- Failure to maintain nothing-by-mouth status
- Radioactive isotopes
- Hemolysis
- Exposure of the specimen to sunlight
- Recent transfusion or vitamin B$_{12}$ therapy

V

| NURSING CARE

Nursing actions are similar to those used in other venipuncture procedures (see Chapter 2), with the following additional measures.

Pretest

- Schedule this test before a radioisotope scan because the radioisotopes of these procedures interfere with the radioimmunoassay method of analysis for this test.
- Schedule this test before a blood transfusion is administered or a trial of vitamin B_{12} treatment is started.

○ *Patient Teaching.* The nurse instructs the patient to fast from food for 8 hours before the test.

Posttest

- Send the specimen to the laboratory without delay. If a delay in analysis occurs, the specimen must be protected from exposure to sunlight.
- The nurse should assess the patient with cobalamin deficiency. The hematologic manifestations associated with this anemia include fatigue, weakness, pallor, and jaundice. In the inspection of the mouth, the tongue is sore and smooth (glossitis) because of a loss of the epithelial surface. The neurologic manifestations are more troubling to the patient because there are changes in the brain, spinal cord, and peripheral nerves. The patient complains of peripheral neuropathy, including symptoms of numbness, tingling, and a loss of vibratory sensation in the hands and feet. There is a loss of position sense and difficulty walking. Brain changes also are present, causing impairment in thinking, change in personality, irritability, and emotional instability.

Vitamin D

Includes: 25(OH)D; [25(OH) calciferol], 1,25(OH)$_2$D; [1,25(OH)$_2$ calciferol]

SPECIMEN OR TYPE OF TEST: Serum, Plasma

PURPOSE OF THE TEST

25(OH)D measures the amount of vitamin D that circulates in the blood.

1,25(OH)$_2$ D , a metabolite of vitamin D, is used to investigate the cause of hypercalcemia (*excess calcium in the blood*), *hypocalcemia*, (decreased calcium in the blood), *hypercalciuria* (excess calcium in the urine), and other bone and mineral disorders.

BASICS THE NURSE NEEDS TO KNOW

Vitamin D is required to enable the calcium absorption in bones. The regular intake of vitamin D in humans comes from two sources. One source is derived from the action of ultraviolet light on a group of provitamins in the skin resulting in absorption of vitamin D into the body. Vitamin D is derived also from vitamin D in food intake. The best natural food sources of Vitamin D are fatty fish (mackerel, salmon, and tuna), as well as fish oil. Other beneficial foods are Vitamin D-enriched, including milk, orange juice, most cereals, and some yogurts.

V

Once the vitamin D (25(OH)D enters the blood, it is metabolized in complex processes by the liver and the kidneys to form various metabolites. The formation of the 1,25(OH)$_2$D in the kidneys is regulated by parathyroid hormone and the serum metabolite level is influenced by calcium and phosphate intake. 1,25(OH)$_2$D is the most active form of vitamin D and it functions to improve intestinal calcium absorption and mobilization in bone growth, remodeling, and bone density.

Variables Affecting Reference Values

The reference values vary among laboratories and standardization of the values is not established (IOM, 2010). The normal values also vary because of differences based on age, skin color (that affects absorption of ultraviolet light), geography (northern latitudes have less ultraviolet B rays), and the season of the year. The winter season may have reference values that are 40% to 50% lower (McPherson & Pinkus, 2007; Wu, 2006).

REFERENCE VALUES | 25(OH)D: 10-50 ng/mL *or* SI: 25-125 nmol/L
1,25(OH)$_2$D: 15-60 pg/mL *or* SI: 39-156 pmol/L

HOW THE TEST IS DONE

Venipuncture is done to obtain a sample of blood.

SIGNIFICANCE OF TEST RESULTS

25(OH)D

Elevated Values

Vitamin D intoxication
Excess sunlight exposure

Decreased Values

Hepatic failure (cirrhosis)
Hyperparathyroidism
Malabsorption syndrome
Osteomalacia
Chronic renal failure

1,25(OH)$_2$D

Elevated Values

Hypoparathyroidism
Calcium-producing tumor
Sarcoidosis

Decreased Values

Chronic renal failure
Hypoparathyroidism
Vitamin D deficient rickets
Osteoporosis, postmenopausal

V

INTERFERING FACTORS

• Recent radioisotope administration

NURSING CARE

The nurse performs actions similar to those in other venipuncture procedures, as described in Chapter 2, with the following additional measures.

Pretest

• Schedule this test before or 3 weeks after a radioisotope scan. The radioactive isotopes of the scan would interfere with the RAI method of lab analysis.

○ *Patient Teaching.* Instruct the patient not to eat for 8 hours before the test.

Posttest

Health Promotion

The newest guidelines from the Institutes of Medicine (2010) recommend a daily intake of vitamin D of 600 IU for all people ages 1 to 70 years. For those who are older than 70, the recommended amount increases to 800 IU /day. For all individuals age 9 and older, the upper limit of daily intake should be no more than 4000 U per day.

• The nurse advises that almost all people can maintain a normal level of vitamin D through food intake and some daily exposure to sunlight. Over-the-counter mega-doses (5000 U per capsule) of a vitamin D supplement can result in an intake that is above the daily maximum limit of 4000 IU. Overdose can result in symptoms of nausea and vomiting, constipation, muscle weakness, and poor appetite. It can also cause elevated levels of calcium in the blood and urine, with formation of kidney stones and possible renal damage.

Water Deprivation Test

Also called: Dehydration Test; Concentration Test

SPECIMEN OR TYPE OF TEST: Urine

PURPOSE OF THE TEST

The water deprivation test is performed to diagnose diabetes insipidus (DI) and to assess the kidney's ability to concentrate urine based on extracellular fluid load.

BASICS THE NURSE NEEDS TO KNOW

Normally, as fluid intake is withheld, blood osmolality increases, urine output decreases, and urinary osmolality increases. The increase in serum osmolality causes an increase in antidiuretic hormone (ADH) secretion. In patients with DI, a normal response to increased plasma osmolality does not occur; instead, little or no increase in ADH occurs, resulting in little or no change in urinary output or osmolality.

DI may be caused by a defect in production, release, or use of ADH. If DI is a result of a problem in production (hypothalamic) or release (pituitary) of ADH, it is called *neurogenic or central* DI. If DI is caused by a failure of the kidney to respond to ADH, it is called *nephrogenic* DI. The water deprivation test supports the diagnosis of diabetes insipidus.

W

As part of the water deprivation test, a *vasopressin stimulation test* or *ADH stimulation test* may be performed to distinguish between neurogenic and nephrogenic DI. This distinction is important in determining appropriate treatment plans.

REFERENCE VALUES   Osmolality: >400 mOsm/kg *or* SI: >400 mmol/kg

HOW THE TEST IS DONE

During the test, the patient is deprived of fluid intake, and periodic urine specimens are obtained to determine osmolality and the specific gravity. The urine is collected in separate clean containers and placed on ice or refrigerated. Strict urinary output measurements are maintained.

If a *vasopressin stimulation* test is included, hypertonic saline or nicotine is given to stimulate ADH release. If complete neurogenic DI is present, no change is noted in urinary output or osmolality. If partial neurogenic DI is present, only minor changes occur.

If desired, a *vasopressin* test may be performed. After vasopressin is given, no change will occur in urinary output or osmolality if nephrogenic DI is present. With central DI, the urine osmolality will increase and the urinary output will decrease.

SIGNIFICANCE OF TEST RESULTS

If no change in urine osmolality exists, the diagnosis of DI is supported.

If the urine osmolarity increased by more than 10% after vasopressin is given, the diagnosis of central/neurogenic DI is supported.

INTERFERING FACTORS

- Noncompliance with fluid restrictions
- Inability to complete test because of hypovolemia
- Glucosuria
- Administration of radiopaque dyes within 7 days

NURSING CARE

Nursing actions related to timed urine collection and pediatric urine collection procedures are presented in Chapter 2, with the following additional measures.

Pretest

- The nurse assesses the patient's hemodynamic status. If a vasopressin test is planned, check for a history of coronary artery disease because vasopressin may cause coronary artery spasm.
- Obtain a history of previous 24-hour periods of fluid intake. Report/document if adequate hydration did not take place.
- Obtain baseline serum and urine specimens to determine osmolality.
- Baseline weight is obtained before the evening meal on the day before testing.

During the Test

- The nurse observes for early signs of hypovolemia (tachycardia, orthostatic hypotension).
- Observe the patient to ensure compliance with nothing-by-mouth status.

W

Continued

| NURSING CARE—cont'd |

- Obtain a urine specimen every 2 hours. Label each specimen with the time and the amount obtained.
- The nurse weighs the patient every 2 to 4 hours. Maintain the patient on nothing-by-mouth status until 2% to 5% of the patient's weight is lost (this takes approximately 6 to 12 hours).
- After 2% to 5% of patient body weight is lost and urinary output continues with urinary osmolality plateauing, an ADH stimulation test may be performed by administering hypertonic saline (3% sodium chloride) or nicotine, as ordered.
- If a vasopressin test is to be performed, check the patient's blood pressure and document it; notify the physician if the patient is hypertensive. Aqueous vasopressin is given subcutaneously or intravenously. One hour after vasopressin administration, collect a urine specimen for amount and osmolality.

▼ **Nursing Response to Critical Values**

Hypovolemia may occur with the water deprivation test. Patients with DI will continue to put out urine, even though they have no intake. If a vasopressin test is performed, the administration of vasopressin may produce the complications of high blood pressure or coronary artery spasms, or both.

Hypovolemia. Tachycardia, restlessness, poor skin turgor, and hypotension are indications of hypovolemia. If these occur, the nurse notifies the physician and anticipates the test being discontinued and fluids being given.

Coronary artery spasms. With spasm of the coronary artery, perfusion will be affected. The patient may complain of chest pain. The physician is informed and the nurse anticipates that the order for vasopressin to be discontinued.

Water-Loading Test

SPECIMEN OR TYPE OF TEST: Plasma, Urine

PURPOSE OF THE TEST

The water-loading test is performed to diagnose the syndrome of inappropriate secretion of the antidiuretic hormone (SIADH).

BASICS THE NURSE NEEDS TO KNOW

Review the discussion of Plasma Vasopressin (pp. 624). Normally, with an increase in fluid intake, urinary output will increase to maintain a normal plasma osmolality. As the urine volume increases, its osmolality decreases. However, patients with syndrome of inappropriate antidiuretic hormone (SIADH) will not respond to increasing fluid intake.

REFERENCE VALUES   Urinary output increases, and plasma and urinary osmolality decrease.

HOW THE TEST IS DONE

With the water-loading test, the patient orally ingests a water load of 20 to 25 mL/kg of body weight. Hourly serum and urine osmolality and urine outputs are recorded for 4 hours.

W

SIGNIFICANCE OF TEST RESULTS

Little or no change in urinary output or plasma and urine osmolality readings supports the diagnosis of SIADH.

INTERFERING FACTORS

- Patient is unable to drink the required volume of fluid.
- Medications such as demeclocycline, diuretics, and lithium carbonate.

NURSING CARE

Pretest
- The nurse assesses the patient for hyponatremia.
- Obtain the patient's cardiac history, the results of which may require that the test be canceled.
- Weigh the patient.

During the Test
- Instruct the patient to drink the required fluid.
- Obtain hourly output measurements and send blood and urine to the laboratory to determine the osmolality. On the requisition slip, indicate the hour the specimen was taken, with zero hour being the time the patient ingested the fluid (see discussion of Osmolality, Plasma [p. 464] and Osmolality, Urine [p. 465] for the nursing procedures associated with the collection of these samples).
- The nurse observes the patient for water intoxication.

Posttest
- Weigh the patient.

▽ **Nursing Response to Critical Values**

When patients with SIADH undergo the water-loading test, their output is not increased. The increased fluid load in the extracellular fluid can cause dilutional hyponatremia, also called water intoxication.

Dilutional hyponatremia. Indications of water intoxication are hyponatremia, lethargy, confusion, muscular twitching, stupor and, eventually, convulsions and death. The nurse will observe closely for changes in mental status and report these to the physician. The nurse should anticipate an order for a serum sodium level. If the sodium level is less than 120 mEq/L, the nurse would notify the physician immediately.

White Blood Cell Count

Also called: WBC, Leukocyte Count, White Count

SPECIMEN OR TYPE OF TEST: Blood

PURPOSE OF THE TEST

The white blood cell count indicates the possible presence and severity of infection or inflammatory response. This test may be part of the complete blood count, performed as a routine screening test or it may be performed separately to evaluate a specific problem. The leukocyte

W

count is a general indicator of infection, tissue necrosis, inflammation, and bone marrow activity.

BASICS THE NURSE NEEDS TO KNOW

White blood cells, called *leukocytes*, maintain the general function of combating infection and inflammation. The white blood cell count includes the five different types of white blood cells (neutrophils, eosinophils, basophils, lymphocytes, and monocytes). Most of the white blood cells are manufactured by the bone marrow. Additional specific diagnostic information is obtained by the White Blood Cell Differential Count (pp. 640-644), which identifies the numbers of each type of white blood cell.

Many of the white blood cells are phagocytic in their action. They are capable of rapid mobility to an area of infection or tissue damage, where they ingest many types of foreign cells, dead cells, or microorganisms. The used white blood cells will self-destruct and must be replaced. In the presence of infection or inflammation, the bone marrow activity increases greatly, and many leukocytes are produced to counteract the invasion by foreign cells or substances.

Variation in Normal Values

The normal value is higher at birth and declines gradually between ages 1 and 15 years. It then rises to a higher normal range in adulthood. In people of African American ancestry, the normal leukocyte count is lower than in whites primarily because of fewer neutrophils in the total white blood count.

Elevated Values

Leukocytosis, an elevated number of white blood cells, occurs in response to infection and usually is directly proportionate to the degree of bacterial invasion. The bone marrow has responded to the infection by producing more neutrophils that will mature into white blood cells. The elevated value may also be caused by inflammation or necrosis of tissue or malignancy of the bone marrow. A white blood cell count of 11,000 to 17,000 cells ($11\text{-}17 \times 10^3/\mu L$ or SI: $11\text{-}17 \times 10^9/L$) is considered to be a mild to moderate leukocytosis.

An elevated white blood cell count will recede and return to normal when the patient is recovering from infection. If the white blood cell count continues to rise, even after antibiotic therapy is administered, it is an indication that the infection is worsening or that there is a noninfectious cause of the elevation. Additional testing may be performed to determine the location of the infection. In noninfectious causes, bone marrow malfunction may be investigated; leukemia is one cause of a dramatic rise in the white blood cell count.

Decreased Values

When the white blood cell count falls to less than normal limits, it is called *leukopenia*. Mild leukopenia is indicated by a white blood cell count of 3000 to 5000 cells ($3\text{-}5 \times 10^3$ cells/mL or SI: $3\text{-}5 \times 10^9$ cells/L). Any marked decrease is usually in neutrophils, although all five forms of leukocytes may be decreased. Decreases in the leukocyte count occur because of the inability of the bone marrow to produce sufficient white blood cells. Leukopenia can be caused by a response to overwhelming infection that has exhausted the supply of neutrophils and bone marrow reserves. It can also be due to leukemia, depression of the bone marrow after radiation treatment or chemotherapy, or because of a toxic reaction to medication.

W

REFERENCE VALUES	Birth: 9.0-30.0 $\times$ 10^3 cells/µL *or* 9-30 $\times$ 10^9 cells/L
	12 months: 6.0-17.5 $\times$ 10^3 cells/µL *or* 6.0-17.5 $\times$ 10^9 cells/L
	6 years: 5.0-14.5 $\times$ 10^3 cells/µL *or* 5.0-14.5 $\times$ 10^9 cells/L
	10 years: 4.5-13.5 $\times$ 10^3 cells/µL *or* 4.5-13.5 $\times$ 10^9 cells/L
	Adult: 4.5-11 $\times$ 10^3 cells/µL *or* SI: 4.5-11 $\times$ 10^9 cells/L
	Adults, African American: 3.6-10.2 $\times$ 10^3 cells/µL *or*
	SI: 3.6-10.2 $\times$ 10^9 cells/L

▽ Critical Values

<2500 cells/mL *or* SI: <2.5 $\times$ 10^9 cells/L
>30,000 cells/mL *or* SI: >30 $\times$ 10^9 cells/L

HOW THE TEST IS DONE

Venipuncture or capillary puncture is done to obtain a specimen of blood.

SIGNIFICANCE OF TEST RESULTS

Elevated Values

Bacterial infection
Lymphoma
Leukemia
Chronic infection
Cancer (liver, bone marrow, intestine)
Leukemoid reaction
Tissue necrosis (burns, gangrene, myocardial infarction)
Mumps
Varicella
Rubeola
Hypersensitivity reaction

Decreased Values

Brucellosis
Typhoid fever
Viral infections (influenza, rubella, hepatitis)
Typhus
Dengue fever
Malaria
Gaucher's disease
Pernicious anemia
Aplastic anemia
Radiation
Antineoplastic drugs
Toxic ingestion of heavy metals or chemical poisons
Systemic lupus erythematosus
Felty syndrome

W

INTERFERING FACTORS

- Strenuous exercise

NURSING CARE

Nursing actions are similar to those used in venipuncture or capillary puncture procedures (see Chapter 2), with the following additional measures.

Pretest

- The specimen should be obtained when the patient is calm and physically still. The nurse organizes the care of the neonate so that minimal disturbance occurs before drawing the blood. The crying infant should be comforted because with stress or distress, the patient's adrenaline causes a rise in the white blood cell count for 15 to 30 minutes.

○ *Patient Teaching.* When the test is planned, the nurse instructs the patient to avoid strenuous exercise for 24 hours before the test. The exercise can cause a very high white blood cell count that is a false positive result.

Posttest

- When infection is suspected or diagnosed, the nurse monitors the patient's temperature and other vital signs every 4 hours, administers extra fluids, encourages the patient to rest, and administers the prescribed medications, such as antipyretics, antibiotics or antimicrobials.

▽ **Nursing Response to Critical Values**

The physician should be notified immediately of either severe elevation or severe decline of the white blood count that is at or beyond the critical values.

Hyperleukocytosis is defined as greater than 100,000 cells/mL (SI: $>100 \times 10^9$ cells/L). It is an extreme elevation of the white blood cell count and is a potential emergency. At this level, the patient may have a fatal hemorrhage in the lung or brain as the leukocytes clump or aggregate in the small blood vessels. Hyperleukocytosis is usually the result of leukemia in the crisis stage. The nurse monitors vital signs frequently and a complete physical assessment is indicated. Particular attention is paid to respiratory and neurologic findings, including levels of consciousness.

Severe leukopenia places the patient at risk because there is little or no defense from infection. Regardless of the medical cause, the patient with leukopenia has diminished ability to defend against infection. The nurse institutes precautionary measures to prevent the patient's exposure to germs. All visitors and employees who enter the patient's room must perform handwashing. Visitors should be limited and no one with an infection should enter the patient's room. If the count declines further, reverse isolation procedures may be instituted.

White Blood Cell Differential Count

Also called: Differential Leukocyte Count; Peripheral Differential; White Blood Cell Morphology; WBC Differential

SPECIMEN OR TYPE OF TEST: Whole Blood

PURPOSE OF THE TEST

The white blood cell differential assesses the ability of the body to respond to and eliminate infection. It also detects the severity of allergic reactions, parasitic and other infections, and identifies various stages of leukemia.

BASICS THE NURSE NEEDS TO KNOW

The white blood cell differential identifies the five different types of leukocytes. The test reports the percentages and cell counts of each type.

Neutrophils are the most active cells and respond to tissue damage or infection. The two types of neutrophils are polymorphonuclear (segmented) neutrophils and bands. Filled with bacteriocidal secretions, these cells are phagocytes that provide an early, rapid removal of cellular debris and a large number of bacteria. Of all the leukocytes, the neutrophils are the largest group.

An elevated value (*neutrophilia*) occurs in response to acute bacterial infection, inflammatory disease, tissue necrosis, and some cancers. A decreased value (*neutropenia*) can be the result of a severe infection that uses up all the reserved supply of neutrophils. It can also be caused by damage or a defect in the bone marrow that results in a decrease in the manufacture of neutrophils. The most common cause of neutropenia is a drug reaction to a specific medication.

The term *left shift* refers to an increase in immature band neutrophils. The increase in band neutrophils is an early indication of infection and the bone marrow's inability to produce sufficient mature segmented neutrophils to keep up with the infection. With decreased numbers of segmented neutrophils, the bone marrow will release proportionately more band neutrophils into the blood. The increase in bands may also be due to malignancy, such as leukemia.

Eosinophils contain antihistamines that kill foreign cells in the blood. The eosinophils also participate in the inflammatory response by phagocytosis. They digest the antigen-antibody complexes and clean up the late stages of inflammation.

Elevated values (*eosinophilia*) occur when extra eosinophils are manufactured to respond to allergic disorders or some parasitic infections in the tissues. Decreased values (*eosinopenia*) occur with most infections that produce purulence.

Basophils are involved in modifying or calming systemic allergic reactions and anaphylaxis. The basophils release histamine, heparin, and serotonin into the circulation during an episode of inflammation.

An elevated value (*basophilia*) occurs during the healing phase of inflammation and in chronic inflammation. It occurs in the presence of hypersensitivity reactions to foods, pollens, injected protein substances, and after radiation therapy. Basophilia often occurs in hematologic disorders, including myeloid leukemia.

Lymphocytes consist of the B cells and T cells that are responsible for the activities of the immune system. The B cells make antibodies and the T cells regulate the immune response.

An elevated lymphocyte count (*lymphocytosis*) occurs in response to viral infection. It also occurs in some hematologic disorders, including lymphocytic leukemia. A decreased value (*lymphopenia or lymphocytopenia*) occurs with impaired lymphatic drainage, long-term drug therapy, and genetically impaired production of lymphocytes. The immunologic deficiency decreases the T lymphocytes.

Monocytes, in the blood, remove debris or foreign particles from the circulation. In the work of phagocytosis, monocytes assist the lymphocytes in an immune response.

W

An elevated value (*monocytosis*) occurs in response to infection of all kinds. An elevated value may be due to a hematologic disease, such as leukemia.

REFERENCE VALUES

Neutrophils
Segmented Neutrophils
Mean percent: 50%-70% *or* SI: 0.50- 0.70 (mean number fraction)
Cell count (range): 2.3-8.1 $\times$ 10^3/μL *or* SI: 2.3-8.1 $\times$ 10^9/L

Bands
Mean percent: 0%-5% *or* SI: 0-0.05 (mean number fraction)
Cell count (range) 0-0.6 $\times$ 10^3/μL *or* SI: 0-0.6 $\times$ 10^9/L

Eosinophils
Mean percent: 1%-3% *or* SI: 0.01-0.03 (mean number fraction)
Cell count (range): 0-0.4 $\times$ 10^3/μL *or* SI: 0-0.4 $\times$ 10^9/L

Basophils
Mean percent: 0%-2% *or* SI: 0-0.02 (mean number fraction)
Cell count (range): 0-0.1$\times$ 10^3/μL *or* SI: 0-0.1 $\times$ 10^9/L

Lymphocytes
Mean percent: 18%-42% *or* SI: 0.18-0.42 (mean number fraction)
Cell count (range): 0.8-4.8 $\times$ 10^3/μL *or* SI: 0.8-4.8 $\times$ 10^9/L

Monocytes
Mean percent: 2%-11% *or* SI: 0.02-0.11 (mean number fraction)
Cell count (range): 0.45-1.3 $\times$ 10^3/μL *or* SI: 0.45-1.3 $\times$ 10^9/L

HOW THE TEST IS DONE

Venipuncture or capillary puncture is performed to obtain a sample of venous blood. For the peripheral blood smear, two slides with coverslips are prepared immediately using drops of venous or capillary blood.

SIGNIFICANCE OF TEST RESULTS

Elevated Values
Neutrophils
Cancer (chronic myelogenous leukemia, sarcoma)
Acute bacterial infection
Severe burns
Trauma
Corticosteroid therapy
Acute inflammatory disease
Ketoacidosis
Uremia

W

Eosinophils
Allergic reaction to some medications
Allergies (hay fever, hives, asthma)
Skin diseases (pemphigus, eczema, exfoliative dermatitis)
Parasitic infection (trichinosis, filariasis, schistosomiasis)
Chronic myelogenous leukemia
Myeloproliferative diseases (Hodgkin's disease, chronic myelogenous leukemia, T-cell lymphoma)
Malignancy
Sarcoidosis
Basophils
Hypersensitivity reactions (allergy to food, medicine, foreign protein)
Ulcerative colitis
Chronic hemolytic anemia
Chronic myeloid leukemia
Infections (varicella)
Polycythemia vera
Lymphocytes
Infectious mononucleosis
Epstein Barr virus infection
Infectious hepatitis
Pertussis
Lymphocytic leukemia
Monocytes
Recovery stage from acute infection
Sarcoidosis
Ulcerative colitis
Leukemia
Myeloproliferative diseases
Multiple myeloma
Hodgkin's disease
Non-Hodgkin's lymphoma
Inflammatory diseases

Decreased Values
Neutrophils
Overwhelming infection
Drug reaction (chloramphenicol, sulfa, antibiotics, benzodiazepine, anticonvulsants, quinine, indomethacin, thiazides, and others)
Rheumatoid arthritis
HIV infection; AIDS
Aplastic anemia
Radiation or chemotherapy
Megaloblastic anemia
Hypersplenism
Cancer of the bone marrow

W

Lymphocytes
Thoracic duct, impaired drainage
Right-sided heart failure
Non-Hodgkin's lymphoma, Hodgkin's disease
Systemic lupus erythematosus
Radiation or chemotherapy
Aplastic anemia
Human immunodeficiency virus infection; AIDS
Infections (tuberculosis, hepatitis, influenza, typhoid fever)
Renal failure
Terminal cancer
Wiskott-Aldrich congenital immunodeficiency

INTERFERING FACTORS

- Exercise
- Pain
- Mental or physical stress
- Heightened emotion

NURSING CARE

Nursing actions are similar to those used in venipuncture or capillary puncture procedures (see Chapter 2), with the following additional measures.

Pretest

- Because the differential count rises falsely in conditions of mental and physical stress, prepare the patient as follows:
- Instruct the physically active patient to avoid strenuous activity for 24 hours before the test because it will cause a false-positive result for neutrophils and lymphocytes.
- Comfort the crying infant. Organize the nursing care of the neonate so that he or she is calm at the time of the test.

Posttest

- Arrange for prompt transport of the blood to the laboratory. Deterioration of the leukocytes begins within 30 minutes.

X-Rays, Conventional

Also called: Plain Film

SPECIMEN OR TYPE OF TEST: Radiography

PURPOSE OF THE TEST

An x-ray film provides a radiographic image of the organs or tissues to detect abnormalities such as tumors, perforations, abscesses, infections, foreign bodies, or fractures of the bone.

X

BASICS THE NURSE NEEDS TO KNOW

Conventional radiographs are low-cost procedures that may be used to provide a preliminary image, with low exposure to radiation for the patient. Computed tomography, magnetic resonance imaging, nuclear scan, and ultrasound have replaced many of the previous uses of radiographs, but the conventional radiograph is still a mainstay of imaging of musculoskeletal tissue, particularly in trauma cases (Renner, 2009).

The source of x-ray emissions are photons created in a special vacuum tube in the x-ray machine. The guided x-ray energy waves are focused on the area of tissue to be imaged. They pass through the patient and onto a photographic plate called an x-ray film. Newer technology is replacing the old method of imaging on film. The new filmless images use computerized digital imaging that is seen on a monitor or display screen.

The varying densities and composition of the tissues permit different amounts of photons to pass through and make photographic images. Dense, thick tissue is more radiopaque, resulting in lighter shades of image. For example, bone contains calcium, a mineral that is radiopaque. Thus bone appears almost white against the contrasting shades of gray of soft tissues and muscles that surround the bones. Conversely, air allows the photons to pass through the tissues or organs such as the lungs, without blockage of the photons. Thus the presence of air (as in the lungs) produces images that are very dark or black. The size, shape, and position of the organs or tissues are accurately visualized because of the differences in the densities and composition of the tissues.

Metal objects absorb or block x-ray emissions and will appear white on the film. Before the radiograph is taken, patients must remove all metal objects and jewelry so that the underlying tissue can be visualized. Radiographs are very useful to image a metallic foreign body that is swallowed, aspirated, or has penetrated the body (Figures 105 and 106).

The radiopacity of metals is useful for protection against unwanted exposure to radiation. The x-ray emissions cannot pass through lead of particular thickness. The patient and staff members wear a lead protective shield or apron to protect reproductive organs and other radio-sensitive tissue. For example, nurses would wear a lead shield in the operating room when radiographs of the patient are taken. Lead is also used to line the walls of the x-ray rooms so that radiation energy cannot pass into the corridors or nearby offices. This protects workers and others from unwanted exposure.

Three-dimensional (3-D) views of the tissue are obtained by filming from the front to the back of the body as well as from the side. In radiology, these views are called anteroposterior and lateral (AP and lateral). Other positions, such as oblique views, may be requested to image a particular section of anatomy that is less visible from a traditional position. All AP x-ray films are viewed as if the patient were facing you. This means that the patient's left side is on your right side. To prevent confusion and possible error in the interpretation of the film, the technician places the letters R and L on the film to indicate the patient's right and left sides.

Chest Radiograph

This film is obtained routinely for preoperative patients to screen for tuberculosis and other serious pulmonary or cardiac diseases. It also provides a preoperative comparison film for the postoperative patient in whom a pulmonary or cardiac complication develops. The chest radiograph is a basic radiologic procedure to identify broken ribs, a pneumothorax, or suspected pulmonary disorder

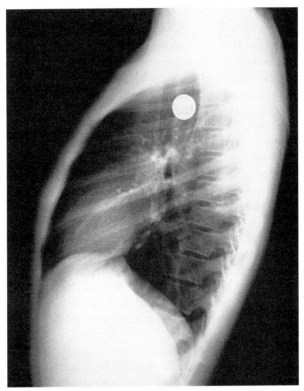

Figure 105. Coin in the esophagus. The coin was swallowed and lodged in a narrowed section of the esophagus. The radiograph *(lateral view)* of the chest shows the metal coin and its location very clearly. (From Mettler FA: *Essentials of radiology,* ed 2, Philadelphia, 2005, Saunders.)

(Figure 107). The chest radiograph also provides data about the heart, including its size and shape. In congenital and acquired cardiac disease, the enlargement of the heart and its atria or ventricles provides information about the improper function of the cardiac valves, pulmonary or aortic arterial hypertension, and venous pulmonary conditions that affect heart size.

Abdominal Radiograph

Various abnormal findings on the abdominal film are useful in obtaining a diagnosis. The patterns of air and gas appear light and bright on the abdominal film. In normal findings, the air remains contained within the intestinal tract. With a perforation of either the stomach or the intestines, the gas escapes into the abdominal cavity. When the patient is seated or in an erect position, the air rises and gathers under the diaphragm, where it is visible on the abdominal x-ray film. In intestinal obstruction, air and fluid collect above the area of obstruction, distending the lumen of the intestine.

Kidney-Ureter-Bladder (KUB) Radiograph

This radiograph images the structure, size, and position of the kidneys, ureters, and bladder, screening for abnormality in these organs and nearby tissues. Calcification of the renal calyces or renal pelvis is visible, as are any radiopaque calculi present in the upper urinary tract.

X

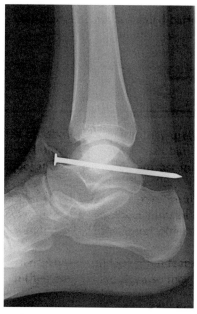

Figure 106. Foreign body. The lateral view of the ankle shows a construction nail that has passed through the talus bone. (From Renner JB. (2009) Conventional radiography in musculoskeletal imaging, *Radiol Clin N Am* 47(3): 357-372.)

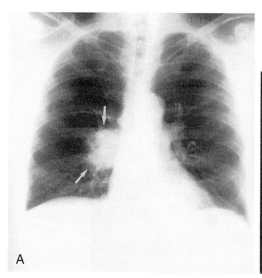

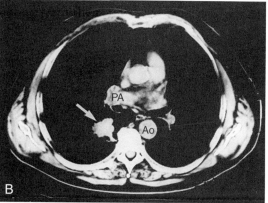

Figure 107. Lung cancer. A, The posteroanterior radiographic view of the lung shows an ill-defined mass *(arrows)*. Its shaggy appearance is very suggestive of carcinoma. **B,** Follow-up with a computed tomography scan on the same patient provides a clear view of the tumor *(arrow)*, its location and relationship to the mediastinal structures, including the pulmonary artery (PA) and aorta (AO). (From Mettler FA: *Essentials of radiology,* ed 2, Philadelphia, 2005, Saunders.)

X

Bone and Joint Radiograph

Radiograph studies are a vital tool in the assessment of bones and joints. In cases of trauma, the radiograph images are used to identify the presence, location, and type of fracture; the potential for injury to the surrounding soft tissue; and the healing activity after the fracture has been treated (Figure 108). Dislocation of a joint, a bone tumor, a bone infection, and a loss of bone mass are also visible. In arthritic disorders or metabolic diseases such as gout, radiograph studies are used to visualize the size and structure of the joints and soft tissues and the alignment of the bones that articulate at the joints.

Child Abuse

When child abuse is suspected as the cause of a skeletal injury, multiple radiograph studies of all parts of the skeleton are performed. In cases of child abuse, the incidence of bone fracture is high, and the sites of skeletal injury are often multiple, particularly in children younger than age 18 months (Figure 109). To differentiate between abuse and other causes of trauma, the radiologist compares the history of how and when the injuries occurred with the radiograph findings. Child abuse or suspected child abuse must be reported to authorities.

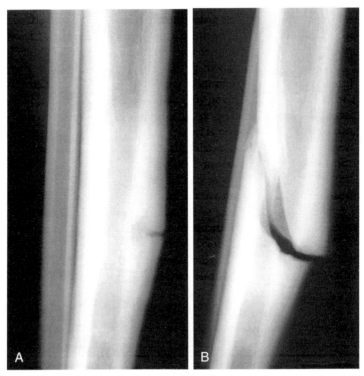

Figure 108. Stress fracture and complete fracture of the tibia. **A,** A runner developed a stress fracture of the tibia, as seen by the linear lucency in the anterior cortex of the bone. **B,** A later radiograph of the same person shows the effect of continued exercise on a long bone that already had a stress fracture. The stress fracture progressed to become a complete fracture. (From Helms CA: *Fundamentals of skeletal radiology*, ed 3, Philadelphia, 2004, Saunders.)

X

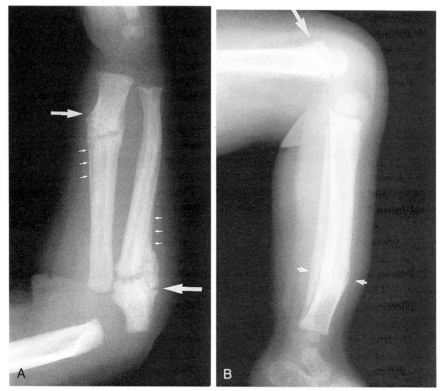

Figure 109. Child abuse. **A,** The forearm of a child, showing extensive periosteal injury *(small arrows)* and transverse fractures *(large arrows)*. Fractures of long bones in children, particularly with different stages of healing, are very suggestive of a battered child. **B,** A lateral view of the lower extremity of the same child also reveals fractures of the fibula and tibia *(small arrows)*, as well as a metaphyseal corner fracture *(large arrow)* of the distal femur. The metaphyseal corner fracture is also typical of child abuse. (From Mettler FA: *Essentials of radiology,* ed 2, Philadelphia, 2005, Saunders.)

REFERENCE VALUES   The size, shape, appearance, thickness, and position of the organs and tissues are within normal limits for the patient's age. No anatomic abnormalities are noted.

HOW THE TEST IS DONE

The patient is positioned so that the correct area of anatomy can be imaged. Several views are taken. The images may be recorded on film or appear as digital images on a computer screen.

SIGNIFICANCE OF TEST RESULTS

Abnormal Values
Chest and Heart
Pneumothorax
Atelectasis
Pleural effusion

X

Pleurisy
Cystic fibrosis
Pulmonary fibrosis
Tumor or cyst
Cor pulmonale
Cardiac hypertrophy
Pneumonia
Tuberculosis
Pulmonary abscess
Chronic obstructive pulmonary disease
Mediastinal nodes
Aortic aneurysm
Congestive heart failure
Adult respiratory distress syndrome
Fracture
Foreign body
Intestinal Tract
Perforation
Obstruction
Paralytic ileus
Volvulus
Intussusception
Subphrenic abscess
Foreign body
Urinary Tract
Renal abscess
Renal tuberculosis
Pyelonephritis
Glomerulonephritis
Polycystic renal disease
Hematoma
Congenital malformation
Tumor or cyst
Renal or ureteral calculus
Hydronephrosis
Amyloidosis
Bones and Joints
Fracture
Dislocation
Subluxation
Bone cyst or tumor
Congenital malformation
Vitamin D deficiency, rickets
Paget's disease
Osteoarthritis
Rheumatoid arthritis

Gout
Osteomyelitis
Osteoporosis
Osteomalacia

INTERFERING FACTORS

- Excessive movement
- Failure to remove jewelry or other metal from the x-ray field
- Improper positioning
- For abdominal and kidney-ureter-bladder films: retained barium or contrast medium, feces, ascites, gas, obesity

NURSING CARE

Pretest

- For the patient who requires an abdominal or kidney-ureter-bladder film, schedule the radiograph study before any radiologic study that uses barium or contrast medium. The contrast medium is radiopaque, and the residual contrast interferes with the visualization of the underlying tissues.
- For most imaging procedures, instruct the patient to remove all clothes and put on a hospital gown. The exceptions are skull radiographs and x-ray films of the distal extremities.
- Instruct the patient to remove all jewelry and metal objects from the area that is to be imaged.
- Provide reassurance to the patient. Young children often fear the equipment, strange room, isolation, and separation from their parents. Adults also may feel somewhat apprehensive.

During the Test

- If the nurse stays with the patient during the imaging, lead protection gear must be worn.
- The patient's safety is a concern at all times, particularly when there is a risk of a fall. The radiography table has no side rails.
- The radiology technician will position the patient for the specific views needed.
- The patient must remain motionless during the imaging. Sometimes the patient is instructed to inhale deeply and hold the breath until the image is taken.
- After the images are completed, the patient waits in the imaging area as the decision is made concerning whether additional x-ray films are needed. A blanket or extra gown for the patient will help prevent a chill in the cool room.

Posttest

- The patient may need assistance in dismounting from the radiography table and getting dressed, as needed.

X

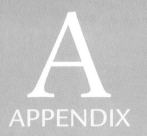

A
APPENDIX

Therapeutic Drug Monitoring

Therapeutic drug monitoring provides exact information about the quantity of medication that is in the blood. This testing is performed for several reasons. In the patient with a normal metabolism, the standard dose and schedule of a particular medication usually results in a therapeutic blood level of the medication within a specific period. In other patients, such as elderly individuals, neonates, and obese persons, the standard dose may produce a diminished or excessive clinical result because of abnormal metabolism or diminished renal or hepatic function. Therapeutic drug monitoring is used to adjust the dose and schedule of medications as needed.

For a variety of reasons, many patients do not take their medication in the same amount or same frequency, as prescribed. This is commonly referred to as "medication nonadherence." Therapeutic drug monitoring provides data to alert the physician or nurse about the need to investigate the problem of a patient's result that is above or below the expected therapeutic range.

Some medications have a narrow range of values for a therapeutic effect. They are known as "narrow therapeutic index" drugs. A small increase beyond that range can have a toxic result. Therapeutic drug monitoring is carried out to protect the patient from the potential harm of excess medication.

With some medications, the therapeutic value and the critical value are reported as peak and trough values. *Peak value* refers to the highest therapeutic level of medication in the blood. This usually occurs at a particular time interval after the medication has been taken or administered. For some drugs, the peak value occurs a few hours after it is taken. Other drugs do not reach their peak value in the blood for days after continuing the medication regimen. The *trough value* identifies the lowest therapeutic level of medication in the blood, usually just before the next dose. Because of the variations of timing, the nurse should consult the laboratory as to when the blood specimen should be drawn for a peak or trough value, as needed.

In the case of overdose (accidental or deliberate), laboratory testing can identify the medication and the amount that is in the blood. The patient may be comatose, psychotic, or agitated from the effect of the overdose and may be unable to identify or describe what was ingested. The test results can also confirm or refute that the drug in question is responsible for the clinical symptoms and condition of the patient. Based on accurate test results, corrective action can be taken.

The following table provides the range of blood values of selected medications to measure for therapeutic effect and for toxicity. For therapeutic drug monitoring, the tests are ordered at planned intervals to establish and maintain an effective medication level in the blood. To identify a critical value or a toxic level of the medication, the laboratory test also may be ordered when the patient demonstrates side effects to the medication or when an unexplained change in behavior, such as agitation, seizures, or loss of consciousness can be caused by toxicity.

The classes of medications that are commonly monitored include: analgesics, antiarrhythmics, antiasthmatics, antibiotics, anticonvulsants, antidepressants, antipsychotics, and immunosuppressants.

Therapeutic Drug Monitoring

Drug	Therapeutic Range	Critical Value (Toxic Value)
Acetaminophen (Tylenol)	10-30 µg/mL SI: 66-199 µmol/L	*4 hours after ingestion* >200 µg/mL SI: >1324 µmol/L *12 hours after ingestion* >50 µg/mL SI: >132 µmol/L
Amikacin (Amikin)	Peak: 25-35 µg/mL SI: 43-60 µmol/L Less severe infection Trough: 1-4 µg/mL SI: 1.7-6.8 µmol/L More severe infection Trough: 4-8 µg/mL SI: 6.8-13.7µmol/L	Peak: >35 µg/mL SI: 60 µmol/L Trough: >10 µg/mL SI: >17 µmol/L
Amiodarone (Cordarone)	1.0-2.0 µg/mL SI: 1.5-3.1 µmol/L	>3.5 µg/mL SI: >5.4 µmol/L
Amitriptyline (Elavil)	80-250 ng/mL SI: 289-903 nmol/L	>500 ng/mL SI: >1805 nmol/L
Amobarbital (Amytal)	1-5 µg/mL SI: >4-22µmol/L	>10 µg/mL SI: >44 µmol/L
Amoxapine (Asendin)	200-600 ng/mL SI: 638-1914 nmol/L	>600 ng/mL SI: >1914 nmol/L
Amphetamine	20-30 ng/mL SI: 148-222 nmol/L	>200 ng/mL SI: >1480 nmol/L
Bupropion (Wellbutrin, Zyban)	25-100 ng/mL SI: 104-417 nmol/L	>100 ng/mL SI: >417 nmol/L
Caffeine	5-25 µg/mL SI: 26-129 µmol/L	>50 µg/mL SI: >258µmol/L
Carbamazepine (Tegretrol)	4-12 µg/mL SI: 17-51 µmol/L	>15 µg/mL SI: >63 µmol/L
Carbenicillin (Geopen)	Dependent on minimum inhibition concentration of specific organism SI: same	>250 µg/mL (neurotoxicity) SI: >660 µmol/L
Chloral hydrate (Noctec), as trichloroethanol	2-12 µg/mL SI: 13-80 µmol/L	>20 µg/mL SI: >134 µmol/L
Chloramphenicol (Chloromycetin)	10-25 µg/mL SI: >25 µmol/L	>20 µg/mL SI: >77 µmol/L
Chlordiazepoxide (Librium)	700-1000 ng/mL SI: 2.3-3.3 µmol/L	>5000 ng/mL SI: >16.7 µmol/L

Continued

Therapeutic Drug Monitoring—cont'd		
Drug	Therapeutic Range	Critical Value (Toxic Value)
Chlorpromazine (Thorazine)	Adult: 50-300 ng/mL SI: 157-942 nmol/L Child: 40-80 ng/mL SI: 126-251 nmol/L	>750 ng/mL SI: 2355 nmol/L
Cimetidine (Tagamet)	Trough: 0.5-1.2 µg/mL SI: 2.0-5.0 µmol/L	>1.3 µg/mL SI: >5.1 µmol/L
Ciprofloxacin	Peak oral dose: 0.5-1.5 µg/mL SI: 1.51-4.53 µmol/L Peak IV dose: <5.0 µg/mL SI: <15.1 µmol/L	>5.0 µg/mL SI: >15.1 µmol/L
Clonidine (Catapres)	1.0-2.0 ng/mL SI: 4.4-8.7 nmol/L	
Clozapine (Clozaril)	100-600 ng/mL SI: 306-1836 nmol/L	>900 ng/mL SI: >27,754 nmol/L
Cyclosporin A (Sandimmune)	12 hours after dose: 100 ng/mL SI: 83-333 nmol/L 24 hours after dose:100-200 ng/mL SI: 83-166 nmol/L	>400 ng/mL SI: >333 nmol/L
Desipramine (Norpramin)	75-300 ng/mL SI: 281-1125 nmol/L	>400 ng/mL SI: >1500 nmol/L
Diazepam (Valium)	100-1000 ng/mL SI: 0.35-3.51 µmol/L	>5000 ng/mL >17 µmol/L
Digoxin (Lanoxin)	0.5-1.5 ng/mL SI: 0.64-1.92 nmol/L	Adult: >2.0 ng/mL SI: >2.6 nmol/L Child: >3.0 ng/mL SI: >3.8 nmol/L
Disopyramide (Norpace)	*For atrial arrhythmia:* 2.0-5.0 µg/mL SI: 5.9-14.8 µmol/L *For ventricular arrhythmia:* 3.3-7.5 0 µg/mL SI: 9.7-22.1 µmol/L	>7 µg/mL SI: >20.6 µmol/L
Ephedrine	0.05-0.10 µg/mL SI: 0.3-0.6 µmol/L	>2 µg/mL SI: >12.1 µmol/L
Ethchlorvynol (Placidyl)	2-8 µg/mL SI: 14-55 µmol/L	>20 µg/mL SI: >138 µmol/L
Flecainide (Tambocor)	0.2-1.0 µg/mL SI: 0.5-2.4 µmol/L	>1.0 µg/mL SI: >2.4 µmol/L
Fluoxetine (Prozac)	90-1150 ng/mL 291-3715 nmol/L	

Therapeutic Drug Monitoring—cont'd

Drug	Therapeutic Range	Critical Value (Toxic Value)
Flurazepam (Dalmane)		>0.2 µg/mL SI: >0.5 µmol/L
Gabapentin (Neurontin)	5.9-21 µg/mL SI: 34.5-123 µmol/L	>85 µg/mL SI: >327 µmol/L
Gentamycin (Garamycin)	*Peak: Less severe infection:* 5-8 µg/mL SI: 10.5-16.7 µmol/L *Peak: severe infection:* 8-10 µg/mL SI:16.7- 20.9 µmol/L *Trough: Less severe infection:* <1.0 µg/mL SI:< 2.0 µmol/L *Trough: severe infection:* <4.0 µg/mL SI:<8.0 µmol/L	Peak: >10µg/mL SI: >21 µmol/L Trough: >2.0µg/mL SI: >4.0 µmol/L
Haloperidol (Haldol)	1-10 ng/mL SI: 2.7-26.6 nmol/L	
Ibuprofen (Motrin)	10-50 µg/mL SI: > 49-243 µmol/L	>100 µg/mL SI: >485 µmol/L
Imipramine (Tofranil)	150-250 ng/mL SI: 536-893 nmol/L	>500 ng/L SI: >1785 nmol/L
Isoniazid (Hyzyd, Nydrazid)	1.0-7.0 µg/mL SI: >7.0-51.0 µmol/L	>20 µg/mL SI: >146 µmol/L
Kanamycin (Kantrex)	*Peak: 25-35µg/mL* SI: 52-72 µmol/L *Trough: Less severe infection:* <1.0-4.0 µg/mL SI: 2.0-8.0 µmol/L *Trough: severe infection:* 4.0-8.0 µg/mL SI: 8.0-17.0 µmol/L	Peak: >35 µg/mL SI: >72 µmol/L Trough: >10.0 µg/mL SI: >21.0 µmol/L
Lidocaine (Xylocaine)	2-6 mg/mL SI: 6.4-25.6 mmol/L	6-8 mg/mL or higher SI: 25.6-34.2 mmol/L or higher
Lithium (Eskalith)	0.6-1.2 mEq/L SI: 0.6-1.2 mmol/L	>2 mEq/L >2 mmol/L
Meprobamate (Equanil)	6-12 µg/mL SI: 28-55 µmol/L	>60 µg/mL SI: >275 µmol/L

Continued

Therapeutic Drug Monitoring—cont'd

Drug	Therapeutic Range	Critical Value (Toxic Value)
Methotrexate	Variable; dosage dependent	*1-2 weeks after low dose therapy* >0.2 µmol/L SI: >0.2 µmol/L *24 hours after high dose therapy* ≥ 5.0 µmol/L SI: ≥ 5.0 µmol/L *72 hours after high dose therapy* ≥ 0.05 µmol/L SI: ≥ 0.05 µmol/L
Methyldopa (Aldomet)	1.0 -5.0 µg/mL SI: >4.7-23.7 µmol/L	>7 µg/mL SI: >33 µmol/L
Nelfinavir (Viracept)	1-3 µg/mL SI: >1.5-4.5 µmol/L	>3 µg/mL SI: >4.5 µmol/L

Nevirapine (Viramune)	Peak: 10-15 µg/mL
	  SI: >37.6-56.4 µmol/L
	Trough: 3-8 µg/mL
	  SI: >11.3-30.1 µmol/L
		>15 µg/mL
		SI: >56.4 µmol/L

Netilmicin (Netromycin)	*Peak: Less severe infection:*
	  5-8 µg/mL
	  SI: 10-17 µmol/L
	  Severe infection:
	  8-10 µmol/L
	  SI 17-21 µmol/L
	Trough: Less severe infection:
	  <1.0 µg/mL
	  SI: <2.0 µmol/L
	Trough: severe infection:
	  < 4.0 µg/mL
	  SI: <8.0 µmol/L
		Peak: >10 µg/mL
		SI: >21 µmol/L
		Trough: >2.0 µg/mL
		SI: >4.0 µmol/L

Nortriptyline (Aventyl)	50-150 ng/mL SI: 190-570 nmol/L	>500 ng/ml SI: >1900 nmol/L
Phenobarbital (Luminal)	Children: 15-35 µg/mL SI: >65-151 µmol/L Adults: 20-40 µg/mL SI: >86-173 µmol/L	35-80 µg/mL SI: >151-345µmol/L
Phenytoin (Dilantin)	10-20 µg/mL SI: >40-79 µmol/L	>20 µg/mL SI: >79 µmol/L
Procainamide (Pronestyl)	4-12 µg/mL SI: >17-51 µmol/L	>10 µg/mL SI: >42 µmol/L
Propranolol (Inderal)	20-100 ng/mL SI: 77-386 nmol/L	

Therapeutic Drug Monitoring—cont'd		
Drug	Therapeutic Range	Critical Value (Toxic Value)
Quinine	5-10 µg/mL SI: 15.4-30.8 µmol/L	>10 µg/mL SI: >30.8 µmol/L
Salicylates as salicylic acid	*For analgesia; antipyresis:* <100 µg/mL SI: <0.72 mmol/L *For antiinflammatory:* 150-300 µg/mL SI: 1.09-2.17 mmol/L	Lethal, 24+ hours after a dose or with chronic ingestion: >500 µg/mL SI: >3.62 mmol/L
Theophylline	10-20 µg/mL SI: 56-111 µmol/L	>20 µg/mL >111 µmol/L
Thioridazine (Mellaril)	1.0-1.5 µg/mL SI: >2.7-4.1 µmol/L	>10 µg/mL SI: >27 µmol/L
Tobramycin (Nebcin)	*Peak: Less severe infection:* 5-8 µg/mL SI: 11-17 µmol/L *Severe infection:* 8-10 µg/mL SI 17-21 µmol/L *Trough: Less severe infection:* <1.0 µg/mL SI: <2.0 µmol/L *Trough: severe infection:* <4.0 µg/mL SI: <9.0 µmol/L	Peak :>10 µg/mL SI: >21 µmol/L Trough: >2.0 µg/mL SI: >4.0 µmol/L
Tolbutamide (Orinase)	90-240 µg/mL SI: >333-888 µmol/L	>640 µg/mL SI: >2368 µmol/L
Vancomycin (Vancocin)	Peak: 20-40 µg/mL SI: >14-28 µmol/L Trough: 5-10 µg/mL SI: >3-7 µmol/L	>80 µg/mL SI: >55 µmol/L
Valproic Acid (Depakene)	50-100 µg/mL SI: >346-693 µmol/L	>100 µg/mL SI: > 693 µmol/L
Warfarin (Coumadin)	1-10 µg/mL SI: >3-32 µmol/L	>10 µg/mL SI: >32 µmol/L
Zidovudine (AZT, Retrovir)	0.02-1.2 µg/mL SI: >0.08-4.49 µmol/L	>1.2 µg/mL SI: >4.49 µmol/L

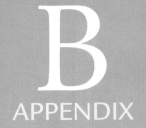

B

APPENDIX

Toxic Substances

Screening for toxic substances is performed to identify the agent responsible for an acute, chronic, or possibly life-threatening illness. Some of these toxic substances are drugs of abuse and have been taken in an unknown quantity. The clinical effect of the substance varies among individuals who are occasional or habitual users. It can also vary with the preparation or mixture that was inhaled, injected, or eaten.

Some toxic substances are ingested by small children. The poisons commonly ingested include rat poison, antifreeze, and insecticide. Other toxic substances that can be identified by laboratory testing are toxic chemicals and metals that poison the individual from an environmental source, including inhalation of poisonous gases from a fire and exposure to hazardous industrial wastes. When the individual is acutely ill from any of these toxic substances, it is essential to identify the cause. Appropriate action can then be taken to reverse the effect and protect the organs from further damage. Some of the toxins pose a long-term threat because they cause mutation and eventual malignancy.

In the following table, the values for the normal range of a toxic substance vary from none to minute amounts. The values for toxicity levels are not always defined. The toxicity may vary among individuals, or its very presence may be considered toxic.

Toxic Substances			
Substance	Specimen	Reference Value	Critical Value (Toxic Level)
Alcohol (ethanol, ETOH)	Blood	Negative	>300 mg/dL SI: 65.1 mmol/L
Amphetamine	Blood	Negative	200 ng/mL* SI: 1480 nmol/L
Arsenic	Blood	2-23 µg/mL SI: 0.03-0.31 µmol/L	Acute poisoning: 6000-9300 µg/L SI:7.98-123.69 µmol/L
	Urine, 24 hours	5-50 µg/day SI: 0.067-0.665 µmol/day	Acute poisoning: 1000-20,000 µg/L/24 hours SI: 13.3-266 µmol/L/24 hours
	Hair	<65 µg/100 g dry weight SI: <8.65 nmol/g dry weight	Acute poisoning: 20,000 µg/100 g dry weight SI: 13.3-266 µmol/L/24 hours

Toxic Substances—cont'd

Substance	Specimen	Reference Value	Critical Value (Toxic Level)
Cadmium	Blood	Nonsmokers: 0.3-1.2 μg/L SI: 2.7-10.7 nmol/L Smokers: 0.6-0.9 μg/L SI: 5.3-34.7 nmol/L	Toxic: 100-3000 μg/L SI: 2660 μmol/L
	Urine	0.5-4.7 μg/L SI: 4.4-41.8 nmol/L	
Carbon Monoxide (Carboxyhemoglobin)	Blood	Nonsmokers: 0.5-1.5 % saturation of Hb SI: 0.005-0.015 fraction of Hb saturation Heavy Smokers: 8-9 % saturation of Hb SI: 0.08-0.09 fraction of Hb saturation	Toxic: >20 % saturation of Hb SI: >0.20 fraction of Hb saturation Lethal: >50% saturation of Hb SI: >0.50 fraction of Hb saturation
Cocaine	Blood	Negative	Toxic: >1000 ng/mL SI: 3300 nmol/L
Cyanide	Serum	Nonsmokers: 0.004 mg//L SI: 0.15 μmol/L Smokers: 0.006 mg//L SI: 0.23 μmol/L	Toxic: >1.00 mg//L SI: >38-40 μmol/L
Ethylene glycol (antifreeze)	Blood	Negative	0.6-4.3 g/L
Fluoride	Plasma	0.01-0.20 mg/L SI: 0.5-10.5 mmol/L	Not well established
	Urine	0.2-3.2 mg/L SI: 10.5-168 mmol/L Occupational exposure: <8.0 mg/L SI: <421 mmol/L	
Lead	Blood	Child: <10 μg/dL SI: <0.48 μmol/L Adult: <25 μg/dL SI: 1.21 μmol/L	Toxic: (Blood): >69 μg/dL SI: >3.33 μmol/L Toxic: (Blood): >99 μg/L SI: >4.78 μmol/L

Continued

Toxic Substances—cont'd			
Substance	Specimen	Reference Value	Critical Value (Toxic Level)
Lysergic Acid Diethylamide (LSD)	Plasma	Negative	Toxic concentration: >1.0 ng/ml SI: >3.09 nmol/L
Manganese	Blood	10.9 ± 0.6 µg/L SI: 198 ± 11 nmol/L	
	Urine	0.5-9.8 µg/L SI: 9.1-178 nmol/L	Toxic: >10 µg/L SI: >182 nmol/L
Mercury	Blood	0.6-59.9 µg/L SI: 3.0-294.4 mmol/L	
	Urine, 24 hour	<20 µg/L SI: <0.10 mmol/L	Toxic: >150 µg/L SI: >0.75 mmol/L Lethal: >800 µg/L SI: >4.0 mmol/L
Methadone	Blood	Negative Therapeutic level: 100-400 ng/mL SI: 0.32-1.29 µmol/L	Toxic: >2000 ng/mL* SI: 6.46 µmol/L
Methanol	Blood	<1.5 mg/L SI:<0.05 mmol/L	Toxic: >200 mg/dL SI: >6.24 mmol/L
Oxycodone (Percodan)	Blood	Negative Therapeutic: 10-100 ng/mL SI: 32-317 nmol/L	Toxic: >200 ng/mL SI: >634 nmol/L
Phencyclidine (PCP)	Blood	Negative	Toxic, nonfatal: 0.02-1.00 µg/mL SI: 0.08-0.41 µmol/L Lethal: 0.5-4.0 µg/mL SI: 2.06-16.44 µmol/L

*The toxic values of amphetamines and methadone may be different for addicts.

Abbreviations Associated with Laboratory Tests

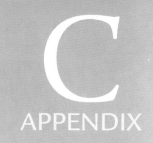

Abbreviation	Complete Name
A-a	Alveolar-arterial
ABI	Ankle-brachial index
ACE	Angiotensin-converting enzyme
ACT	Activated clotting time
ACTH	Adrenocorticotrophic hormone
ADH	Antidiuretic hormone
AFAFP	Amniotic fluid alpha fetoprotein
AFP	Alpha fetoprotein
A/G	Albumin/globulin ratio
AGT	Antiglobulin test
ALB	Albumin
ALP	Alkaline phosphatase
ALT	Alanine aminotransferase
ANA	Antinuclear antibody
Anti-HAV	Hepatitis A antibody
Anti-HBc	Hepatitis B core antibody
Anti-Be	Hepatitis Be antibody
Anti-HCV	Hepatitis C virus antibody
APTT	Activated partial thromboplastin time
ART	Automated reagin test
AST	Aspartate aminotransferase
BAO	Basal acid output
BE	Barium enema
BUN	Blood urea nitrogen
C&S	Culture and susceptibility
Ca, Ca^{2+}	Calcium
Ca_i	Calcium, ionized
CA 19-9	Carbohydrate antigen 19-9
CA 125	Cancer antigen 125
CAT	Computed axial tomography
CBC	Complete blood count
CCr	Creatinine clearance
CEA	Carcinoembryonic antigen
CH_{50}	Complement, total
CK	Creatine kinase

Continued

Abbreviation	Complete Name
Cl^-	Chloride ion
CO_2	Carbon dioxide
CPK	Creatine phosphatase
CRH	Corticotropin releasing hormone
CRP	C-reactive protein
CSF	Cerebrospinal fluid
CT	Calcitonin
CT	Computed tomography
cTnI	Cardiac troponin I
cTnT	Cardiac troponin T
CVS	Chorionic villus sampling
DAT	Direct antiglobulin test
DOPAC	Dihydroxyphenyl acetic acid
DSA	Digital subtraction angiography
DVI	Digital vascular imaging
E_2	Estradiol
E_3	Estriol
EA	Early antigen
EBNA	Epstein-Barr nuclear antigen
ECG	Electrocardiogram
ECHO	Echocardiogram
ECT	Emissions computed tomography
EEG	Electroencephalogram
EGD	Esophagogastroduodenoscopy
EIA	Enzyme immunoassay
EKG	Electrocardiogram
ELISA	Enzyme-linked immunoassay
EMG	Electromyography
EP	Erythropoietin
EPS	Electrophysiologic studies
ERC	Endoscopic retrograde cholangiography
ERCP	Endoscopic retrograde cholangiopancreatography
ER/PGR	Estrogen/progesterone assay
ERV	Expiratory reserve volume
ESR	Erythrocyte sedimentation rate
EUG	Excretory urogram
EUS	Endoscopic ultrasound
FBP	Fibrin breakdown products
FBS	Fasting blood glucose
FDP	Fibrin degradation products
FEF	Forced expiratory flow
FEV	Forced expiratory volume
fFN	Fetal fibronectin
FNA	Fine needle aspiration

Abbreviation	Complete Name
FNB	Fine needle biopsy
FOB	Fetal occult blood
FRC	Functional residual capacity
FSH	Follicle stimulating hormone
FSP	Fibrin-split products
FT_3	Free triiodothyronine
FT_4	Free thyroxine
FTA-ABS	Fluorescent treponemal antibody absorption test
FVC	Forced vital capacity
GB	Gallbladder
GEST	Graded exercise testing
GGT	Gamma-glutamyltransferase
GGPT	Gamma-glutamyltranspeptidase
GH	Growth hormone
GHb	Glycohemoglobin
GLU	Glucose
GPT	Glutamic pyruvic transaminase
G-6-PD	Glucose-6-phosphate dehydrogenase
GTP	Glutamyl transpeptidase
HAA	Hepatitis associated antigen
HAP	Haptoglobin
HAV, Ab	Hepatitis A virus antibody
HAVAB	Hepatitis A virus antibody
Hb	Hemoglobin
HBA_1	Glycosylated hemoglobin
HBcAb	Hepatitis B core antibody
HBeAb	Hepatitis Be antibody
HBeAg	Hepatitis Be antigen
HbF	Fetal hemoglobin
Hbg	Hemoglobin
HBsAb	Hepatitis B surface antibody
HBsAg	Hepatitis B surface antigen
hCG	Human chorionic gonadotrophin
HCO_3	Bicarbonate
Hct	Hematocrit
HDL	High density lipoprotein
HLA	Human leukocyte antigen
HSV	Herpes simplex virus
IADSA	Intraarterial subtraction angiography
I-ALP	Alkaline phosphatase isoenzymes
IAT	Indirect antiglobulin test
IC	Inspiratory capacity
IF	Intrinsic factor
IgG	Immunoglobulin G

Continued

Abbreviation	Complete Name
IgM	Immunoglobulin M
INR	International normalized ratio
IRV	Inspiratory reserve volume
ITT	Insulin tolerance test
IUG	Intravenous urography
IVDSA	Intravenous digital subtraction angiography
IVFA	Intravenous fluorescent angiography
IVP	Intravenous pyelography
IVU	Intravenous urography
IVUS	Intravascular ultrasound
K^+	Potassium ion
17-KGS	17-Ketogenic steroid
17-KS	17-Ketosteroid
LAP	Leucine aminopeptidase
LATS	Long-acting thyroid stimulator
LDH	Lactate dehydrogenase
LDL	Low-density lipoprotein
LDM	Low-dose myelography
LH	Luteinizing hormone
LP	Lumbar puncture
L/S	Lecithin-sphingomyelin
Mb	Myoglobin
MBC	Maximum breathing capacity
MCH	Mean corpuscular hemoglobin
MCHC	Mean corpuscular hemoglobin concentration
MCV	Mean corpuscular volume
MDCT	Multidetector computed tomography
Mg, Mg^{2+}	Magnesium, magnesium ion
MHA-TP	Microhemagglutinin assay-Treponema pallidum
MMEF	Forced midexpiratory flow
MPV	Mean platelet volume
MRI	Magnetic resonance imaging
MUGA	Multiple gated acquisition angiography
MV	Minute volume
MVV	Maximum voluntary ventilation
5'N	5'-Nucleotidase
Na^+	Sodium ion
NAP	Neutrophil alkaline phosphatase
NCS	Nerve conduction study
NH_3	Ammonia
NPO	Nothing by mouth
NST	Nonstress testing
O & P	Ova and parasites
O_2 sat	Oxygenation saturation

Abbreviation	Complete Name
OF	Osmotic fragility
OGTT	Oral glucose tolerance test
P_4	Progesterone
PAP	Papanicolaou smear
PAP	Prostatic acid phosphatase
PCA	Parietal cell antibody
pCO_2	Partial pressure of carbon dioxide
P_{cr}	Plasma creatinine
PCR	Polymerase chain reaction
PCV	Packed cell volume
Pdi	Transdiaphragmatic pressure
PET	Positron emission tomography scan
PET_{CO_2}	End tidal partial pressure of carbon dioxide
pH	Partial pressure of hydrogen
Phe	Phenylalanine
Pimax	Maximum intrathoracic pressure
PKU	Phenylketonuria
PNB	Percutaneous needle biopsy
pO_2	Partial pressure of oxygen
PO_4^{3-}	Phosphate
PRA	Plasma renin activity
PSA	Phosphate specific antigen
PT	Prothrombin time
PTC	Percutaneous transhepatic cholangiography
PTH	Parathyroid hormone
PTT	Partial thromboplastin time
PUBS	Percutaneous umbilical cord sampling
pvO_2	Partial pressure of oxygen in the venous system
RAIU	Radioactive iodine uptake
RBC	Red blood cell, erythrocyte
RDW	Red cell distribution width
RF	Rheumatoid factor
RIA	Radioimmunoassay
RPR	Rapid plasma reagin
RT_3U	Resin triiodothyronine uptake
RV	Residual volume
SACE	Serum angiotensin-converting enzyme
SAECG	Signal-averaged electrocardiogram
SAo_2	Arterial oxygen saturation
SBGM	Self-blood glucose monitoring
SGOT	Serum glutamic-oxaloacetic transaminase
SGPT	Serum glutamate-pyruvate transaminase
SHBD	Serum hydroxybutyrate dehydrogenase
SI	Système International (International System of Units)

Continued

Abbreviation	Complete Name
SMUG	Self-monitoring of urinary glucose
SPECT	Single positron emission computed tomography
STH	Growth hormone; somatotropin
Svo_2	Oxygen saturation in the venous system
T & C	Type and crossmatch
T-ALP	Total alkaline phosphatase
T_3	Triiodothyronine
T_4	Thyroxine
TBG	Thyroxine-binding globulin
tCO_2	Total carbon dioxide
TEE	Transesophageal echocardiography
TIBC	Total iron-binding capacity
TLC	Total lung capacity
TP	Total protein
TRH	Thyroid-releasing hormone
TSH	Thyroid-stimulating hormone
TUS	Transluminal ultrasound
TV	Tidal volume
UA	Urinalysis
VBN	Virtual bronchoscopic navigator
VC	Vital capacity
VCA	Viral capsid antigen
VCG	Vectorcardiogram
Vds	Dead space volume
VDRL	Venereal Disease Research Laboratory
VMA	Vanillylmandelic acid
V/Q	Ventilation/perfusion
WBC	White blood cell

Common Laboratory and Diagnostic Tests for Frequently Occurring Medical Diagnoses

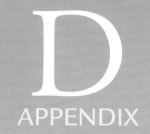

D
APPENDIX

When caring for the patient, there are a number of laboratory tests and diagnostic procedures that the physician or nurse practitioner uses to make a diagnosis as to what has caused the illness and to determine the seriousness or extent of the disease. In the table below, common medical conditions are listed with the tests that are specific to that diagnosis. Generally, when specific tests can confirm or support the diagnosis, the list is somewhat shorter. In conditions where there are no specific tests, there is a longer list of tests that provides partial information.

Essential parts of the diagnostic process begin with the patient's history and the physical examination. The physician or nurse practitioner uses this important, initial information as a guide to determine what is wrong. The diagnostic procedures and laboratory tests that are selected confirm or support the diagnosis by providing measurable, objective data. The physician or nurse practitioner uses all of the data, in totality, to arrive at a definitive diagnosis.

There are some tests that may provide similar information regarding the disease. For example, CT scan, MRI, ultrasound, and nuclear imaging all provide visualization of the particular organ. In cases of infection, culture, antigen/antibody tests, and PCR-DNA identification of the organism all identify or help identify the microbial cause of the infection. The physician or nurse practitioner selects some of the tests because they are the most useful or specific in the individual patient's circumstance. If the tests do not identify the cause, or they provide partial data only, additional tests or procedures will be ordered.

The nurse notes that there are some tests and procedures that are used to exclude or rule out other conditions that have presented similar symptoms. Additionally, some tests may be ordered that are supportive of the diagnosis or used to identify possible complications. In the following table, the tests listed are specific to the medical diagnosis and do not include tests to exclude other diagnoses or verify complications.

Clinical Guides to Diagnoses	
Common Medical Diagnoses	Common Tests Used
Acquired immune deficiency syndrome	Rapid HIV antibody test, blood, saliva, urine Western Blot antibody test P24 antigen HIV-RNA CD4 (T) lymphocyte count Viral load (RT-PCR)

Continued

Clinical Guides to Diagnoses—cont'd	
Common Medical Diagnoses	**Common Tests Used**
Addison's disease	Adrenocorticotrophic hormone, plasma
	Corticotrophic stimulation test
	Cortisol, serum, plasma
	Electrolytes, serum
	Growth hormone, serum
	Osmolarity, urine
	Sodium, urine
	Thyroid stimulating hormone, serum
	Thyroxine, serum
Aldosteronism	Adrenal vein catheterization for renin
	Aldosterone, serum or plasma
	Computed tomography scan, abdomen
	Electrolytes, serum
	Potassium, urine
	Renin, plasma
	Sodium, urine
Alzheimer's disease	Lumbar puncture
	Cerebrospinal analysis
	Beta amyloid (1-42)
	PET scan
Anemia	Complete blood count (CBC)
	Hemoglobin
	Hematocrit
	Red blood cell morphology, peripheral blood
	Red blood cell indices
	Reticulocyte count
	Bone marrow aspiration and biopsy
Anemia, iron deficiency	CBC
	Red blood cell morphology, peripheral blood
	Ferritin, serum
	Iron, serum
	Transferrin, serum
	Total iron binding capacity
	Biopsy, bone marrow
	Occult blood, feces
Anemia, sickle cell	Sickle cell testing, newborn screening test, peripheral blood
	Hemoglobin electrophoresis
	CBC
	Red blood cell morphology, peripheral blood
	In pregnancy, amniocentesis for chromosomal and genetic analysis

Clinical Guides to Diagnoses—cont'd

Common Medical Diagnoses	Common Tests Used
Aneurysm, aortic	Computed tomography
	Computed tomography arteriogram (CTA)
	B-mode ultrasonography
	Magnetic resonance angiography (MRA), as needed
Angina	Cardiac markers
	Cardiac catheterization
	Echocardiogram
	Electrocardiogram
	Holter monitoring
	Lipids, serum
	Thallium stress testing
Appendicitis	Computed tomography, abdomen
	Complete blood count
	White blood cell count
	White blood cell count differential
Arthritis, rheumatoid	Complete blood count
	Erythrocyte sedimentation rate
	C-reactive protein
	Rheumatoid factor
	Arthrocentesis, with synovial fluid analysis
	Radiograph, affected joints
Ascariasis	Stool for ova and parasites
	Complete blood count
	Eosinophil count
Asthma	Allergen identification
	Arterial blood gases
	Eosinophil count
	Culture, sputum
	Pulmonary function studies
	Radiograph, chest
Bronchitis	Arterial blood gases
	Culture, bacterial, sputum
	Culture, viral, sputum
	Radiograph, chest
Cancer, bone	Radiograph, bone
	Bone scan, nuclear
	Computed tomography, bone
	Magnetic resonance imaging, bone, extremity
	Bone biopsy
Cancer, bone marrow	*See* Leukemia

Continued

Clinical Guides to Diagnoses—cont'd	
Common Medical Diagnoses	**Common Tests Used**
Cancer, breast	Mammography
	Biopsy, breast
	Estrogen receptor and progesterone receptor assay, breast biopsy specimen
	Her-2*neu*, breast biopsy specimen, serum
	Carcinogenic embryonic antigen, serum
	Bone scan
Cancer, cervix	Papanicolaou smear
	Cervicovaginal cytology
	Carcinogenic embryonic antigen, serum
	Human papilloma virus-DNA
	Colposcopy
	Ultrasound, pelvis
Cancer, colorectal	Occult blood, feces
	Colonoscopy
	Sigmoidoscopy
	Anoscopy
	Barium enema
	Carcinoembryonic antigen, serum
Cancer, esophagus, stomach	Occult blood, feces
	Esophagogastroduodenoscopy (EGD), with biopsy of gastric cytology
	Upper gastrointestinal series
	Esophagogram
	Carcinoembryonic antigen, serum
	Computed tomography, chest, abdomen
Cancer, liver	Liver biopsy, with cytology studies
	Ultrasound, abdomen
	Computed tomography scan
	Alkaline phosphatase, serum
	Aspartate aminotransferase, serum
	Alkaline phosphatase, serum
	Alanine, aminotransferase, serum
	Carcinoembryonic antigen, serum
	PET scan
Cancer, lung	Bronchial brushings for cytology
	Bronchial washings for cytology
	Cytology, sputum
	Computed tomography, chest
	Fine needle biopsy, lung
	Open lung biopsy
	Transbronchial fine needle aspiration
	Radiograph, chest
	PET scan

Clinical Guides to Diagnoses—cont'd

Common Medical Diagnoses	Common Tests Used
Cancer, pancreas	Percutaneous needle aspiration biopsy of pancreas, with cytology
	Endoscopic ultrasound, pancreas
	ERCP, with biopsy
	Computed tomography, abdomen
	Magnetic resonance, imaging
	CA 19-9, serum
	Alanine aminotransferase (ALT), serum
	Gamma glutamyl transpeptidase (GGT), serum
	Aspartate aminotranspeptidase (AST), serum
	Bilirubin, serum, urine
	Amylase, serum
	Lipase, serum
Cancer, prostate	Prostatic specific antigen (PSA), serum
	Transrectal-guided biopsy of prostate gland
	Urinalysis
	Blood, urea nitrogen, serum
	Creatinine, serum
Cancer, renal	Urinalysis
	Ultrasound, renal
	Computed tomography, abdomen, chest
	Fine needle aspiration biopsy, kidney
	Electrolytes, serum
	Urea, nitrogen, blood (BUN)
	Creatinine, serum
Cancer, testicular	Ultrasound, testis
	Alpha fetoprotein, serum
	β-human chorionic gonadotrophin, serum
	Lactate dehydrogenase, serum
	Biopsy, testis
	Chest radiograph
	Computed tomography, abdomen, pelvis
Cancer, thyroid	Ultrasound, thyroid gland
	Fine needle aspiration biopsy, thyroid gland, with cytology
	Thyroid stimulating hormone, serum
	Thyroglobin, serum
	Calcitonin, serum or plasma

Continued

Clinical Guides to Diagnoses—cont'd	
Common Medical Diagnoses	**Common Tests Used**
Cholecystitis/cholelithiasis	Ultrasound, gallbladder
	Radionuclide scan, gallbladder (HIDA scan)
	Computed tomography scan, abdomen
	MRI, cholangiography
	Endoscopic retrograde cholangiopancreatography (ERCP)
	Percutaneous transhepatic cholangiography
	White blood cell count
	Bilirubin, serum
	Alkaline phosphatase
	Alanine aminotransferase, serum
	Aspartate aminotransferase, serum
	Amylase, serum
	Lipase, serum
Chronic obstructive lung disease (COPD)	Radiograph, chest
	Pulmonary function studies
	Arterial blood gases
	Complete blood count (CBC)
	Electrocardiogram
	Culture, sputum
Cirrhosis, liver	Alanine aminotransferase (ALT), serum
	Aspartate aminotransferase, (AST), serum
	Protein, total, serum
	Albumin, serum
	Prothrombin time, serum
	Sodium, serum
	Bilirubin, total, direct, indirect, serum
	Liver biopsy
	Nuclear scan, liver-spleen
	Paracentesis, with peritoneal fluid analysis
	Ultrasound, abdomen
	Computed tomography, abdomen
Colitis, ulcerative	Occult blood, feces
	Complete blood count
	Sigmoidoscopy, or colonoscopy, with biopsy and cytology studies
	Radiograph, abdominal plain film
	Erythrocyte sedimentation rate, serum
	Albumin, serum
	Electrolytes, serum
	Liver function tests, serum
	Anti-*Saccharomyces cerevisiae* antibody (ASCA)
	Perinuclear antineutrophil cytoplasmic antibody (p-ANCA)

Clinical Guides to Diagnoses—cont'd

Common Medical Diagnoses	Common Tests Used
Coronary artery disease (CAD)	Cardiac catheterization
	Cardiac markers
	Electrocardiogram
	Stress testing, cardiac
Coronary artery disease, risk for	Cholesterol, total, serum or plasma
	C-reactive protein
	Homocysteine, plasma
	Lipids, serum
Crohn's disease	Colonoscopy with ileoscopy and biopsy
	Upper gastrointestinal series, with small bowel follow through (small bowel series)
	Computed tomography, abdominal, with oral contrast
	Radiograph, abdominal
	Anti-*Saccharomyces cerevisiae* antibody (ASCA)
	Perinuclear antineutrophil cytoplasmic antibody (p-ANCA)
	Stool examination, ova and parasites, *Clostridium difficile* toxin and cytomegalovirus
	Complete blood count
	Erythrocyte sedimentation rate, serum
	Electrolytes, serum
	Urea nitrogen, blood (BUN)
	Albumin, serum
	Liver function tests, serum
	Vitamin B_{12} level
Cushing syndrome	Cortisol, free, urine
	Cortisol, serum or plasma
	Metyrapone test
	Magnetic resonance imaging, head
	Potassium, urine
Cystic fibrosis	Chloride sweat test
	Cystic fibrosis DNA amplification
	Fat, fecal
	Radiograph, chest
	Computed tomography scan, chest
	Pulmonary function tests
	In pregnancy, amniocentesis with amniotic fluid analysis with chromosomal analysis of fetal cells
Deep vein thrombosis	*See* thrombophlebitis

Continued

Clinical Guides to Diagnoses—cont'd

Common Medical Diagnoses	Common Tests Used
Dehydration	Electrolyte panel, serum
	Sodium, urine
	Urea nitrogen, (BUN), serum
	Creatinine, serum
	Urinalysis
	Specific gravity, urine
	Osmolarity, serum, urine
	Complete blood count, blood
	Hemoglobin
	Hematocrit
Diabetes insipidus	Albumin, serum
	Antidiuretic hormone, plasma
	Electrolytes, serum
	Fluid deprivation test
	Magnetic resonance imaging, pituitary, hypothalamus
	Osmolarity, serum
	Osmolarity, urine
	Specific gravity, urine
Diabetes mellitus	Glucose, fasting, whole blood
	Glycosylated hemoglobin assay
	Anion gap
	Electrolytes, serum
	Ketone bodies, blood
	Ketones, urine
	Osmolarity, plasma
Disseminated intravascular coagulation (DIC)	Disseminated intravascular coagulation screen
	D-dimer and fibrin split products
	Fibrinogen
	Partial thromboplastin time
	Prothrombin time
	Complete blood count
	Platelet count
	Chest radiograph
Gastritis	*Helicobacter pylori* antibody, serum
	H. pylori antigen, serum
	Esophagogastroduodenoscopy (EGD) with biopsy and cytology
	Esophagography
	Esophageal manometry
	pH monitoring
	Electrocardiogram

Clinical Guides to Diagnoses—cont'd	
Common Medical Diagnoses	**Common Tests Used**
Gonorrhea	Gram stain of secretions to identify *Neisseria gonorrhoeae*
	Culture, genital, anal, throat, conjunctiva
	Rapid test for DNA amplification, urine, vaginal or urethral secretions
	Rapid test for antigen of *Neisseria gonorrhoeae*, urine, vaginal or urethral secretions
Gout	Uric acid, serum, urine
	Urinalysis
	Arthrocentesis, with synovial fluid analysis
Heart failure	B-type natriuretic peptide (BNP)
	Complete blood count
	Creatinine, serum or plasma
	Electrolytes, serum
	Electrolytes, urine
	Albumin, serum
	Radiograph, chest
	Transthoracic echocardiography
	Thyroid stimulating hormone
	Liver function tests
Hepatitis	Alanine aminotransferase (ALT)
	Aspartate aminotransferase (AST)
	Bilirubin, total, direct, indirect, serum
	Hepatitis A antibody, IgM, IgG, serum
	Hepatitis B surface antigen, serum
	Hepatitis B surface antibody, serum
	Hepatitis B core antibody, serum
	Hepatitis Be antibody, serum
	Hepatitis B Virus DNA assay, serum
	Hepatitis C antibody, serum
	Hepatitis C-RNA assay, serum
	Hepatitis C core antigen, serum
	Hepatitis D antigen, serum
	Hepatitis D antibody, serum
	Hepatitis E antigen, serum
	Hepatitis E antibody, serum
	Liver biopsy, with cytology examination

Continued

Clinical Guides to Diagnoses—cont'd	
Common Medical Diagnoses	**Common Tests Used**
Histoplasmosis infection	Histoplasma antigen, urinary
	Radiograph, chest
	Computed tomography, chest
	Fungal culture, blood, sputum, bronchial lavage, cerebrospinal fluid, urine
	Cytology studies of ulcers or sores
	Bronchoscopy with transbronchial biopsy, fine needle aspiration and cytology
	Pulmonary function studies
HIV infection	*See* AIDS
Hodgkin disease	Complete blood count
	White blood cell count, with WBC differential
	Erythrocyte sedimentation rate
	Liver function tests
	Protein tests, serum
	Biopsy, lymph node(s)
	Radiograph chest
	Computed tomography scan, neck, thorax, abdomen, and/or pelvis
	PET scan
Hyperosmolar coma (HHNK)	Anion gap
	Arterial blood gases
	Electrolytes, serum
	Glucose, fasting, plasma
	Ketones, serum
	Ketones, urine
	Osmolarity, serum
	Osmolarity, urine
Hyperparathyroidism	Calcium, serum
	Parathyroid hormone, serum
	Phosphorus serum
	Calcium, urine
	25-hydroxyvitamin D, serum
	Technetium-99m-sestamibi scanning
Hypertension	Creatinine serum or plasma
	Protein, urine
	Renal biopsy
	Renin, plasma
	Urea nitrogen (BUN), serum or plasma
	Sodium, serum or plasma
	Urinalysis

Clinical Guides to Diagnoses—cont'd	
Common Medical Diagnoses	**Common Tests Used**
Hyperthyroidism	Thyroid stimulating hormone (TSH)
	Thyroxine, free (free T_4), serum
	Thyroxine, total, serum
	Triiodothyronine (free T_3)
	T_3 resin uptake, serum, serum
	Radioactive iodine uptake (^{123}I)
	Thyroid scan
	Thyroid autoantibodies, serum
	Erythrocyte sedimentation rate
Hypoparathyroidism	Calcium, serum
	Calcium, urine
	Parathyroid hormone, serum
	Phosphorus, plasma
Hypopituitarism	Adrenocorticotropic hormone
	Cortisol, free, serum or plasma
	Computed tomography, head
	Magnetic resonance imaging, head
	Follicle stimulating hormone
	Luteinizing hormone
	Metyrapone stimulation test
	Thyroid stimulating hormone (TSH)
Hypothyroidism	Thyroid stimulating hormone (TSH)
	Thyroxine, free, serum (T_4)
	Thyroxine, total, serum
	Triiodothyronine, serum (T_3)
	Ultrasound, thyroid
	Cholesterol, serum, plasma
Kidney stones	Computed tomography, kidneys
	Ultrasound, renal
	Urinalysis
	Kidney stone analysis
	Calcium, serum
	Phosphorus, serum
	pH, urine
	Uric acid, serum
	Uric acid, urine
Leukemia	Complete blood count
	Peripheral blood film, with microscopic analysis of cells
	White blood cell count
	White blood cell, differential
	Platelet count
	Bone marrow aspiration and biopsy
	Chromosomal analysis, bone marrow tissue

Continued

Clinical Guides to Diagnoses—cont'd	
Common Medical Diagnoses	**Common Tests Used**
Lymphoma, non-Hodgkin's	Complete blood count
	White blood cell count, with WBC differential
	Liver function tests, serum
	Lactate dehydrogenase (LDH), serum
	Renal function tests, serum
	Biopsy, lymph node(s)
Melanoma	Biopsy of the lesion, with histopathology examination and chromosomal analysis of the tumor
	Biopsy, sentinel lymph node
	Computed tomography scan
	PET scan
Meningitis, bacterial	Cultures, blood
	Computed tomography, brain
	Lumbar puncture with Gram stain of cerebrospinal fluid (CSF) and microscopic analysis
	Culture, cerebrospinal fluid, fungal, bacterial
	Complete blood count
	Antigen testing, cryptococcal, serum, CSF
	Antigen testing, streptococcus pneumonia, serum, CSF
	Lactate dehydrogenase, serum
Multiple myeloma	Complete blood count
	Urea creatinine, (BUN) serum
	Electrolytes, serum
	Total protein, albumin, globulin, serum
	Calcium, serum
	Alkaline phosphatase (ALP), serum
	Erythrocyte sedimentation rate (ESR), serum
	Protein electrophoresis, serum, 24-hour urine
	Immunofixation electrophoresis, serum, urine
	Bone marrow biopsy
	Radiograph, skeletal survey
Multiple sclerosis	Magnetic resonance imaging, head and/or spine
	Lumbar puncture, with cerebrospinal fluid analysis
Myocardial infarction, acute	Cardiac markers
	Electrocardiogram
	Echocardiogram, heart
	Perfusion scan
	Erythrocyte sedimentation rate (ESR)

Clinical Guides to Diagnoses—cont'd

Common Medical Diagnoses	Common Tests Used
Myocarditis	Radiograph, chest
	Electrocardiogram
	Echocardiogram
	Cardiac catheterization and angiography
	Biopsy, myocardium
	Magnetic resonance imaging, with contrast
	White blood cell count
	Erythrocyte sedimentation rate (ESR)
	Culture, blood, nasopharyngeal secretions, rectal swab
	Autoimmune serum markers
Nephrotic syndrome	Complete blood count
	Urea nitrogen, (BUN), serum
	Creatinine, serum
	Electrolytes, serum
	Albumin, serum
	Protein, serum
	Cholesterol, serum
	Urinalysis
	Creatinine clearance, urine
	Proteinuria, 24-hour urine
	Protein electrophoresis, serum, urine
	Antinuclear antibodies (ANA), serum
	Double-stranded DNA antibodies
	Complement components (C3, C4, CH50)
	Antineutrophil cytoplasmic antibodies (C-ANCA, P-ANCA)
	Ultrasound
	Biopsy, renal
Osteoporosis	Bone density scan (dual x-ray absorptiometry, DXA scan)
	Calcium, serum, urine, 24-hour
	Complete blood count
	25-hydroxyvitamin D, serum
	Phosphate, blood
	Parathyroid hormone, serum
	Thyroid stimulating hormone, serum
	Alkaline phosphatase, serum
	Creatinine, serum
	Protein electrophoresis, serum, urine
	Testosterone, total and free, (in men)

Continued

Clinical Guides to Diagnoses—cont'd	
Common Medical Diagnoses	**Common Tests Used**
Pancreatitis	Complete blood count
	White blood count (WBC)
	Amylase, serum, urine
	Lipase, serum
	Calcium, serum
	Liver function tests, serum
	Glucose, serum
	Radiograph, abdominal, chest
	Computed tomography, abdomen
	Ultrasound, abdomen
Peptic ulcer	*H. pylori* antibodies, serum
	Urea breath test
	H. pylori antigen test, stool
	Esophagogastroduodenoscopy (EGD), with gastric cytology, biopsy, rapid urease test of tissue
	Upper gastrointestinal series
Peripheral arterial occlusive disease	Duplex Doppler ultrasound
	Plethysmography, arterial, with ankle-brachial index
	Magnetic resonance angiography (MRA), extremity
	Computed tomography angiography (CTA)
	Lipids, serum
	Cholesterol, total, serum
Peritonitis, acute	Complete blood count
	Electrolytes, serum
	Culture, blood
	Amylase, serum
	Radiograph, abdomen, chest
	Computed tomography
	Paracentesis with peritoneal fluid aspiration and analysis
	Ultrasound, abdomen
	Arterial blood gases
Pheochromocytoma	Catecholamines, plasma
	Free catecholamines, 24-hour urine
	Metanephrines, plasma
	Free metanephrines, 24-hour urine
	Vanillylmandelic acid, 24-hour urine
	Clonidine suppression test
	Computed tomography, abdomen/pelvis
	Magnetic resonance imaging, abdomen/pelvis
	Nuclear scan, 131-iodine-metaiodobenzylguanidine (MBIB)

Clinical Guides to Diagnoses—cont'd	
Common Medical Diagnoses	**Common Tests Used**
Pneumonia	Complete blood count
	Pulse oximetry
	Arterial blood gases
	Culture, bacterial (tissue biopsy, blood, sputum)
	Culture, (influenza, viral), sputum
	Gram stain, sputum
	Cytology, sputum
	Radiograph, chest
	Rapid antigen tests, urine, nasopharyngeal secretions
Preeclampsia	Complete blood count (hemoglobin, hematocrit, platelet count)
	Creatinine, serum
	Albumin, serum
	Protein, 24-hour urine
	Prothrombin time, serum
	Coagulation profile, serum
	Alanine aminotransferase, serum
	Aspartate aminotransferase, serum
	Lactic dehydrogenase, serum
Prostatitis	Bacterial culture, urine, blood, prostatic secretions
	Complete blood count
	Computed tomography, pelvis, if needed
	Transrectal ultrasound with biopsy, if needed
Pulmonary embolism	D-dimer
	Multidimensional computed tomography (MDCT)
	Nuclear scans, ventilation/perfusion
Renal failure; end stage renal disease (ESRD)	Urinalysis
	Microscopy, urinary sediment (for red blood cells, red blood cell casts, and white blood cell casts)
	Specific gravity, urine
	Complete blood count
	Anion gap
	Erythropoietin, serum
	Urea nitrogen, blood (BUN)
	Protein, 24-hour urine
	Creatinine clearance, urine
	Creatinine, serum, plasma
	Electrolytes, serum
	Calcium, serum
	Potassium, serum

Continued

Clinical Guides to Diagnoses—cont'd	
Common Medical Diagnoses	**Common Tests Used**
	Protein, serum
	Albumin, serum
	Albumin, urine
	25-hydroxyvitamin D
	Chest radiograph
	Ultrasound, renal
	Biopsy, renal
Sarcoidosis	Biopsy, affected organ, with culture, stain and microscopic analysis
	Magnetic resonance imaging, distal bones and joints
	Radiograph, chest
	Pulmonary function tests
	Electrocardiogram
	Liver function tests
	Renal function tests
	Calcium, serum
	Calcium, 24-hour urine
Seizure	Electroencephalogram, with video monitoring
	Magnetic resonance imaging, brain
	PET scan
	Computed tomography, brain
	Glucose, plasma
	Sodium, serum
	Magnesium, serum
	Calcium, serum
	Urea nitrogen, blood (BUN)
	Osmolarity, serum
	Toxicology, screen, urine
	Lumbar puncture, with cerebrospinal analysis and culture (bacterial, viral)
Syndrome of inappropriate secretion of antidiuretic hormone	Antidiuretic hormone, plasma
	Electrolytes, serum
	Osmolarity, serum
	Osmolarity , urine
	Sodium, urine
	Specific gravity, urine
	Urea nitrogen, blood (BUN)
	Uric acid, serum

Clinical Guides to Diagnoses—cont'd

Common Medical Diagnoses	Common Tests Used
Syphilis	Venereal Disease Research Laboratory (VDRL)
	Rapid plasma reagin test (RPR)
	Fluorescent treponemal antibody absorption test (FTA-ABS)
	Treponema pallidum passive particle agglutination (TP-PA)
	Immunofluorescent staining, exudates or tissue biopsy with microscopic examination
	Lumbar puncture with cerebrospinal fluid analysis
Systemic lupus erythematosus	Complete blood count
	Erythrocyte sedimentation rate (ESR)
	C-reactive protein
	Liver function tests, serum
	Renal function tests
	Antinuclear antibody (ANA) and subtypes, serum
	Antibody to double-stranded DNA (dsDNA)
	Extractable nuclear antibodies (ENA panel: Anti-anti-Ro (SS-A), anti-La (SS-B), anti-Smith, and anti-RNP antibodies
	Antiphospholipid antibody
	Complement screen, (C3, C4), serum
	Urinalysis
	Partial thromboplastin time
	Radiograph, chest, joints
	Electromyography and nerve conduction velocity
	Electrocardiogram
Thalassemia	Complete blood count
	Red blood cell morphology
	Hemoglobin electrophoresis
	Bilirubin, serum
	Urobilinogen, urine
	Ferritin, iron-binding capacity, transferrin, serum
Thrombophlebitis	D-dimers
	Duplex ultrasound
	Venography, with radiograph, computed tomography, or magnetic resonance imaging
	Plethysmography, venous
	Hypercoagulation panel: protein C, protein S

Continued

Clinical Guides to Diagnoses—cont'd

Common Medical Diagnoses	Common Tests Used
Toxoplasmosis	Complete blood count
	Toxoplasma gondii antibodies (IgM, IgG), serum
	Biopsy, lymph node, muscle, or endomyocardial, with tissue culture
	PCR-DNA, blood, body fluids
Tuberculosis	Tuberculin test, skin
	Acid-fast stain, sputum, with microscopic examination
	Rapid test PCR-DNA (and RNA) TB, sputum
	Culture, sputum
	Bronchoscopy, fiberoptic
	Transbronchial biopsy/washing
	Radiograph, chest
Urinary tract infection	Urinalysis
	Bacterial culture, bacterial with susceptibility testing
	Gram stain, urine
	Computed tomography
	Cystoscopy for recurrent infection
Valvular heart disease	Cardiac catheterization
	Echocardiogram
	Transthoracic
	Transesophageal
	Electrocardiogram
	Radiograph, chest
Wilson's disease	Ceruloplasmin
	Copper, serum, urine
	Liver biopsy
	Alanine aminotransferase
	Alkaline phosphatase
	Aspartate aminotransferase
	Bilirubin, total, serum

Bibliography

Abou-Diwan, C., Young, A.N., & Molinaro, R.J. (2009). Hemoglobinopathies and clinical laboratory testing. *Medical Laboratory Observer, 41*(8), 8, 10–16, 18.

ACOG Committee on Practice Bulletins (2007). ACOG practice bulletin No 77: Screening for fetal abnormalities. *Obstetrics and Gynecology, 109*(1), 217–227.

Alcaide, M.L. & Bisno, A.L. (2007). Pharyngitis and epiglottitis. *Infectious Disease Clinics of North America, 21*(2), 449–469.

American Diabetes Association. (2010). Standards of medical care in diabetes. *Diabetes Care, 33*(Suppl 1), S4–S10.

Anderson, C.L. & Brown, C.E. (2009). Fetal chromosomal abnormalities: Antenatal screening and diagnosis. *American Family Physician, 79*(2), 117–123.

Apgar, B.S., Brotzman, G.L., & Spitzer, M. (2008). *Colposcopy: Principles and practice,* (2nd ed.) Philadelphia: Saunders.

Arnold, L.M. (2010). The pathophysiology, diagnosis and treatment of fibromyalgia. *Psychiatric Clinics of North America, 33*(2), 375–408.

Arnoldi, E. and others. (2010). Evaluation of plagues and stenosis. *Radiology Clinics of North America, 48*(4), 729–744.

Asano, F. (2010). Virtual bronchoscopic navigation. *Clinics in Chest Medicine, 31*(1), 75–85.

Ault, P. & Jones, K. (2009). Understanding iron overload: Screening, monitoring, and caring for patients with transfusion-dependent anemias. *Clinical Journal of Oncology Nursing, 13*(5), 511–517.

Bahado-Singh, R.O., & Argoti, P. (2010). An overview of first-trimester screening for chromosomal abnormalities. *Clinics in Laboratory Medicine, 30*(3), 545–556.

Baldwin, S.L. (2008). Gallbladder disease: Imaging and treatment. *Radiologic Technology, 80*(2), 131–148, 195–198.

Bashir, K., Hussain, N., Hasnain, S., & Elhai, S. (2009). Seroprevalence of hepatitis E virus immunoglobin G and M in adults: A hospital based study. *Indian Journal of Medical Microbiology, 27*(2), 139–141.

Bates, S.E., Comeau, D., Robertson, R., Zurakowski, D., & Netzke-Doyle, V. (2010). Brain magnetic resonance image quality initiative for pediatric examinations: Sedated versus nonsedated children. *Journal of Radiology Nursing, 29*(1), 25–28.

Bazaco, M.C., Albrecht, S.A., & Malek, A.M. (2008). Preventing foodborne infection in pregnant women and infants. *Nursing for Women's Health, 12*(1), 46–55.

Beaty, A.D., Lieberman, P.L., & Slavin, R.G. (2008). Seafood allergy and radiocontrast media: Are physicians propagating a myth? *The American Journal of Medicine, 121*(2), 158.e1–e4.

Becker, H.D. (2010). Bronchoscopy: The past, the present and the future. *Clinics in Chest Medicine, 31*(1), 1–18.

Bekos, V. & Marini, J.J. (2007). Monitoring the mechanically ventilated patient. *Critical Care Clinics, 23*(3), 575–611.

Beller, G.A. (2010). Recent advances and future trends in multimodality cardiac imaging. *Heart, Lung and Circulation, 19*(3), 193–209.

Bennett, N. (2007). Laboratory-based investigations of IM and Epstein-Barr virus. *MLO: Medical Laboratory Observer, 39*(1), 10–12, 14–17.

Berde, C.B. & Stevens, B. (2009). Blood sampling and other needle procedures: The Achilles heel of newborn intensive care. *Pain, 147*(1–3), 15–16.

Bockwoldt, D. (2010). Antithrombosis management in community-dwelling elderly: Improving safety. *Geriatric Nursing, 31*(1), 28–36.

Boekholdt, S.M. & Kostelein, J.J. (2010). C-reactive protein and cardiovascular risk: More fuel to the fire. *Lancet, 375*(9709), 95–96.

Bolejko, A., Sarvik, C., Hagell, P., & Brinck, A. (2008). Meeting informational needs before magnetic resonance imaging: Development and evaluation of an information booklet. *Journal of Radiology Nursing, 27*(3), 96–102.

Bonham, P.A. (2009). Identifying and treating wound infection: Topical and systemic therapy. *Journal of Gastrointestinal Nursing, 35*(10), 12–16.

Bonifacio, E. & Ziegler, A.G. (2010). Advances in the prediction and natural history of type 1 diabetes. *Endocrinology and Metabolism Clinics, 39*(3), 513–525.

Booker, R. (2009). Interpretation and evaluation of pulmonary function tests. *Nursing Standard, 23*(39), 46–56.

Bradbury, M.J.E. (2008). A comparative study of anticoagulant control in patients on long-term warfarin using house and hospital monitoring of the international normalized ratio. *Archives of Disease in Childhood, 93*(4), 303–306.

Brietzke, S.A. (2007). Controversy in diagnosis and management of the metabolic syndrome. *Medical Clinics of North America, 91*(6), 1041–1061.

Brockow, K. (2009). Immediate and delayed reactions to radiocontrast media: Is there an allergic mechanism? *Radiologic Clinics of North America, 29*(3), 453–468.

Brown, A.F.T., Cullen, L., & Than, M. (2010). Future developments in chest pain diagnosis and management. *Medical Clinics of North America, 94*(2), 375–400.

Buclovec, J.J., Pollema, M., & Grogan, M. (2010). Update on the multilinear detector computed tomography angiography of the abdominal aorta. *Radiologic Clinics of North America, 48*(2), 283–309.

Bruining, N., de Winter, S., & Serruys, P.W. (2009). Intravascular ultrasound registration/integration with coronary angiography. *Cardiology Clinics, 27*(3), 531–540.

Burtis, C.A., Ashwood, E.R., & Bruns, D.E. (Eds). (2006). *Tietz textbook of clinical chemistry and molecular diagnostics*, (4th ed.). Philadelphia: Saunders.

Cardella, J. and others. (2008). Compliance, attitudes, and barriers, to post-operative colorectal cancer follow-up. *Journal of Evaluation in Clinical Practice, 14*, 407–415.

Carlson, N. E. and others. (2009). Hypogonadism on admission to acute rehabilitation is related with lower functional status at admission and discharge. *Brain Injury, 23*(4), 336–344.

Carrera-Bueno, F.J. and others. (2009). Dobutamine stress echocardiography identifies patients with angina and dynamic left ventricular outflow obstruction in physiological exercise. *Echocardiography, 26*(3), 272–276.

Casaletto, J.J. (2010). Is salt, vitamin, or endocrinopathy causing this encephalopathy? A review of endocrine and metabolic causes of altered level of consciousness. *Emergency Medicine Clinics of North America, 28*(3), 633–662.

Cederholm, M., Haglund, B., & Axelsson, O. (2009). Infant mortality following amniocentesis and chorionic villus sampling for prenatal karyotyping. *BJOG: An International Journal of Obstetrics and Gynecology, 112*(4), 394–402.

Centers for Disease Control and Prevention. (CDC). (2009). Adult blood lead epidemiology and surveillance–United States, 2005-7. *MMWR: Morbidity and Mortality Weekly Report, 58*(14), 365–369.

Centers for Disease Control and Prevention. (CDC). (2009). Clinic-based testing for rectal and pharyngeal Neisseria gonorrheae and Chlamydia trachomatis infections by community-based organizations-five cities, United States. *MMWR: Morbidity and Mortality Weekly Report, 58*(26), 716–769.

Centers for Disease Control and Prevention. (CDC). (2010). FDA licensure of bivalent human papillomavirus vaccine (HPV2, Cervarix) for use in females and updated HPV vaccination recommendations from the advisory committee on immunization practices (ACIP). *MMWR: Morbidity and Mortality Weekly 59*(20), 626–629.

Chansky, M.E., Corbett, J.G., & Cohen, E. (2009). Hyperglycemic emergencies in athletes. *Clinics in Sports Medicine, 28*(3), 469–478.

Chasen, S.T. (2010). Clinical implications of first semester screening. *Clinics in Laboratory Medicine, 30*(3), 605–611.

Chen, S.J., Hansgen, A.R., & Carroll, J.D. (2009). The future cardiac cauterization laboratory. *Cardiology Clinics, 27*(3), 541–548.

Chinnaiyan, K.M., Raff, G.L., & Goldstein, J.A. (2009). Cardiac CT in the emergency department. *Cardiology Clinics, 27*(4), 587–596.

Choby, B.A. (2009). Diagnosis and treatment of streptococcal pharyngitis. *American Family Physician, 79*(5), 383–390.

Choyke, P.L. (2008). Radiologic evaluation of hematuria: Guidelines from the American College of Radiology's appropriateness criteria. *American Family Physician, 78*(3), 347–352.

Cleri, D.J. & Ricketti, A.J. (2010). Severe acute respiratory syndrome (SARS). *Infectious Disease Clinics of North America, 24*(1), 175–202.

Collier, R. (2009). Prenatal DNA test raises both hopes and worries. *CMAJ: Canadian Medical Association Journal, 180*(7), 705–706.

Collins, L. (2009). Examination of body fluids: Evaluating gross appearance; performing cell counts. *Clinical Laboratory Science, 22*(1) 46–48.

Colton, J.B. & Curran, C.C. (2009). Quality indicators, including complications, of ERCP in a community setting: A prospective study. *Gastrointestinal Endoscopy, 70*(3), 457–467.

Contraceptive Technology Update. (2010). Check the new screening guidelines for cervical and breast cancer: Guidelines may change schedules for mammography, Pap smears. *Contraceptive Technology Update 31*(1), 1–3.

Cooper, C.A. (2010). Centesis studies in critical care. *Critical Care Nursing Clinics of North America, 22*(1), 95–108.

Cornea, V., Jaffer, S., Bleiweiss, I.J., & Nagi, C. (2009). Adequate histologic sampling of breast magnetic resonance imaging-guided core needle biopsy. *Archives of Pathology & Laboratory Medicine, 133*(12), 1961–1964.

Cox, L. and others. (2008). Pearls and pitfalls of allergy diagnostic testing: Report from the American College of Allergy, Asthma, and Immunology/American Academy of Allergy, Asthma, and Immunology Specific Test Task Force. *Annals of Allergy, Asthma, & Immunology, 101*, 580–592.

Cuckle, H. (2010). Monitoring quality control of nuchal translucency. *Clinics in Laboratory Medicine, 30*(3), 593–604.

Cummings, K.W. & Bjalla, S. (2010). Multidetector tomographic pulmonary angiography: Beyond acute pulmonary embolism. *Radiologic Clinics of North America, 48*(1), 81–87.

Cury, R.C. and others. (2010). Dipyridamole stress and rest myocardial perfusion by 64-detector row computed tomography in patients with suspected coronary artery disease. *The American Journal of Cardiology, 106*(3), 310–315.

Dasgupta, A. (2009). False-positive DOA testing results due to prescription medication. *Medical Laboratory Observer, 41*(10), 24, 26.

Dasher, L.G., Newton, C.D., & Lenchick, L. (2010). Dual x-ray absorptiometry in today's clinical practice. *Radiologic Clinics of North America, 48*(3), 541–560.

Daube, J.R. & Rubin, D.I. (2009). Needle electromyography. *Muscle and Nerve, 39*(2), 244–270.

Delgado Almandoz, J.E., Romero, J.M., Pomerantz, S.R., & Lev, M.H. (2010). Computed tomography angiography of the carotid and cerebral circulation. *Radiologic Clinics of North America, 48*(2) 265–281.

Devdhar, M., Ousman, Y.H., & Burman, K.D. (2007). Hypothyroidism. *Endocrinology and Metabolism Clinics, 36*(3), 595–615.

DeWitt, J.M. (2008). Endoscopic ultrasound-guided fine-needle aspiration of right adrenal masses: report of 2 cases. *Journal Ultrasound Medicine, 27*(2), 261–267.

Diaz-Guzman, E. and others. (2010). Frequency and causes of combined obstruction and restriction identifies in pulmonary function tests in adults. *Respiratory Care, 55*(3), 310–316.

Dimopoulos, G. (2009). Approach to the febrile patient in the ICU. *Infectious Disease Clinics of North America, 23*(3), 471–484.

Dirckx, J.H. (2009). From the bench: Skin biopsy. *Health Data Matrix, 28*(3), 12–15.

Dolan, S.M. (2009). Prenatal genetic testing. *Pediatric Annals, 38*(8), 426–430.

Draznin, M.B. (2010). Managing the adolescent athlete with type 1 diabetes mellitus. *Pediatric Clinics of North America, 57*(3), 829–847.

Drueke, T.B. (2008). Is parathyroid hormone measurement useful for the diagnosis of renal bone disease? *Kidney International, 73*, 674–676.

Edell, E. & Krier-Morrow, D. (2010). Navigational bronchoscopy. *Chest, 137*(2), 450–454.

Ehrmeyer, S.S. & Laessig, R.H. (2009). Regulatory compliance for point-of-care testing: 2009 United States perspective. *Clinics in Laboratory Medicine, 29*(3), 463–478.

Ellison, D. (2010). Electrodiagnostic studies. *Critical Care Nursing Clinics of North America, 22*(1), 1–18.

Farley, A., & McLafferty, E. (2008). Lumbar puncture . . . art & science clinical skills: 35. *Nursing Standard, 22*(22), 46–48.

Ferri, F.F. (2011). *Practical guide to the care of the medical patient*, (8th ed.). Philadelphia: Mosby.

Findki, S. and others. (2008). Massive pulmonary emboli and CT pulmonary angiography. *Respiration, 76*(4), 403–412.

Fitzgerald, M.A. (2006). Lab logic: A case of acute drug-induced hepatitis. *The Nurse Practitioner, 31*(4), 7, 11.

Flanagan, J. & Jones, D. (2009). High frequency nursing diagnoses following same-day knee arthroscopy. *International Journal of Nursing Terminologies & Classifications, 20*(2), 89–95.

Flicker, L. (2010). Cardiovascular risk factors, cerebrovascular disease burden, and healthy brain aging. *Clinics in Geriatric Medicine, 26*(1), 17–27.

Flint, P.W. and others. (2010). *Cummings otolaryngology: Head and neck surgery*, (5th ed.). St Louis: Mosby.

Foley, W.D. & Stonely, T. (2010). CT angiography of the lower extremities. *Radiologic Clinics of North America, 48*(2), 367–396.

Forbes, B.A., Sahm, D.F., & Weissfeld, A.S. (2007). *Bailey & Scott's diagnostic microbiology*, (12th ed.). St Louis: Mosby.

Frank, E.D., Long, B., & Smith, B.J. (2007). *Merrill's Atlas of radiographic positioning and procedures*, St Louis: Mosby.

Fransen, M.P., Hajo,W., Vogel, I., Mackenbach, J., Steegers, E., & Essink-Bol, M.L. (2009). Information about pre-natal screening for Down syndrome: Ethnic differences in knowledge. *Patient Education & Counseling, 77*(2), 279–288.

Fromm, A.L. (2009). Care of the older populations diagnosed with *Helicobacter pylori*: A review of current literature. *Gastroenterology Nursing, 32*(6), 393–400.

Gilbert-Barness, E., Kapur, R., Oligny, L.L., & Siebert, J. (2007). *Potter's pathology of the fetus, infant and child*, (2nd ed.). St Louis: Mosby.

Gill, E.A. & Liang, D.H. (2007). Interventional three-dimensional echocardiography: using real-time three-dimensional echocardiography to guide and evaluate intracardiac therapies. *Cardiology Clinics, 25*(2), 335–340.

Glenn, A.L. & Raine, A. (2008). The neurobiology of psychopathy. *Psychiatric Clinics of North America, 31*(3), 463–475.

Goetzinger, K.R. & Cahill, A. (2010). An update on cystic fibrosis screening. *Clinics in Laboratory Medicine, 30*(3), 533–543.

Goldberg, A. & Litt, H.I. (2010). Evaluation of the patient with acute chest pain. *Radiologic Clinics of North America, 48*(4), 745–755.

Goldstein, M. (2008). Carbon monoxide poisoning. *Journal of Emergency Nursing, 34*(6), 538–542.

Gothard, J.W.W. (2008). Anesthetic considerations for patients with anterior mediastinal masses. *Anesthesiology, 26*(2), 305–314.

Greenwald, D.S. (2007). Periprocedure pharmaco-therapy, preparation and infection control. *Gastrointestinal Endoscopy Clinics of North America, 17*(1), 29–40.

Grenache, D.G. & Karon, B.B. (2009). The ABCs of pre-, neo-, and post natal testing. *Medical Laboratory Observer, 41*(9), 10, 12, 14–18.

Grimshaw-Mulcahy, L.J. (2008). Now I know my STDs part II: Bacterial and protozoal. *The Journal of Nurse Practitioners, 4*(4), 271–281.

Goetz, C.G. (Ed.). (2007). *Textbook of clinical neurology*, (3rd ed.). Philadelphia: Saunders.

Gooch, C.L. & Weimer, L.H. (2007). The electrodiagnosis of neuropathy: Basic principles and common pitfalls. *Neurologic Clinics, 25*(1), 1–28.

Haddad, F. & Patel, R. (2008). Technique of knee joint aspiration. In Haddad, F., Oussedik, S., & Patel, R. (Eds.). *Orthopedic trauma: A systematic approach*, London: Quay Books.

Hall, J.M. (2008). Identifying a research-based post-procedure observation period for outpatients undergoing percutaneous liver biopsy. *Journal of Radiology Nursing, 27*(3), 90–95.

Hant, F.N., Herpel, L.B., & Silver, R.M. (2010). Pulmonary manifestations of scleroderma and mixed connective tissue disease. *Clinics in Chest Medicine, 31*(3), 433–449.

Hawthorne, F. & Ahern, K. (2009). "Holding our breath." The experiences of women contemplating nuchal translucency screening. *Applied Nursing Research, 22*(4) 236–242.

Herman, L. (2009). What's new in . . . allergy testing: A simple new blood test for allergy triggers. *Journal of the American Academy of Physician Assistants, 22*(6), 52, 54.

Higgins, C. (2008). Capillary blood gases: To arterialize or not. *MLO: Medical Laboratory Observer, 40*(11), 42, 44–47.

Hill, G.E., Ogunnaike, B., & Nasirn, D. (2010). Patients presenting with acute toxin ingestion. *Anesthesiology Clinics, 28*(1), 117–137.

Hohnloser, S.H. (2008). Risk factor assessment: Defining populations and individuals risk. *Cardiology Clinics, 26*(3), 355–366.

Horton, K.M. & Fishman, E.K. (2010). CT angiography of the mesenteric circulation. *Radiologic Clinics of North America, 48*(2), 331–345.

Hunt, K.J. and others. (2010). Inflammation in aging part 1: Physiology and immunological mechanisms. *Biological Research in Nursing, 11*(3), 245–252.

Institute of Medicine. (2010). Dietary reference intakes for calcium and vitamin D. *Institute of Medicine Report of November 30, 2010*. Washington DC: The National Academy Press.

Jackson, B.R. (2008). The dangers of false-positive and false-negative test results: False-positive results as a function of pretest probability. *Clinics in Laboratory Medicine, 28*(2), 305–319.

Jain, S. & Kamat, D. (2009). Evaluation of microcytic anemia. *Clinical Pediatrics, 48*(1), 7–13.

Jantz, M.A. (2009). The old and the new of sedation for bronchoscopy. *Chest, 135*(1), 4–6.

Jenkins C., Karunanithi, K., & Hewanama, S. (2008). Examination of the bone marrow. *British Journal of Hospital Medicine, 69*(8), M124–M127.

Jessee, M.A. (2010). Stool studies: Tried, true and new. *Critical Care Nursing Clinics of North America, 22*(1), 129–145.

Johnson, K. & Merok, J. (2009). What is the sensitivity and specificity of the cosyntropin (ACTH) stimulation test for adrenal insufficiency? *Evidence-Based Practice, 12*(8), 9.

Joshi, S.B. and others. (2009). CT applications in electrophysiology. *Cardiology Clinics, 27*(4), 619–631.

Kaferle, J. & Strzoda, C.E. (2009). Evaluation of macrocytosis. *American Family Physician, 79*(3), 203–208.

Kamai, A.H., Tefferi, A., & Pruthi, R.K. (2007). How to interpret and pursue an abnormal prothrombin time, activated partial thromboplastin time, and bleeding time in adults. *Mayo Clinic Proceedings, 82*(7), 864–873.

Kapoor, D. & Thompson, R.C. (2009). Diagnostic accuracy of CT coronary angiography. *Cardiology Clinics, 27*(4), 563–571.

Kazory, A. (2010). Emergence of blood urea nitrogen as a biomarker of neurohormonal activation in heart failure. *The American Journal of Cardiology, 106*(5), 694–700.

Kelley, R.E. & Minagar, A. (2009). Memory complaints and dementia. *Medical Clinics of North America, 93*(2), 389–406.

Ketelsen, D. and others. (2010). Computed tomography evaluation of cardiac valves: A review. *Radiologic Clinics of North America, 48*(4), 783–797.

Khor, B. & Van Cott, E.M. (2009). Laboratory evaluation of hypercoagulability. *Clinics in Laboratory Medicine, 29*(2), 339–366.

Kim, J.Y., & Hofstetter, W.L. (2010). Tumors of the mediastinum and chest wall. *Surgical Clinics of North America, 90*(5), 1019–1040.

Klein, M. and others. (2009). Recent consensus statements in pediatric endocrinology: A selective review. *Endocrinology and Metabolism Clinics, 38*(4), 811–825.

Kline, J.A. and others. (2009). Incidence and predictors of repeated computed tomographic pulmonary angiography in emergency department patients. *Annals of Emergency Medicine, 54*(1), 41–48.

Knudtson, M. (2009). Osteoporosis: Background and overview. *The Journal for Nurse Practitioners, 5*(6), S4–S12.

Kopans, D.B. (2010). The 2009 US Preventive Services Taskforce (USPSTF) guidelines are not supported by science: The scientific support for mammography screening. *Radiologic Clinics of North America, 48*(5), 843–857.

Kramer, B.J. (2009). Arterial blood gases. *RN, 72*(4), 22–24.

Kranke, B. & Aberer, W. (2009). Skin testing for IgE-mediated drug allergy. *Immunology & Allergy Clinics of North America, 29*(3), 503–516.

Krantz, D.A., Hallahan, T.W., & Sherwin, J.E. (2010). Screening for open neural tube defects. *Clinics in Laboratory Medicine, 30*(3), 721–725.

Krau, S.D. & McInnis, L.A. (2010). Allergy skin testing: What nurses need to know. *Critical Care Nursing Clinics of North America, 22*(1), 75–82.

Kreuder, M.E. and others. (2007). Complications of video-assisted thoracoscopic lung biopsy in patients with interstitial lung disease. *The Annals of Thoracic Surgery, 84*(6), 2136–2137.

Krishnam, M. and others. (2008). CT-guided percutaneous transpulmonary adrenal biopsy: A technical note. *The British Journal of Radiology, 81*(967), e191–e193.

Krishnamurthy, R. (2009). Pediatric body MR angiography. *Magnetic Resonance Imaging Clinics of North America, 17*(1), 133–144.

Kulstad, C. & Hannafin, B. (2010). Dizzy and confused: A step-by-step evaluation of the clinician's favorite chief complaint. *Emergency Medicine Clinics of North America, 28*(3), 453–469.

Kumamaru, K.K., Hoppel, B.E., Mather, R.T., & Rybicki, F.J. (2010). CT angiography: Current technology and clinical use. *Radiologic Clinics of North America, 48*(2), 213–235.

Kwon, K.T. & Tsai, V.W. (2007). Metabolic emergencies. *Emergency Medicine Clinics of North America, 25*(4), 1041–1060.

Laio, M., Chen, P., Chen, S., & Chen Y. (2009). Supportive care for Taiwanese women with suspected breast cancer during the diagnostic period: Effect on health-care and support needs. *Oncology Nursing Forum, 36*(5), 585–592.

Lang, T.F. (2010). Quantitative computed tomography. *Radiologic Clinics of North America, 48*(3), 589–600.

Lau, J.F. & Smith, D.A. (2009). Advanced lipoprotein testing: Recommendations based on current evidence. *Endocrinology and Metabolism Clinics, 38*(1), 1–31.

Lee, Y.Z., McGrefor, J., & Chong, W.K. (2009). Ultrasound-guided kidney biopsies. *Ultrasound Clinics, 4*(1), 45–55.

Lerma, E.V. (2009). Anatomic and physiologic changes of the aging kidney. *Clinics in Geriatric Medicine, 25*(3), 325–329.

Lewandrowski, K. (2009a). Point of care testing: An overview and a look to the future (circa 2009), United States. *Clinics in Laboratory Medicine, 29*(3), 421–423.

Lewandrowski, K. (2009b). Point-of-care testing for cardiac markers in acute coronary syndromes and heart failure. *Clinics in Laboratory Medicine, 29*(3), 561–571.

Lewandrowski, K. (2009c). Selected topics in point of care testing: Whole blood creatinine, influenza testing, fetal fibronectin, and patient self-testing in the home. *Clinics in Laboratory Medicine, 29*(3), 607–614.

Lindahi, B., Venge, P., & James, S. (2010). The new high-sensitivity cardiac troponin T assay improves risk assessment in acute coronary syndromes. *American Heart Journal, 160*(2), 224–229.

Linder, J.M.B. & Schiska, A.D. (2008). Radiologic advances in the diagnosis of breast cancer. *Journal of Radiology Nursing, 27*(4), 118–122.

Liu, P.S. & Platt, J.F. (2010). CT angiography of the renal circulation. *Radiologic Clinics of North America, 48*(2), 347–365.

Loughlin, K.R. (2007). Urologic radiology during pregnancy. *Urologic Clinics of North America, 34*(1), 23–26.

Luk, A. (2009). Do clinical diagnoses correlate with pathological diagnoses in cardiac transplant patients? The importance of endomyocardial biopsy. *Canadian Journal of Cardiology, 25*(2), e48–e54.

Mahon, C.R., Lehman, D.C., & Manuselis, G. (2011). *Textbook of diagnostic microbiology*, Philadelphia: Saunders.

Mahon, S.M. (2009). Prevention and screening of gastrointestinal cancers. *Seminars on Oncology Nursing, 25*(1), 15–31.

Majeroni, B.A., & Ukkadam, S. (2007). Screening and treatment for sexually transmitted infections in pregnancy. *American Family Physician, 76*(2), 265–270.

Major, N.M. (2006). *A practical approach to radiology*, Philadelphia: Saunders.

Manco, M. and others. (2007). Massive weight loss decrease corticosteroid-binding globulin levels and increase free cortisol in healthy obese patients: An adaptive phenomenon? *Diabetes Care, 30*(6), 1494–1500.

Manning, W.J. and others. (2007). Coronary magnetic resonance imaging. *Cardiology Clinics, 25*(1), 141–170.

Mannino, D.M. (2009). Setting standards for pulmonary function measurements: What is reasonable? *Respiratory Care, 54*(9), 1161–1162.

Marrelli, D. and others. (2009). CA 19-9 serum levels in obstructive jaundice: Clinical value in benign and malignant conditions. *The American Journal of Surgery, 198*, 333–339.

Maxime, V., Lesur, O., & Annane, D. (2009). Adrenal insufficiency in septic shock. *Clinics in Chest Medicine, 30*(1), 17–27.

Maziak, D.E. and others. (2009). Positron emission tomography plus computed tomography in staging early lung cancer: A randomized trial. *Annals of Internal Medicine, 151*, 221–228.

Mc Clean, P. (2008). Recognizing liver disease in jaundiced infants. *British Journal of Midwifery, 16*(2), 106–109.

McGee, S. (2007). *Evidence-based physical diagnosis*, (2nd ed.). Philadelphia: Saunders.

Mc Innes, L.A., Krau, A.D., & Parsons, L. (2010). Angiography: From the patient's perspective. *Critical Caring Nursing Clinics of North America, 22*(1), 51–60.

Mc Innes, L.A., Revell, M.A., & Smith, T.L. (2010). Nuclear scan studies in critical care. *Critical Caring Nursing Clinics of North America, 22*(1), 61–74.

McKenzie, T.J. and others. (2009). Aldosteronomas: State of the art. *Surgical Clinics of North America, 89*(5), 1241–1253.

McPherson, R.A. & Pincus, M.R. (Eds.). 2007). *Henry's clinical diagnosis and management by laboratory methods,* (21st ed.). Philadelphia: Saunders.

McRae, M.E., Chan, A., & Imperial-Perez, F. (2010). Cardiac surgical nurses' use of atrial electrograms to improve diagnosis of arrhythmia. *American Journal of Critical Care, 19*(2), 124–128, 130–133.

Medford, A.L. and others. (2010). Current status of medical pleuroscopy. *Clinics in Chest Medicine, 31*(1), 165–172.

Medta, S.N. & Wolfsdorf, J.I. 2010). Contemporary management of patients with type 1 diabetes. *Endocrinology and Metabolism Clinics, 39*(3), 573–593.

Melanson, S.E.F. (2009). Drug-of-abuse testing at the point of care. *Clinics of Laboratory Medicine, 29*(2), 503–509.

Melis, D M. and others. (2007). Increased prevalence of thyroid autoimmunity and hypothyroidism in patients with glycogen storage disease type 1. *Journal of Pediatrics, 150*(3), 300–305.

Mettler, F.A. (2005). *Essentials of radiology,* (2nd ed.). Philadelphia: Saunders.

Mettler, F.A,. & Guiberteau, M.J. (2006). *Essentials of nuclear medicine imaging,* (5th ed.). Philadelphia: Saunders.

Mittendorf, E.A. and others. (2007). Pheochromocytoma: advances in genetics, diagnosis, localization, and treatment. *Hematology/Oncology Clinics of North America, 21*(3), 509–525.

Moitra, V. & Sladen, R.N. (2009). Monitoring endocrine function. *Anesthesiology Clinics, 27*(2), 355–364.

Montgomery, K., & Bloch, J.R. (2010). The human papilloma virus in women over 40: Implications for practice and recommendations for screening. *Journal of the American Academy of Nurse Practitioners, 22*(2), 92–100.

Moran, G.J., Talan, D.A., & Abrahamian, F.M. (2008). Diagnosis and management of pneumonia in the emergency department. *Infectious Disease Clinics of North America, 22*(1), 53–72.

Mori, A. and others. (2008). Autonomic nervous function in upper gastrointestinal endoscopy: A prospective randomized comparison between transnasal and oral procedures. *Journal of Gastroenterology, 43*(1), 38–44.

Moviat, M. and others. (2008). Contribution of various metabolites to the "unmeasured" anions in critically ill patients with metabolic acidosis. *Critical Care Medicine, 36*(3), 752–758.

Murgo, S., Wyshoff, H., Faverly, D., Crener, K., & Lenaerts, L. (2008). Computed tomography-guided localization of breast lesions. *Breast Journal, 114*(2), 169–175.

National Osteoporosis Foundation. (2010). *Clinician's guide to prevention and treatment of Osteoporosis,* Washington, DC: National Osteoporosis Foundation.

Nayak, N., Van Cleaves, M., &Thune, N. (2009). Better respiratory outcomes via allergy testing. *Medical Laboratory Observer, 41*(12), 16, 18.

Ng, V.L. (2009). Anticoagulation monitoring. *Clinics in Laboratory Medicine, 29*(2), 283–304.

Ng, V.L. (2009). Liver disease, coagulation and hemostasis. *Clinics in Laboratory Medicine, 29*(2), 265–282.

Nguyen, N.C., Akduman, I., & Osman, M.M. (2008). F-18 FDG-PET and PET/CT imaging of cancer patients. *Geriatric Nursing, 27*(2), 61–69.

Nichols, J.H. (2007). Point of care testing. *Clinics in Laboratory Medicine, 27*(4), 893–908.

Nosov, V. and others. (2009). Validation of serum biomarkers for detection of early-stage ovarian cancer. *American Journal of Obstetrics and Gynecology, 200*(639) e1–e5.

Omtand, T. (2009). Natriuretic peptides: Physiologic & analytic considerations. *Heart Failure Clinics, 5*(4), 471–487.

O'Sullivan, B.P., & Freedman, S.D. (2009). Cystic fibrosis, *Lancet, 373*(9678), 1891–1904.

Ouyang, H., & Quinn, J.H. (2010). Diagnosis and evaluation of syncope in the emergency room department. *Emergency Medicine Clinics of North America, 28*(3), 471–485.

Pack- Maybien, A. & Haynes, J. (2009). A primary care provider's guide to preventive and acute care management of adults and children with sickle cell disease. *Journal of the American Academy of Nurse Practitioners, 21*(5), 250–257.

Palmer, B.F. (2008). Approach to fluid and electrolyte disorders and acid-bas problems. *Primary Care: Clinics in Office Practice, 35*(2), 195–213.

Papazian, L. and others. (2007). A contributive result of open-lung biopsy improves survival in acute respiratory distress syndrome. *Critical Care Medicine, 35*(3), 755–762.

Peart, O. (2009). Technical query. It takes gall to spot a stone. *Radiologic Technology, 80*(5), 486.

Peláez, L.M., Fox, N.S., & Chasen, S.T. (2008). Negative fetal fibronectin: Who is still treating preterm labor and does it help? *Journal of Perinatal Medicine, 36*(2), 202–205.

Perez-Johnson, R., Lenhart, D.K., & Sahani, D.V. (2010). CT angiography of the hepatic and pancreatic circulation. *Radiologic Clinics of North America, 48*(2), 311–330.

Pergament, E. (2010). First trimester genetic counseling: Perspectives and considerations. *Clinics in Laboratory Medicine, 30*(3), 557–564.

Peteiro, J. and others. (2010). Prognostic value of exercise echocardiographin patients with left ventricular systolic dysfunction and known or suspected coronary disease. *American Heart Journal, 160*(2), 301–307.

Peterson, C.C. (2006). A review of biochemical and ultrasound markers in the detection of Down syndrome. *Journal of Perinatal Education, 15*(1), 19–25.

Petrini, J. and others. (2010). The feasibility of velocity vector imaging by transesophageal echocardiography for assessment of elastic properties of the descending aorta in aortic valve disease. *Journal of the American Society of Echocardiography, 23*(9), 985–992.

Pfenniger, J.L. (2010). *Pfenniger and Fowler's procedures for primary care,* St Louis: Mosby.

Pollart, SM., Warniment, C., & Mori, T. (2009). Latex allergy. *American Family Physician, 80*(12), 1413–1419.

Poulios, P.D. & Beaulieu, C.F. (2010). Current techniques in the performance, interpretation, and reporting of CT colonography. *Gastrointestinal Endoscopy Clinics, 20*(2), 169–192.

Raymond, D.P. & Watson, T.L. (2010). Endoscopic evaluation of the tracheobronchial tree and mediastinal lymph nodes. *Surgical Clinics of North America, 90*(5), 1053–1063.

Reisch, N., & Arlt, W. (2009). Fine tuning for the quality of life: 21st century approach to treatment of Addison's disease. *Endocrinology and Metabolism Clinics, 38*(2), 407–418.

Renner, J.B. (2009). Conventional radiography in musculoskeletal imaging. *Radiologic Clinics of North America, 47*(3), 357–372.

Revell, M.A., Pugh, M., Smith, T.L., & McInnes, L.A. (2010). Radiographic studies in the critical care environment. *Critical Caring Nursing Clinics of North America, 22*(1), 41–50.

Ribichini, F. and others. Early creatinine shifts predict contrast-induced nephropathy and persistent renal damage after angiography. *The American Journal of Medicine, 123*(8), 755–763.

Ringman, J.M. and others. Biochemical markers in persons with preclinical familial Alzheimer disease. *Neurology, 71*(2), 85–92.

Robinsin, J., Hanke, C.W., Seigel, D., & Fratila, A. (2010). *Surgery of the skin,* St Louis: Mosby.

Rodak, B.F., Fritsma, G.A., & Doig, K. (2007). *Hematology clinical principles and applications,* (3rd ed.). Philadelphia: Saunders.

Rogalla, P., Kloeters, C., & Hein, P.A. (2009). CT technology overview: 64 slice and beyond. *Radiologic Clinics of North America, 47*(1), 1–11.

Romanelli, F. & Matheny, S.C. (2009). HIV infection: The role of primary care. *American Family Physician, 80*(9), 946–952.

Rossi, G.P. and others. (2008). Adrenal vein sampling for primary aldosteronism: The assessment of selectivity and lateralization of aldosterone excess baseline and after adrenocorticotropic hormone (ACTH) stimulation. *Journal of Hypertension, 26*(5), 989–997.

Rudnek, T., & Sacco, R.L. (2008). Risk factor management to prevent first stroke. *Neurologic Clinics, 26*(4), 1007–1045.

Ruegg, TA., Curran, CR., & Lamb, T. (2009). Use of buffered lidocaine in bone marrow biopsies: A randomized, controlled trial. *Oncology Nursing Forum, 36*(1), 52–60.

Rumack, C.M., Wilson, S.R., & Carboneau, J.W. (2005). *Diagnostic ultrasound,* (3rd ed.). St Louis: Mosby.

Sachdeva, A., Horwich, T.B., & Fonarow, G.C. (2010). Comparison of usefulness of each of five predictors of mortality and urgent transplantation in patients with advanced heart failure. *The American Journal of Cardiology, 106*(6), 830–835.

Sakharova, O.V. & Inzucchi, S.E. (2007). Endocrine assessments during critical illness. *Critical Care Clinics, 23*(3), 467–490.

Sanford, K.W. & McPherson, R.A. (2009). Fecal occult blood testing. *Clinics in Laboratory Medicine, 29*(3), 523–541.

Schade, G.R. & Faerber, G.J. (2010). Urinary tract stones. *Primary Care: Clinics in Office Practice, 37*(3), 565–581.

Scholten, S.R. (2010). Endoscopy: A guide for the registered nurse. *Critical Care Clinics of North America, 22*(1), 19–32.

Sharp, D.B., Santos, L.A., & Cruz, M.L. (2009). Fatty liver in adolescents on the U.S.-Mexico border. *Journal of the American Academy of Nurse Practitioners, 21*(4), 225–230.

Sidani, M. & Ziegler, C. (2008). Preventing heart disease: who needs to be concerned and what to do. *Primary Care: Clinics in Office Practice, 35*(4), 589–607.

Siddiqui, S. & Patel, D.R., (2010). Cardiovascular screening of adolescent athletes. *Pediatric Clinics of North America, 57*(3), 635–647.

Silverstein, M.J. and others. (2009). Image-detected breast cancer: State-of the-art diagnosis and treatment. *Journal of the American College of Surgeons, 209*(4), 504–520.

Singh, M. (2007). Risk stratification following acute myocardial infarction. *Medical Clinics of North America, 91*(4), 603–606.

Smellie, W.S. (2009). Liver function tests. *British Journal of Hospital Medicine, 70*(2), M26–M28.

Sonek, J. & Nicolaides, K. (2010). Additional first trimester ultrasound markers. *Clinics in Laboratory Medicine, 30*(3), 573–593.

Spritzer, C.E. (2009). Progress in MR imaging of the venous system. *Perspectives in Vascular Surgery & Endovascular Therapy, 21*(2), 105–116.

Stebbins, W.G., Garibyan, L., & Sober, A.J. (2010). Sentinel lymph node biopsy and melanoma: 2010 update, part I. *Journal of the American Academy of Dermatology, 62*(5), 723–734.

Stern, L. (2010). Navigating the evidence about cancer screening. *The Clinical Advisor, 13*(5), 20, 23, 25, 29–30, 33–34.

Steward, L. & Norton, C. (2009). Improving bowel preparation for colonoscopy: A literature review. *Gastrointestinal Nursing, 7*(4), 28–35.

Strasinger, S.K. & DiLorenzo, M.S. (2008). *Urinalysis and body fluids*, (5th ed.). Philadelphia: FA Davis.

Sundaram, B., Kremi, R., & Patel, S. (2010). Imaging of coronary artery anomalies. *Radiologic Clinics of North America*, 48(4), 711–727.

Takakuwa, K.M. and others. (2007). Preferences for cardiac tests and procedures may partially explain sex but not race disparities. *The American Journal of Emergency Medicine*, 26(5), 545–550.

Taler, S.J. (2008). Secondary causes of hypertension. *Primary Care: Clinics in Office Practice*, 35(3), 489–500.

Taylor, D.L. (2010). Bronchoscopy: What critical care nurses need to know? *Critical Caring Nursing Clinics of North America*, 22(1), 33–40.

Teffert, A., Hanson, C.A., & Inward, D.J. (2005). How to interpret and pursue an abnormal complete blood cell count in adults. *Mayo Clinic Proceedings*, 80(7), 923–936.

The American College of Obstetricians and Gynecologists. (2010). Cervical cytology screening. *The Practice Bulletin 109*, December 2009 1–12.

The Joint Commission. (2010). NPSG chapter outline and overview: Laboratory; *Author*. Prepublication version. Retrieved on September 9, 2010 from http://www.jointcommission.org/patientsafety/nationalpatientsafetygoals.

Tognini, S. and others. (2010). Non-thyroidal illness syndrome and short-term survival in a hospitalized older population. *Age and Aging*, 39(1), 46–50.

Toogood, A.A. & Stewart, P.M. (2008). Hypopituitarism: Clinical features, diagnosis, and management. *Endocrinology and Metabolism Clinics*, 37(1), 235–261.

Udani, S.M. & Koyner, J.L. (2010). The effects of heart failure on renal function. *Cardiology Clinics*, 28(3), 453–465.

Unger, J. (2007). Diagnosis and management of type 2 diabetes and prediabetes. *Primary Care Clinics in Office Practice*, 34(4), 731–759.

US Preventive Services Task Force. (2007). Screening for sickle cell disease: US Preventive Services Task Force recommendation statement. *Agency for Healthcare Research and Quality*, Rockville, MD: AHRQ Publication No 07-05104-EF-2.

US Preventive Services Task Force. (2008). Screening for colorectal cancer: US Preventive Services Task Force recommendation statement. *Annals of Internal Medicine*, 149(9), 627–637.

US Preventive Services Task Force. (2009). Screening for breast cancer: US Preventive Services Task Force recommendation statement. *Annals of Internal Medicine*, 151(10), 716–727.

US Preventive Services Task Force. (2011). Screening for osteoporosis, topic page. January, 2011. Retrieved on January 17, 2011 from: http://www.uspreventiveservicestaskforce.org/uspsoste.htm

Uyeda, J.W., Andersen, S.W., Sakai, O., & Soto, J.A. (2010). CT angiography in trauma. *Radiologic Clinics of North America*, 48(2), 423–438.

Vento, S. & Nobili, V. (2008). Aminotransferases as predictors of mortality. *Lancet*, 371(9627), 1822–1823.

Vernon, C., & LeTourneau, J.L. (2010). Lactic acidosis: Recognition, kinetics and associated prognosis. *Critical Care Clinics*, 26(2), 255–283.

Villemagne, V.L. & Rowe, C. (2010). Amyloid PET ligands for dementia. *PET Clinics*, 5(1), 33–53.

Vora, S.R., Zheng, H., Zsofia, K., Stadler, K., Fuchs, C.S., & Zhu, A.X. (2009). Serum α-fetoprotein response as a surrogate for clinical outcome in patients receiving systemic therapy for advanced hepatocellular carcinoma. *The Oncologist*, 14, 717–725.

Wangenman, B.J., Townsend, K.T., Mathew, P., & Crookston, K.P. (2009). The laboratory approach to inherited and acquired coagulation factor deficiencies. *Clinics in Laboratory Medicine*, 29(2) 229–252.

Watson, R.C. (2009). Hyperbilirubinemia. *Critical Care Clinics of North America*, 21(1), 97–120.

Wax, J.R., Caryin, A., & Pinette, M.G. (2010). Biophysical and biochemical screening for the risk of preterm labor. *Clinics in Laboratory Medicine*, 30(3), 693–707.

Weidner, N., Cote, R., Suster, S., & Weiss, L. (2009). *Modern surgical pathology*, (2nd ed.) Philadelphia: Saunders.

Wexler, J.A. & Sharretts, J. (2007). Thyroid and bone. *Endocrinology and Metabolism Clinics*, 36(3), 673–705.

Wilkins T. & Reynolds, P.L. (2008). Colorectal cancer: A summary of the evidence for screening and prevention. *American Family Physician*, 78(12), 1385–1392.

Willatt, J.M. (2010). Radiologic evaluation of incidental discovered adrenal mass. *American Family Physician*, 81(911), 1361–1366.

Williams, J., Lye, D.B.C., & Umapathi, T. (2008). Diagnostic lumbar puncture: Minimizing complications. *Internal Medicine Journal*, 38(7), 587–591.

Williams, M.L., Elleison, D., Moodt, G., & Farron, F.C. (2010). Electrodiagnostic studies. *Critical Caring Nursing Clinics of North America*, 22, 7–18.

Williams, R., Haag, R., Lopez, R., Baker, W., Osborne, L., & Pelligrini, J. (2008). A comparison of 3 anesthetic techniques for outpatient knee arthroscopy: General anesthesia, spinal anesthesia, and intra-articular infiltration of local anesthetic. *AANA Journal*, 76(5), 393.

Winchester, DE. and others. (2010). Responsible use of computed tomography in the evaluation of coronary artery disease and chest pain. *Mayo Clinic Proceedings*, 85(4), 358–364.

Woo, K.C. & Schneider, J.I. (2009). High-risk chief complaints: Chest pain-the big three. *Emergency Medicine Clinics of North America*, 27(4), 685–712.

Wu, A.H.B. (2006). *Tietz clinical guide to laboratory tests*, (4th ed.) Philadelphia: Saunders.

Yao, S., Bangalore, S., & Chaudry, F.A. (2010). Prognostic implications of stress echocardiography and the impact on patient outcomes: An effective gatekeeper for coronary angiography and revascularization. *Journal of the American Society of Echocardiography*, *23*(8), 832–839.

Yee, J. (2009). CT colonography: Techniques and applications. *Radiologic Clinics of North America*, *4*(1), 133–145.

Zhang, K. (2010). The comparison of clonidine, arginine and both combined: A growth hormone stimulation test to differentiate multiple system atrophy from idiopathic Parkinson's disease. *Journal of Neurology*, *257*(9), 1486–1491.

Zhao, C., Li, L., Harrison, T., Wang, Q., Song, A., Fan, J., Ma, H., Zhang, C., & Wang, Y. (2009). Relationships among viral diagnostic markers and markers of liver function in hepatitis E. *Journal of Gastroenterology*, *44*, 139–145.

Index

A

Abdomen, CT scan of, 217-218, 218f
Abdominal aorta scan, 594b
Abdominal paracentesis. *See* Paracentesis and ascitic fluid analysis
Abdominal radiograph, 646
Abdominal scan, 594b
Abdominal tap. *See* Paracentesis and ascitic fluid analysis
Abdominal trauma, amylase values elevated with, 74
Abdominal ultrasound, 594-595, 595f
ABG. *See* Blood gases, arterial
ABI. *See* Ankle-brachial index
ABO system, erythrocyte and antibodies in, 591t
Abortion
    spontaneous, AFP decreased with, 64
    threatened, human chorionic gonadotropin decreased with, 195
Abscess, CT scan, abnormal values with, 220
ACE. *See* Angiotensin-converting enzyme
Acetaminophen (Tylenol), 653-657t
Acetoacetate. *See* Ketones, urinary
Acetones. *See* Ketones, urinary
Acetylcholinesterase, amniotic fluid analysis with, 67, 70
ACOG. *See* American College of Obstetricians and Gynecologists
Acquired immune deficiency syndrome (AIDS). *See* Human immunodeficiency virus tests
Acromegaly
    ALP values elevated with, 57
    glucose (capillary) values elevated with, 337
    glucose (fasting) values elevated with, 338
    growth hormone values elevated with, 353
    pCR values elevated with, 235
ACT. *See* Activated clotting time
ACTH. *See* Adrenocorticotropic hormone

ACTH stimulation test. *See* Adrenocorticotropic hormone stimulation test
ACTH-producing tumor, androstenedione elevated with, 77
Activated clotting time (ACT), 40-41
    interfering factors with, 41
    knowledge needed by nurse for, 40
    nursing care for, 41b
    nursing response to critical values in, 41
    point-of-care testing available for, 6b
    procedure for, 40
    purpose of, 40
    reference values for, 40b
    results significance for, 40
    specimen collected by, 40
    type of test, 40
Activated coagulation time. *See* Activated clotting time
Activated partial thromboplastin time (APTT), 42-43
    decreased values for, 43
    elevated values for, 42
    interfering factors with, 43
    knowledge needed by nurse for, 42
    nursing care for, 43b
    nursing response to critical values in, 43
    procedure for, 42
    purpose of, 42
    reference values for, 42b
    results significance for, 42-43
    specimen collected by, 42
    type of test, 42
Acute illness, total cortisol values elevated with, 228
Addison's disease
    ACTH stimulation test values unchanged with, 47
    aldosterone, decreased values with, 53
    glucose (capillary) values decreased with, 338
    glucose (fasting) values decreased with, 341
    serum chloride values decreased with, 189

Addison's disease *(Continued)*
    17-OHCS decreased values with, 390
    total cortisol values decreased with, 228
    urinary aldosterone values decreased with, 55
Adenocarcinoma
    barium enema with, 106
    CA 125 values elevated for, 164
ADH. *See* Vasopressin
Adrenal adenoma (Conn's syndrome)
    primary aldosteronism with, 53
    urinary aldosterone values elevated with, 55
Adrenal atrophy, ACTH stimulation test values unchanged with, 47
Adrenal cancer, 17-OHCS elevated values with, 390
Adrenal hyperfunction, total cortisol values elevated with, 228
Adrenal hyperplasia
    primary aldosteronism with, 53
    urinary aldosterone values elevated with, 55
Adrenal insufficiency, total calcium values elevated with, 160
Adrenocortical hyperfunction, serum chloride values elevated with, 189
Adrenocorticotropic hormone (ACTH), 44-46
    decreased values for, 45
    elevated values for, 45
    interfering factors with, 45-46
    knowledge needed by nurse for, 44, 45f
    nursing care for, 46b
    procedure for, 44
    purpose of, 44
    reference values for, 44b
    results significance for, 45
    specimen collected by, 44
    type of test, 44
Adrenocorticotropic hormone stimulation test, 46-47
    elevated values for, 47
    interfering factors with, 47
    knowledge needed by nurse for, 46-47

694